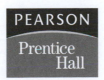

# Guide to Health Claims Examining

## An Honors Certification™ Textbook

### Second Edition

## ICDC Publishing, Inc.

**PEARSON**
Prentice
Hall

**Upper Saddle River, New Jersey 07458**

**Library of Congress Cataloging-in-Publication Data**

Guide to health claims examining : an honors certification textbook / ICDC
Publishing, Inc.—2nd ed.

    p. cm.

ISBN 0-13-219408-2

1. Health insurance claims.   I. ICDC Publishing, Inc.

HG9386.5.G854 2007

368.38'2014—dc22

2006019007

**Publisher:** Julie Levin Alexander
**Publisher's Assistant:** Regina Bruno
**Executive Editor:** Joan Gill
**Assistant Editor:** Bronwen Glowacki
**Director of Marketing:** Karen Allman
**Senior Marketing Manager:** Harper Coles
**Marketing Coordinator:** Michael Sirinides
**Marketing Assistant:** Wayne Celia, Jr.
**Managing Production Editor:** Patrick Walsh
**Production Liaison:** Julie Li
**Production Editor:** Assunta Petrone, Preparé, Inc.
**Manufacturing Manager:** Ilene Sanford
**Manufacturing Buyer:** Pat Brown
**Senior Design Coordinator:** Maria Guglielmo
**Interior Designer:** Amy Rosen
**Cover Designer:** Solid State Graphics
**Composition:** Preparé, Inc.
**Printing and Binding:** Bind Rite Graphics
**Cover Printer:** Phoenix Color Corporation

Pearson Education Ltd.
Pearson Education Singapore Pte. Ltd.
Pearson Education Canada, Ltd.
Pearson Education—Japan
Pearson Education Australia Pty. Limited

Pearson Education North Asia Ltd.
Pearson Educación de Mexico, S.A. de C.V.
Pearson Education Malaysia Pte. Ltd.
Pearson Education Inc., Upper Saddle River, New Jersey

10  9  8  7  6  5  4  3  2  1

ISBN 0-13-219408-2

# Disclaimer

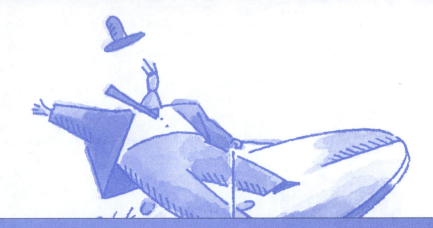

This text is a guide for learning health claims examining. Decisions should not be based solely on information within this guide. Decisions impacting the practice of health claims examining must be based on individual circumstances including legal/ethical considerations, local conditions, and payer policies.

The information contained in this text is based upon experience and research. However, in the complex, rapidly changing insurance environment, this information may not always prove correct. Data used is widely variable and can change at any time. Readers should follow current coding regulations as outlined by official coding organizations.

Any five-digit numeric *Current Procedural Terminology*, (CPT®) codes, services, and descriptions, instructions and/or guidelines are copyright 2006 (or such other date of publication of CPT® as defined in the federal copyright laws) American Medical Association. All Rights Reserved.

CPT® is a listing of descriptive terms and five-digit numeric identifying codes and modifiers for reporting medical services performed by physicians. This presentation includes only CPT® descriptive terms, numeric identifying codes and modifiers for reporting medical services and procedures that were selected by ICDC Publishing, Inc. for inclusion in this Publication. The most current CPT® is available from the American Medical Association. No fee schedules, basic unit values, relative value guides, conversion factors or scales or components thereof are included in the CPT®.

ICDC Publishing, Inc. has selected certain CPT® codes and service/procedure descriptions and assigned them to various specialty groups. The listing of a CPT® service or procedure description and its code number in this Publication does not restrict its use to a particular specialty group. Any procedure or service in this Publication may be used to designate the services rendered by any qualified physician.

The American Medical Association assumes no responsibility for the consequences attributable to, or related to, any use or interpretation of any information or views contained in or not contained in this Publication.

All alphanumeric five-digit Current Dental Terminology (CDT) codes, services descriptions, instructions and/or guidelines are copyright 2006 (or such other date of publication of CDT as defined in the federal copyright laws) American Dental Association. All Rights Reserved.

All codes contained in the dental services section of this text are copyright © by the American Dental Association. All Rights Reserved.

Claims and forms contained in this text are examples only. The publisher and author do not accept responsibility for any adverse outcome from undetected errors, opinion and analysis contained in this manual that may prove inaccurate or incorrect, or from the reader's misunderstanding of an extremely complex topic. All names used in this book are completely fictitious. Any resemblance to persons or companies, current or no longer existing is purely coincidental.

All rights reserved. No part of this Publication may be reproduced, stored in a retrieval system, or transmitted, in any form or by any means, electronic, mechanical, photocopying, recording or otherwise, without prior written permission from the publisher.

# Contents

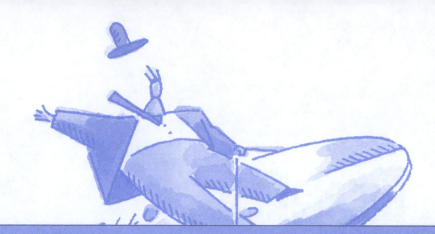

# Preface

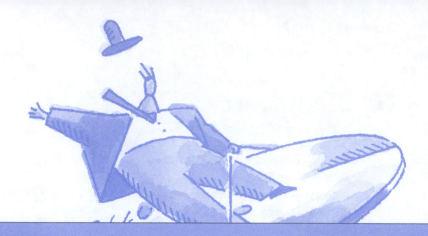

## Introduction

Health claims examining is the study of health claims examining procedures from the time a claim is billed through the moment the claim is processed.

Health claims examining and medical billing are two of the fastest-growing employment opportunities in the United States today. Insurance companies, medical offices, hospitals and other health care providers are in great need of trained personnel to create and process claims.

The most important ingredient for success is the desire to learn, without which the learning process is ineffective. The desire to learn can lead to a rewarding career in the health claims examining field.

## Writing Style

The straightforward easy-to-understand writing style presents information clearly and concisely. Patient and provider names, diagnoses, exercises, and examples in this training material have been designed to incorporate a lighthearted humorous context. We have found that humorous writing improves the ability to comprehend and retain information.

## Text Features

Special features of the text, such as learning objectives, key terms and definitions, end of chapter exercises, and Honors Certification™ challenges, enhance understanding and retention of the material.

**Learning Objectives** Each chapter begins with a bulleted list of learning objectives to help focus the student on the most pertinent topics, key skills, and concepts covered in that chapter.

**Key Terms and Definitions** Key terms are listed at the beginning of the chapter and defined within the text. Key terms are bolded and defined when initially introduced, thus allowing for quick identification. This structural element allows the student to read the term in context with the related material. In addition, the student can remain focused on reading the material without having to stop and refer to the glossary for a definition.

**On the Job Now Exercises** These in-text exercises allow the student to immediately practice concepts as they are learned. They are professional practice exercises that will prepare the student for "real life" job duties.

**Practice Pitfalls** This special feature provides the student with a professional insider's point of view. These practice pitfalls provide additional information for professional success and ideas, shortcuts, and good habits to follow in the office, as well as the bad work habits, the outcomes of sloppy work, and common mistakes that the student can avoid.

**Summaries** Each chapter ends with a bulleted list of key concepts. These summaries are useful study tools that enable the student to assess their level of knowledge and are also useful as a quick study reference.

**End of Chapter Exercises** Questions for Review located at the end of the chapter helps to reinforce key concepts. Answering questions without looking back at the chapter will help students determine if they have grasped the principles within the chapter or will allow them to determine if there is a need for further study. They also serve to prepare students for examinations. **Vocabulary Words** and **Other Exercises** give students the opportunity to put their knowledge into practice. These hands-on exercises help to ensure competence in health claims examining. Answers are contained in the Instructor Resource Guide for this textbook.

**Honors Certification™ Challenges** Our trademarked Honors Certification™ Challenges are presented at the end of every chapter. These challenges provide an opportunity for students to obtain "honors certification" by passing a series of additional examinations. These challenges focus on the skills learned in each chapter, and give students a chance to prove that they have mastered the material, and are capable of performing these skills in the workplace. These requirements are the same skills the student will be asked to perform on the job. Taking and passing these exams will not only earn the student the certification, but will also prepare them for the real working world. This extra distinction allows students and schools to certify that the student has achieved mastery of the skills needed to succeed. Employers find this certification useful in recruiting and employing the best students. The Honors Certification™ Challenges are located in the Instructor Resource Guide.

**Pedagogy** The *Guide to Health Claims Examining* will aid the student in learning the skills necessary to become a successful health claims examiner. The material is designed to be comprehensive, yet user-friendly. The text follows a logical learning format by beginning with a broad base of information and then, step by step, following the course for learning the specific health claims examiner job duties.

# Organization of the Text

*Guide to Health Claims Examining* provides students with all the theoretical knowledge and practical skills needed to achieve success as a health claims examiner. The text introduces the student to health claims examining, before proceeding on to the more in-depth procedures and practices of receiving, reviewing, and processing claims. All aspects of health claims exam-

ining procedures are covered. Content includes a variety of subjects such as billing forms and resource manuals, contract plan provisions, contract benefit structures, claims administration, physician's services, hospital services, workers' compensation, as well as effective communication and job search preparation.

# Ancillary and Program Material

When designing a curriculum and related materials, ICDC does extensive research regarding the skills employers consider essential for job performance. The curriculum and related books and materials are then written to ensure that students learn each of these essential skills. Many schools have gained state and accrediting agency approval with these materials. ICDC's material provide instructors and training institutions with all the materials needed to quickly and easily start and run a new program.

Both *The Practice of Health Claims Examining* and the *Guide to Health Claims Examining Instructor Resource Guide* are designed to reinforce the concepts learned in the *Guide to Health Claims Examining,* and also provide students an opportunity to practice and sharpen their skills.

**The Practice of Health Claims Examining** *The Practice of Health Claims Examining* is a **Real Life™** exercise book that helps the student master skills learned in the *Guide to Health Claims Examining. The Practice of Health Claims Examining* is designed as an exciting, interactive simulated work program and helps the student make the transition from student to actual employee. Health claims examining, insurance, and related business skills are taught in a simulated health insurance office environment. These experiential learning activities allow the student to develop critical skills and "work" from the classroom or at home. The exercise book facilitates confidence and skill building by allowing the practicing of skills in a virtual setting which closely mimics being "on-the-job." The exercise book contains simulation exercises, cases, all documents, and forms packaged in realistic scenarios.

**Guide to Health Claims Examining Instructor Resource Guide** This all-inclusive combined performance evaluator and curriculum gives the instructors the necessary tools to both run and manage a medical billing program, and assess the student's progress at critical points in the program. The Instructor Resource Guide includes the following components:

- **Program Overview**—Provides the instructor with general information on the program's structure, and details how to obtain maximum benefits from the program materials.
- **Modularization of the Program**—The program modules are structured to be small, individual, and topic-specific in order to emphasize the importance of learning through participation and practice. The modules also follow the sequence of the *Guide to Medical Billing and Coding* textbook. The flexible modular design allows schools to easily alter the program's length and sequence, and to have concurrent enrollments. The Modularization of the Program includes:
  - Module Objectives.
  - Program Prerequisites.
  - Chapters Covered.
- **Transparency Masters**—Forms and documents for the program are provided for in-class presentations.
- **Program Marketing Materials**—Twenty-plus sample marketing letters and brochures are provided for marketing the program including a labor market survey form and health claims examiner job analysis.
- **Professional Achievement of Certification and Educational Requirements (PACER™) Curriculum**—Provides the instructor with all the necessary materials needed to quickly and easily start a new program. The PACER™ curriculum includes the following:
  - **Daily Lesson Plans**
    - Topics/Lessons Covered.
    - Performance Objectives.
    - Required Materials.
    - Discussion and Investigation Questions.
    - Teaching Methodologies/Evaluation.
- **Performance Evaluators and Answer Keys (PEAK™)**—Provides the instructor with the necessary tools to assess the student's progress at critical stages in the program. The PEAK™ are categorized by chapter and include the following:
  - On the Job Now Exercise Answers.
  - End-of-chapter Exercise Answers.

- Honors Certification™ Challenges.
- Honors Certification™ Challenges Answers.
- **Test Banks**—The questions and exams are developed from module objectives. Test Banks include the following:
  - Fill-in Questions.
  - Multiple Choice Questions.
  - Short Answers.
  - True or False Questions.
  - Matching Exercises.
  - Problem Solving.
  - Test Bank Answer Keys.

To purchase *The Practice of Health Claims Examining* or the *Guide to Health Claims Examining Instructor Resource Guide,* call Prentice Hall at (800) 526-0485 or visit their website at www.prenhall.com.

**The Practice of Health Claims Examining Instructor Resource Guide** This all-inclusive performance evaluator gives the instructor the necessary tools to assess the student's progress at critical points in the program. The *Guide to Health Claims Examining* "Performance Evaluators and Answer Keys" Instructor Resource Guide (PEAK™ IRG) provides the instructor with the following:

- In-text On the Job Now Exercise Answers,
- End-of-chapter Exercise Answers,
- Honors Certification™ Challenges, and
- Honors Certification™ Challenges Answers

Call Prentice Hall at (800) 526-0485 to inquire about purchasing *The Practice of Health Claims Examining* and the PEAK™ Instructor Resource Guide.

## Additional Resources

The following additional resources are available to accompany this text:

- *CPT© (Current Procedural Coding) Manuals*
- *ICD-9-CM (International Classification of Diseases) Manuals*
- *HCPCS (Healthcare Common Procedure Coding System) Manual*
- *Taber's Medical Dictionary*
- *PDR (Physician's Desk Reference)*
- *Merck Manual*

For more information on Ancillary and Program aterials or Additional Resources, please contact Prentice Hall at (800) 526-0485 or www.prenhall.com.

# Before You Start

**Claims** Claims may contain notations on them such as "Prescription on File"; "Pre-Certification Received"; "Network Provider" etc. These notations have been placed on the claim to facilitate claims processing and inform the claims examiner that the necessary documents and/or information noted has been received by the insurance carrier. The claims should be processed based on the information noted, and it is not necessary for the claims examiner to request this information. In addition, any associated penalties for noncompliance should not be taken.

**Dates** Please note that when YY is used in reference to a date, YY indicates the current year (12/01/YY). When PY is used in reference to a date, PY indicates the prior year or last year (12/01/PY). When NY is used in reference to a date, NY indicates the next year (12/01/NY).

**Birth Dates** Birth dates will be referenced with CCYY-##. This means that the ## should be subtracted from the current year to determine the birth year.

> **Example:** What is the birth date for 10/04/CCYY-14, if **CCYY = 2006?**
>
> 2006 – 14 = 1992, therefore the birth date is **10/04/1992**

**Forms** The forms needed for processing claims in this text are located in Appendix D. These forms should be copied and used as needed.

**Relative Value Study, Contracts, and UCR Conversion Factor Report** A Relative Value Study, Contracts and a UCR Conversion Factor Report are included in Appendices A and B. These materials are to be used for processing the claims in this text.

# About the Author

ICDC Publishing, Inc. has been writing and creating vocational school materials since 1989. As a training center, Insurance Career Development Center (ICDC) trained students in various vocational occupations. ICDC authors are all professionals who have worked and have extensive training and knowledge in the field of the particular area of study for which they write.

# Acknowledgements

Many people have contributed to the development and success of *Guide to Health Claims Examining*. We extend our thanks and deep appreciation to the many students and classroom instructors who have provided us with helpful suggestions for this edition of the text.

We would like to express our thanks to the following individuals:

Linda Jepson; Janet Grossfeld, Adelante Career Institute, Van Nuys, CA; Hollis Anglin and Michael Coffin, Dawn Training Institute, New Castle, DE; Michael Williams and Timothy McGraw, 4-D College, Colton, CA; Anna McCracken and Lynn Russell, American Career College, Los Angeles, CA; Evelyn S. Wyskiel CPC, Branford Hall Institute, Southington, CT; Annie Rackley, Western Technical Institute, El Paso, TX; Tabari Jeffries; Krisia J. Hernandez; Sean Adams; Sydney Adams; Floree Brown; Nathaniel Brown Sr.; Celia R. Luna; Teresa Aguilar; Anita M. Garcia; Alexandra Fratkin; Sandra Yu Kim; Nicole Ghio; Edward Blancarte; Sharon E. Brown; and CarolAnn Jeffries, PA-C, MHS.

Thanks to the CPA firm of Miller, Kaplan, Arase and Company, LLP especially Mannon Kaplan, CPA; Gail Freeman; and Kathy Gartland.

We would also like extend our appreciation to the following reviewers for providing valuable feedback throughout the review process:

Edwin H. Bayne, CPC, PMCC, ETM-P
Palm Beach Community College
Lake Worth, FL

Robin Berenson, EdD, JCTC
Spartanburg Technical College
Spartanburg, SC

Susan DeGirolamo, RMA, NCPT, NCICS
CHI Institute
Southampton, PA

Shirley Jelmo, CMA
PIMA Medical Institute
Colorado Springs, CO

Karen S. Mooney, CPC, CMSCS, CHI
Thompson Institute
Harrisburg, PA

# SECTION 1

## INTRODUCTION TO HEALTH CLAIMS EXAMINING

# 1

# Introduction to Technical
## and Legal Issues

## After completion of this chapter
**you will be able to:**

- Explain what insurance is and how it works.
- Explain the reasons for the rising cost of healthcare.
- Identify and explain the various types of insurance available.
- Identify and explain various types of health benefit plans.
- Identify and explain the duties of a health claims examiner.
- Recognize the different departments in an insurance company and discuss their functions.

- Identify the responsibilities of the Department of Insurance.
- Explain what disclaimers are and how to use them appropriately.
- List HIPAA guidelines regarding privacy issues.
- List several examples of what constitutes fraud in a medical environment.
- List items that may indicate fraud or embezzlement in various situations (i.e., provider fraud).
- List the appropriate procedures to be followed for a subpoena of records.

## Keywords and concepts
**you will learn in this chapter:**

- Actuarial Statistics
- Benefit
- Claim
- Compensatory Damages
- Department of Insurance
- Disclaimer
- Embezzlement
- Employee Benefit
- Fraud
- Group Insurance

- Individual Insurance
- Insurance
- Insurance Policy
- Insurance Speculation
- Investigation
- Lapse in Coverage
- Legal Damages
- Malice
- Oppression
- Premiums

- Products
- Punitive Damages
- Reinsurance
- Renewal
- Self-Funded Plan
- Stoploss Insurance
- Subpoena
- Third-Party Administrator (TPA)

Because of the rising costs of healthcare and replacement of personal property, it is virtually impossible for each person to have the necessary funds available to cover his or her expenses in a disaster, whether it is a large-scale disaster or a personal one. For this reason, insurance has become a necessary part of life in American society.

Essentially, **insurance** is an agreement whereby insurance companies collect fees or **"premiums"** from individuals or companies on a regular basis. In return, they agree to pay for specific benefits. A **benefit** is an item covered by an insurance policy, or something paid to or on behalf of a recipient. These benefits can be the payment of healthcare expenses, the replacement or repair of personal property, or the payment for expenses of others who may have been injured by you or your property.

A person does not have insurance until they complete an insurance application, pay the premium, and have their application accepted by the insurance company. Some policies specify a waiting period before coverage begins. All policies have an effective date of coverage and most have a termination date. To have the coverage continue, premiums must be paid and eligibility qualifications must be maintained. Also, the insured must renew their insurance before the coverage expires in order to remain insured. **Renewal** means paying a premium in order to continue coverage after the initial policy period has expired.

If the insured does not do so, they may have a lapse in coverage, and in some cases will not be able to purchase insurance even by paying the premium. A **lapse in coverage** is a break in continuous insurance coverage. It is best to pay premiums as agreed to avoid complications ranging from having no coverage at all, to a large increase in premiums.

After enrolling in an insurance plan, the insurance company will send the member an insurance identification card or policy. The card or policy remains valid only as long as the member continues to pay their insurance premiums.

The member must file a claim to be reimbursed for any benefits available under his or her insurance policy. A **claim** is a written request by the insured individual for payment by the insurance company of expenses that are covered under the insurance policy. Filing a claim notifies the insurance company of the member's loss or entitlement to reimbursement for any losses incurred. Failure to notify the insurance carrier in a timely manner could result in denial or a reduction of benefits. Therefore, it is wise to file a claim as soon as possible.

Insurance companies operate on the principle that most of those who pay premiums will not need services, or that the services they need will cost less than the premiums paid. As you can see, it becomes very important for an insurance company to place restrictions on the amount and type of benefits that will be paid. These restrictions can include eligibility requirements, deductibles, maximum benefits, exclusions to a policy, and many other policy provisions. The health claims examiner is responsible for ensuring that each claim or request for payment is within the guidelines set by the company or the policy.

## The Rising Cost of Healthcare

The inflation that has affected so many areas of the American economy has probably most severely impacted the cost of healthcare. National health expenditures are expected to continue to rise steadily in the next decade.

This has prompted the Federal Government to introduce major changes in the healthcare system in an effort to control costs and to help insure a higher percentage of Americans.

There are a number of reasons for the enormous increase in the cost of healthcare. The eight most significant factors are:

1. More people are seeking healthcare now compared to 20 years ago.

2. Medical treatments are more extensive and sophisticated than ever before. Additionally, the equipment required for many treatments is extremely expensive. For example, one MRI unit can easily cost $1 million or more.

3. The cost of training healthcare professionals, such as physicians, nurses, and laboratory technicians is much greater than ever before.

4. The price that healthcare professionals pay for malpractice insurance has increased dramatically because of the increase in lawsuits.

5. When a significant part of a person's medical expenses are paid for by a health plan, neither the patient nor the healthcare provider has much incentive to control costs or limit the utilization of services.

6. There is little competition among healthcare providers. Consequently, the marketplace does not place restraints on costs.

7. As people live longer, they require more healthcare, thus prolonging the need for care and increasing costs.

8. Fraud by both providers and members (insured persons) is increasing.

For these reasons and many others, the cost of healthcare has been rising steadily and quickly for the past few decades. Unless major steps are taken to curb this increase, many Americans will find themselves unable to afford healthcare, and many companies will no longer be able to afford to insure their employees.

# On the Job Now

**Directions:** Answer the following question without looking back at the material just covered. Write your answers in the space provided.

Give five reasons for the rising cost of healthcare.

1. _____

_____

2. _____

_____

3. _____

_____

4. _____

_____

5. _____

_____

# Types of Insurance

There are various types of insurance coverage. The following list includes some of the most common:

- **Accidental Death and Dismemberment Insurance** pays a benefit to the beneficiary in the event of the insured person's death by accidental means. It also pays a benefit to the insured when an accident causes the loss of a limb.

- **Disability Insurance** covers an employee's salary, or a percentage of it, while the employee is on disability leave. There is short-term disability insurance, usually up to 12 weeks, and long-term disability insurance.

- **Health Insurance** covers medical and hospital services. Such policies are sold as individual or group policies.

- **Life Insurance** is coverage on a person's life. In the event of the insured person's death, a benefit is paid to the named beneficiary.

- **Medicaid** is a federal program established under Title XIX of the Social Security Act of 1965. Its purpose is to provide the needy with access to medical care.

- **Medicare** is the Federal Health Insurance Benefit Plan for the Aged and Disabled under Title XVIII of Public Law 89-97 of the Social Security Act. This program is for people 65 years of age and older and certain individuals who are totally disabled.

- **Workers' Compensation** is a medical and disability reimbursement program that provides 100% medical coverage and a scheduled weekly disability benefit for job-related injuries, illnesses, or conditions arising out of or in the course of employment.

Numerous other types of coverage may be purchased from insurance companies. It is possible to be insured against almost any loss if you are willing to pay the premium.

In addition, the term insurance is often incorrectly used to refer to all types of health coverage. In reality, insurance is only one type of health coverage. As part of this course, you will be expected to learn the correct terminology for referring to the various benefit plans.

# Individual vs. Group Insurance

Insurance coverage is categorized as being either individual or group. **Individual insurance** is issued to insure the life or health of a named person or persons, rather than the life or health of the members of a group. That means premiums are usually higher because of the higher risks associated with insuring individuals on a case-by-case basis. With individual insurance, there is nowhere to spread risks, and the chance that losses may exceed the premiums collected is greater than in group insurance. The number of participants in a plan does not distinguish whether or not the plan is individual or group. The difference is defined by the type of contract, not the number of participants.

**Group insurance** provides coverage for several people under one contract, called a master contract. It is available to all people who qualify on a class basis, regardless of individual considerations. A group consists of any number of people who have a common purpose other than obtaining insurance coverage. Under this definition, members of unions, trade associations, and other organizations are able to purchase insurance as a group.

**Example:** *Group Insurance:* A company purchases insurance for all its employees, or a club or organization offers insurance to its members through a specified insurance company. All members of the group or organization may buy the policy which the organization has chosen.

*Individual Insurance:* A person purchases an insurance policy from an insurance carrier that is customized based on their specifications (i.e., auto insurance where the insured may choose the amount of coverage, deductible, and other factors).

Often individuals only purchase insurance when they feel there is a reasonable chance of needing the benefits. Therefore, there is often a greater risk to the insurance carrier since healthy people will tend not to purchase coverage.

However, there is less risk for the insurance carrier in a group coverage situation since an employer will purchase coverage for all the employees, not just those likely to be ill. Thus, the premiums for the healthy employees help cover the costs of those employees who need benefits.

## Conventional Insurance

In a conventional insurance arrangement, an employer or individual purchases an insurance plan and agrees to pay premiums to the insurance company. In return, the insurance company agrees to pay specific benefits. The premium cost is based on the "experience" of the plan, which includes the actuarial statistics, inflation, and administrative expenses of the company. **Actuarial statistics** are studies that an insurance company uses. For a carrier which covers health insurance, these can include statistics covering average life span, number of days in hospital per year for each age group, number of doctor visits, costs of all medical services, and so on.

In the past few years, the rise in healthcare costs has affected the increase in premiums. As a result, it has become almost prohibitively expensive for small employers and individuals to purchase coverage. For many larger employers, benefits have been decreased, the portion paid by the employee has been increased, or the plan has become self-funded.

## Self-Funded Plans

In a **self-funded plan**, the total and ultimate responsibility for providing all plan benefit payments rests solely with the employer, group, or association. In self-funding the risk of loss is assumed by the funding entity. Because of this economic risk, it is not uncommon for portions of the benefits to be self-funded (employer, group or association provides payment for benefits), and others portions to be insured (insurance company provides payment for benefits). For example, the medical benefits may be self-funded, and the dental benefits may be insured. This potential risk may be decreased by the employer purchasing **reinsurance** or **stoploss insurance**. Such insurance would reimburse the employer when losses exceed a specific amount agreed on by the employer and the reinsurance carrier.

In this book, the term "plan benefits" is used to refer to coverages—medical or dental—with no distinction made as to whether those benefits are insured or self-funded. Such a distinction is irrelevant for our purposes, because handling and processing of claims within both arrangements are nearly identical.

**Example:** The Giant-Mega Corporation has 10,000 employees. The company determines that the yearly insurance premiums for all its employees would be approximately $10 million. However, the company does not expect the employees to receive $10 million in benefits during the year. Thus, the company chooses to become self-funded. The $10 million is placed in an account, and the company pays the benefits to the employees directly.

## Third-Party Administrators

A **Third-Party Administrator (TPA)** is a professional firm that is under contract to deal solely with administering the eligibility and claim payment services including all of the paperwork (along with various other administrative services) for self-funded benefit plans. The administrator provides all of the equipment and personnel required to meet the plan's needs. In turn, the plan supplies the funds or monies needed for payment of the administrator's services and for amounts paid out for claims. In contrast, the insurance company handles all plan administration, provides all of the equipment and personnel required, and supplies the funds for claim payments.

In response to the increase in the number of self-funded plans, many insurance companies now offer what are known as Administrative Services Only (ASO) contracts. These contracts basically work the same way as a TPA insofar as all of the funding is provided by the client, and the expertise, equipment, and personnel are provided by the insurance company. As with all areas of the benefit industry, a multitude of variations are possible on both of these concepts.

**Example:** The Giant-Mega Corporation has decided that it takes too much time and effort for their claims department to process the claims submitted by its employees. They hire a TPA to process the claims and pay the benefits out of the account they have set up.

## Employee Benefits

Auto, home, and most other personal property insurance is purchased by individuals. However, healthcare insurance is often supplied (partly or fully) by a person's employer. The supplying of healthcare insurance comes under the heading of an employee benefit. Healthcare benefits are an extremely important part of almost everyone's economic security. These benefits were once considered to be fringe benefits by employers. Today, many employees consider them to be a major consideration when seeking a job.

Benefits account for almost 40 percent of an employee's total compensation. In actuality, there are many definitions of employee benefits. In the broadest view, **employee benefits** are virtually any form of compensation other than direct wages paid or given to an employee. Other benefits include paid vacations, sick leave, pension plans, tuition reimbursement or payment plans, yearly bonuses, and many other perks that employers offer to attract employees.

# Types of Health Benefit Plans

There are many different types of insurance health plans that provide medical benefits. However, most people in the United States are insured under one of the following systems:

**1. Indemnity Plan**—Traditional indemnity plans are almost nonexistent today, but they used to be the most common type of benefit plan. Under an indemnity insurance plan, the member pays an insurance premium and the insurance pays a fixed percentage of covered expenses. The policy would require the member to pay deductibles and copayments (a portion of the payment); however, the member can choose their own physician and other healthcare providers and specialists, and can otherwise make independent decisions about what type of care to seek.

**2. Preferred Provider Organization (PPO)**—A preferred provider organization operates much like an indemnity plan, except the plan provides incentives for insured individuals to seek care from providers who are on a list provided by the insurance company. A PPO plan is one type of managed care plan. Under a PPO plan, the insurance company will generally cover a higher percentage of the cost, and sometimes require the member to pay a lower deductible, if a preferred provider is chosen. However, a PPO lets the member seek services from providers outside the network if the member is willing to pay a larger portion of the cost, sometimes called open paneled.

**3. Health Maintenance Organization (open access)**—A Health Maintenance Organization (HMO) with open access provides coverage for many services but requires that the member seek care first from either a Gatekeeper or a Primary Care Provider (PCP) before they go to any other physicians or health facilities. The

HMO will provide the member with a list of physicians from which to select a primary care provider. The insurance will provide coverage for visits to the primary care provider and most services that the PCP recommends. Services that are sought independently (without consulting the PCP) are generally not covered. If the member needs to see a specialist, be hospitalized, or have lab or x-ray work, the member's PCP must refer them to a provider or facility. The member's PCP must give authorization for these services to be covered by the HMO.

**4. Health Maintenance Organization (closed panel)**—An HMO with closed panel is one in which the physicians and other practitioners work directly for the HMO. All services must be provided directly by the HMO and its staff. Services which are sought by the member outside the HMO are generally not covered.

**5. Point-Of-Service (POS)**—These plans combine characteristics of HMOs and PPOs. The member chooses a PCP who controls all aspects of care, including referrals to specialists. All care received under that physician's guidance (including referrals) is fully covered. Care received by out-of-network providers is reimbursed, but the member must pay a significant copayment or deductible. So basically, the member decides each time they need medical care whether they want to use their plan as an HMO or a PPO.

**6. Dental Plan**—Dental insurance covers preventive and therapeutic services of the teeth and gums. Dental plans come in almost as many forms as health coverage. This coverage can be included as a benefit under an indemnity, PPO, or HMO plan, or can be an entirely separate plan. Some HMOs have dental practices associated with them. Other companies provide the same kind of in-network low-pay and out-of-network/higher-pay options as they do with their healthcare. Still others opt for a traditional indemnity approach allowing members to go to the dentist of their choice, pay up front, and wait for reimbursement. Basic dental coverage in managed care plans usually includes 100% payment for annual checkups with the member being responsible for a percentage of other necessary treatments (x-rays, surgeries, etc.).

**7. Vision Coverage**—This coverage can be included as a benefit under an indemnity, PPO, or HMO plan, or can be an entirely separate plan. Some plans offer coverage for annual eye exams and a percentage of the frame and prescription lens or contact lens costs every 24 months. HMOs usually have eye care professionals on site; other types of plans may have in-network and out-of-network restrictions.

**8. Prescription Drug Plan**—This coverage can be included as a benefit under an indemnity, PPO, or HMO plan, or can be an entirely separate plan. One of the highest costs of healthcare today is prescription drugs. Some health plans do not cover prescription drugs at all. HMOs generally have pharmacies on site that fill prescriptions from doctors in the network. Other plans cover a specific list of approved medications for a small copayment, while still others reimburse the member for a percentage of the costs after they have purchased the prescription drug.

# Departments in an Insurance Company

Within each insurance company, there are a number of departments with varying responsibilities. Depending on the size of the company, a department may consist of a number of people or only one person. In fact, one person may perform the functions of several departments. Most insurance companies have the following departments; however, the name of the department may vary.

The **Human Resources Department**, also called the Personnel Department, is responsible for matters relating to the company's employees. The Human Resources Department formulates company policy with respect to hiring, training, compensation, and ensuring company compliance with federal, state, and local employment laws and regulations. It also administers employee benefit plans, such as group insurance, tuition refund plans, and employee pensions.

**Example:** Innocuous Insurers, Inc. sells health and life insurance coverage. The personnel department makes sure that there are enough people working in each department to meet the needs of the company, and handles all matters relating to hiring, termination, payroll, and benefits for the employees.

The **Marketing Department** is responsible for presenting insurance products to the company's customers. **"Products"** within the insurance industry refers to various benefit plans. This department normally conducts market research, works with other departments to develop new products and revise current ones to meet the changing needs of the company's customers, prepares advertising campaigns, designs promotional materials, and establishes and maintains distribution systems for the company's products. Marketing is also in charge of selling the products.

**Example:** Innocuous Insurers, Inc. decides to offer a policy which covers 20% of medical costs, up to their limits. Their research has shown that there are a lot of people who do not have health insurance coverage and they want to create a health insurance plan to sell to these people.

The **Actuarial Department** is responsible for ensuring that the company's operations are conducted on a mathematically sound basis. In conjunction with other departments, it designs and revises the company's products. The Actuarial Department is also chiefly responsible for establishing premium rates based on research performed to predict the profitability of the company's products. Research includes the use of a number of studies such as morbidity rates, life expectancy studies, cost of service studies, and others. These studies can help companies to determine the cost of premiums according to how long a person is expected to live, the types of services the average person will need as they grow older, and the cost of these services.

**Example:** The Innocuous Insurers Actuarial Department determines whether or not the company can afford to offer new health insurance coverage. They use reports to determine the amount that can reasonably be expected to be paid out on the new health insurance policy the marketing department wants to sell. Together the Actuarial Department and the Underwriting Department determine the premium amount for the new policy.

The **New Business Department** does just what its name states—it processes new business acquired by the company. This department's primary responsibilities are to determine and verify that all information and forms submitted by the sales agents are complete and accurate. The New Business Department also schedules physical examinations for policies that require evidence of insurability.

**Example:** The New Business Department checks over all the forms submitted by people who want to purchase the new health insurance to make sure they are accurate and complete. It then sends out the complete information on the policy and any policy cards or identification needed by policyholders.

All policies issued require premium payments to be made to keep the policy in force. The **Premium Services Department** handles and processes all premium payments received. This department handles the billing of premium notices and overdue statements to policyholders.

**Example:** The Premium Services Department keeps track of all the people who have signed up for the new health insurance policy and makes sure that they are paying their premiums each month. If someone misses a premium payment, they cancel the policy and make sure that the claims department stops paying benefits to those people who have not paid their premiums.

The **Underwriting Department** is responsible for making sure that the premium rates are accurate and that claim payments do not exceed the amount assumed when the premium rates were calculated. The Underwriting Department makes determinations as to the insurability of applicants, both individuals and employer groups, based on their present experience and medical status.

**Example:** The Underwriting Department keeps a close eye on how much money the new health insurance policy is bringing in, and how much it is paying out. If they determine that too much is being paid out, or that too many people with extended illnesses are signing up for the policy, they may change the rules regarding who is eligible. They may also decide that the policy is only available to people who are under a certain age and reasonably healthy, or may require a physical before they allow coverage.

The **Accounting Department** maintains the records to show if the company is being run in a profitable manner. This department is responsible for maintaining the company's general accounting records, preparing financial statements, controlling receipts and disbursements, overseeing the budgeting process, administering the payroll program, and working with the Legal Department to ensure that the company is complying with government regulations and tax laws.

**Example:** The Accounting Department keeps track of all the money coming in and going out. They also create all the reports needed for tax filings each year. If they determine that the company does not have enough money, or is paying out too much in relation to what is coming in, they will discuss it with the Underwriting Department and suggest that the premium amount for all policies be raised to bring in more money.

The primary responsibility of the **Claims Department** is the processing of claims in a correct and timely manner. The claims examiner reviews the claims submitted by members or providers of service for the correct application of plan benefits. This area also includes a support staff of clerical and customer service personnel and often includes nurses and physicians for the administration of cost-containment programs.

**Example:** The Claims Department looks at each claim (bill) sent in for people covered under the new health insurance policy. They look at the contract and determine how much to pay after subtracting amounts for unreasonable fees, deductibles, non-covered services, items over a limit, and the portion the insured person is supposed to cover (i.e., if the policy covers 80% of reasonable fees, the insured is responsible for 20%). Once they determine the proper amount to pay on each claim, they will issue payment.

The **Legal Department** makes sure that the company's operations comply with federal, state, and local laws and with the Department of Insurance regulations. It studies current and proposed legislation to determine the effects on future operations and advises the Claims Department when claim disputes are received. This department also works with the Accounting Department in determining tax liabilities and represents the company in legal matters.

# On the Job Now

**Directions:** Answer the following questions without looking back at the material just covered. Write your answers in the space provided.

1. What studies does the Actuarial Department of an insurance company use to help determine premiums? _____

    _____

2. What work does the Underwriting Department of an insurance company do? _____

    _____

3. What is the primary responsibility of the Claims Department? _____

    _____

4. What other types of professionals will the Claims Department use as support staff and why? _____

    _____

## Claims Examiner's Responsibilities

The conduct of all claims personnel is extremely important. Claims personnel are more visible because most of the public interfaces with either the customer service representative or directly with claims processing personnel. The public's opinion of the payer is based primarily on their contacts with claims personnel. Therefore, it is important for claims examining personnel to establish and adhere to basic principles. The claims examiner's guiding philosophy should be to provide timely, competent, fair, and friendly claims service to all members. A proposed workflow model is illustrated in **Figure 1–1**. Reviewing this model periodically will ensure that you have taken the basic steps toward proper claims processing. Keep in mind that this is a basic outline, and the specifics may vary from company to company.

When mail comes in, it is opened, sorted, and stamped with the receipt date. If the mail is a response to a pended claim, the letter is matched with the original claim. The claims examiner then enters the claims and processes them, pends them, or refers them for review.

If the claim is to be processed (**see Figure 1–1, Column 1**), it is either paid or denied, according to the terms of the contract. A check or statement is then generated. The claim is stored in a daily batch with the file copy. The clerk then mails out the check or statement and files the file copy.

If additional information is needed, the claim is pended (**see Figure 1–1, Column 2**). A letter is generated by the system or the claims examiner manually fills out a form letter identifying the additional information needed. The pended claim is stored in the pended file for 30 days. If a response has not been received within 30 days, a follow-up letter is sent. A maximum of two follow-up letters should be sent. If the reply has not been received within 30 days of the last follow-up letter, the pended claim should be denied for lack of information.

If the claims examiner is unable to make a decision based on his or her own expertise, the claim is referred for review (column three). Many insurance companies have a listing of certain types of claims that should be referred for review. These claims are then reviewed by the consultant for appropriateness. The reviewer will inform the claims examiner of the action to be taken, and the claim is processed accordingly. Reviewing the consultant's decision helps the claims examiner to improve their claims processing abilities.

Since the examiner's main responsibility is to determine the payer's obligation in accordance with policy provisions and to discharge those obligations fairly and promptly, each examiner is expected to have exemplary integrity and to demonstrate forthrightness in dealing with the public.

# Proposed Workflow Model

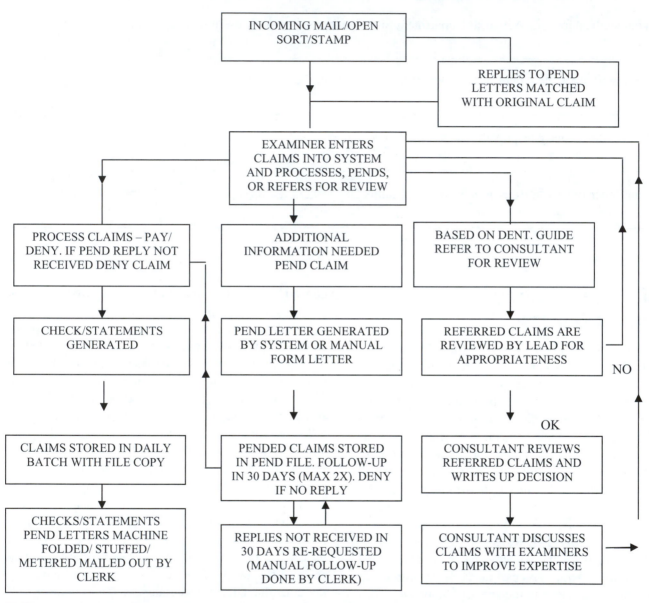

**■ Figure 1–1** Sample Workflow Model

## Practice
# Pitfalls

The following is a list of nine guiding principles to assist the examiner in adopting a professional claims philosophy:

1. Know the plan provisions of the contracts you are responsible for handling.

2. Be sure you understand the application of the provisions. If you are not sure, ask before processing claims.

3. Conduct claim investigations that reflect a prompt and diligent search for the facts.

4. If additional information or clarification is required, review the claim and ask for all information needed at one time. Re-pending claims and asking for additional information is extremely irritating to members and providers.

5. Conclude each claim, large or small, on the basis of its own merits, in light of the facts, the law, and the coverage afforded.

6. Give a prompt, courteous, and forthright explanation to each claimant about the company's position with respect to the claim.

7. Respond promptly when a response is indicated to all communications from policyholders, claimants, attorneys, and other involved persons. (Or refer the claim promptly to the designated person responsible for responding in those situations.)

8. Seek and support new methods designed to provide improved claims service.

9. Suggest or help establish procedures and practices to:

    a. Prevent misrepresentation of the pertinent facts or policy provisions.

    b. Avoid unfair advantage by reason of superior knowledge.

    c. Maintain accurate claim records as privileged and confidential.

# The Department of Insurance

The entire insurance industry is overseen by a larger body called the **Department of Insurance**. The Department of Insurance for each state holds the primary legal authority over the operations of all insurance companies within that state. Therefore, it has influence over insured benefit plans but generally does not have authority over self-funded plans. The many responsibilities of the Department of Insurance include:

- Issuing certificates and licenses authorizing insurance companies to operate and insured products to be sold in the state.

- Licensing agents to sell insurance and revoking licenses when warranted.

- Reviewing the annual statements of insurance companies for verification of solvency.

- Ensuring that policy forms include the required provisions and are printed in the proper format.

- Performing on-site inspections of insurance companies.

- Maintaining an office for receiving and acting on consumer complaints.

- Ensuring that insurance companies observe the rules affecting policy reserve maintenance and investment activities.

# On the Job Now

**Directions:** Answer the following question without looking back at the material just covered. Write your answers in the space provided.

List five responsibilities of the Department of Insurance.

1. _____

_____

2. _____

_____

3. _____

_____

4. _____

_____

5. _____

_____

## Legal Issues Pertaining to Disclaimers

There are several legal issues that affect the health claims examiner on a daily basis. One of the most common is disclaimers. Insurance companies are in the business of providing healthcare benefits to their members. However, there are times when a health claims examiner may quote benefits to a provider or member, but based on changes in circumstances the benefits quoted may not be available when the claim is received (i.e., it is found that the member's coverage has terminated since the benefits were quoted, the group has not paid their premiums, or some other extenuating circumstance). Because of this it is highly advised that the health claims examiner use a disclaimer when giving benefit information.

A **disclaimer** is defined as a denial or renunciation of responsibility. In the health claims examiner's world, it means to use words and phrases that refuse to promise an outcome.

Disclaimers are one of the best ways to protect yourself from possible legal action. Disclaimers use words such as "It appears that" or "This may be."

These words allow a general answer to a question without making any type of promise. If the examiner makes a statement that is later found to be in error, it can cause numerous problems both in customer satisfaction and in possible legal issues.

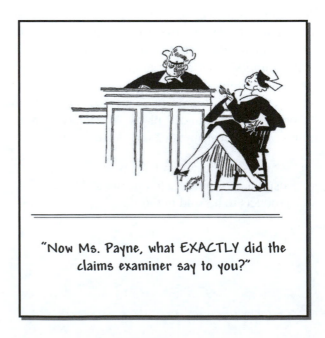

"Now Ms. Payne, what EXACTLY did the claims examiner say to you?"

**Example:** Ms. Smith called the claims examiner in charge of her claim and was told, "Yes, you are covered for a hysterectomy." It was later discovered that there was no medical reason to perform the hysterectomy, but instead Ms. Smith wanted it as a form of foolproof contraception. Since contraceptive devices and procedures were not covered by the contract, the claim was later denied. Ms. Smith insisted that she had been told that the procedure would be covered, and therefore the insurance carrier must pay, regardless of what it said in the contract. She insisted she had a verbal agreement from the insurance carrier that they would pay for the procedure.

All claims examiners should practice using disclaimers in their conversations. When confirming a member's eligibility and benefits, disclaimers should always be included. The following are disclaimers that may be used in your verbal and written responses:

Eligibility—We show that _____ is currently effective on group _____. To receive benefits, he or she must be eligible at the time services are rendered.

Benefits—These are the benefits now in effect for this contract. To receive benefits, your membership must be in good standing on the dates services are rendered.

Remember that your main purpose when using disclaimers is to clarify an issue or answer a customer's question without making a promise that the company may be held to later. This does not mean that you want to mislead the customer in any way, or neglect to answer their questions. It simply means that disclaimers should be used to ensure that you are not making any promises the company will be held to later.

# On the Job Now

**Directions:** Reword the statements below to include the use of a disclaimer in the sentence.

1. Yes, your plan does include that coverage. _____
   _____

2. Yes, you are a member of that plan. _____
   _____

3. Yes, that is a covered service and we will be paying for it. _____
   _____

4. Your check will arrive in five days. _____
   _____

5. Your deductible and stoploss have been met so you will not have to put out any more money on this bill. ____
   _____

6. You have worked for over 90 days so your company's insurance should cover the services. _____
   _____

7. Do not worry; your insurance will cover the bill. _____
   _____

**8.** All hospitalization expenses are covered under your plan. _____

_____

**9.** We pay 80% of the billed amount. _____

_____

**10.** All preventive care is covered under your contract. _____

_____

**11.** Your insurance will cover the cost of these services. _____

_____

**12.** Your policy includes coverage for those services, so we will pay a portion of the cost. _____

_____

**13.** We process all claims upon receipt, so you should have your payment within 10 working days. _____

_____

**14.** Yes, your child is an eligible dependent. _____

_____

**15.** If your claim reaches us by the 15th, it should be paid by the end of the month. _____

_____

# Legal Issues Pertaining to Privacy Guidelines

In addition to disclaimers, privacy guidelines are another common legal issue that affects the health claims examiner on a daily basis. The very nature of health benefits administration requires a great deal of personal information to be gathered and maintained about many individuals. Therefore, the needs of the company must be carefully weighed against the person's right to privacy so as to avoid unwarranted invasions of that right.

In particular, claims information is considered to be privileged and confidential in the context of the administrator-member relationship. Unauthorized disclosure of information may represent a violation of that confidentiality and may be prosecuted under the confidentiality of Medical Information Privacy and Security Act (MIPSA).

The confidentiality of claims records has assumed a new importance for several reasons:

**1.** People are becoming more litigation-minded.

**2.** Health plans are reimbursing for more sensitive services that were excluded in the past, for example, alcohol detoxification, mental health treatment, and AIDS-related illnesses.

**3.** More employers are self-administering or self-funding their health plans, which means that highly personal medical information is in some instances routinely handled by fellow employees.

**4.** New HIPAA regulations require that all personnel involved in the healthcare process respect the patient's right to privacy and confidentiality.

## HIPAA

In 1996, President William Clinton signed into law the Health Insurance Portability and Accountability Act (HIPAA). The portability issues will be addressed in another chapter. Here we will discuss the patient privacy and fraud and abuse issues.

The Act encompasses two main issues:

**1.** Portability, or the ability to transfer insurance companies and still be covered for pre-existing conditions (which will be discussed in more depth in a later chapter).

**2.** Accountability, generally dealing with the patient's right to privacy from the medical provider, health insurer, and any other parties required in the healthcare process (i.e., billers, clearinghouses, and so on).

Regarding the Privacy section of HIPAA, the Department of Health and Human Services states:

The privacy requirements limit the release of patient Protected Health Information (PHI) without the patient's knowledge and consent beyond that required

# Practice
# Pitfalls

Following are the general rules for ensuring that privacy guidelines are met:

**1.** Always obtain an authorization to release information before releasing any information. Most releases routinely signed in the medical practice only authorize the physician to release information necessary to process a patient's claim. Additional authorization should be obtained to release any information to other parties. These releases should state exactly what information is to be released, the dates of any services provided which fall within the release, the person to whom the information may be released, the signature of the patient, the date of the signature, and the date the release expires.

**2.** Make sure that a release was signed by the member prior to processing a claim. If possible, ask the provider for a copy of the patient's signature on the release form. This will ensure that you have the right to look at the information contained on the claim.

**3.** Gather only the information that is necessary and relevant to the billing or processing of the claim.

**4.** Use only legal and ethical means to collect the information required. Whenever permission is necessary, obtain written authorization from the insured or claimant (guardian or parent if the claimant is a minor).

**5.** When requested, and subject to any applicable legal or ethical prohibition or privilege, the insured or claimant concerned should be advised of the nature and general uses to be made of the information.

**6.** Make every reasonable effort to ensure that the information upon which an action is based is accurate, relevant, timely, and complete.

**7.** Upon request, the claimant or insured should be given the opportunity to correct or clarify the information given by or about him or her, and the file should be amended to the extent that it is fair to both the insurer and the member or claimant. Requests for review or clarification of medical information will be accepted only from the healthcare provider from whom the information was obtained.

**8.** In general, disclosures of information to a third party (other than those described to the insured or claimant) should be made only with the written authorization of the member or claimant. This includes disclosure to employers, family members, or former spouses.

**9.** All practical precautions should be taken to ensure that claim files are physically secure and that access to the use of such files is limited to authorized personnel. This includes not leaving files out, locking all files, and even turning your computer screen away from where it might be seen by other persons. Security passwords and other security measures may also be required, depending on your office situation.

**10.** All personnel involved in the processing of claims should be advised of the need to protect the Right of Privacy in obtaining required information and the need to treat all individually identifiable information as confidential. Willful abuse of the privacy of any insured or claimant by the employee may be cause for dismissal.

**11.** The disclosure of a diagnosis should never be made to a member or his or her family. If the member requests this information, refer the member to the physician. There may be a reason the patient does not know his or her diagnosis.

**12.** Never release any information to an ex-spouse. This includes the member's address, phone number, when a claim was paid, to whom, and other information. The ex-spouse should be instructed to contact the member directly.

**13.** Do not leave files, members' records, or appointment books open on your desk or in an area where they may be seen by others. This includes member files or information that may be displayed on a computer screen. The best way to handle this is to be sure that all files are closed or are turned over on your desk. Computer screens must be placed in such a way that they cannot be seen by anyone passing by. If necessary, use a screen saver or other unrestricted document that can be clicked on to replace the one you are working on instantaneously.

**14.** If a minor patient has the legal right to authorize treatment for services, then disclosure to the parents, legal guardians of the minor, or to other persons may be a violation of HIPAA or the confidentiality of Medical Information Privacy and Security Act (MIPSA).

**15.** Be cautious about releasing information to a patient's employer, even if an authorization to release information has been obtained.

for patient care. Patient's personal information must be more securely guarded and more carefully handled when conducting the business of health care.

All healthcare entities were required to meet the standards set in the privacy issues section of HIPAA on April 14, 2003.

If in doubt as to whether specific information should be released, check with your supervisor before, not after, releasing it.

These guidelines cover some of the basic aspects of HIPAA privacy regulations. For detailed information regarding HIPAA guidelines, complete rules and regulations regarding HIPAA are printed in the Federal Register.

# On the Job Now

**Directions:** Answer the following question without looking back at the material just covered. Write your answers in the space provided.

List 10 privacy guidelines that should be followed.

1. _____

   _____

2. _____

   _____

3. _____

   _____

4. _____

   _____

5. _____

   _____

6. _____

   _____

7. _____

   _____

8. _____

   _____

9. _____

   _____

10. _____

   _____

## Faxing

When faxing items, be aware of sensitive information on a fax document. All faxes should contain a cover sheet which announces who the fax is to, who it is from, and a notation that the enclosed information is personal and confidential. Information regarding diagnoses, treatments, sexually transmitted diseases, HIV, drug or alcohol abuse, or financial information should never be faxed. Following is sample wording for the fax confidentiality statement:

> The enclosed information is intended exclusively for the individual or entity to which it is addressed and contains information which is privileged, confidential or exempt from disclosure under federal or state laws. If the reader of this message is not the recipient or the agent or employee responsible for delivering this facsimile transmission to the intended recipient you are hereby notified that any dissemination, distribution or copying of the information contained in this facsimile is strictly prohibited. If you have received this facsimile in error, please notify our office immediately by telephone and return the original facsimile to us at the above address.

When faxing other information, consider asking the receiving party for a code number (i.e., the patient's ID number or birthdate), then black out all pertinent identifying information regarding the patient and replace it with the code number.

Also, a good practice to help in maintaining confidentiality is to call ahead to ensure that the recipient is near the fax machine if it is in a public area.

Items should only be faxed in an emergency. Otherwise, regular or certified mail should be used.

## Legal Issues Pertaining to Fraud

Legal issues pertaining to fraud commonly affect the health claims examiner on a daily basis. **Fraud** is defined as deception to cause a person to give up property or something of lawful right. Fraud is synonymous with deceit, trickery, cheat, and imposter. Schemes for gain involve almost every conceivable form of deception, from a subtle omission of fact to the most flagrant lie.

Fraud can be perpetrated by anyone and involves every type of claim. Doctors, lawyers, hospitals, claimants, beneficiaries, and claims handlers working for an insurance company are capable of committing fraud. It is estimated that millions of dollars annually are paid out by the health benefits industry on fraudulent claims. Regardless of who or how the expenses are submitted for payment, the overall impact on claim payments, premiums, administrative costs, and other expenses is devastating.

## Practice Pitfalls

The following scenarios may be of assistance in identifying fraudulent situations:

1. A member is covered for group hospital benefits as both an employee and a dependent. This fact is concealed to avoid reduced payments by one or more insurers.

2. A prospective insured has been receiving medical treatment for hypertension. This question is answered negatively on an application for life insurance in an effort to obtain coverage not otherwise available or at a more favorable rate.

3. A member has a condition that requires prescription medication. Dates on the bills are altered and photocopies plus the originals are filed to receive multiple payments for the same charges.

4. An employee copies another claimant's bills, replacing the actual claim data with his own. The bills are marked "paid" and the fake claims are submitted as his own.

5. The insured's attending physician signs a return to work release. Discarding this, the insured shops for another doctor who will extend disability.

6. The insured stages an intentional injury to appear accidental.

7. A worker strains his back lifting a TV set at home. The next day, coworkers find the insured lying at the bottom of a flight of stairs complaining of back pain. A workers' compensation claim for loss of wages and medical expenses is filed.

8. The member's spouse sustains a stroke and requires constant custodial care at home. The member's stable, chronic condition suddenly becomes acute, thus rendering the member unable to continue working and enabling the member to remain home and care for the spouse.

## Forms of Fraud

Fortunately, most claims are legitimate and forthright. Therefore, a claims examiner should not automatically assume fraud. However, awareness of the possibility is necessary to properly recognize and detect those instances of fraud. The two major areas of fraud concern are:

1. **Internal fraud**, which involves the employees of the company against which the fraud is perpetrated. The employee may act alone or with another or other employees.

2. **External fraud**, which involves people outside the company that it is directed against. Claims personnel are often the innocent parties that discover the existence of fraud during routine claim-paying activities.

Fraud can assume many different shapes and forms and is as limitless as the creativity of the human mind. Some forms are more obvious than others. With training and experience, a competent examiner develops a sense about claims that do not appear just right. In such cases, the examiner needs to listen to that intuition and take steps to explore such a possibility.

Although the list of potential fraud situations is endless, an attitude of alertness and thorough, conscious efforts can curb the success of the various scenarios.

The following four procedures can assist in establishing a case of fraud and subsequent successful prosecution.

**1.** If the file is out of the ordinary in any way or contains discrepancies, be inquisitive. Try to determine why file statements or circumstances conflict with expected conclusions. The claim should be filed in a timely manner. Information about other insurance, the how, when, and where of the accident, and the names and addresses of all attending physicians and witnesses should be freely available from the claimant. Appearance of undue anxiety or anger on the part of the claimant or beneficiary for a prompt payment could be a fraud indicator. Any alteration of a claim form or bill is to be questioned.

Sometimes routine, in-depth reviews of original claim files disclose questionable elements or trends. Suspicious elements should not be ignored and should be pursued and developed.

A questionable element in one area of a claim file often points to further discrepancies in other areas until an entire series of payments may be found to have been made but not owed. Follow through on all leads and clues. Be sure claims are handled promptly. Use tact in pursuing possible fraud indicators.

Attempts to recognize and deal with fraud are a basic part of an overall philosophy of good claim practices. There is not only a contractual obligation to properly handle possible fraudulent situations, but a social obligation as well. Like any other crime, insurance fraud is detrimental to society in many ways, including the influence it may have in increasing the overall price of benefit coverage.

**2.** Although investigation of fraudulent claims may be thorough and complete and the documentation may seem irrefutable, fraud is often difficult to prove in court. In some cases, depending on the nature of the fraud, the insurance company or administrator may be hesitant to prosecute because of the possibility of a countersuit on the charge of libel. This does not mean that efforts to resolve fraudulent claims should be restricted. Rather, this emphasizes the need for in-depth investigation and development of a complete, accurate claim file so that any fraud case that is prosecuted will be as solid as possible. Thorough investigation increases the chances that the case will be prosecuted in the courts, that prosecution will be successful, and that the occurrence of countercharges for libel will be reduced.

**3.** Although each examiner must recognize and investigate each case of potential fraud, actual and overall control should be retained by management. In the process of prosecuting fraud, many persons have certain definite responsibilities. Cooperation among and between several different departments is essential. Communication plays a critical role in the investigation process.

**4.** In identifying possible fraud, some indicators may help to isolate situations. No single indicator is necessarily suspicious, nor is it evidence that fraud has occurred. The claims examiner must assume an identity of an investigator and put all of the facts and indicators together to see whether fraud is actually present. Following are some indicators that have been put into categories for easier reference.

## Fraud Indicators

Indicators associated with the claimant or insured (employee) are as follows:

1. Claimant is overly pushy and demanding of a quick claim settlement.

2. Claimant is unusually familiar with insurance terminology or claims procedures.

3. Claimant handles business in person or by phone, apparently avoiding use of the mail. (Using the mail for such purposes is a federal offense.)

4. Attorney or claimant is willing to accept less than the actual claim estimate just to help out and resolve the matter quickly.

5. Insured/claimant contacts the insurance agent to verify coverage or extent of coverage just before loss.

6. Attorney representation is coincident with or shortly after injury date, and threatens a bad-faith lawsuit unless the carrier or administrator agrees to settle quickly.

7. No police report was made or only an over-the-counter report occurred when police would usually investigate the actual scene.

8. Claimants or witnesses use post office box or a hotel address.

9. Claimant has multiple policies covering the same loss.

10. Unwitnessed, one-car or hit-and-run accidents.

11. Medical treatment is declined at the time of the accident, but the injured party is later hospitalized for extensive injuries.

12. History of previous loss with similar treatment exists, or the same doctor or attorney repeatedly handles medical or lost earnings claims following minor accidents.

13. Claimant has a history of numerous past questionable claims.

14. Trends can be observed on billing statements or treatments by providers that appear to show excessive charges. These may include same fees and treatment regardless of condition, and differences between amounts billed to patient and amounts on claim forms.

## Claim Processing and Claim Inflation Indicators

During claim review, discrepancies seem to exist. Often, these are flags that should warn the claims examiner to go over the claim papers more thoroughly or to check past history at length. Rather than being obvious, these indicators are often seen only after a number of payments have occurred. Things to look for include:

1. A minor accident produces major accident costs, lost wages, and so on.

2. Medical bills indicate routine treatment being provided on Sundays, holidays, or on a doctor's day off.

3. Summary medical bills are submitted without itemization of office visits or treatments.

4. Photocopies of medical, prescription, or dental bills; third or fourth generation bills are especially suspect. Photocopies of claim forms contain alterations or corrections.

5. Receipts or bills are submitted without provider's letterhead.

6. Several different typefaces, handwritings, or colors of ink are on claim forms or bills.

7. Unusually high number of treatments is noted for relatively minor conditions. Such ailments persist for weeks or months.

8. Insurance effective or employment commenced just a short time before the claim.

9. Condition is diagnosed subjectively as nausea, fatigue, inability to sleep, headaches, low back pain, sprain, whiplash, and so on.

10. Patient's statement that services were not received as shown on the billing.

11. Provider accepts claim payment as payment in full for services rendered, regardless of the billed amount.

12. Unassigned benefits are seen on large medical claim amounts with questionable evidence to support payment in full and with a claim form as the only information submitted. Supporting bills are seldom, if ever, included.

13. Incorrect or incomplete forms are submitted. For example, there are questionable signatures from providers (i.e., doctor's name is signed Doctor J. Jones instead of J. Jones, MD).

14. Unusual or unfamiliar medical terms, misspelled medical words, or a nonexistent diagnosis are found.

15. The claim file indicates that the insured does not have other coverage, but photocopies of unassigned medium or large dollar-amount claims are frequently submitted.

16. Improbable, impossible treatment or unlikely surgery (i.e., second appendectomy, hysterectomy on a male, two gallbladder removals) is listed.

17. Doctor's specialty is not related to the patient's diagnosis (i.e., male treated by an obstetrician, severe heart problem treated by a chiropractor).

## Insurance Speculation Indicators

**Insurance Speculation** means buying insurance or coverage for the purpose of making a profit. It may include staging a fake death or accident to file claims under more than one policy. Collusion with others may occur. Things to look for are as follows:

1. An attorney demand or threat of lawsuit even before a claimant files a claim.
2. Claims reported late.
3. Instant pressure from the claimant or provider to pay quickly.
4. Multiple hospital indemnity coverage held by claimant or combined hospital, medical, accident, and hospital indemnity policies.
5. Denial or omission of information about other insurance coverage.

## Other Indicators of Fraud

Indicators pointing to employee embezzlement usually apply to employees within or even outside the claim operation. Access to claim files is usually involved. Things to look for include:

1. Payee name and address does not match claim form, bills, or other pertinent material.
2. Change in lifestyle or lifestyle is inconsistent with expected income level.
3. Undocumented claim file actions are found, such as voids, reversals, or reissued payments by employee.
4. Provider bills and claim forms do not match explanation of benefits; unusual payee, questionable assignments/non-assignments are noted.
5. Claim payments are split by examiner to allow payment to be within dollar authorized levels.
6. No documentation is located for many payments on a claimant's file. System production records and manual counts of work do not match and claim papers are missing from daily correspondence files.
7. Overutilization of certain benefits: claims are for hospitalization or extensive treatment indicating total disability even though the claimant was not observed to have been absent or ill from work.
8. Pattern of accident claims by an individual or family is found.
9. The patient name is altered to that of another family member to allow payment under another member's history and avoid deductible, and so on.

# On the Job Now

**Directions:** Answer the following question without looking back at the material just covered. Write your answers in the space provided.

List 10 items or situations that may indicate fraud (either internal or external).

1. _____
   _____

2. _____
   _____

3. _____
   _____

4. _____
_____

5. _____
_____

6. _____
_____

7. _____
_____

8. _____
_____

9. _____
_____

10. _____
_____

## HIPAA and Fraud and Abuse

The new HIPAA fraud statutes have greatly broadened the scope of the federal government for prosecuting fraud and abuse in the healthcare industry. HIPAA defines four new criminal healthcare fraud offenses: Healthcare Fraud, Theft or Embezzlement in Connection with Healthcare, False Statements Relating to Healthcare Matters, and Obstruction of Criminal Investigations of Healthcare Offenses.

HIPAA now defines a healthcare benefit program as: any public or private plan or contract, affecting commerce, under which any medical benefit, item, or service is provided to any individual, and includes any individual or entity who is providing a medical benefit, item, or service for which payment may be made under the plan or contract. By including private health benefit plans and any individual or entity, they have effectively given themselves the right to prosecute anyone involved in the healthcare industry for fraud or abuse.

The following four sections further define the HIPAA statutes:

**"Health Care Fraud (18 USC 1347):** Whoever knowingly and willfully executes, or attempts to execute, a scheme or artifice to defraud any healthcare benefit program; or to obtain, by means of false or fraudulent pretenses, representations, or promises, any of the money or property owned by, or under the custody or control of, any healthcare benefit program, in connection with the delivery of or payment for healthcare benefits, items, or services, shall be fined under this title [up to $250,000 per offense] or imprisoned not more than 10 years, or both."

The health claims examiner needs to keep in mind that if he processes a health claim which he knows to be fraudulent, he may be held liable under this portion of the statute.

**"Theft or Embezzlement in Connection with Health Care (18 USC 669):** Whoever knowingly and willfully embezzles, steals, or otherwise without authority converts to the use of any person other than the rightful owner, or intentionally misapplies any of the moneys, funds, securities, premiums, credits, property, or other assets of a healthcare benefit program, shall be fined under this title or imprisoned not more than 10 years, or both; but if the value of such property does not exceed the sum of $100 the defendant shall be fined under this title or imprisoned not more than one year, or both."

Any health claims examiner that does any of the following: pays on claims which they know to be fraudulent; takes home office supplies, equipment, or other items with the intent to keep; and drafts unauthorized checks to himself, may be held liable under this portion of the statute.

**"False Statements Relating to Health Care Matters (18 USC 1035):** Whoever, in any matter involving a healthcare benefit program, knowingly and willfully falsifies, conceals, or covers up by any trick, scheme, or device a material fact; or makes any materially false, fictitious, or fraudulent statements or representations, or makes or uses any materially false writing or document knowing the same to contain any materially false, fictitious, or fraudulent statement or entry, in connection with the delivery of or payment for healthcare benefits, items, or services, shall be fined under this title or imprisoned not more than five years, or both."

A health claims examiner that creates false claims or claim documents, alters or falsifies claim information, lies about claims situations, and does not come forward to disclose fraudulent situations that they are aware of, may be held liable under this portion of the statute.

**"Obstruction of Criminal Investigations of Health Care Offenses (18 USC 1518):** (a) Whoever willfully prevents, obstructs, misleads, delays or attempts to prevent, obstruct, mislead or delay the communication of information or records relating to a violation of a Federal healthcare offense to a criminal investigator shall be fined under this title or imprisoned not more than five years, or both. (b) As used in this section the term criminal investigator means any individual duly authorized by a department, agency, or armed force of the United States to conduct or engage in investigations for prosecutions for violations of healthcare offenses."

Destroying records, not turning over files or documents when asked, lying to investigators, and generally being uncooperative during an investigation may cause a health claims examiner to be liable under this portion of the statute.

While it may seem that these statutes apply mostly to those who are billing healthcare claims, it is important for the health claims examiner to be aware of these issues. If you discover a possibly fraudulent claim, it is important to bring it to your supervisor's attention as soon as possible. Additionally, if an investigation is initiated, you should cooperate fully with the investigators. Not doing so could be construed as hindering their investigation, making you liable for fines and imprisonment of up to five years. It is important to note that the statutes are written in such a way that you can be found guilty of hindering an investigation even if that investigation later fails to turn up fraud.

Additionally, health claims examiners need to be cautious about the statements or comments they make regarding a claim, especially written comments which are placed in a file. If those comments turn out to be fraudulent, the health claims examiner may be held liable.

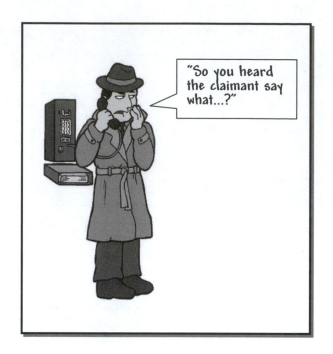

# Investigation

**Investigation** means an organized effort to discover the facts or truth of the matter. Legitimate claims should be paid promptly and in accordance with scheduled allowances. The handling of such claims should reflect a positive service attitude. The same amount of effort and determination should go into the denial of every illegitimate claim. The claims examiner cannot accomplish this purpose without exercising investigative efforts whenever claim discrepancies occur.

During review of every claim, the examiner must be alert to items that do not look right. Because most claims are payable without further questions, it is only necessary to investigate claims that raise questions.

Although investigation of facts takes time, it is absolutely necessary to properly document the claim file. Threats of contacting a State Department of Insurance or threat of a lawsuit should not deter continued investigation as long as the examiner and his or her supervisor are relatively sure that the claim investigation is justified. The claimant or the provider should be kept well informed of the claim's status regarding what has been requested and what items are necessary or outstanding in order to complete the processing of the claim. Be aware of legal time standards required in responding to claimants and in communicating regularly during investigation.

Be candid with persons inquiring about the claim to a point. Do not hesitate to let him or her know that the claim needs further research to determine the validity of the facts presented. Avoid words that can be damaging to a case, such as "crook" and "thief"; and never make accusations (**see Table 1–1**).

| Words to avoid | Words to use |
|---|---|
| Investigation | Clarification of charges, services, etc. |
| Fraud | Incomplete/omitted information |
| Lied | Inconsistency in information reported |
| Any other derogatory remark/term | It appears that… |

**Table 1–1   Investigation Terminology**

Prompt, cautious contact with information sources is essential in every investigation. When possible fraud indicators are present, a greater degree of caution must be exercised and the source of suspected fraud must be taken into account when various contacts are made.

Remember that all plans have the right to investigate and confirm the validity of the submitted information.

## Inside Sources of Fraud

Whenever a company's employees within or outside the claim processing area appear to be involved in questionable activity, the claims examiner should contact his or her supervisor, personnel director, or others in management.

Under no circumstances should the matter be discussed with anyone other than management personnel in a secluded area. It is then up to management to decide how the matter will be handled.

## Outside Sources of Fraud

Whenever insureds, members, claimants, or other persons (not including the provider of service) appear to be involved in fraud, careful contact with providers of services should be made. These contacts involve the verification of dates, type of service rendered, and amounts charged to the patient. Verification of disability and accident-related information should also be investigated. The use of an outside investigator may be required to expedite the investigation. All contacts should be documented in writing. If possible, the information should be requested in writing, and the reply should also be given in writing with the name and the title of the person supplying the information.

When providers of services appear to be involved in fraud, careful contact with the member/claimant should be made. Limit verification to dates and types of treatment and to amounts of charges for those services. Avoid discussions regarding diagnoses. As previously indicated, all information requested and received should be documented in writing whenever possible.

## Building the Claim File

The following five steps should be taken to build evidence in a claim file.

1. Carefully document all discrepancies, conflicting facts, and omissions. Do not write on any of the original submitted claim documents. Make notes on a note pad or separate pieces of paper.

2. Make a written record of pertinent points of phone conversations. Summarize conflicting facts that were obtained by phone and note any new information carefully. Include dates of conversations, names, and phone numbers of contacts.

3. Place all documents in the order in which they occurred or were received. Keep a log that clearly shows the dates of all communications and whom they were with.

4. Retain the envelopes for all documents mailed to the office. Attach the envelope to the back of the documentation received.

5. Coordinate the investigation with the insurance company's or administrator's legal department or counsel.

## Practice
# Pitfalls

Every claims examiner should be aware of the possibility of fraud and check each claim for fraudulent indicators. The following checklist should alert you to the need for further investigation, although one or more of these factors do not prove that fraud exists. Look carefully for the following situations:

- The insured lists no insurance coverage on hospital admissions forms.

- The insured does not assign benefits on inpatient hospital bills.

- Proof of accident or illness includes photocopies of documents, forms, or bills with altered dates or receipts with serialized numbers.

- Prescription bills submitted for payment are consecutively numbered.

- Claimants say that the insurance company is being billed for services not received or treatment not provided.

- Claims are submitted for injuries not reported or not witnessed.

- The doctor's portion of the bill or claim form has erasure or strikeovers.

# Embezzlement

**Embezzlement** is the act of an employee illegally taking funds from a company they work for. Embezzlement can be committed by anyone in a firm.

To protect against embezzlement:

**1.** Accurate records must be kept of all transactions. Be sure to follow all procedures when issuing claim payment checks.

**2.** Any amounts paid out should be clearly notated, including the payee, the amount, the date, the check number, and the reason for payment.

**3.** Any discrepancies should be reported immediately to a supervisor.

**4.** If embezzlement is suspected, the proper person should be notified. In the case of a coworker, this is usually their supervisor. If an employee knows of embezzlement by a coworker and says nothing, they are guilty of being an accomplice to the crime.

**5.** A bond (insurance against embezzlement) should be obtained for each member of the company who deals directly with the company's receipts or processes payments.

**6.** If you notice poor bookkeeping or inaccurate records that were kept by a previous employee or a current coworker, this should be brought to the attention of your supervisor or employer. You should then document the problems in writing and ask the supervisor or employer to initial a copy for you to keep. This may provide minimal protection in case the problems with the records were found to conceal embezzlement or mismanagement of funds.

Insurance carriers are responsible for the acts of their employees. If embezzlement is found, the insurance carrier may be considered guilty and may be responsible for monies embezzled by their employees.

# Legal Damages

**Legal damages** are monetary awards above and beyond the benefits provided by the group plan that a plan member may attempt to recover.

In the legal climate today, it is not uncommon for plan members to seek legal channels to obtain benefits or to obtain greater benefits than provided by a plan. Usually, such cases are based on what is known as "bad faith."

An **insurance policy** or a health and welfare plan is considered a legal contract. Under contract law, the claimant can only recover benefits up to the policy or plan limits.

However, with the development of consumerism, the courts have become more liberal. In some states a body of law has developed that says there is an implied obligation of good faith and fair dealings in every contract. A breach of this obligation is termed bad faith. Generally, the law of bad faith allows an insured to attempt to recover various types of damages above and beyond the benefits provided by the plan. The courts will look at two concepts to determine whether a plan has met the obligation of good faith and fair dealing:

**1.** Did the plan give the claimant's interest equal consideration with that given the company's interest?

**2.** Was the claim handled or denied in accordance with the plan provisions and in a timely manner?

The following are examples of how courts often view policy interpretations:

**1.** The meaning of a plan of benefits is determined by the member's reasonable expectations of coverage.

**2.** Uncertain wording that could be subject to more than one interpretation will usually be resolved against the plan and in favor of the member.

**3.** When two equally believable interpretations may be made, the one that gives the greatest amount of protection to the member will prevail.

There are two types of damages that a court may award: compensatory damages and punitive damages.

**Compensatory damages** are designed to compensate an insured for all of the actual losses or damages to make that person whole again. For example, if a person has not been able to pay his or her home mortgage or car payment because they did not receive a monthly disability check and, therefore, the person's home and car are repossessed, he or she may be able to recover equity for the home and car, attorney fees, and damages for emotional stress.

**Punitive damages** are often the larger of the two awards and are intended primarily to punish wrongdoing by the defendant and make an example of them to help deter such actions in the future. Unlike compensatory damages, punitive damages are not automatically recoverable if bad faith is found. In addition to bad faith, a plan member in California, for example, must prove the plan to be guilty of fraud, oppression, or malice. **Malice** is defined as intentional conduct to cause injury or conduct that is carried on with the conscious disregard of the rights of others. **Oppression** is defined as putting a person through cruel and unjust hardships with conscious disregard of rights.

## Bad Faith Awards

The dollar amount of a bad faith award is based on two concepts: (1) the degree of wrongfulness and (2) the wealth of the defendant.

All lawsuits are expensive not only in the dollar cost of the damages, but in other costs as well. These costs remain even if the case is settled out of court. If the case is settled out of court, the plaintiff's attorney costs, miscellaneous costs, the attorney costs for the plan, and the benefit not originally paid must be paid. Additionally, substantial pain and suffering costs may be included. The value of the claim usually has no correlation to the amount of restitution (award) sought.

Part of the reason for the continuing escalation of premium costs is the necessity to be prepared for lawsuits, because whether the case is settled in court or out of court, the monetary damage to the plan is usually significant and often preventable.

In light of the foregoing information, it is important that every claim be handled quickly, correctly, and fairly. This responsibility falls on each and every claims examiner. To fulfill this responsibility, the following four guidelines should be incorporated into the routine handling and processing of claims.

1. Every customer and claimant is entitled to courteous, fair, and just treatment. An acknowledgment of all communications with respect to a claim or bill should be received with reasonable promptness.

2. Customers and claimants should be treated equally and without outside considerations other than those dictated by the office policy or plan provisions.

3. Every claim is entitled to prompt investigation of all pertinent facts and objective evaluation in the fair and equitable settlement of the claim.

4. The obligation to pay all just claims promptly should be recognized.

# On the Job Now

**Directions:** Answer the following questions without looking back at the material just covered. Write your answers in the space provided.

1. Name and explain the two types of damages that may be awarded in bad faith actions.

    1. _____

    _____

    2. _____

    _____

2. The dollar amount of a bad faith award is based on these two concepts:

    1. _____

    2. _____

# Maintenance of Records

Records should be accurate and contain details of the claims processing history. If information is to be changed on a record, a single line should be drawn through the old information and the corrected data should be placed above or beside it. The date of the change should be notated and initialed by the person responsible for the change.

All records should be kept as long as they are needed. Most insurance carriers put their medical records on microfiche and keep them indefinitely.

There are local and state laws governing how long claims records should be preserved. These usually range from seven to 10 years.

# Subpoenas

Occasionally, the records of a member may be needed in a court action. In such a case a subpoena is issued requesting the records. A **subpoena** is a demand for a witness or a document to appear. Sometimes a witness will need to turn the records over to the court personally. At other times they may be mailed.

One person in the office should be designated in charge of handling subpoenas. This person should be the only person to accept a subpoena of claims records. If you are designated as that person, the subpoena must be served in person. It cannot be laid on a desk or sent through the mail. No one else should accept the subpoena in your absence.

A witness fee or mileage amount may be given to a witness. You should request any payable fees at the time the subpoena is served.

Usually, you are given a specified amount of time to produce the records. Occasionally the records will need to be turned over at the time of the subpoena. In all cases, consult with your supervisor before turning over the records. If your supervisor is unavailable, let the server know that you are unable to turn over the records without proper authorization and let them know when they can come back and serve the subpoena directly on your supervisor. This will give you time to be sure that the record is complete, accurate, and in good order. Also be sure all signatures are identifiable and make copies.

In most cases the original record must be sent. Always keep a copy of all records sent. This allows you to check for changes in the records and protects against loss of information if the records are lost. Number the pages before copying so you can determine if any pages are missing.

If you are unable to accept the subpoena and no one is present who is authorized to accept it, explain the situation to the person serving the subpoena. Suggest a time when they can come back or ask them to contact the insurance carrier's legal department. Then inform the legal department of the situation.

Once a subpoena has been served, check over the records to be sure they are accurate and complete, then number the pages and make the copy. The original file should then be sent out immediately (if delivery by certified mail is allowed), or placed under lock and key to avoid tampering. Find out the day of the trial and comply with all orders given by the court. Be sure not to allow anyone to see the records or tamper with them. The records should only be turned over to the judge and should only be left in the care of the judge or jury, never in the care of an attorney. Be sure to obtain a receipt for the records if leaving them.

## Subpoena Notification

If a subpoena is served to request claims records, many insurance carriers will notify the member in writing that the records have been requested. This allows the member's attorney to file papers with the court to block the subpoena.

If there is very little time between the date the subpoena was served and the date the records have been requested, the letter may be faxed or the member may be contacted by phone. In either case, be sure to let the member know that they do not have the authority to stop you from releasing the records. They must have their attorney file a petition with the court in order to have the subpoena rescinded. For a sample of a subpoena notification see **Figure 1–2**.

---

**MEMBER NOTIFICATION OF SUBPOENA**

Date:


To:
Address:


Dear Member and your Attorney of Record:

Please note that records pertaining to you are being sought by _____; as shown in the subpoena attached to this Notice.

**If you object to us furnishing any part of the records described in this action, you must file papers with the court prior to our release of these records.** This subpoena requires that we furnish the records on or by (date).

You or your attorney of record may contact the attorney for the party seeking to examine such records and determine whether they are willing to agree to cancel or limit this subpoena. If no such agreement is reached and you are not already represented by an attorney in this action, **you should consult an attorney to advise you of your rights in this matter.**

If we do not have notification in writing regarding the cancellation or limitation of this subpoena at least 24 hours prior to the above date, we will assume you have no objection to us releasing this information.


Signed: _____  Date: _____

---

**■ Figure 1–2** Subpoena Notification

# On the Job Now

**Directions:** Answer the following questions without looking back at the material just covered. Write your answers in the space provided.

1. (True or False?) When someone enters the office with a subpoena you should immediately turn over all records that are requested. _____

2. What should you do if the person who handles subpoenas is not in the office and someone attempts to serve a subpoena? _____

_____

# CHAPTER REVIEW

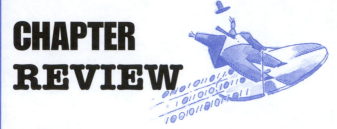

## Summary

- There are several types of insurance companies, and each provides benefits in exchange for premium payments from its members.

- Insurance companies are overseen by the Department of Insurance, which holds the primary legal authority over the operations of insurance companies within that state.

- As a health claims examiner, you need to understand the principles that underlie the Claims Department's primary objective, which is to deliver timely, competent, fair, and friendly claim service. When conscientiously and consistently applied, these principles enable a company to build and maintain a respectable image with its customers and the general public.

- The maintenance of strong customer good will and the creation of a favorable public position are vital to the progress of a company, as well as to each individual employee.

- Disclaimers should always be used when speaking to patients or providers. This can help prevent the insurance carrier from being held liable for a promise made by a claims examiner.

- Submission of fraudulent claims has hit epidemic levels. Payments for fraudulent claims cost administrators millions of dollars annually.

- One of the qualities of a good claims examiner is the ability to use good judgment in making claim decisions.

- Fraud is a very sensitive issue, and the guidelines we have just covered should be practiced along with your company guidelines to ensure accurate and fair claims decisions.

- Records should be maintained properly and requests for subpoenas should be answered promptly and correctly.

## Assignments

Complete the Questions for Review.
Complete Exercises 1–1 through 1–3.

## Questions for Review

**Directions:** Answer the following questions without looking back at the material just covered. Write your answers in the space provided.

1. What is insurance? _____

   _____

2. What are the two categories of insurance plans and how do they differ?

   1. _____

   2. _____

3. What does TPA stand for and what do these companies do? _____

   _____

4. What are employee benefits? _____

   _____

5. What does the word "disclaimer" mean? _____

   _____

6. What is insurance speculation? _____

   _____

7. Define Fraud. _____

   _____

**8.** Define Embezzlement. _____

_____

**9.** What are the two main areas of fraud concern?

    **1.** _____

    **2.** _____

**10.** What is an investigation? _____

_____

If you were unable to answer any of these questions, refer back to that section and then fill in the answers.

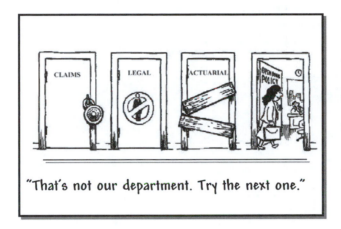

"That's not our department. Try the next one."

# Exercise 1-1

**Directions:** Find and circle the words listed below. Words can appear horizontally, vertically, diagonally, forward, or backward.

```
Z L P X L E E G Q M M I H E V S I S E I
T I F E N E B E E Y O L P M E N K T C T
F S J E A O F F E L B E R Z S I R O N B
N M E I M S I C F E D O P U H H O P A L
F C E G C B N S N S T S R C C L W L R O
A N W I A A E E S A Q A C K F R T O U F
J R R I R M F Z R E N A C O I E E S S L
I X K U X I A T Z C R O E Z K N N S N E
G C S F C V S D E L K P U T O I N I I G
Y N Y I I I I C E H E D P G C Q I N P A
I M A L N J O L C V O M F O O C U S U L
G R Z I S M J L X O I B E Y C G I U O D
Y D M P P T F P C X Z T C N M H P R R A
H D G A I N E O S W G I I I T R K A G M
A P N E L B I T C U D E D N N Q C N I A
J Y G P T M U Q B P N G W I U S B C T G
I N V E S T I G A T I O N Q S P U E L E
V O Q O X G X G U A S T Q W I N T R H S
S Q V B V J W O X Y Y B F R Y S V J E K
E Y Q A C A C A K P R E M I U M S O D D
```

**1.** Embezzlement

**2.** Employee Benefit

**3.** Group Insurance

**4.** Insurance

**5.** Investigation

**6.** Legal Damages

**7.** Oppression

**8.** Premiums

**9.** Punitive Damages

**10.** Stoploss Insurance

# Exercise **1-2**

**Directions:** Complete the crossword puzzle by filling in a word from the keywords that fits each clue.

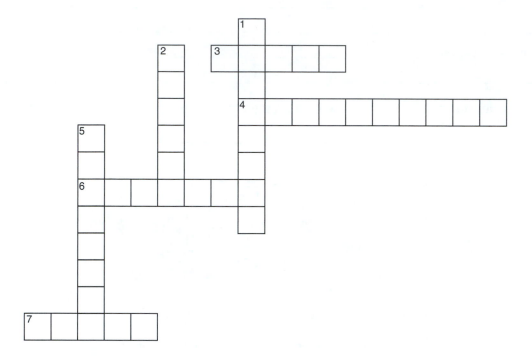

**Across**

3. Deception to cause a person to give up property or something of lawful right.
4. A denial or renunciation, as of responsibility.
6. An item covered by an insurance policy, or something paid to or on behalf of a recipient.
7. A written request by the insured individual for payment by the insurance company of covered expenses under the insurance policy.

**Down**

1. Items or services offered for sale by a company. In the case of insurance carriers, the products are the various policies they offer.
2. Intentional conduct to cause injury, or conduct that is carried on with the conscious disregard of the rights of others.
5. A written legal order directing a person or document to appear in court to testify.

# Exercise 1-3

**Directions:** Match the following terms with the proper definition by writing the letter of the correct definition in the space next to the term.

1. _____ Actuarial Statistics

2. _____ Compensatory Damages

3. _____ Department of Insurance

4. _____ Individual Insurance

5. _____ Insurance Policy

6. _____ Insurance Speculation

7. _____ Lapse in Coverage

8. _____ Reinsurance

9. _____ Renewal

10. _____ Self Funded Plan

11. _____ Third-Party Administrator

a. A person or entity buying insurance or maintaining coverage for the purpose of making a profit.

b. A plan administration firm that deals solely with administering the eligibility and claim payment services (along with various other administrative services) for self-funded plans.

c. A break in continuous insurance coverage, usually resulting from nonpayment of premium.

d. When the total and ultimate responsibility for providing all plan benefit payments rests solely with the employer, group, or association.

e. An insurance that covers expenses when the benefit payments on a self-funded plan exceed a certain amount.

f. Paying a premium in order to continue coverage after the initial policy period has expired.

g. An insurance policy issued to insure the life or health of a named person or persons, rather than the life or health of the members of a group.

h. Damages designed to compensate an insured for all of the actual losses or damages to make that person whole again.

i. Studies that an insurance company uses. For a carrier that covers health insurance, these can include statistics covering average life span, number of days in hospital per year for each age group, number of doctor visits, costs of all medical services, and so on.

j. A written contract defining the insurance plan, its coverage, exclusions, eligibility requirements, and all benefits and conditions that apply to individuals insured under the plan.

k. The legal entity that oversees the operations of all insurance companies.

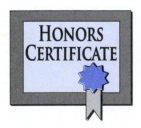

## Honors Certification™

The Honors Certification™ challenge for this chapter consists of a written test of the information contained within this chapter. In the second test you will also be presented with several scenarios and asked to respond to the situations using the guidelines in this chapter. Each incorrect answer will result in a deduction of up to 5% from your grade. You must achieve a score of 80% or higher to pass this test. If you fail the test on your first attempt, you may retake the test one additional time. The items included in the second test may be different from those in the first test.

# 2 Resource Manuals
## and Billing Forms

## After completion of this chapter
**you will be able to:**

- Recognize the reference books commonly used by health claims examiners (*CPT*®, *ICD-9-CM*, *CDT*, *Merck Manual*, *Physician's Desk Reference (PDR)*, medical dictionaries, and *Red Book* and *Blue Book*) and explain their uses.

- Properly identify various information on a completed CMS-1500 form.

- Properly identify various information on a completed UB-92 billing form.

- Properly look up the meaning of a hospital revenue code.

## Keywords and concepts
**you will learn in this chapter:**

- CMS-1500
- *Current Dental Terminology (CDT)*
- Healthcare Common Procedure Coding System (HCPCS)
- *International Classification of Disease – 9th Revision*
- *Clinical Modification (ICD-9-CM)*
- Medical Dictionary
- *Merck Manual*
- Modifier Codes
- *Physicians' Current Procedure Terminology (CPT*®*)*
- *Physicians' Desk Reference (PDR)*
- Procedure Code
- *Red Book* and *Blue Book*
- *Relative Value Study (RVS)*
- UB-92

A resource manual or reference book is a source of information to which a reader is referred. In health claims billing, coding, and examining, there are a number of books that are utilized as reference books. These include the *International Classification of Diseases—9th Revision—Clinical Modification (ICD-9-CM)*, *Physician's Current Procedure Terminology (CPT®)*, *Relative Value Study (RVS)*, *Current Dental Terminology (CDT)*, *Health Care Common Procedure Coding System (HCPCS)*, *Physicians' Desk Reference (PDR)*, various medical dictionaries, the *Merck Manual*, and the *Red Book* and *Blue Book*. We will discuss each of these books briefly in this chapter.

## ICD-9-CM

The **International Classification of Diseases–9th Revision Clinical Modification (ICD-9-CM)** is an indexing of conditions that serves a dual purpose for health benefits personnel. Mainly, it enables the medical biller and the claims examiner to convert English language descriptions of an illness, injury, or other condition into a numerical code. Secondly, it allows for the classification of diseases for statistical purposes. Symptoms, diseases, injuries, and routine services are identified with either a three-, four-, or five-digit code, which may be entirely numerical or a combination of letters and numbers.

The *ICD-9-CM* consists of three volumes:

- Volume I – A tabular listing of diseases.
- Volume II – An alphabetical listing of diseases by English language description.
- Volume III – A numerical and alphabetical listing of surgical or nonsurgical procedures that may be performed by a physician.

The order of use and the degree of use of each of these volumes varies. However, Volume III is not widely used by health claims personnel.

### Volume I

Volume I is structured numerically according to body system. It is used when:

1. An *ICD-9-CM* code is provided, but there is no language description of the diagnosis.

2. A language diagnosis is included, but an *ICD-9-CM* is not indicated and the terms used by the provider cannot be found in Volume II. If you can identify the body system, you may be able to locate an appropriate *ICD-9-CM* code.

Volume I is categorized as follows:

| BODY # | SYSTEM/ CLASSIFICATION |
|---|---|
| 001-139 | Infectious and Parasitic Diseases |
| 140-239 | Neoplasms |
| 240-279 | Endocrine, Nutritional, Metabolic Diseases and Immunity Disorders |
| 280-289 | Diseases of the Blood and Blood-Forming Organs |
| 290-319 | Mental Disorders |
| 320-389 | Diseases of the Nervous System and Sense Organs |
| 390-459 | Diseases of the Circulatory System |
| 460-519 | Diseases of the Respiratory System |
| 520-579 | Diseases of the Digestive System |
| 580-629 | Diseases of the Genitourinary System |
| 630-679 | Complications of Pregnancy, Childbirth, and the Puerperium |
| 680-709 | Diseases of the Skin and Subcutaneous Tissue |
| 710-739 | Diseases of the Musculoskeletal System and Connective Tissue |
| 740-759 | Congenital Anomalies |
| 760-779 | Certain Conditions Originating in the Perinatal Period |
| 780-799 | Symptoms, Signs, and Ill-Defined Conditions |
| 800-899 | Injury and Poisoning |

**SUPPLEMENTARY CLASSIFICATION**

| V-Codes | Supplementary Classification of Factors Influencing Health Status and Contact with Health Services |
|---|---|
| E-Codes | Supplementary Classification of External Causes of Injury and Poisoning |

A number in parentheses after a code is the page number in Volume II that can be checked to verify the code.

### Volume II

Volume II is the alphabetical listing of diagnoses. This section is most commonly used first. It is divided into four sections:

1. An alphabetical index of diseases and injuries.
2. A table of drugs and chemicals.
3. An alphabetical index of external causes of injuries and poisonings (accidents) (E codes).
4. A listing of factors affecting the health status of an individual (V codes).

## Volume III

Volume III of the *ICD-9-CM* is used for coding diagnoses and procedures performed in a hospital. Volume III contains both a tabular listing and index. The tabular listing has procedures arranged according to body sections. The body sections are arranged as follows:

1. Operations on the Nervous System
2. Operations on the Endocrine System
3. Operations on the Eye
4. Operations on the Ear
5. Operations on the Nose, Mouth, and Pharynx
6. Operations on the Respiratory System
7. Operations on the Cardiovascular System
8. Operations on the Hemic and Lymphatic System
9. Operations on the Digestive System
10. Operations on the Urinary System
11. Operations on the Male Genital Organs
12. Operations on the Female Genital Organs
13. Obstetrical Procedures
14. Operations on the Musculoskeletal System
15. Operations on the Integumentary System
16. Miscellaneous Diagnostic and Therapeutic Procedures

The index has procedures listed in alphabetical order. Thus, it is the easiest way to look up a procedure. The health claims examiner should confirm that the correct code has been selected by looking in the tabular listing and checking all referrals, exclusions, and notes included.

# CPT®/RVS

The ***Physicians' Current Procedure Terminology (CPT®)*** is a systematic listing for coding the procedures or services performed by a physician. Within this text the word "physician" is used generically to apply to any provider of services other than a hospital or other facility. A **procedure code** is a five-digit numer-

ical code used to designate medical services according to standardized, industry accepted methods, usually reflected in the *CPT®* manual. The purpose of the *CPT®* is to provide a uniform method of accurately describing medical, surgical, and diagnostic services, which facilitates an effective means of communication among physicians, patients, and claim administrators. **Modifier codes** are two-digit numerical codes attached to a *CPT®* code to indicate special circumstances for that particular service.

The ***Relative Value Study (RVS)*** is another reference book used for coding physician services. The studies assign unit values to a particular procedure code. The *RVS* preceded the *CPT®* and was, in fact, the basis on which the *CPT®* was designed. Consequently, the purpose of the *RVS* is the same as that of the *CPT®*. These two manuals are referred to interchangeably even though the rules guiding their usage differ somewhat. Therefore, it is important for the medical biller and claims examiner to know which standard is specified by the plan being processed so that the appropriate rules can be used. The *CPT®* and *RVS* each have six major sections:

1. Evaluation and Management  99201–99499
2. Medicine  90281–99199, 99500–99602
3. Surgery  10040–69990
4. Anesthesiology, *CPT®* 00100–01999, 99100–99140
5. *RVS*  99100–99140 (same as surgery but add anesthesia modifier)
6. Radiology  70010–79999
7. Pathology & Laboratory  80048–89356

To properly code using the *CPT®*, choose the number code associated with the English-language description of the procedure performed. Sometimes the procedure will be phrased in different terminology (i.e., testectomy is found under orchiectomy even though both are legitimate medical terms). Therefore, it is important to check all related codes and alternate terminology for a procedure. It may also be necessary to consult a medical dictionary for alternate terminology for a specified procedure.

Each section of the *CPT®* has specific instructions relating to that section prior to the first codes. It is important that you read each of these instructions in order to properly code the procedures contained in that section.

Some descriptions in the *CPT®* are subprocedures of other descriptions. These subheading descriptions will be indented under the main procedure. To properly read an indented procedure, read the description of the main procedure (the one not indented) up to the semicolon. Then add the remaining description found in the indented wording.

For example, codes 21208 and 21209 read as follows:

21208　　Osteoplasty, facial bones; augmentation

21209　　　　　reduction

Therefore, the correct description for 21209 is Osteoplasty, facial bones; reduction. It is important to carefully read the full description of all related procedures before choosing the one which best describes the procedure performed. A slight change in the main description can significantly alter the meaning of the indented procedure.

## Using the *CPT*® Index

The *CPT*® index lists all main procedures, often with a choice of several codes. Once again, some procedures are indented, indicating that the unindented procedure listed directly above them is part of the description.

Listings in the *CPT*® are arranged by the procedure done, then by the site of the procedure. For example, the heading Transplantation then lists numerous portions of the body which can be transplanted, and their related codes. Some portions of the body also have a heading. Thus, the code for transplantation of the liver can be located by looking under either Transplantation and Liver or Liver and Allotransplantation. In most cases it is best to check both descriptions since there may be additional codes located under one of the descriptions.

## *CDT*

The *Current Dental Terminology (CDT)* is a reference manual published by the American Dental Association that contains dental procedure codes. Dental procedure codes are comprised of the letter "D" followed by four numbers. The codes provide the dental profession with a standardized coding system to document and to communicate accurate information about dental treatment procedures and services to agencies involved in adjudicating insurance claims. *CDT* codes are used in dental offices and by the dental benefits industry for purposes of keeping patient records, reporting procedures on patients and processing and reporting of dental insurance claims, and in developing, marketing, and administering dental benefit products.

## HCPCS

The **Health Care Common Procedure Coding System (HCPCS)** (Commonly referred to as 'hicpics' in the medical community) came about because of the limitations in the *CPT*® and *RVS* for billing injections, medication, supplies, and durable medical equipment. These codes are most often used for billing Medicare claims but may also be used for Medicaid claims and for some carriers. The HCPCS system actually includes three levels of coding:

- Level I utilizes the current *CPT*® codes for most procedures.
- Level II utilizes the HCPCS codes listed in the HCPCS manual.
- Level III utilizes codes which are specific to the local Medicare carrier.

To properly code using the HCPCS system, you should check Level III codes first. If no code exists for the service or item you are billing, check the Level II codes. Only if there is no Level III or Level II code should you use the appropriate *CPT*® code.

To use the HCPCS manual:

1. If you have a code number, but need the English language equivalent, look in the front section of the HCPCS. HCPCS codes have a letter, then several numbers. The codes are listed by the letter, then the numbers within that letter (i.e., V2100, V2101, V2102, etc.). Additionally, codes are assigned within groups. Therefore the items within a group will be found near each other (i.e., medications, orthopedic devices, etc.).
2. If you have an English language equivalent and need to look up a HCPCS code, look up the item in the index.

## Physicians' Desk Reference

*Physicians' Desk Reference (PDR)*—A manual that provides information on prescription drugs, including usage, dosage, appearance, prescription status, makeup, and other factors. Among other things the *PDR* enables a person to determine whether a pharmaceutical product is a prescription or nonprescription drug. This is a very important distinction since most health plans do not cover nonprescription drugs.

The *PDR* is divided into six sections:

1. **Manufacturer's Index (white)** arranged alphabetically by manufacturer, then by drug

name. The name and address of the manufacturer are included. This section includes prescription and nonprescription drugs. The related information has been provided by the manufacturer.

2. **Product Name Index (pink)** arranged alphabetically by brand name or generic name (if provided). Prescription and nonprescription drugs are included. This section is usually used first to locate the manufacturer's name and the page number for further information.

3. **Product Category Index (blue)** arranged alphabetically by drug action category, that is, according to the most common use of the drug. If the drug is an antidepressant, it is listed under the antidepressant category. If it is an antacid, it is listed under the antacid category.

4. **Product Identification Section (gray)** arranged alphabetically by manufacturer, then by brand name. This section contains the actual size and full-color reproductions. Only the reproductions submitted by the manufacturer are included.

5. **Product Information Section (white)** arranged alphabetically by manufacturer, then brand name. Most pharmaceuticals are described by indications and usage, dosage, administration, description, clinical pharmacology, supply warnings, contraindications, adverse reactions, overdosage precautions, and other information.

6. **Diagnostic Product Information (green)** arranged alphabetically by manufacturer, then by product. This section provides a description of diagnostic products only.

Claims examiners use the Product Information Section (white) the most. However, since generic drugs are cheaper than brand name medications, many plans encourage their members to purchase generically and offer increased payment incentives. Therefore, use of the Product Name Index (which includes both brand names and generic names) is increasing. For instance, instead of paying for generic drugs at the plan's regular coinsurance rate of 80%, 100% may be payable. As with all benefits, this varies widely by plan.

# Medical Dictionary

**Medical dictionaries** list medical terms and their definitions, synonyms, illustrations, and supplemental information. Numerous medical dictionaries are

on the market. These dictionaries can be very helpful in assisting the examiner to identify diagnoses, their symptoms, prognoses, and common treatment protocols. The use of a dictionary can assist the claims examiner in both coding the claim and determining whether or not the diagnosis or service is allowable under a plan.

As a rule, this manual should be used mainly for verifying a diagnosis or affected body area or checking definitions and the spelling of terms. For greater detail on symptomatology and treatment protocols, the *Merck Manual* is more definitive. As with most dictionaries, entries are arranged alphabetically.

When using the medical dictionary, it is important that you first read through the foreword and any instructions or general guidelines contained in the front of the book. Since each publisher uses different symbols and information, you must read these instructions to understand the symbols and terms and their meanings.

# Merck Manual

Even the most experienced examiner occasionally has questions regarding the appropriateness of services for a reported diagnosis. The *Merck Manual* is relied on within the medical profession to assist in identifying the symptomatology, prognosis, treatment protocols, etiology, and other miscellaneous information regarding diagnoses.

When an examiner receives a claim with unusual services based on the diagnosis, using the *Merck Manual* may assist in identifying whether or not the treatment is appropriate for the reported diagnosis or symptoms.

The *Merck Manual* has two main sections: a listing of diseases and an index. The index is arranged alphabetically by disease. To look something up, simply turn to the index to find out what page the disease information is on.

The information provided includes the diagnosis, symptoms, prognosis, and treatment. If the treatment provided is not consistent with the diagnosis, it may be forwarded to a medical review board or a consultant, causing a delay in the processing of the claim.

# Red Book and Blue Book

The ***Red Book*** and ***Blue Book*** are manuals which list drug product information, along with prevailing wholesale prices.

# Practice
# Pitfalls

In addition to basic definitions, many medical dictionaries include other information regarding the word or term. These can include the following 14 pieces of information:

1. The etymology of the word (i.e., the original language and meaning).

2. The pronunciation of the word.

3. Biographical information on diseases, symptoms, conditions, procedures, or cures that have been given an eponym (named after a person, such as Addison's disease).

4. Synonyms. Often diseases or conditions are known by more than one name. In these instances, they are listed as synonyms in the dictionary (i.e., Addison's disease: adrenocortical hypofunction).

5. Abbreviations. If a word or term has a standard abbreviation in the medical community, this abbreviation is often listed in the medical dictionary.

6. Etiology. The causes of the disease.

7. Treatment. Common medical treatments are stated for some diagnoses or conditions. It is understood that this may not be the only effective medical treatment and that specifics of the treatment are not given.

8. Cross-reference. Cross-references for treatments may be included, allowing the user to locate possible drugs or treatments that may prove to be effective.

9. Prognosis. A generalized prognosis for the disease is given. At times it will include a prognosis for patients who are not treated and for those who are.

10. Nursing implications. The implications of care of the patient are listed. This may include the need for monitoring of certain conditions or vital signs.

11. Nursing diagnosis cross-reference. Some dictionaries list an appendix of nursing diagnoses and implications. Certain diseases or conditions will be cross-referenced to this section.

12. Subentries. Subentries contain more specific information regarding a term or condition and list some of the different types of conditions that can occur. For example, the subentries under the term "acid" can include acetic a., boric a., citric a., fatty a., and sulfuric a., as well as many others. It is understood that a small letter followed by a period refers to a repetition of the original term or condition. In the example above, the "a." would stand for the word "acid."

13. Illustration cross-reference. An illustration can occur in the dictionary—placed either near the word or under another heading—that illustrates either the term or a portion of the definition. The user is directed to the correct page or term under which the illustration can be found.

14. Cautions or warnings. Certain terms or conditions have a warning placed within the definition. This is most often used with drugs and treatments. This warning can include any side effects or adverse reactions or conditions that can occur from use of the drug or treatment. Often this caution or warning is in boldface or marked off within a section to help call attention to it.

When using the medical dictionary, it is imperative that the health claims examiner read through the entire entry. If terms are used in the definition that the health claims examiner does not understand, the unknown word should also be looked up, either in the medical dictionary (if it is a medical term) or in a standard dictionary (if it is not).

There are numerous diseases, conditions, or terms that are very similar to each other in spelling or pronunciation, but vastly different in meaning. It is important to use the proper term and its proper spelling when billing, coding, and examining a claim.

Some plans have a separate drug coverage. Drugs on these plans are often paid according to a set price schedule, regardless of the amount charged by the pharmacy or dispensing physician. These schedules are often based upon the *Blue Book* or the *Red Book*. These two books list wholesale prices of drugs.

Often the plan provisions will specify payment at 150% or 175% of the *Blue Book* or *Red Book* price.

# On the Job Now

**Directions:** Determine the correct resource manual needed to answer the question, and then use that reference to find the answer. Do not be concerned if you do not understand all the words in the description or answer.

1. What is the English language description for diagnosis codes 460 and 487.1? _____

_____

2. Describe diagnosis 1 (code 460) from question 1. _____

_____

3. Define catarrhal. _____

_____

4. Is fever most commonly a symptom of diagnosis 1 or diagnosis 2? _____

5. What is a synonym for the common cold? _____

6. How long is a person contagious with this disease? _____

_____

7. Name two symptoms or signs of diagnosis 1. _____

_____

8. What causes the condition from diagnosis 1? _____

_____

9. What is the incubation period for this disease? _____

10. What is the procedure code 87070 for and is it appropriate for diagnosis code 460? _____

_____

## CMS-1500 Form

There are two types of forms most commonly used for billing claims, the CMS-1500 and the UB-92. The **CMS-1500** (Health Care Finance Administration) claim form is a standardized form, approved by the American Medical Association for use as a "universal" form for billing professional services (**see Figures 2–1 and 2–2**). Many providers' offices use only the CMS-1500 for billing; however, a few still use alternate forms unique to their office (called "superbills").

As you use this form, you will become familiar with the various blocks and know where to obtain the information required for completing and processing claim forms. The following listing will assist in explaining the uses of the various blocks. It contains the block number along with the name of the block and a brief description of the information needed. The word "same" refers to a description that is the same as the title of the block. Explanations which are too lengthy to be included here have been recorded after this brief listing.

# On the Job Now

**Directions:** Determine the correct resource manual needed to answer the question, and then use that reference to find the answer. Do not be concerned if you do not understand all the words in the description or answer.

1. What is the English Language description for diagnosis code 696.1? _____

_____

2. Describe the disease from question 1. _____

_____

3. What are erythematous papules? _____

_____

4. What is the cause of the disease in question 1? _____

_____

5. Name two symptoms or signs of this disease. _____

_____

6. Name two possible treatments for this disease. _____

_____

7. What is the English language description for procedure code 97028? _____

_____

8. Is procedure code 97028 a valid treatment for diagnosis code 696.1? _____

9. Should a patient with this disease expose themselves to sunlight? _____

10. Does smoking affect this condition? If so, in what way? _____

_____

Since it is easier to remember information in groups, we have broken the CMS-1500 into sections. These sections include information about the patient, the insured, the secondary insurance, third party liability, authorization signature, the illness, the procedures performed, and the provider of services.

## Block # and Block Name/Description

Following are the numbers, titles, and descriptions of the blocks found on the CMS-1500.

## Information About the Patient

These blocks contain information about the patient.

1  **Medicare, Medicaid, TRICARE (CHAMPUS), CHAMPVA, FECA Black Lung or Other.** Check the box of the organization to which you are submitting this claim for payment if you are submitting the form to one of those organizations listed.

2  **Patient's Name.** Same.

PLEASE
DO NOT
STAPLE
IN THIS
AREA

BALL INSURANCE CARRIERS
3895 BUBBLE BLVD STE 283
BUXWOOD CO 85926

APPROVED MOB-0938-0008

□□□ PICA

# HEALTH INSURANCE CLAIM FORM

PICA □□□

| 1. MEDICARE  MEDICAID  CHAMPUS  CHAMPVA  GROUP HEALTH PLAN  FECA BLK LUNG  OTHER | 1a. INSURED'S I.D NUMBER  (FOR PROGRAM IN ITEM 1) |
|---|---|
| ☐ (Medicare #)  ☐ (Medicaid #)  ☐ (Sponsor's SSN)  ☐ (VA File #)  ☒ (SSN or ID)  ☐ (SSN)  ☐ (ID) | 777 77 XYZ |

| 2. PATIENT'S NAME (Last, First, Middle Initial). | 3. PATIENT'S BIRTH DATE  MM DD  SEX | 4. INSURED'S NAME (Last, First, Middle Initial) |
|---|---|---|
| NORMAL NANCY N | 07 02 CCYY-28  M ☐ F ☒ | SAME |

| 5. PATIENT'S ADDRESS (No., Street) | 6. PATIENT'S RELATIONSHIP TO INSURED | 7. INSURED'S ADDRESS (No., Street) |
|---|---|---|
| 707 NATIONAL STREET | Self ☒ Spouse ☐ Child ☐ Other ☐ | |
| CITY  NANDO  STATE  NV | 8. PATIENT STATUS  Single ☒ Married ☐ Other ☐ | CITY  STATE |
| ZIP CODE  89577  TELEPHONE (Include Area Code)  (775) 555 3377 | Employed ☒ Full-Time ☐ Part-Time ☐  Student Student | ZIP CODE  TELEPHONE (INCLUDE AREA CODE) |

| 9. OTHER INSURED'S NAME (Last, First, Middle Initial) | 10. IS PATIENT'S CONDITION RELATED TO: | 11. INSURED'S POLICY GROUP OR FECA NUMBER:  62958XYZ |
|---|---|---|
| a. OTHER INSURED'S POLICY OR GROUP NUMBER | a. EMPLOYMENT? (CURRENT OR PREVIOUS)  ☐ YES ☒ NO | a. INSURED'S DATE OF BIRTH  MM DD YY  SEX  M ☐ F ☐ |
| b. OTHER INSURED'S DATE OF BIRTH  MM DD YY  SEX  M ☐ F ☐ | b. AUTO ACCIDENT?  PLACE (State)  ☐ YES ☒ NO |_____| | b. EMPLOYER'S NAME OR SCHOOL NAME  XYZ CORPORATION |
| c. EMPLOYER'S NAME OR SCHOOL NAME | c. OTHER ACCIDENT?  ☐ YES ☒ NO | c. INSURANCE PLAN NAME OR PROGRAM NAME  BALL INSURANCE CARRIERS |
| d. INSURANCE PLAN NAME OR PROGRAM NAME | 10d. RESERVED FOR LOCAL USE | d. IS THERE ANOTHER HEALTH BENEFIT PLAN?  ☐ YES ☒ NO  if yes, return to and complete item 9 a-d |

READ BACK OF FORM BEFORE COMPLETING & SIGNING THIS FORM
12. PATIENT'S OR AUTHORIZED PERSON'S SIGNATURE I authorize the release of any medical or other information necessary to process this claim. I also request payment of government benefits either to myself or to the party who accepts assignment below.

SIGNED  SIGNATURE ON FILE   DATE

13. INSURED'S OR AUTHORIZED PERSON'S SIGNATURE I authorize payment of medical benefits to the undersigned physician or supplier for services described below.

SIGNED  SIGNATURE ON FILE

| 14. DATE OF CURRENT:  MM DD YY  ◄ ILLNESS (1st symptom)  INJURY (Accident)  PREGNANCY (LMP)  02 03 YY | 15. IF PATIENT HAS HAD SAME OR SIMILAR ILLNESS, GIVE FIRST DATE  MM DD YY | 16. DATES PATIENT UNABLE TO WORK IN CURRENT OCCUPATION  MM DD YY  MM DD YY  FROM  TO |
|---|---|---|
| 17. NAME OF REFERRING PHYSICIAN OR OTHER SOURCE | 17a. I.D. NUMBER OF REFERRING PHYSICIAN | 18. HOSPITALIZATION DATES RELATED TO CURRENT SERVICES  MM DD YY  MM DD YY  FROM  TO |
| 19. RESERVED FOR LOCAL USE | | 20. OUTSIDE LAB?  $ CHARGES  ☐ YES ☐ NO |

| 21. DIAGNOSIS OR NATURE OF ILLNESS OR INJURY, (RELATE ITEMS 1,2,3, OR 4 TO ITEM 24E BY LINE) | 22. MEDICAID RESUBMISSION  CODE  ORIGINAL REF. NO. |
|---|---|
| 1. |_079_._3_|  3. |_____.___| | 23. PRIOR AUTHORIZATION NUMBER |
| 2. |_____.___|  4. |_____.___| | |

| 24. A  DATE(S) OF SERVICE  From    To  MM DD YY  MM DD YY | B  Place of Service | C  Type of Service | D  PROCEDURES, SERVICES, OR SUPPLIES  (Explain Unusual Circumstances)  CPT/HCPS | MODIFIER | E  DIAGNOSIS CODE | F  $ CHARGES | G  DAYS OR UNITS | H  EPSDT Family Plan | I  EMG | J  COB | K  RESERVED FOR LOCAL USE |
|---|---|---|---|---|---|---|---|---|---|---|---|
| 02 05 YY 02 05 YY | 11 | 1 | 99201 | | 1 | 220 00 | 1 | | | | |
| 02 05 YY 02 05 YY | 11 | 1 | 85025 | | 1 | 40 00 | 1 | | | | |
| 02 05 YY 02 05 YY | 11 | 1 | 87040 | | 1 | 30 00 | 1 | | | | |
| | | | | | | | | | | | |
| | | | | | | | | | | | |

| 25. FEDERAL TAX I.D. NUMBER  SSN EIN | 26. PATIENT'S ACCOUNT NO. | 27. ACCEPT ASSIGNMENT?  (For govt. claims, see back) | 28. TOTAL CHARGE | 29. AMOUNT PAID | 30. BALANCE DUE |
|---|---|---|---|---|---|
| 70 7759777  ☐ ☒ | NANNR001  737 | ☒ YES ☐ NO | $ 290 00 | $ 200 00 | $ 90 00 |

| 31. SIGNATURE OF PHYSICIAN OR SUPPLIER INCLUDING DEGREES OR CREDENTIALS  (I certify that the statements on the reverse apply to this bill and are made a part thereof.)  SIGNED  Dee N Aee MD  DATE 02/18/YY | 32. NAME AND ADDRESS OF FACILITY WHERE SERVICES WERE RENDERED (If other than home or office) | 33. PHYSICIAN'S, SUPPLIERS BILLING NAME, ADDRESS, ZIP CODE & PHONE #  DEE N AEE MD  2577 NONE STREET STE 575N  NOLTY NV 89578  (775) 555 0077  PIN# D44444  GRP# |
|---|---|---|

(APPROVED BY AMA COUNCIL ON MEDICAL SERVICE 8/88)   **PLEASE PRINT OR TYPE**

FORM CMS-1500 (12-90)
FORM OWCP-1500  FORM RRB-1500
FORM AMA-OP050591

■ **Figure 2–1** Front of CMS-1500

BECAUSE THIS FORM IS USED BY VARIOUS GOVERNMENT AND PRIVATE HEALTH PROGRAMS, SEE SEPARATE INSTRUCTIONS ISSUED BY APPLICABLE PROGRAMS.

NOTICE: Any person who knowingly files a statement of claim containing any misrepresentation or any false, incomplete or misleading information may be guilty of a criminal act punishable under law and may be subject to civil penalties.

### REFERS TO GOVERNMENT PROGRAMS ONLY

MEDICARE AND CHAMPUS PAYMENTS: A patient's signature requests that payment be made and authorizes release of any information necessary to process the claim and certifies that the information provided in Blocks 1 through 12 is true, accurate and complete. In the case of a Medicare claim, the patient's signature authorizes any entity to release to Medicare medical and nonmedical information, including employment status, and whether the person has employer group health insurance, liability, no-fault, worker's compensation or other insurance which is responsible to pay for the services for which the Medicare claim is made. See 42 CFR 411.24(a). If item 9 is completed, the patient's signature authorizes release of the information to the health plan or agency shown. In Medicare assigned or CHAMPUS participation cases, the physician agrees to accept the charge determination of the Medicare carrier or CHAMPUS fiscal intermediary as the full charge, and the patient is responsible only for the deductible, coinsurance and noncovered services. Coinsurance and the deductible are based upon the charge determination of the Medicare carrier or CHAMPUS fiscal intermediary if this is less than the charge submitted. CHAMPUS is not a health insurance program but makes payment for health benefits provided through certain affiliations with the Uniformed Services. Information on the patient's sponsor should be provided in those items captioned in "Insured"; i.e., items 1a, 4, 6, 7, 9, and 11.

### BLACK LUNG AND FECA CLAIMS

The provider agrees to accept the amount paid by the Government as payment in full. See Black Lung and FECA instructions regarding required procedure and diagnosis coding systems.

### SIGNATURE OF PHYSICIAN OR SUPPLIER (MEDICARE, CHAMPUS, FECA AND BLACK LUNG)

I certify that the services shown on this form were medically indicated and necessary for the health of the patient and were personally furnished by me or were furnished incident to my professional service by my employee under my immediate personal supervision, except as otherwise expressly permitted by Medicare or CHAMPUS regulations.

For services to be considered as "incident" to a physician's professional service, 1) they must be rendered under the physician's immediate personal supervision by his/her employee, 2) they must be an integral, although incidental part of a covered physician's service, 3) they must be of kinds commonly furnished in physician's offices, and 4) the services of nonphysicians must be included on the physician's bills.

For CHAMPUS claims, I further certify that I (or any employee) who rendered services am not an active duty member of the Uniformed Services or a civilian employee of the United States Government or a contract employee of the United States Government, either civilian or military (refer to 5 USC 5536). For Black-Lung claims, I further certify that the services performed were for a Black Lung-related disorder.

No Part B Medicare benefits may be paid unless this form is received as required by existing law and regulations (42 CFR 424.32).

NOTICE: Any one who misrepresents or falsifies essential information to receive payment from Federal funds requested by this form may upon conviction be subject to fine and imprisonment under applicable Federal laws.

### NOTICE TO PATIENT ABOUT THE COLLECTION AND USE OF MEDICARE, CHAMPUS, FECA, AND BLACK LUNG INFORMATION
### (PRIVACY ACT STATEMENT)

We are authorized by HCFA, CHAMPUS and OWCP to ask you for information needed in the administration of the Medicare, CHAMPUS, FECA, and Black Lung programs. Authority to collect information is in section 205(a), 1862, 1872 and 1874 of the Social Security Act as amended, 42 CFR 411.24(a) and 424.5(a) (6), and 44 USC 3101;41 CFR 101 et seq and 10 USC 1079 and 1086; 5 USC 8101 et seq; and 30 USC 901 et seq; 38 USC 613; E.O. 9397.

The information we obtain to complete claims under these programs is used to identify you and to determine your eligibility. It is also used to decide if the services and supplies you received are covered by these programs and to insure that proper payment is made.

The information may also be given to other providers of services, carriers, intermediaries, medical review boards, health plans, and other organizations or Federal agencies, for the effective administration of Federal provisions that require other third parties payers to pay primary to Federal program, and as otherwise necessary to administer these programs. For example, it may be necessary to disclose information about the benefits you have used to a hospital or doctor. Additional disclosures are made through routine uses for information contained in systems of records.

FOR MEDICARE CLAIMS: See the notice modifying system No. 09-70-0501, titled, 'Carrier Medicare Claims Record,' published in the Federal Register, Vol. 55 No. 177, page 37549, Wed. Sept. 12, 1990, or as updated and republished.

FOR OWCP CLAIMS: Department of Labor, Privacy Act of 1974, "Republication of Notice of Systems of Records," Federal Register Vol. 55 No. 40, Wed Feb. 28, 1990, See ESA-5, ESA-6, ESA-12, ESA-13, ESA-30, or as updated and republished.

FOR CHAMPUS CLAIMS: PRINCIPLE PURPOSE(S): To evaluate eligibility for medical care provided by civilian sources and to issue payment upon establishment of eligibility and determination that the services/supplies received are authorized by law.

ROUTINE USE(S): Information from claims and related documents may be given to the Dept. of Veterans Affairs, the Dept. of Health and Human Services and/or the Dept. of Transportation consistent with their statutory administrative responsibilities under CHAMPUS/CHAMPVA; to the Dept. of Justice for representation of the Secretary of Defense in civil actions; to the Internal Revenue Service, private collection agencies, and consumer reporting agencies in connection with recoupment claims; and to Congressional Offices in response to inquiries made at the request of the person to whom a record pertains. Appropriate disclosures may be made to other federal, state, local, foreign government agencies, private business entities, and individual providers of care, on matters relating to entitlement, claims adjudication, fraud, program abuse, utilization review, quality assurance, peer review, program integrity, third-party liability, coordination of benefits, and civil and criminal litigation related to the operation of CHAMPUS.

DISCLOSURES: Voluntary; however, failure to provide information will result in delay in payment or may result in denial of claim. With the one exception discussed below, there are no penalties under these programs for refusing to supply information. However, failure to furnish information regarding the medical services rendered or the amount charged would prevent payment of claims under these programs. Failure to furnish any other information, such as name or claim number, would delay payment of the claim. Failure to provide medical information under FECA could be deemed an obstruction.

It is mandatory that you tell us if you know that another party is responsible for paying for your treatment. Section 1128B of the Social Security Act and 31 USC 3801-3812 provide penalties for withholding this information.

You should be aware that P.L. 100-503, the "Computer Matching and Privacy Protection Act of 1988", permits the government to verify information by way of computer matches.

### MEDICAID PAYMENTS (PROVIDER CERTIFICATION)

I hereby agree to keep such records as are necessary to disclose fully the extent of services provided to individuals under the State's Title XIX plan and to furnish information regarding any payments claimed for providing such services as the State Agency or Dept. of Health and Humans Services may request.

I further agree to accept, as payment in full, the amount paid by the Medicaid program for those claims submitted for payment under that program, with the exception of authorized deductible, coinsurance, copayment or similar cost-sharing charge.

SIGNATURE OF PHYSICIAN (OR SUPPLIER): I certify that the services listed above were medically indicated and necessary to the health of this patient and were personally furnished by me or my employee under my personal direction.

NOTICE: This is to certify that the foregoing information is true, accurate and complete. I understand that payment and satisfaction of this claim will be from Federal and State funds, and that any false claims, statements, or documents, or concealment of a material fact, may be prosecuted under applicable Federal or State laws.

Public reporting burden for this collection of information is estimated to average 15 minutes per response, including time for reviewing instructions, searching existing date sources, gathering and maintaining data needed, and completing and reviewing the collection of information. Send comments regarding this burden estimate or any other aspect of this collection of information, including suggestions for reducing the burden, to HCFA, Office of Financial Management, P.O. Box 26684, Baltimore, MD 21207; and to the Office of Management and Budget, Paperwork Reduction Project (OMB-0938-0008), Washington, D.C. 20503.

■ **Figure 2–2**  Back of CMS-1500

**3** **Patient's Birth Date and Sex.** All dates should be recorded as Month/Day/Year. Check the box for the appropriate sex.

**5** **Patient's Address and Phone Number.** Same.

**6** **Patient's Relationship to Insured.** Same.

**8** **Patient's Status.** Check applicable boxes.

## Information About the Insured

These blocks contain information on the insured, their insurance, and their employment.

**1a** **Insured's ID Number.** Social Security number, ID number, or policy number of insured.

**4** **Insured's Name.** Subscriber's Name.

**7** **Insured's Address and Phone Number.** Same.

**11** **Insured's Policy Group or FECA Number.** Subscriber's Group Number. This number refers to primary insured listed in 1a above.

**11a** **Insured's Date of Birth.** Same.

**11b** **Employer's Name or School Name.** Employer or school name of insured party.

**11c** **Insurance Plan Name or Program Name.** Name of insurance company or group plan.

**11d** **Is There Another Health Benefit Plan?** Check appropriate box. If "YES" is checked, then items 9a-9d must be completed.

## Information About the Secondary Insurance

These blocks contain information about a secondary insurance policy (if any), which may provide coverage on this patient.

**9** **Other Insured's Name.** Other insured whose coverage may be responsible, in whole or in part, for the payment of this claim.

**9a** **Other Insured's Policy or Group Number.** Same.

**9b** **Other Insured's Date of Birth and Sex.** Same.

**9c** **Employer's Name or School Name.** Employer or School Name of other insured party.

**9d** **Insurance Plan Name or Program Name.** Name of insurance company or group plan for other insured.

## Information About Third Party Liability

These blocks contain information on whether a third party may be liable for payment on this claim.

**10a** **Was Condition Related to: Employment?** If "YES" is marked, then there is Worker's Compensation Insurance involved. If "NO" is marked, then Worker's Compensation is not involved. Circle whether employment is current or previous.

**10b** **Was Condition Related to: Auto Accident?** If "YES" is marked, then check for an injury date (Block 14) and an injury diagnosis (Block 21). The state the accident occurred in should also be indicated. If "NO" is marked then the claim may not be for an auto accident injury.

**10c** **Was Condition Related to: Other Accident?** If "YES" is marked, then check for an injury date (Block 14) and an injury diagnosis (Block 21). If "NO" is marked then the claim may not be for an accident injury.

**10d** **Reserved for Local Use.** Same.

## Authorization Signatures

These blocks should be signed by the insured, or a permanent release of information and assignment of benefits should be kept on file. If there is a permanent release of information or assignment of benefits on file, the words SIGNATURE ON FILE should be placed in these boxes.

**12** **Patient's or Authorized Person's Signature.** Patient's release of medical information.

**13** **Assignment of Benefits.** This block should always be signed by the patient to allow the insurer to pay the physician directly instead of paying the patient and waiting for the patient to pay the provider.

## Information About the Illness

These blocks contain information about the current illness.

**14** **Date of Illness, Injury, Accident or Pregnancy.** All injury claims (i.e., injury diagnosis) must have an injury or accident date. If the patient's condition is a pregnancy, the date of the last menstrual period should be indicated.

**15** **If Patient Has Had Same Or Similar Illness, Give First Date.** Same.

**16** **Dates Patient Unable To Work in Current Occupation.** Same.

**17** **Name Of Referring Physician or Other Source.** If this patient was referred to the current physician by another physician, hospital, or clinic, the referring party should be listed here.

**17a    I.D. Number of Referring Physician.** Same.

**18    Hospitalization Dates Relating to Current Services.** Same.

**19    Reserved for Local Use.** Leave blank

**20    Outside Lab.** Was laboratory work performed outside your office? If so, check the yes box and indicate the total of the charges.

**21    Diagnosis or Nature of Illness or Injury.** The diagnosis states why the patient went to see the provider. Both an ICD-9-CM code and a description should be indicated.

**22    Medicaid Resubmission Code.** Leave blank.

## Information About the Procedures Performed

These blocks contain information about the procedures which were performed.

**23    Prior Authorization Number.** Authorization number for services which were approved prior to being rendered.

**24a    Date of Service.** The date service was rendered by the provider. A complete date must be given.

**24b    Place of Service.** The location where the services were performed (see following section for further information).

**24c    Type of Service.** Leave blank.

**24d    Procedure Code.** The five-digit procedure code as found in the *CPT*®/RVS and HCPCS manuals. These are codes that have been assigned to each procedure the provider can perform. By selecting the proper code, billers can describe the type of service performed with a few numbers. This eliminates the confusion that used to arise from various abbreviations and descriptions of a procedure. It also allows for easy computer tabulation of the different procedures performed.

**24d    Modifier Code.** The two-digit modifier from the *CPT*®/RVS further describing the procedure code.

**24e    Diagnosis Code.** This is used in conjunction with block 21. The number placed in block 24e (i.e., 1, 2, 3, 4) refers to diagnosis 1, 2, 3, or 4 in block 21. In other words, the doctor can perform different services for different illnesses or injuries on different dates and submit them all on one claim form.

**24f    Charges.** The charge per line of service.

**24g    Days or Units.** The number of times a service was performed.

**24h    EPSDT Family Plan.** Leave blank.

**24i    EMG.** If service was rendered in the hospital emergency room, this should match the service code in block 24b.

**24j    COB.** Coordination of Benefits. Are there other insurance policies or plans which may be responsible for payment on this claim? Indicate a "Y" for yes, an "N" for no.

**24k    Reserved for Local Use.** Leave blank.

**28    Total Charge.** The total charge of the claim.

**29    Amount Paid.** The amount paid by the patient or subscriber.

**30    Balance Due.** The difference between the total charge and the amount paid by the patient or subscriber (if any).

## Information About the Provider of Services

These blocks contain information about the provider of services.

**25    Federal Tax ID Number.** If the provider of service is a physician or an individual, his/her Social Security Number should be used. If the provider of service is a facility, an Employer Identification Number should be used.

**26    Patient's Account Number.** Same.

**27    Accept Assignment for Government Claims.** Refers only to TRICARE or Medicare. Do not use to assign payment on this claim to the provider. Use block 13 only for your assignment of payment.

**31    Signature of Physician or Supplier of Service.** Must be signed by the provider indicating that the said services have indeed been rendered. Degrees or credentials (i.e., M.D., D.O., etc.) should follow the name.

**32    Name and Address of Facility Where Services Rendered.** If this information is the same as block 33, it may be left blank.

**33    Physician's/Supplier's Billing Name, Address, Zip Code And Phone #.** The name, address and phone number of the physician or supplier of service. This is the address that payments will be addressed to if assignment of benefits has been signed for in block 13.

## Block 24b, Place of Service

This item needed further description for which space was not available in the above text. This is a numerical code to indicate the place where the service was rendered (**see Table 2–1**).

| Code | Description |
|------|-------------|
| | **Place of Service Codes** |
| 01 | **Pharmacy** (A facility or location where drugs and other medically related items and services are sold, dispensed, or otherwise provided directly to patients). |
| 02 | **Unassigned** N/A |
| 03 | **School** (A facility whose primary purpose is education). |
| 04 | **Homeless Shelter** (A facility or location whose primary purpose is to provide temporary housing to homeless individuals (e.g., emergency shelters, individual or family shelters). |
| 05 | **Indian Health Service Free-standing** (A facility or location, owned and operated by the Indian Health Service, which provides diagnostic, therapeutic (surgical and nonsurgical), and rehabilitation services to American Indians and Alaska Natives who do not require hospitalization). |
| 06 | **Indian Health Service Provider-based Facility** (A facility or location, owned and operated by the Indian Health Service, which provides diagnostic, therapeutic (surgical and nonsurgical), and rehabilitation services rendered by, or under the supervision of, physicians to American Indians and Alaska Natives admitted as inpatients or outpatients). |
| 07 | **Tribal 638 Free-standing Facility** (A facility or location owned and operated by a federally recognized American Indian or Alaska Native tribe or tribal organization under a 638 agreement, which provides diagnostic, therapeutic (surgical and nonsurgical), and rehabilitation services to tribal members who do not require hospitalization). |
| 08 | **Tribal 638 Provider-based Facility** (A facility or location owned and operated by a federally recognized American Indian or Alaska Native tribe or tribal organization under a 638 agreement, which provides diagnostic, therapeutic (surgical and non-surgical), and rehabilitation services to tribal members). |
| 09-10 | **Unassigned** (N/A). |
| 11 | **Office** (Location other than a hospital, Skilled Nursing Facility [SNF], Military Treatment Facility, Community Health Center, State or Local Public Health Clinic or Intermediate Care Facility [ICF], where the health professional routinely provides health examinations, diagnosis, and treatment of illness or injury on an ambulatory basis). |
| 12 | **Home** (Location other than a hospital or other facility where the patient received care in a private residence). |
| 13 | **Assisted Living Facility** (Congregate residential facility with self-contained living units providing assessment of each resident's needs and on-site support 24 hours a day, seven days a week, with the capacity to deliver or arrange for services, including some healthcare and other services). |
| 14 | **Group Home (non-facility)** (Congregate residential foster care setting for children and adolescents in state custody that provides some social, healthcare, and educational support services and that promotes rehabilitation and reintegration of residents into the community). |
| 15 | **Mobile Unit** (A facility/unit that moves from place to place, equipped to provide preventive, screening, diagnostic, and/or treatment services.) |
| 16-19 | **Unassigned** |
| 20 | **Urgent Care Facility** (Location, distinct from a hospital emergency room, an office, or a clinic, whose purpose is to diagnose and treat illness or injury for unscheduled, ambulatory patients seeking immediate medical attention.) |
| 21 | **Inpatient Hospital** (A facility other than psychiatric, which primarily provides diagnostic, therapeutic (both surgical and nonsurgical), and rehabilitation services by, or under the supervision of, physicians to patients admitted for a variety of medical conditions). |
| 22 | **Outpatient Hospital** (A portion of a hospital which provides diagnostic, therapeutic (both surgical and nonsurgical), and rehabilitation services to sick and injured persons who do not require hospitalization or institutionalization.) A patient who is not admitted to a hospital (i.e., one who is under 24-hour supervision) is an outpatient. |
| 23 | **Emergency Room - Hospital** (A portion of a hospital where emergency diagnosis and treatment of illness or injury is provided.) Patients in the emergency room are considered to be facility outpatients. (Remember to also complete block 24I.) |

**Table 2–1** Place of Service Codes

| 24 | **Ambulatory Surgical Center (ASC)** (A freestanding facility, other than a physician's office, where surgical and diagnostic services are provided on an ambulatory basis.) When this code is used, the facility must be a CMS-approved ASC. |
|---|---|
| 25 | **Birthing Center** (A facility other than a hospital's maternity facilities or a physician's office that provides a setting for labor, delivery, and immediate postpartum care, as well as immediate care of newborn infants.) |
| 26 | **Military Treatment Facility** (MTF) (A medical facility operated by one or more of the Uniformed Services. MTF also refers to certain former U.S. Public Health Service facilities now designated as Uniformed Service Treatment Facilities (USTF). |
| 27-30 | **Unassigned** |
| 31 | **Skilled Nursing Facility** (A facility that primarily provides inpatient skilled nursing care and related services to patients who require medical, nursing, or rehabilitative services but does not provide the level of care or treatment available in a hospital). |
| 32 | **Nursing Facility** (A facility which provides skilled nursing care and related services for the rehabilitation of injured, disabled, or sick persons or on a regular basis health-related care services above the level of custodial care to other than mentally retarded individuals.) |
| 33 | **Custodial Care Facility** (A facility which provides room, board and personal assistance services, generally on a long-term basis, and which does not include a medical component.) |
| 34 | **Hospice** (A facility, other than a patient's home, in which palliative and supportive care for terminally ill patients and their families is provided.) |
| 35-40 | **Unassigned** |
| 41 | **Ambulance -- Land** (A land vehicle specifically designed, equipped and staffed for lifesaving and transporting the sick or injured.) |
| 42 | **Ambulance -- Air or Water** (An air or water vehicle specifically designed, equipped and staffed for lifesaving and transporting the sick or injured.) |
| 43-48 | **Unassigned** |
| 49 | **Independent Clinic (non-facility)** (A location, not part of a hospital and not described by any other Place of Service code, that is organized and operated to provide preventive, diagnostic, therapeutic, rehabilitative, or palliative services to outpatients only.) |
| 50 | **Federally Qualified Health Center** (A facility located in a medically underserved area that provides Medicare beneficiaries preventive primary medical care under the general direction of a physician.) |
| 51 | **Inpatient Psychiatric Facility** (A facility that provides inpatient psychiatric services for the diagnosis and treatment of mental illness on a 24-hour basis, by or under the supervision of a physician.) |
| 52 | **Psychiatric Facility-Partial Hospitalization** (A facility for the diagnosis and treatment of mental illness that provides a planned therapeutic program for patients who do not need full-time hospitalization, but who need broader programs than are possible from outpatient visits in a hospital-based or hospital-affiliated facility.) |
| 53 | **Community Mental Health Center** (A facility that provides comprehensive mental health services on an ambulatory basis, primarily to individuals residing or employed in a defined area. Includes a physician-directed mental health facility.) |
| 54 | **Intermediate Care Facility/Mentally Retarded** (A facility which primarily provides health-related care and services above the level of custodial care of mentally retarded individuals but does not provide the level of care or treatment available in a hospital or SNF.) |
| 55 | **Residential Substance Abuse Treatment Facility** (A facility which provides treatment for substance (alcohol and drug) abuse to live-in residents who do not require acute medical care. Services include individual and group therapy and counseling, family counseling, laboratory tests, drugs and supplies, psychological testing, and room and board.) |
| 56 | **Psychiatric Residential Treatment Center** (A facility or distinct part of a facility for psychiatric care which provides a total 24-hour therapeutically planned and professionally staffed group living and learning environment.) |
| 57 | **Non Residential Substance Abuse Treatment Facility (non-facility)** (A location which provides treatment for substance (alcohol and drug) abuse on an ambulatory basis. Services include individual and group therapy and counseling, family counseling, laboratory tests, drugs and supplies, and psychological testing.) |

**Table 2–1** (*continued*)

| 58-59 | Unassigned |
|---|---|
| 60 | **Mass Immunization Center** (A location where providers administer pneumococcal pneumonia and influenza virus vaccinations and submit these services as electronic media claims, paper claims, or using the roster billing method. This generally takes place in a mass immunization setting, such as a public health center pharmacy or mall, but may include a physician office setting.) |
| 61 | **Comprehensive Inpatient Rehabilitation Facility** (A facility that provides comprehensive rehabilitation services under the supervision of a physician to inpatients with physical disabilities. Services include rehabilitation nursing, physical therapy, occupational therapy, speech pathology, social or psychological services, and orthotics and prosthetics services. There are specific licensing requirements for these facilities.) |
| 62 | **Comprehensive Outpatient Rehabilitation Facility** (A facility that provides comprehensive rehabilitation services under the supervision of a physician to inpatients with physical disabilities. Services include physical therapy, occupational therapy, and speech pathology services. There are specific licensing requirements for these facilities.) |
| 63-64 | Unassigned |
| 65 | **End Stage Renal Disease Treatment Facility** (A facility other than a hospital, which provides dialysis treatment, maintenance and/or training to patients or caregivers on an ambulatory or home-care basis.) |
| 66-70 | Unassigned |
| 71 | **State or Local Public Health Clinic** (A facility maintained by either State or local health departments that provides ambulatory primary medical care under the general direction of a physician. Such facilities must be physician-directed.) |
| 72 | **Rural Health Clinic** (A certified facility which is located in a rural medically underserved area that provides ambulatory primary medical care under the general direction of a physician. Qualified facilities do not bill Part B of Medicare for items or services except for DME and orthotics and prosthetics.) |
| 73-80 | Unassigned |
| 81 | **Independent Laboratory** (A laboratory certified to perform diagnostic and/or clinical tests independent of an institution or a physician's office.) <br> With the exception of hospital inpatients, the place of service for lab tests will be based on where "drawn" instead of where the test is actually performed. If the physician is billing for a lab service performed in his/her own office, then use the appropriate code for provider's office. If an independent laboratory is billing, show the place where the sample is drawn. An independent laboratory drawing a sample in its laboratory shows the code for independent laboratory as the place of service. If an independent laboratory is billing for a test on a sample drawn on a hospital inpatient, then the appropriate code for hospital inpatient is entered as the place of service. If the independent laboratory is billing for a test on a sample drawn in a physician's office, then the appropriate code is for provider's office. |
| 82-98 | Unassigned |
| 99 | **Other Unlisted Facility** (Other service facilities not identified above.) |

**Table 2–1** (*continued*)

## Practice Pitfalls

**Tips on Understanding the CMS-1500**

Properly using the CMS-1500 is vital to paying the proper reimbursement on claims. The following tips will help to minimize errors and speed processing of a claim.

1. Be sure the patient information contained on the claim matches that in your records.

2. Be sure that all necessary blocks are filled in.

3. Be sure that all diagnoses have related procedures, and all procedures have a related diagnosis.

4. Do not write on the form. Instead, attach a separate paper for comments.

5. Do not sign or write in red ink. Many scanners used by insurance carriers are programmed to pass over everything in red on the form and just pick up the data. Therefore, anything in red will not be picked up by the scanner.

6. Do not use a highlighter on the form. Some scanners will pick up the highlighter and turn it into a black mark, thus obliterating the information in that field.

# On the Job Now

**Directions:** Look at the CMS-1500 form in **Figure 2–1**, and then answer the following questions.

1. What is the patient's name? _____

2. What is the name of the insured person on this claim? _____

3. What is the procedure code for the procedure performed? _____

4. What is the diagnosis code given? _____

5. What is the patient's marital status? _____

6. What insurance plan is the patient covered under? _____

7. Has the authorization to release information been signed? _____

8. Is this patient covered under more than one insurance policy? _____

9. Have benefits been assigned on this claim? _____

10. What is the name of the provider on this claim? _____

## 1500 Health Insurance Claim Form (Version 08/05)

The National Uniform Claim Committee (NUCC) was formed in the mid 1990s to establish a standardized data set for use in the submission of both paper and electronic health insurance claims for physicians, suppliers, and ambulance services. NUCC replaces the Uniform Claim Form Task Force.

Minor changes have been made to the 1500 Health Insurance Claim Form (version 08/05) in order to accommodate the National Provider Identifier (NPI), to comply with HIPAA regulations, and to address the needs of electronic claim submission. The 1500 Health Insurance Claim Form was approved by the NUCC in November, 2005 and will replace the CMS-1500 (version 12/90). Finalization of the 1500 Health Insurance Form (version 08/05) is expected to take place in the spring of 2006, so changes to this form are anticipated.

The following is a sample of the new 1500 Health Insurance Claim Form (version 08/05), and is for informational purposes only (**see Figures 2–3 and 2–4**).

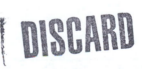
DISCARD

1500

HEALTH INSURANCE CLAIM FORM

APPROVED BY NATIONAL UNIFORM CLAIM COMMITTEE 08/05

[ ] [ ] PICA
PICA [ ] [ ]

1. MEDICARE (Medicare #)   MEDICAID (Medicaid #)   TRICARE CHAMPUS (Sponsor's SSN)   CHAMPVA (Member ID#)   GROUP HEALTH PLAN (SSN or ID)   FECA BLK LUNG (SSN)   OTHER (ID)
1a. INSURED'S I.D. NUMBER   (For Program in Item 1)

2. PATIENT'S NAME (Last Name, First Name, Middle Initial)
3. PATIENT'S BIRTH DATE   MM  DD  YY   SEX   M [ ]  F [ ]
4. INSURED'S NAME (Last Name, First Name, Middle Initial)

5. PATIENT'S ADDRESS (No., Street)
6. PATIENT RELATIONSHIP TO INSURED   Self [ ]  Spouse [ ]  Child [ ]  Other [ ]
7. INSURED'S ADDRESS (No., Street)

CITY   STATE
8. PATIENT STATUS   Single [ ]  Married [ ]  Other [ ]
CITY   STATE

ZIP CODE   TELEPHONE (Include Area Code)  (   )
Employed [ ]  Full-Time Student [ ]  Part-Time Student [ ]
ZIP CODE   TELEPHONE (Include Area Code)  (   )

9. OTHER INSURED'S NAME (Last Name, First Name, Middle Initial)
10. IS PATIENT'S CONDITION RELATED TO:
11. INSURED'S POLICY GROUP OR FECA NUMBER

a. OTHER INSURED'S POLICY OR GROUP NUMBER
a. EMPLOYMENT? (Current or Previous)   YES [ ]  NO [ ]
a. INSURED'S DATE OF BIRTH   MM  DD  YY   SEX   M [ ]  F [ ]

b. OTHER INSURED'S DATE OF BIRTH   MM  DD  YY   SEX   M [ ]  F [ ]
b. AUTO ACCIDENT?   PLACE (State)   YES [ ]  NO [ ]
b. EMPLOYER'S NAME OR SCHOOL NAME

c. EMPLOYER'S NAME OR SCHOOL NAME
c. OTHER ACCIDENT?   YES [ ]  NO [ ]
c. INSURANCE PLAN NAME OR PROGRAM NAME

d. INSURANCE PLAN NAME OR PROGRAM NAME
10d. RESERVED FOR LOCAL USE
d. IS THERE ANOTHER HEALTH BENEFIT PLAN?   YES [ ]  NO [ ]   If yes, return to and complete item 9 a-d.

READ BACK OF FORM BEFORE COMPLETING & SIGNING THIS FORM.
12. PATIENT'S OR AUTHORIZED PERSON'S SIGNATURE I authorize the release of any medical or other information necessary to process this claim. I also request payment of government benefits either to myself or to the party who accepts assignment below.
SIGNED_____   DATE_____

13. INSURED'S OR AUTHORIZED PERSON'S SIGNATURE I authorize payment of medical benefits to the undersigned physician or supplier for services described below.
SIGNED_____

14. DATE OF CURRENT:   MM  DD  YY   ILLNESS (First symptom) OR INJURY (Accident) OR PREGNANCY(LMP)
15. IF PATIENT HAS HAD SAME OR SIMILAR ILLNESS. GIVE FIRST DATE   MM  DD  YY
16. DATES PATIENT UNABLE TO WORK IN CURRENT OCCUPATION   FROM  MM  DD  YY  TO  MM  DD  YY

17. NAME OF REFERRING PROVIDER OR OTHER SOURCE
17a.
17b. NPI
18. HOSPITALIZATION DATES RELATED TO CURRENT SERVICES   FROM  MM  DD  YY  TO  MM  DD  YY

19. RESERVED FOR LOCAL USE
20. OUTSIDE LAB?   YES [ ]  NO [ ]   $ CHARGES

21. DIAGNOSIS OR NATURE OF ILLNESS OR INJURY (Relate Items 1, 2, 3 or 4 to Item 24E by Line)
1. |___.___
2. |___.___
3. |___.___
4. |___.___
22. MEDICAID RESUBMISSION CODE   ORIGINAL REF. NO.

23. PRIOR AUTHORIZATION NUMBER

24. A. DATE(S) OF SERVICE | B. PLACE OF SERVICE | C. EMG | D. PROCEDURES, SERVICES, OR SUPPLIES (Explain Unusual Circumstances) CPT/HCPCS  MODIFIER | E. DIAGNOSIS POINTER | F. $ CHARGES | G. DAYS OR UNITS | H. EPSDT Family Plan | I. ID QUAL. | J. RENDERING PROVIDER ID. #
From  MM DD YY  To  MM DD YY

1   NPI
2   NPI
3   NPI
4   NPI
5   NPI
6   NPI

25. FEDERAL TAX I.D. NUMBER   SSN EIN [ ] [ ]
26. PATIENT'S ACCOUNT NO.
27. ACCEPT ASSIGNMENT? (For govt. claims, see back)   YES [ ]  NO [ ]
28. TOTAL CHARGE  $
29. AMOUNT PAID  $
30. BALANCE DUE  $

31. SIGNATURE OF PHYSICIAN OR SUPPLIER INCLUDING DEGREES OR CREDENTIALS (I certify that the statements on the reverse apply to this bill and are made a part thereof.)
SIGNED_____   DATE_____
32. SERVICE FACILITY LOCATION INFORMATION
a. NPI   b.
33. BILLING PROVIDER INFO & PH # (   )
a. NPI   b.

NUCC Instruction Manual available at: www.nucc.org
OMB APPROVAL PENDING

**■ Figure 2–3** Sample of Front of 1500 Health Insurance Claim Form

BECAUSE THIS FORM IS USED BY VARIOUS GOVERNMENT AND PRIVATE HEALTH PROGRAMS, SEE SEPARATE INSTRUCTIONS ISSUED BY APPLICABLE PROGRAMS.

NOTICE: Any person who knowingly files a statement of claim containing any misrepresentation or any false, incomplete or misleading information may be guilty of a criminal act punishable under law and may be subject to civil penalties.

### REFERS TO GOVERNMENT PROGRAMS ONLY

MEDICARE AND CHAMPUS PAYMENTS: A patient's signature requests that payment be made and authorizes release of any information necessary to process the claim and certifies that the information provided in Blocks 1 through 12 is true, accurate and complete. In the case of a Medicare claim, the patient's signature authorizes any entity to release to Medicare medical and nonmedical information, including employment status, and whether the person has employer group health insurance, liability, no-fault, worker's compensation or other insurance which is responsible to pay for the services for which the Medicare claim is made. See 42 CFR 411.24(a). If item 9 is completed, the patient's signature authorizes release of the information to the health plan or agency shown. In Medicare assigned or CHAMPUS participation cases, the physician agrees to accept the charge determination of the Medicare carrier or CHAMPUS fiscal intermediary as the full charge, and the patient is responsible only for the deductible, coinsurance and noncovered services. Coinsurance and the deductible are based upon the charge determination of the Medicare carrier or CHAMPUS fiscal intermediary if this is less than the charge submitted. CHAMPUS is not a health insurance program but makes payment for health benefits provided through certain affiliations with the Uniformed Services. Information on the patient's sponsor should be provided in those items captioned in "Insured"; i.e., items 1a, 4, 6, 7, 9, and 11.

### BLACK LUNG AND FECA CLAIMS

The provider agrees to accept the amount paid by the Government as payment in full. See Black Lung and FECA instructions regarding required procedure and diagnosis coding systems.

### SIGNATURE OF PHYSICIAN OR SUPPLIER (MEDICARE, CHAMPUS, FECA AND BLACK LUNG)

I certify that the services shown on this form were medically indicated and necessary for the health of the patient and were personally furnished by me or were furnished incident to my professional service by my employee under my immediate personal supervision, except as otherwise expressly permitted by Medicare or CHAMPUS regulations.

For services to be considered as "incident" to a physician's professional service, 1) they must be rendered under the physician's immediate personal supervision by his/her employee, 2) they must be an integral, although incidental part of a covered physician's service, 3) they must be of kinds commonly furnished in physician's offices, and 4) the services of nonphysicians must be included on the physician's bills.

For CHAMPUS claims, I further certify that I (or any employee) who rendered services am not an active duty member of the Uniformed Services or a civilian employee of the United States Government or a contract employee of the United States Government, either civilian or military (refer to 5 USC 5536). For Black-Lung claims, I further certify that the services performed were for a Black Lung-related disorder.

No Part B Medicare benefits may be paid unless this form is received as required by existing law and regulations (42 CFR 424.32).

NOTICE: Any one who misrepresents or falsifies essential information to receive payment from Federal funds requested by this form may upon conviction be subject to fine and imprisonment under applicable Federal laws.

### NOTICE TO PATIENT ABOUT THE COLLECTION AND USE OF MEDICARE, CHAMPUS, FECA, AND BLACK LUNG INFORMATION
(PRIVACY ACT STATEMENT)

We are authorized by CMS, CHAMPUS and OWCP to ask you for information needed in the administration of the Medicare, CHAMPUS, FECA, and Black Lung programs. Authority to collect information is in section 205(a), 1862, 1872 and 1874 of the Social Security Act as amended, 42 CFR 411.24(a) and 424.5(a) (6), and 44 USC 3101;41 CFR 101 et seq and 10 USC 1079 and 1086; 5 USC 8101 et seq; and 30 USC 901 et seq; 38 USC 613; E.O. 9397.

The information we obtain to complete claims under these programs is used to identify you and to determine your eligibility. It is also used to decide if the services and supplies you received are covered by these programs and to insure that proper payment is made.

The information may also be given to other providers of services, carriers, intermediaries, medical review boards, health plans, and other organizations or Federal agencies, for the effective administration of Federal provisions that require other third parties payers to pay primary to Federal program, and as otherwise necessary to administer these programs. For example, it may be necessary to disclose information about the benefits you have used to a hospital or doctor. Additional disclosures are made through routine uses for information contained in systems of records.

FOR MEDICARE CLAIMS: See the notice modifying system No. 09-70-0501, titled, 'Carrier Medicare Claims Record,' published in the Federal Register, Vol. 55 No. 177, page 37549, Wed. Sept. 12, 1990, or as updated and republished.

FOR OWCP CLAIMS: Department of Labor, Privacy Act of 1974, "Republication of Notice of Systems of Records," Federal Register Vol. 55 No. 40, Wed Feb. 28, 1990. See ESA-5, ESA-6, ESA-12, ESA-13, ESA-30, or as updated and republished.

FOR CHAMPUS CLAIMS: PRINCIPLE PURPOSE(S): To evaluate eligibility for medical care provided by civilian sources and to issue payment upon establishment of eligibility and determination that the services/supplies received are authorized by law.

ROUTINE USE(S): Information from claims and related documents may be given to the Dept. of Veterans Affairs, the Dept. of Health and Human Services and/or the Dept. of Transportation consistent with their statutory administrative responsibilities under CHAMPUS/CHAMPVA; to the Dept. of Justice for representation of the Secretary of Defense in civil actions; to the Internal Revenue Service, private collection agencies, and consumer reporting agencies in connection with recoupment claims; and to Congressional Offices in response to inquiries made at the request of the person to whom a record pertains. Appropriate disclosures may be made to other federal, state, local, foreign government agencies, private business entities, and individual providers of care, on matters relating to entitlement, claims adjudication, fraud, program abuse, utilization review, quality assurance, peer review, program integrity, third-party liability, coordination of benefits, and civil and criminal litigation related to the operation of CHAMPUS.

DISCLOSURES: Voluntary; however, failure to provide information will result in delay in payment or may result in denial of claim. With the one exception discussed below, there are no penalties under these programs for refusing to supply information. However, failure to furnish information regarding the medical services rendered or the amount charged would prevent payment of claims under these programs. Failure to furnish any other information, such as name or claim number, would delay payment of the claim. Failure to provide medical information under FECA could be deemed an obstruction.

It is mandatory that you tell us if you know that another party is responsible for paying for your treatment. Section 1128B of the Social Security Act and 31 USC 3801-3812 provide penalties for withholding this information.

You should be aware that P.L. 100-503, the "Computer Matching and Privacy Protection Act of 1988", permits the government to verify information by way of computer matches.

### MEDICAID PAYMENTS (PROVIDER CERTIFICATION)

I hereby agree to keep such records as are necessary to disclose fully the extent of services provided to individuals under the State's Title XIX plan and to furnish information regarding any payments claimed for providing such services as the State Agency or Dept. of Health and Human Services may request.

I further agree to accept, as payment in full, the amount paid by the Medicaid program for those claims submitted for payment under that program, with the exception of authorized deductible, coinsurance, co-payment or similar cost-sharing charge.

SIGNATURE OF PHYSICIAN (OR SUPPLIER): I certify that the services listed above were medically indicated and necessary to the health of this patient and were personally furnished by me or my employee under my personal direction.

NOTICE: This is to certify that the foregoing information is true, accurate and complete. I understand that payment and satisfaction of this claim will be from Federal and State funds, and that any false claims, statements, or documents, or concealment of a material fact, may be prosecuted under applicable Federal or State laws.

According to the Paperwork Reduction Act of 1995, no persons are required to respond to a collection of information unless it displays a valid OMB control number. The valid OMB control number for this information collection is 0938-0008. The time required to complete this information collection is estimated to average 10 minutes per response, including the time to review instructions, search existing data resources, gather the data needed, and complete and review the information collection. If you have any comments concerning the accuracy of the time estimate(s) or suggestions for improving this form, please write to: CMS, Attn: PRA Reports Clearance Officer, 7500 Security Boulevard, Baltimore, Maryland 21244-1850. This address is for comments and/or suggestions only. DO NOT MAIL COMPLETED CLAIM FORMS TO THIS ADDRESS.

**■ Figure 2–4** Sample of Back of 1500 Health Insurance Claim Form

## UB-92

The **Uniform Bill-1992 (UB-92)** is intended to be used by hospitals or other hospital-type facilities for inpa-

tient and outpatient billing **(see Figures 2–5 and 2–6)**. The data elements and the design of the form were determined by the National Uniform Billing Committee (NUBC). This form was designed to provide the basic

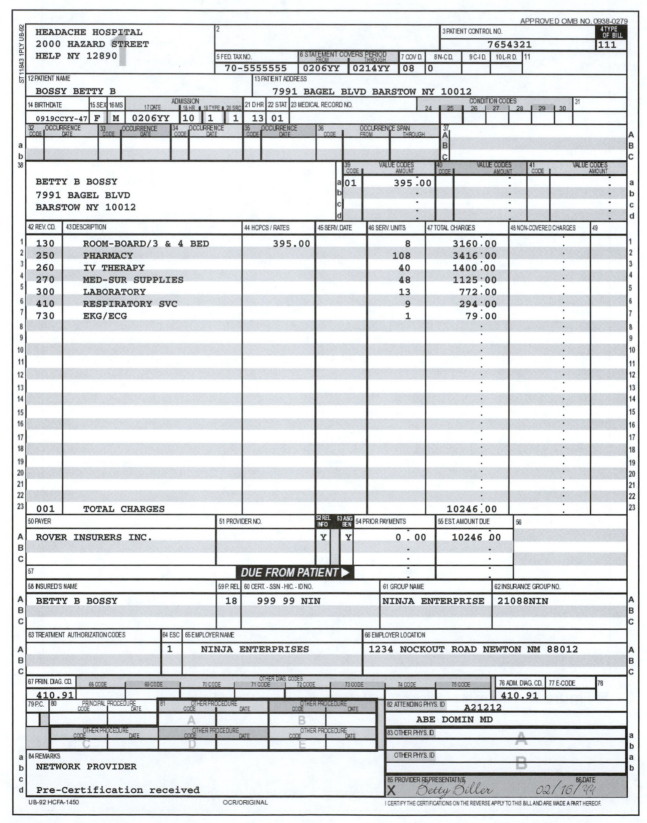

■ **Figure 2–5** Front of UB-92

data needed by most payers to adjudicate a large majority of their claims. The objective was to accommodate a wide range of needs while eliminating the need for attachments.

As you use this form, you will become familiar with the various boxes and know where to obtain the information required for completing and processing claim forms. The following list will assist in explaining the uses of the various fields. It contains the field number along with the name of the field and a brief description of the information needed. The word "same" refers to a description that is the same as the title of the box. Explanations that are too lengthy to be included here have been recorded after this brief listing.

---

UNIFORM BILL:    NOTICE: ANYONE WHO MISREPRESENTS OR FALSIFIES ESSENTIAL INFORMATION REQUESTED BY THIS FORM MAY UPON CONVICTION BE SUBJECT TO FINE AND IMPRISONMENT UNDER FEDERAL AND/OR STATE LAW.

Certifications relevant to the Bill and Information Shown on the Face Hereof:   Signatures on the face hereof incorporate the following certifications or verifications where pertinent to this Bill:

1. If third party benefits are indicated as being assigned or in participation status, on the face thereof, appropriate assignments by the insured/beneficiary and signature of patient or parent or legal guardian covering authorization to release information are on file. Determinations as to the release of medical and financial information should be guided by the particular terms of the release forms that were executed by the patient or the patient's legal representative. The hospital agrees to save harmless, indemnify and defend any insurer who makes payment in reliance upon this certification, from and against any claim to the insurance proceeds when in fact no valid assignment of benefits to the hospital was made.

2. If patient occupied a private room or required private nursing for medical necessity, any required certifications are on file.

3. Physician's certifications and re-certifications, if required by contract or Federal regulations, are on file.

4. For Christian Science Sanitoriums, verifications and if necessary re-verifications of the patient's need for sanitorium services are on file.

5. Signature of patient or his/her representative on certifications, authorization to release information, and payment request, as required be Federal law and regulations (42 USC 1835f, 42 CFR 424.36, 10 USC 1071 thru 1086, 32 CFR 199) and any other applicable contract regulations, is on file.

6. This claim, to the best of my knowledge, is correct and complete and is in conformance with the Civil Rights Act of 1964 as amended. Records adequately disclosing services will be maintained and necessary information will be furnished to such governmental agencies as required by applicable law.

7. For Medicare purposes:

If the patient has indicated that other health insurance or a state medical assistance agency will pay part of his/her medical expenses and he/she wants information about his/her claim released to them upon their request, necessary authorization is on file. The patient's signature on the provider's request to bill Medicare authorizes any holder of medical and non-medical information, including employment status, and whether the person has employer group health insurance, liability, no-fault, workers' compensation, or other insurance which is responsible to pay for the services for which this Medicare claim is made.

8. For Medicaid purposes:

This is to certify that the foregoing information is true, accurate, and complete. I understand that payment and satisfaction of this claim will be from Federal and State funds, and that any false claims, statements, or documents, or concealment of a material fact, may be prosecuted under applicable Federal or State Laws.

9. For CHAMPUS purposes:

This is to certify that:

(a) the information submitted as part of this claim is true, accurate and complete, and, the services shown on this form were medically indicated and necessary for the health of the patient;

(b) the patient has represented that by a reported residential address outside a military treatment center catchment area he or she does not live within a catchment area of a U.S. military or U.S. Public Health Service medical facility, or if the patient resides within a catchment area of such a facility, a copy of a Non-Availability Statement (DD Form 1251) is on file, or the physician has certified to a medical emergency in any assistance where a copy of a Non-Availability Statement is not on file;

(c) the patient or the patient's parent or guardian has responded directly to the provider's request to identify all health insurance coverages, and that all such coverages are identified on the face the claim except those that are exclusively supplemental payments to CHAMPUS-determined benefits;

(d) the amount billed to CHAMPUS has been billed after all such coverages have been billed and paid, excluding Medicaid, and the amount billed to CHAMPUS is that remaining claimed against CHAMPUS benefits;

(e) the beneficiary's cost share has not been waived by consent or failure to exercise generally accepted billing and collection efforts; and,

(f) any hospital-based physician under contract, the cost of whose services are allocated in the charges included in this bill, is not an employee or member of the Uniformed Services. For purposes of this certification, an employee of the Uniformed Services is an employee, appointed in civil service (refer to 5 USC 2105), including part-time or intermittent but excluding contract surgeons or other personnel employed by the Uniformed Services through personal service contracts. Similarly, member of the Uniformed Services does not apply to reserve members of the Uniformed Services not on active duty.

(g) based on the Consolidated Omnibus Budget Reconciliation Act of 1986, all providers participating in Medicare must also participate in CHAMPUS for inpatient hospital services provided pursuant to admissions to hospitals occurring on or after January 1, 1987.

(h) if CHAMPUS benefits are to be paid in a participating status, I agree to submit this claim to the appropriate CHAMPUS claims processor as a participating provider. I agree to accept the CHAMPUS-determined reasonable charge as the total charge for the medical services or supplies listed on the claim form. I will accept the CHAMPUS-determined reasonable charge even if it is less than the billed amount, and also agree to accept the amount paid by CHAMPUS, combined with the cost-share amount and deductible amount, if any, paid by or on behalf of the patient as full payment for the listed medical services or supplies. I will make no attempt to collect from the patient (or his or her parent or guardian) amounts over the CHAMPUS-determined reasonable charge. CHAMPUS will make any benefits payable directly to me, if I submit this claim as a participating provider.

ESTIMATED CONTRACT BENEFITS

■ **Figure 2–6** Back of UB-92

## Form Locator #, Name, and Description

1 **Provider Name, Address, and Telephone Number.** Name, address, and telephone number of hospital or clinic where services were rendered.

2 **Reserved (untitled).** All unlabeled fields are reserved for state or national use. Their use may be assigned by either the state or National Uniform Billing Committee.

3 **Patient Control Number.** Patient's account number.

4 **Type of Bill.** Three-digit code providing information regarding what type of bill is being submitted. (**see Table 2–3** for further information.)

5 **Federal Tax Number.** Provider's identification number or Social Security Number.

6 **Statement Covers Period.** The dates of service that this billing statement represents. Dates should match those on the itemized billing statement. For services rendered on the same day, both dates should be the same.

7 **Covered Days.** Number of days that services are covered by the primary payer.

8 **Noncovered Days (inpatient only).** Number of days that services are not covered by the primary payer. For Medicare, the reason for noncoverage should be explained by occurrence codes, PSRO fields, or in remarks.

9 **Coinsurance Days.** Number of days for which the patient must pay a portion of the costs of services. For Medicare, the inpatient Medicare days occurring after the 60th and before the 91st day in a single spell of illness.

10 **Lifetime Reserve Days.** Under Medicare, each beneficiary has a lifetime reserve of 60 additional days of inpatient hospital services after using 90 days of inpatient hospital services during a spell of illness.

11 **Reserved for State Assignment.** Leave blank

12 **Patient's Name.** Same.

13 **Patient's Address.** Same.

14 **Birth Date.** Patient's date of birth.

15 **Sex.** Patient's sex. (**see Table 2–2** for further information.)

16 **Marital Status.** Patient's marital status. (**see Table 2–2** for further information.)

17 **Date of Admission.** Date patient was admitted to hospital.

18 **Hour of Admission.** Hour patient admitted to hospital according to a 24-hour clock. 99 = unknown.

19 **Type of Admission.** Numerical code denoting the priority of this admission (**see Table 2–2** for further information.).

20 **Source of Admission.** Numerical code denoting the source of this admission (**see Table 2–2** for further information.).

21 **Discharge Hour.** Time patient was discharged from inpatient care. Time should be written according to a 24-hour clock. 99 = unknown. This element is not necessary for outpatient care.

22 **Patient Status.** Numerical code denoting the status of the patient as of the statement-through date. This element is necessary only for inpatient care (**see Table 2–2** for further information.).

23 **Medical Record Number.** Number assigned by the provider to the medical record.

24–30 **Condition Codes.** Codes used to identify conditions relating to the claim that may affect payer processing (**see Table 2–2** for further information.). No specific date is associated with this code.

31 **Reserved for National Assignment.** Leave blank.

32–35 **Occurrence Codes.** The code and associated date defining a significant event relating to this bill that may effect payer processing.

36 **Occurrence Span.** The code and the related dates that identify an event that relates to the payment of the claim. These codes identify occurrences that happened over a span of time.

37 **Internal Control Number.** The control number assigned to the original bill by the payer or the payer's intermediary.

38 **Responsible Party Name and Address.** Name and address of person ultimately responsible for ensuring payment of the bill. This is usually the patient, or the parent or legal guardian if the patient is a minor.

39–41 **Value Codes and Amounts.** Codes and the related dollar amount that identify data of a monetary nature that is necessary for the processing of this claim.

**42   Revenue Code.**  Revenue code referencing the type of services provided.

**43   Revenue Description.**  A description of the services provided. Abbreviations may be used. Accommodation (room) descriptions must be entered first on the bill and must be in chronologic order of appearance (i.e., 03/01/YY ICU, 03/02/YY semi-private room).

**44   HCPCS/Rates.**  The accommodation rate for inpatient bills, or the *CPT®* or HCPCS code for ancillary or outpatient services. Outpatient Worker's Compensation and Medicaid require HCPCS coding in this space.

**45   Service Date.**  The date the service was provided if this is a series bill where the date of service differs from the from/through date on the bill.

**46   Units of Service.**  Quantitative measure of services, days, miles, pints of blood, units, or treatments (i.e., if a patient was hospitalized for three days, a 3 would be placed here).

**47   Total Charges.**  Total charges for that line of services.

**48   Noncovered Charges.**  The amount per line of service that is not covered by the primary payer.

**49   Reserved for National Assignment.**  Leave blank.

**50   Payer Identification.**  Name of Insurer(s) covered by the patient who may be responsible for payment on this bill. Insurers should be listed in order of Primary Payer, Secondary Payer, and Tertiary Payer(s). If required, numbers identifying each payer organization should be listed.

**51   Provider Number.**  The number assigned to the provider by the listed payer.

**52   Release Information.**  A "Y" (yes) or "N" (no) designation stating whether or not patient's signature is on file authorizing the release of information. An "R" may also be entered to show that a hospital has restricted authorization to release information. In such a case, the authorization should be attached. If no Authorization to Release Information is on file, one must be obtained before sending in the claim (**see Table 2–2** for further information.).

**53   Assignment of Benefits.**  A "Y" (yes) or "N" (no) designation stating whether or not patient's signature is on file authorizing the insurer to pay the provider of service directly instead of the patient. If a "Y" is placed in this box, you must have an assignment of benefits, signed by the insured, on file in your office.

**54   Prior Payments.**  The amount that has been paid toward this bill prior to the current billing date. These can include payments by the patient, other payers, and so on.

**55   Estimated Amount Due.**  The amount estimated by the provider to be due from the indicated payer. This is usually the total amount due minus any previous payments.

**56   Reserved for State Assignment.**  Leave blank.

**57   Reserved for National Assignment.**  Leave blank.

**58   Insured's Name.**  Name of the person listed on the insurance forms (subscriber's name). This may be a spouse or parent of the patient.

**59   Patient's Relationship to Insured.**  Numerical code designation indicating the relationship between the patient and the insured (**see Table 2–2** for further information.).

**60   Subscriber's Certificate Number.**  The policy number under which the insured is covered if it is an individual policy. If the insured is covered under a group policy (such as one offered by his/her employer), often the insured's social security number is used as the subscriber number.

**61   Insured Group Name.**  The name of the group or company that holds the insured's policy. Often this is the employer of the insured. This information is required by Medicare when Medicare is not the primary payer.

**62   Insurance Group Number.**  The group number denoting the group policy or plan under which the insured is covered.

**63   Treatment Authorization Code.**  A number indicating that the treatment described by this bill has been authorized by the payer.

**64   Employment Status Code.**  A code denoting the employment status of the person in block 63 (**see Table 2–2** for further information.).

**65   Employer Name.**  Name of the employer of the insured person.

**66   Employer Location.**  Address of the employer of the insured or responsible party.

**67   Principal Diagnosis Code.**  *ICD-9-CM* code for the diagnosis of the patient's condition.

**68–75** **Other Diagnosis Codes.** *ICD-9-CM*, V, and E codes for any additional diagnosis of the patient's condition.

**76** **Admitting Diagnosis.** The *ICD-9-CM* code provided at the time of admission.

**77** **External Cause of Injury Code (E Code).** The *ICD-9-CM* code for an external cause of injury, poisoning, or adverse effect.

**78** **Reserved for State Assignment.** Leave blank.

**79** **Procedure Coding Method Used.** A code that identifies the method used for procedure coding.

**80** **Principal Procedure Codes and Date.** *CPT®* code for principal procedure rendered and the date that procedure was rendered. For Medicare, *ICD-9-CM* codes must be entered here.

**81** **Other Procedure Codes and Dates.** *CPT®* code for additional procedures rendered and the dates of those procedures.

**82** **Attending Physician ID.** Name and license number of the physician who is primarily responsible for the patient.

**83** **Other Physician ID.** Name and license number of secondary physician, assistant surgeon, and so on.

**84** **Remarks.** Pertinent data for which there is no other specific place on the form. Often this space is used to record the nature of an accident (i.e., fell and hit head on concrete, 06/09/PY). Also, multiple visits to the ER on the same day should be recorded.

**85** **Provider Representative Signature.** Signature of provider representative. In the case of a hospital billing, it is not necessary for the attending physician to sign, as long as a representative of the hospital signs the form certifying that the information entered is in conformance with the certifications specified on the reverse of the bill.

**86** **Date Bill Submitted.** Date the bill was signed and submitted for payment.

# Uniform Bill (UB-04)

The UB-92 will be replaced by the UB-04. Minor changes have been made to the UB-04 in order to accommodate the National Provider Identifier (NPI), to comply with HIPAA regulations, and to address the needs of electronic claim submission. The UB-04 was approved by the NUBC in February, 2005 and will replace the UB-92. There may be additional changes to the UB-04.

The following is a sample of the UB-04, and is for informational purposes only (**see Figures 2–7 and 2–8**).

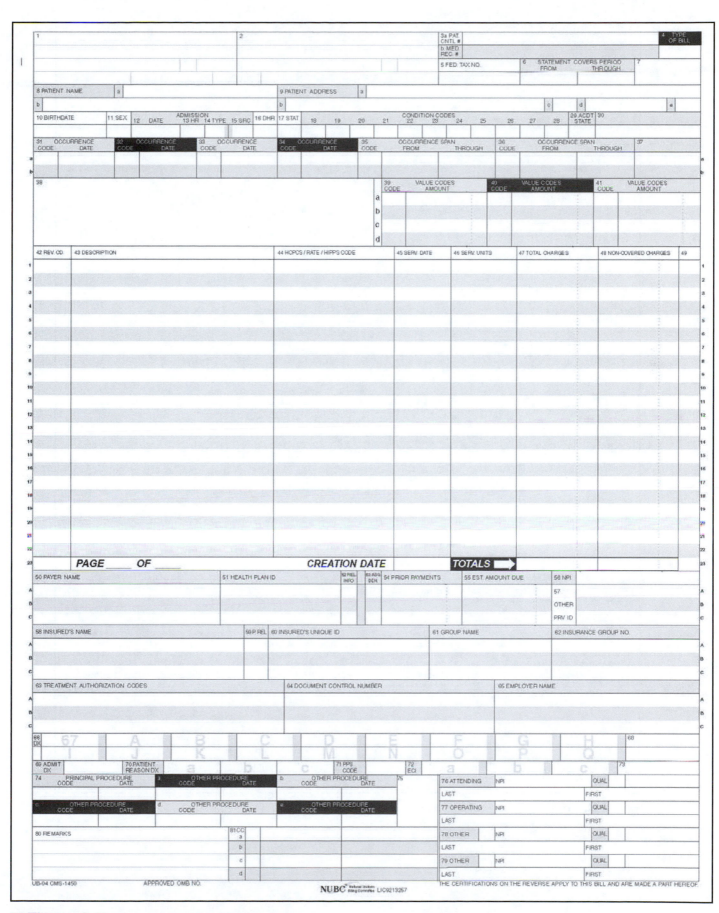

BECAUSE THIS FORM IS USED BY VARIOUS GOVERNMENT AND PRIVATE HEALTH PROGRAMS, SEE SEPARATE INSTRUCTIONS ISSUED BY APPLICABLE PROGRAMS.

NOTICE: Any person who knowingly files a statement of claim containing any misrepresentation or any false, incomplete or misleading information may be guilty of a criminal act punishable under law and may be subject to civil penalties.

REFERS TO GOVERNMENT PROGRAMS ONLY

MEDICARE AND CHAMPUS PAYMENTS: A patient's signature requests that payment be made and authorizes release of any information necessary to process the claim and certifies that the information provided in Blocks 1 through 12 is true, accurate and complete. In the case of a Medicare claim, the patient's signature authorizes any entity to release to Medicare medical and nonmedical information, including employment status, and whether the person has employer group health insurance, liability, no-fault, worker's compensation or other insurance which is responsible to pay for the services for which the Medicare claim is made. See 42 CFR 411.24(a). If item 9 is completed, the patient's signature authorizes release of the information to the health plan or agency shown. In Medicare assigned or CHAMPUS participation cases, the physician agrees to accept the charge determination of the Medicare carrier or CHAMPUS fiscal intermediary as the full charge, and the patient is responsible only for the deductible, coinsurance and noncovered services. Coinsurance and the deductible are based upon the charge determination of the Medicare carrier or CHAMPUS fiscal intermediary if this is less than the charge submitted. CHAMPUS is not a health insurance program but makes payment for health benefits provided through certain affiliations with the Uniformed Services. Information on the patient's sponsor should be provided in those items captioned in "Insured"; i.e., items 1a, 4, 6, 7, 9, and 11.

BLACK LUNG AND FECA CLAIMS

The provider agrees to accept the amount paid by the Government as payment in full. See Black Lung and FECA instructions regarding required procedure and diagnosis coding systems.

SIGNATURE OF PHYSICIAN OR SUPPLIER (MEDICARE, CHAMPUS, FECA AND BLACK LUNG)

I certify that the services shown on this form were medically indicated and necessary for the health of the patient and were personally furnished by me or were furnished incident to my professional service by my employee under my immediate personal supervision, except as otherwise expressly permitted by Medicare or CHAMPUS regulations.

For services to be considered as "incident" to a physician's professional service, 1) they must be rendered under the physician's immediate personal supervision by his/her employee, 2) they must be an integral, although incidental part of a covered physician's service, 3) they must be of kinds commonly furnished in physician's offices, and 4) the services of nonphysicians must be included on the physician's bills.

For CHAMPUS claims, I further certify that I (or any employee) who rendered services am/is not an active duty member of the Uniformed Services or a civilian employee of the United States Government or a contract employee of the United States Government, either civilian or military (refer to 5 USC 5536). For Black-Lung claims, I further certify that the services performed were for a Black Lung-related disorder.

No Part B Medicare benefits may be paid unless this form is received as required by existing law and regulations (42 CFR 424.32).

NOTICE: Any one who misrepresents or falsifies essential information to receive payment from Federal funds requested by this form may upon conviction be subject to fine and imprisonment under applicable Federal laws.

NOTICE TO PATIENT ABOUT THE COLLECTION AND USE OF MEDICARE, CHAMPUS, FECA, AND BLACK LUNG INFORMATION
(PRIVACY ACT STATEMENT)

We are authorized by CMS, CHAMPUS and OWCP to ask you for information needed in the administration of the Medicare, CHAMPUS, FECA, and Black Lung programs. Authority to collect information is in section 205(a), 1862, 1872 and 1874 of the Social Security Act as amended, 42 CFR 411.24(a) and 424.5(a) (6), and 44 USC 3101;41 CFR 101 et seq and 10 USC 1079 and 1086; 5 USC 8101 et seq; and 30 USC 901 et seq; 38 USC 613; E.O. 9397.

The information we obtain to complete claims under these programs is used to identify you and to determine your eligibility. It is also used to decide if the services and supplies you received are covered by these programs and to insure that proper payment is made.

The information may be given to other providers of services, carriers, intermediaries, medical review boards, health plans, and other organizations or Federal agencies, for the effective administration of Federal provisions that require other third parties payers to pay primary to Federal program, and as otherwise necessary to administer these programs. For example, it may be necessary to disclose information about the benefits you have used to a hospital or doctor. Additional disclosures are made through routine uses for information contained in systems of records.

FOR MEDICARE CLAIMS: See the notice modifying system No. 09-70-0501, titled, 'Carrier Medicare Claims Record,' published in the Federal Register, Vol. 55 No. 177, page 37549. Wed. Sept. 12, 1990, or as updated and republished.

FOR OWCP CLAIMS: Department of Labor, Privacy Act of 1974, "Republication of Notice of Systems of Records," Federal Register Vol. 55 No. 40, Wed Feb. 28, 1990, See ESA-5, ESA-6, ESA-12, ESA-13, ESA-30, or as updated and republished.

FOR CHAMPUS CLAIMS: PRINCIPLE PURPOSE(S): To evaluate eligibility for medical care provided by civilian sources and to issue payment upon establishment of eligibility and determination that the services/supplies received are authorized by law.

ROUTINE USE(S): Information from claims and related documents may be given to the Dept. of Veterans Affairs, the Dept. of Health and Human Services and/or the Dept. of Transportation consistent with their statutory administrative responsibilities under CHAMPUS/CHAMPVA; to the Dept. of Justice for representation of the Secretary of Defense in civil actions; to the Internal Revenue Service, private collection agencies, and consumer reporting agencies in connection with recoupment claims; and to Congressional Offices in response to inquiries made at the request of the person to whom a record pertains. Appropriate disclosures may be made to other federal, state, local, foreign government agencies, private business entities, and individual providers of care, on matters relating to entitlement, claims adjudication, fraud, program abuse, utilization review, quality assurance, peer review, program integrity, third-party liability, coordination of benefits, and civil and criminal litigation related to the operation of CHAMPUS.

DISCLOSURES: Voluntary; however, failure to provide information will result in delay in payment or may result in denial of claim. With the one exception discussed below, there are no penalties under these programs for refusing to supply information. However, failure to furnish information regarding the medical services rendered or the amount charged would prevent payment of claims under these programs. Failure to furnish any other information, such as name or claim number, would delay payment of the claim. Failure to provide medical information under FECA could be deemed an obstruction.

It is mandatory that you tell us if you know that another party is responsible for paying for your treatment. Section 1128B of the Social Security Act and 31 USC 3801-3812 provide penalties for withholding this information.

You should be aware that P.L. 100-503, the "Computer Matching and Privacy Protection Act of 1988", permits the government to verify information by way of computer matches.

MEDICAID PAYMENTS (PROVIDER CERTIFICATION)

I hereby agree to keep such records as are necessary to disclose fully the extent of services provided to individuals under the State's Title XIX plan and to furnish information regarding any payments claimed for providing such services as the State Agency or Dept. of Health and Human Services may request.

I further agree to accept, as payment in full, the amount paid by the Medicaid program for those claims submitted for payment under that program, with the exception of authorized deductible, coinsurance, co-payment or similar cost-sharing charge.

SIGNATURE OF PHYSICIAN (OR SUPPLIER): I certify that the services listed above were medically indicated and necessary to the health of this patient and were personally furnished by me or my employee under my personal direction.

NOTICE: This is to certify that the foregoing information is true, accurate and complete. I understand that payment and satisfaction of this claim will be from Federal and State funds, and that any false claims, statements, or documents, or concealment of a material fact, may be prosecuted under applicable Federal or State laws.

According to the Paperwork Reduction Act of 1995, no persons are required to respond to a collection of information unless it displays a valid OMB control number. The valid OMB control number for this information collection is 0938-0008. The time required to complete this information collection is estimated to average 10 minutes per response, including the time to review instructions, search existing data resources, gather the data needed, and complete and review the information collection. If you have any comments concerning the accuracy of the time estimate(s) or suggestions for improving this form, please write to: CMS, Attn: PRA Reports Clearance Officer, 7500 Security Boulevard, Baltimore, Maryland 21244-1850. This address is for comments and/or suggestions only. DO NOT MAIL COMPLETED CLAIM FORMS TO THIS ADDRESS.

**■ Figure 2–8** Sample of Back of UB-04 Billing

# Hospital Revenue Codes

| Major Category | Subcategory (Standard Abbreviation) |
|---|---|
| 001 | **Total Charges.** To reflect the total of all charges on this bill. |
| 01X | **Reserved for internal payer use.** Leave blank. |
| 02X-06X | **Reserved for National Assignment.** Leave blank. |
| 07X-09X | **Reserved for State Assignment.** Leave blank. |
| 10X | **All-inclusive Rate.** Flat fee charge incurred on either a daily basis or total stay basis for services rendered. Charge may cover room and board plus ancillary services or room and board only.<br>0    All-inclusive room and board plus ancillary  (ALL-INCL R&B/ANC)<br>1    All-inclusive room and board (ALL-INCL R&B) |
| 11X | **Room and Board--Private (Medical or General).** Routine service charges for single-bed rooms.<br>0    General Classification (R&B/PVT)<br>1    Medical/Surgical/Gyn (MED-SER-GYN/PVT)<br>2    OB (OB/PVT)<br>3    Pediatric (PEDS/PVT)<br>4    Psychiatric (PSYCH/PVT)<br>5    Hospice (HOSPICE/PVT)<br>6    Detoxification (DETOX/PVT)<br>7    Oncology (ONCOLOGY/PVT)<br>8    Rehabilitation (REHAB/PVT)<br>9    Other )OTHER/PVT) |
| 12X | **Room and Board--Semiprivate Two-Bed (Medical or General).** Routine service charges incurred for accommodations with two beds.<br>0    General Classification (R&B/SEMI)<br>1    Medical/Surgical/Gyn (MED-SUR-GYN/2 Bed)<br>2    OB (OB/2 Bed)<br>3    Pediatric (PED/ 2 Bed)<br>4    Psychiatric (PSYCH/2 Bed)<br>5    Hospice (HOSPICE/2 Bed)<br>6    Detoxification (DETOX/2 Bed)<br>7    Oncology (ONCOLOGY/2 Bed)<br>8    Rehabilitation (REHAB/2 Bed)<br>9    Other (OTHER/2 Bed) |
| 13X | **Semiprivate--Three and Four Beds.** Routine service charges incurred for accommodations with three and four beds.<br>0    General Classification (R&B/3&4 Bed)<br>1    Medical/Surgical/Gyn (MED-SUR-GYN/3&4 Bed)<br>2    OB (OB/3&4 Bed)<br>3    Pediatric (PED/3&4 Bed)<br>4    Psychiatric (PSYCH/3&4 Bed)<br>5    Hospice (HOSPICE/3&4 Bed)<br>6    Detoxification (DETOX/3&4 Bed)<br>7    Oncology (ONCOLOGY/3&4 Bed)<br>8    Rehabilitation (REHAB/3&4 Bed)<br>9    Other (OTHER/3&4 Bed) |

**Table 2–2  Hospital Revenue Codes** *(continued on next page)*

| | |
|---|---|
| 14X | **Private (Deluxe).** Deluxe rooms are accommodations with amenities substantially in excess of those provided to other patients.<br>0   General Classification (R&B/PVT/DLX)<br>1   Medical/Surgical/Gyn (MED-SUR-GYN/DLX)<br>2   OB (OB/DLX)<br>3   Pediatric (PED/DLX)<br>4   Psychiatric (PSYCH/DLX)<br>5   Hospice (HOSPICE/DLX)<br>6   Detoxification (DETOX/DLX)<br>7   Oncology (ONCOLOGY/DLX)<br>8   Rehabilitation (REHAB/DLX)<br>9   Other (OTHER/DLX) |
| 15X | **Room and Board—Ward (Medical or General).** Routine service charge for accommodations with five or more beds.<br>0   General Classification (R&B/WARD)<br>1   Medical/Surgical/Gyn (MED-SUR-GYN/WARD)<br>2   OB (OB/WARD)<br>3   Pediatric (PED/WARD)<br>4   Psychiatric (PSYCH/WARD)<br>5   Hospice (HOSPICE/WARD)<br>6   Detoxification (DETOX/WARD)<br>7   Oncology (ONCOLOGY/WARD)<br>8   Rehabilitation (REHAB/WARD)<br>9   Other (OTHER/WARD) |
| 16X | **Other Room and Board.** Any routine service charges for accommodations that cannot be included in the more specific revenue center codes.<br>0   General Classification (R&B)<br>4   Sterile Environment (R&B/STRL)<br>7   Self-Care (R&B/SELF)<br>9   Other (R&B/Other) |
| 17X | **Nursery.** Charges for nursing care to newborn and premature infants in nurseries.<br>0   General Classification (NURSERY)<br>1   Newborn (NURSERY/NEWBORN)<br>2   Premature (NURSERY/PREMIE)<br>5   Neonatal ICU (NURSERY/ICU)<br>9   Other (NURSERY/OTHER) |
| 18X | **Leave of Absence.** Charges for holding a room while the patient is temporarily away from the provider.<br>0   General Classification (LOA)<br>1   Reserved (RESERVED)<br>2   Patient Convenience (LOA/PT CONV)<br>3   Therapeutic Leave (LOA THER)<br>4   ICF/MR--any reason (LOA/ICF/ MR)<br>5   Nursing Home (for hospitalization) (LOA/NURS HOME)<br>6   Other Leave of Absence (LOA/OTHER) |
| 19X | **Not Assigned.** |
| 20X | **Intensive Care.** Routine service charge for medical or surgical care provided to patients who require a more intensive level of care than is rendered in the general medical or surgical unit.<br>0   General Classification (ICU)<br>1   Surgical (ICU/SURGICAL)<br>2   Medical (ICU/MEDICAL)<br>3   Pediatric (ICU/PEDS)<br>4   Psychiatric (ICU/PSYCH)<br>6   Post-ICU (POST ICU)<br>7   Burn Care (ICU/BURN CARE)<br>8   Trauma (ICU/TRAUMA)<br>9   Other Intensive Care (ICU/OTHER) |

**Table 2–2** *(continued)*

| 21X | **Coronary Care.** Routine service charge for medical or surgical care provided to patients with coronary illness who require a more intensive level of care than is rendered in the general medical care unit. |
|---|---|
| | 0   General Classification (CCU) |
| | 1   Myocardial Infarction (CCU/MYO INFARC) |
| | 2   Pulmonary Care (CCU/PULMON) |
| | 3   Heart Transplant (CCU/TRANS-PLANT) |
| | 4   Post-CCU (POST CCU) |
| | 9   Other Coronary Care (CCU/OTHR) |
| 22X | **Special Charges.** Charges incurred during an inpatient stay or on a daily basis for certain services. |
| | 0   General Classification (SPCL CHGS) |
| | 1   Admission Charge (ADMIT CHG) |
| | 2   Technical Support Charge (TECH SUPPT CHG) |
| | 3   UR Service Charge (UR CHG) |
| | 4   Late Discharge, Medically Necessary (LATE DISCH/MED NEC) |
| | 9   Other Special Charges (OTHER SPEC CHG) |
| 23X | **Incremental Nursing Charge Rate.**   Charge for nursing service assessed in addition to room and board. |
| | 0   General Classification (NURSING INCREM) |
| | 1   Nursery (NUR INCR/NURSERY) |
| | 2   OB (NUR INCR/OB) |
| | 3   ICU (NUR INCR/ICU) |
| | 4   CCU (NUR INCR/CCU) |
| | 5   Hospice (NUR INCR/HOSPICE) |
| | 9   Other (NUR INCR/OTHER) |
| 24X | **All-Inclusive Ancillary.** A flat rate incurred on either a daily basis or total stay basis for ancillary services only. |
| | 0   General Classification (ALL INCL ANCIL) |
| | 9   Other Inclusive Ancillary (ALL INCL ANCIL/OTHER) |
| 25X | **Pharmacy.** Charges for medication produced, manufactured, packaged, controlled, assayed, dispensed, and distributed under the direction of a licensed pharmacist. This category includes blood plasma, other components of blood, and IV solutions. |
| | 0   General Classification (PHAR) |
| | 1   Generic Drugs (DRUGS/GENRC) |
| | 2   Nongeneric Drugs (DRUGS/ NONGENRC) |
| | 3   Take Home Drugs (DRUGS/ TAKEHOME) |
| | 4   Drugs Incident to Other Diagnostic Services (DRUGS/INCIDENT OTHER DX) |
| | 5   Drugs Incident to Radiology (DRUGS/INCIDENT RAD) |
| | 6   Experimental Drugs (DRUGS/ EXPERIMT) |
| | 7   Nonprescription (DRUGS/ NONPSCRPT) |
| | 8   IV Solutions (IV SOLUTIONS) |
| | 9   Other Pharmacy (DRUGS/OTHER) |
| 26X | **IV Therapy.** Administration of intravenous solution by specially trained personnel to individuals requiring such treatment. |
| | 0   General Classification (IV THER) |
| | 2   Infusion Pump (IV THER/INFSN PUMP) |
| | 3   IV Therapy--Pharmacy Services (IV THER/PHARM/ SVC) |
| | 4   IV Therapy/Drug/Supply Delivery (IV THER/DRUG/ SUPPLY DELV) |
| | 9   Other IV Therapy (IV THERP/ OTHER) |
| | NOTE: Providers billing for home IV therapy should use the HCPCS code that describes the pump in Item 44. |
| 27X | **Medical/Surgical Supplies and Devices.** Charges for supply items required for patient care. |
| | 0   General Classification (MED-SUR SUPPLIES) |
| | 1   Nonsterile Supply (NON-STER SUPPLY) |
| | 2   Sterile Supply (STERILE SUPPLY) |
| | 3   Take Home Supplies (TAKE HOME SUPPLY) |
| | 4   Prosthetic/Orthotic Devices (PROSTH/ORTH DEV) |
| | 5   Pacemaker (PACE MAKER) |
| | 6   Intraocular Lens (INTRA OC LENS) |
| | 7   Oxygen-Take Home (O2/ TAKEHOME) |
| | 8   Other Implants (SUPPLY/ IMPLANTS) |
| | 9   Other Supplies/Devices (SUPPLY/ OTHER) |

**Table 2–2** *(continued)*

| | |
|---|---|
| 28X | **Oncology.** Charges for the treatment of tumors and related diseases.<br>0 General Classification ONCOLOGY<br>9 Other Oncology (ONCOLOGY/ OTHER) |
| 29X | **Durable Medical Equipment (Other Than Renal).** Charges for medical equipment that can withstand repeated use (excluding renal equipment).<br>0 General Classification (DME)<br>1 Rental (MED EQUIP/RENT)<br>2 Purchase of new DME (MED EQUIP/NEW)<br>3 Purchase of used DME (MED EQUIP/USED)<br>4 Supplies/Drugs for DME Effectiveness (Home Health Agency Only) (MED EQUIP/SUPPLIES/ DRUGS)<br>9 Other Equipment (MED EQUIP/ OTHER) |
| 30X | **Laboratory.** Charges for the performance of diagnostic and routine clinical laboratory tests.<br>0 General Classification (LAB)<br>1 Chemistry (LAB/CHEMISTRY)<br>2 Immunology (LAB/IMMUNLGY)<br>3 Renal Patient (Home) (LAB/RENAL HOME)<br>4 Nonroutine Dialysis (LAB/NR DIALYSIS)<br>5 Hematology (LAB/HEMAT)<br>6 Bacteriology & Microbiology (LAB/BACT-MICRO)<br>7 Urology (LAB/UROLOGY)<br>9 Other Laboratory (LAB/OTHER) |
| 31X | **Laboratory Pathological.** Charges for diagnostic and routine lab tests on tissues and culture.<br>0 General Classification (PATH LAB)<br>1 Cytology (PATHOL/CYTOLOGY)<br>2 Histology (PATHOL/HYSTOL)<br>4 Biopsy (PATHOL/BIOPSY)<br>9 Other (PATHOL/OTHER) |
| 32X | **Radiology--Diagnostic.** Charges for diagnostic radiology services provided for the examination and care of patients. Includes taking, processing, examining, and interpreting radiographs and fluorographs.<br>0 General Classification (DX X-RAY)<br>1 Angiocardiography (DX X-RAY/ ANGIO)<br>2 Arthrography (DX X-RAY/ARTH)<br>3 Arteriography (DX X-RAY/ ARTER)<br>4 Chest X-Ray (DX X-RAY/CHEST)<br>9 Other (DX X-RAY/OTHER) |
| 33X | **Radiology--Therapeutic.** Charges for therapeutic radiology services and chemotherapy that are required for care and treatment of patients. Included therapy by injection or ingestion of radioactive substances.<br>0 General Classification (RX X-RAY)<br>1 Chemotherapy--Injected (CHEMOTHER/INJ)<br>2 Chemotherapy--Oral (CHEMOTHER/ORAL)<br>3 Radiation Therapy (RADIATION RX)<br>5 Chemotherapy--IV (CHEMOTHERP-IV)<br>9 Other (RX X-RAY/OTHER) |
| 34X | **Nuclear Medicine.** Charges for procedures and tests performed by a radioisotope laboratory utilizing radioactive materials as required for diagnosis and treatment of patients.<br>0 General Classification (NUC MED)<br>1 Diagnostic (NUC MED/DX)<br>2 Therapeutic (NUC MED/RX)<br>9 Other (NUC MED/OTHER) |
| 35X | **CT Scan.** Charges for computed tomographic scans of the head and other parts of the body.<br>0 General Classification (CT SCAN)<br>1 Head Scan (CT SCAN/HEAD)<br>2 Body Scan (CT SCAN/BODY)<br>9 Other CT Scans (CT SCAN/OTHR) |
| 36X | **Operating Room Services.** Charges for services provided to patients in the performance of surgical and related procedures during and immediately following surgery.<br>0 General Classification (OR SERVICES)<br>1 Minor Surgery (OR/MINOR)<br>2 Organ Transplant--Other than kidney (OR/ORGAN TRANS)<br>7 Kidney Transplant (OR/KIDNEY TRANS)<br>9 Other Operating Room Services (OR/OTHER) |

**Table 2–2** (*continued*)

| 37X | **Anesthesia.** Charges for anesthesia services in the hospital. |
| --- | --- |
| | 0  General Classification (ANESTHE) |
| | 1  Anesthesia Incident to Radiology (ANESTHE/INCIDENT RAD) |
| | 2  Anesthesia Incident to Other Diagnostic Services (ANESTHE/ INCDNT OTHER DX) |
| | 4  Acupuncture (ANESTHE/ ACUPUNC) |
| | 9  Other Anesthesia (ANESTHE/ OTHER) |
| 38X | **Blood.** |
| | 0  General Classification (BLOOD) |
| | 1  Packed Red Cells (BLOOD/PKD RED) |
| | 2  Whole Blood (BLOOD/WHOLE) |
| | 3  Plasma (BLOOD/PLASMA) |
| | 4  Platelets (BLOOD PLATELETS) |
| | 5  Leucocytes (BLOOD/ LEUCOCYTES) |
| | 6  Other Components (BLOOD/ COMPONENTS) |
| | 7  Other Derivatives (Cryoprecipitates) (BLOOD/DERIVATIVES) |
| | 9  Other Blood (BLOOD/OTHER) |
| 39X | **Blood Storage and Processing.** Charges for storage and processing of whole blood. |
| | 0  General Classification (BLOOD/ STOR-PROC) |
| | 1  Blood Administration (BLOOD/ ADMIN) |
| | 9  Other Blood Storage and Processing (BLOOD/OTHER STOR) |
| 40X | **Other Imaging Services.** |
| | 0  General Classification (IMAGE SVS) |
| | 1  Diagnostic Mammography (DIAG MAMMOGRAPHY) |
| | 2  Ultrasound (ULTRASOUND) |
| | 3  Screening Mammography (SCRN MAMMOGRAPHY) |
| | 4  Positron Emission Tomography (PET SCAN) |
| | 9  Other Imaging Services (OTHER IMAGE SVS) |
| | NOTE:  High-risk beneficiaries should be noted by the inclusion of one of the following ICD-9CM diagnosis codes: |
| | V10.3  Personal History--Malignant neoplasm breast cancer |
| | V16.3  Family History--Malignant neoplasm breast cancer (mother, sister or daughter with breast cancer) |
| | V15.89  Other specified personal history representing hazards to health (not given birth prior to 30, a personal history of biopsy proven breast disease). Must be coded to the appropriate 4th or 5th digit. |
| 41X | **Respiratory Services.** Charges for administration of oxygen and certain potent drugs through inhalation or positive pressure and other forms of rehabilitative therapy through measurement of inhaled and exhaled gases and analysis of blood and evaluation of the patient's ability to exchange oxygen and other gases. |
| | 0  General Classification (RESPIR SVC) |
| | 2  Inhalation Services (INHALATION SVC) |
| | 3  Hyperbaric Oxygen Therapy (HYPERBARIC O2) |
| | 9  Other Respiratory Services (OTHER RESPIR SVS) |
| 42X | **Physical Therapy.** Charges for therapeutic exercises, massage, and utilization of light, heat, cold, water, electricity, and assistive devices for diagnosis and rehabilitation of patients who have neuromuscular, orthopedic, and other disabilities. |
| | 0  General Classification (PHYS THERP) |
| | 1  Visit Charge (PHYS THERP/ VISIT) |
| | 2  Hourly Charge (PHYS THERP/ HOUR) |
| | 3  Group Rate (PHYS THERP/ GROUP) |
| | 4  Evaluation or Reevaluation (PHYS THER/EVAL) |
| | 9  Other Physical Therapy (OTHER PHYS THERP) |

**Table 2–2**  *(continued)*

| | |
|---|---|
| 43X | **Occupational Therapy.** Charges for teaching manual skills and independent personal care to stimulate mental and emotional activity on the part of patients.<br>0     General Classification (OCCUP THERP)<br>1     Visit Charge (OCCUP THERP/ VISIT)<br>2     Hourly Charge (OCCUP THERP/ HOUR)<br>3     Group Rate (OCCUP THERP/ GROUP)<br>4     Evaluation or Reevaluation (OCCUP THER/EVAL)<br>9     Other Occupational Therapy (OTHER OCCUP THERP) |
| 44X | **Speech-Language Pathology.** Charges for services provided to persons with impaired functional communications skills.<br>0     General Classification (SPEECH PATHOL)<br>1     Visit Charge (SPEECH PATH/ VISIT)<br>2     Hourly Charge (SPEECH PATH/ HOUR)<br>3     Group Rate (SPEECH PATH/ GROUP)<br>4     Evaluation or Reevaluation (SPEECH PATH/EVAL)<br>9     Other Speech-Language Pathology (OTHER SPEECH PAT) |
| 45X | **Emergency Room.** Charges for emergency treatment to those ill and injured persons who require immediate unscheduled medical or surgical care.<br>0     General Classification (EMERG ROOM)<br>9     Other Emergency Room (OTHER EMER ROOM) |
| 46X | **Pulmonary Function.** Charges for tests that measure inhaled and exhaled gases and analysis of blood and for tests that evaluate the patient's ability to exchange oxygen and other gases.<br>0     General Classification (PULMON FUNC)<br>9     Other Pulmonary Function (OTHER PULMON FUNC) |
| 47X | **Audiology.** Charges for the detection and management of communication handicaps centering in whole or in part on the hearing function.<br>0     General Classification (AUDIOL)<br>1     Diagnostic (AUDIOLOGY/DX)<br>2     Treatment (AUDIOLOGY/RX)<br>9     Other Audiology (OTHER AUDIOL) |
| 48X | **Cardiology.** Charges for cardiac procedures rendered in a separate unit within the hospital. Such procedures include but are not limited to heart catheterization, coronary angiography, Swan-Ganz catheterization, and exercise stress test.<br>0     General Classification (CARDIOL)<br>1     Cardiac Cath Lab (CARDIAC CATH LAB)<br>2     Stress Test (STRESS TEST)<br>9     Other Cardiology (OTHER CARDIOL) |
| 49X | **Ambulatory Surgical Care.**<br>0     General Classification (AMBUL SURG)<br>9     Other Ambulatory Surgical Care (OTHER AMBL SURG) |
| 50X | **Outpatient Services.** Outpatient charges for services rendered to an outpatient who is admitted as an inpatient before midnight of the day following the date of service. These charges are incorporated on the inpatient bill of Medicare patients.<br>0     General Classification (OUTPATIENT SVS)<br>9     Other Outpatient Services (OUTPATIENT/OTHER) |
| 51X | **Clinic.** Clinic (nonemergency/scheduled outpatient visit) charges for providing diagnostic, preventive, curative, rehabilitative, and education services on a scheduled basis to ambulatory patients.<br>0     General Classification (CLINIC)<br>1     Chronic Pain Center (CHRONIC PAIN CL)<br>2     Dental Clinic (DENTAL CLINIC)<br>3     Psychiatric Clinic (PSYCH CLINIC)<br>4     OB-GYN Clinic (OB-GYN CLINIC)<br>5     Pediatric Clinic (PEDS CLINIC)<br>9     Other Clinic (OTHER CLINIC) |
| 52X | **Free-Standing Clinic.**<br>0     General Classification (FR/STD CLINIC)<br>1     Rural Health--Clinic (RURAL/ CLINIC)<br>2     Rural Health--Home (RURAL/ HOME)<br>3     Family Practice (FAMILY PRAC)<br>9     Other Freestanding Clinic (OTHER FR/STD CLINIC) |

**Table 2–2** *(continued)*

| | |
|---|---|
| 53X | **Osteopathic Services.** Charges for a structural evaluation of the cranium, entire cervical, dorsal, and lumbar spine by a doctor of osteopathy.<br>0    General Classification (OSTEOPATH SVS)<br>1    Osteopathic Therapy (OSTEOPATH RX)<br>9    Other Osteopathic Services (OTHER OSTEOPATH) |
| 54X | **Ambulance.** Charges for ambulance service, usually unscheduled, to the ill/ injured who require immediate medical attention.<br>0    General Classification (AMBUL)<br>1    Supplies (AMBUL/SUPPLY)<br>2    Medical Transport (AMBUL/MED TRANS)<br>3    Heart Mobile (AMBUL/ HEARTMOBL)<br>4    Oxygen (AMBUL/OXY)<br>5    Air Ambulance (AIR AMBUL)<br>6    Neonatal Ambulance Services (AMBUL/NEONAT)<br>7    Pharmacy (AMBUL/PHARMACY)<br>8    Telephone Transmission EKG (AMBUL/TELEPHONIC EKG)<br>9    Other Ambulance (OTHER AMBULANCE)<br>NOTE: Units may be either miles or trips.<br>NOTE: On items 55-58, charges should be reported to the nearest hour. |
| 55X | **Skilled Nursing.** Charges for nursing services that must be provided under the direct supervision of a licensed nurse to ensure the safety of the patient and to achieve the medically desired result. This code may be used for nursing home services or a service charge for home health billing.<br>0    General Classification (SKILLED NURS)<br>1    Visit Charge (SKILLED NURS/ VISIT)<br>2    Hourly Charge (SKILLED NURS/ HOUR)<br>9    Other Skilled Nursing (SKILLED NURS/OTHER) |
| 56X | **Medical Social Services.** Charges for services such as counseling patients, interviewing patients, and interpreting problems of social situation rendered to patients on any basis.<br>0    General Classification (MED SOCIAL SVS)<br>1    Visit Charge (MED SOC SERVS/ VISIT)<br>2    Hourly Charge (MED SOC SERVS/HOUR)<br>9    Other Medical Social Services (MED SOCIAL SERVS/OTHER) |
| 57X | **Home Health Aide (Home Health).** Charges made by a home health agency for personnel that are primarily responsible for the personal care of the patient.<br>0    General Classification (AIDE/ HOME HEALTH)<br>1    Visit Charge (AIDE/HOME HLTH/ VISIT)<br>2    Hourly Charge (AIDE/HOME HLTH/HOUR)<br>9    Other Home Health Aide (AIDE/ HOME HLTH/OTHER) |
| 58X | **Other Visits (Home Health).** Charges by a home health agency for visits other than physical therapy, occupational therapy or speech therapy, which must be specifically identified.<br>0    General Classification (VISIT/ HOME HEALTH)<br>1    Visit Charge (VISIT/HOME HLTH/ VISIT)<br>2    Hourly Charge (VISIT/HOME HLTH/HOUR)<br>9    Other Home Health (VISIT/HOME HLTH/OTHER) |
| 59X | **Units of Service (Home Health).** Revenue code used by a home health agency that bills on the basis of units of service.<br>0    General Classification (UNIT/ HOME HEALTH)<br>9    Home Health Other Units (UNIT/ HOME HLTH/OTHER) |
| 60X | **Oxygen Home Health.** Charges by a home health agency for oxygen equipment, supplies, or contents, excluding purchased items. If a beneficiary has purchased a stationary oxygen system, and oxygen concentrator or portable equipment, revenue codes 292 or 293 apply. DME other than oxygen systems is billed under codes 291, 292, or 293.<br>0    General Classification (O2/HOME HEALTH)<br>1    Oxygen--Stationary Equipment, Supplies or Contents (O2/STAT EQUIP/SUPPL/CONT)<br>2    Oxygen--Stationary Equipment or Supplies Under 1 LPM (O2/STAT EQUIP/UNDER 1 LPM)<br>3    Oxygen--Stationary Equipment or Supplies Over 4 LPM (O2/STAT EQUIP/OVER 4 LPM)<br>4    Oxygen--Portable Add-on (O2/ PORTABLE ADD-ON) |

**Table 2–2** (*continued*)

| | |
|---|---|
| 61X | **MRI.** Charges for Magnetic Resonance Imaging of the brain and other parts of the body.<br>0    General Classification (MRI)<br>1    Brain (including brain stem) (MRI-BRAIN)<br>2    Spinal Cord (including spine) (MRI-SPINE)<br>9    Other MRI (MRI-OTHER) |
| 62X | **Medical/Surgical Supplies.** Charges for supplies required for patient care. This code is an extension of code 27X and allows for the reporting of additional breakdown, if needed. Subcategory 1 is for providers who are not able to bill supplies used for radiology procedures under radiology. Subcategory 2 is for providers who are not able to bill supplies used for other diagnostic procedures under diagnostic procedures.<br>1    Supplies Incident to Radiology (MED-SUR SUPP/INCDNT RAD)<br>2    Supplies Incident to Other Diagnostic Services (MED-SUR UPP/INCDNT ODX) |
| 63X | **Drugs Requiring Specific identification.** Charges for drugs and biologicals requiring specific identification required by the payer. If you are using HCPCS to identify the drug, the HCPCS code should be entered in Item 44.<br>0    General Classification (DRUGS)<br>1    Single Source Drug (DRUG/ SNGLE)<br>2    Multiple Source Drug (DRUG/ MULT)<br>3    Restrictive Prescription (DRUG/ RSTR)<br>4    Erythropoietin (EPO) less than 10,000 units (DRUG/EPQ10,000 Units)<br>5    Erythropoietin (EPO) more than 10,000 units (DRUG/EPQ10,000 Units)<br>6    Drugs requiring detailed coding (DRUGS/DETAIL CODE)<br>NOTE:  Revenue Code 636 relates to a HCPCS code. Therefore, the appropriate HCPCS code should be entered in Item 44. The specific units of services to be reported should be in hundreds (100s) rounded to the nearest hundred. |
| 64X | **Home IV Therapy Services.** Charge for IV drug therapy services that are done in the patient's home. For home IV providers, the appropriate HCPCS code must be entered for all equipment and covered therapy.<br>0    General Classification (IV THER SVC)<br>1    Nonroutine Nursing, Central Line (NON RT NURSING/CENTRAL)<br>2    IV Site Care, Central Line, HCPCS related(IV SITE CARE/CENTRAL)<br>3    IV Start/Change Peripheral Line (IV STRT/CHNG/PERIPHRL)<br>4    Nonroutine Nursing Peripheral Line (NON RT NURSING/PERIPHRL)<br>5    Training Patient/Caregiver, Central Line (TRNG PT/CAREGVR/ CENTRAL)<br>6    Training Disabled Patient, Central Line (TRNG DSBLPT/CENTRAL)<br>7    Training Patient/Caregiver, Peripheral Line (TRNG PT/ CAREGVR/PERIPHRL)<br>8    Training Disabled Patient, Peripheral Line (TRNG DSBLPT/ PERIPHRL)<br>9    Other IV Therapy Services (OTHER IV THERAPY SVC)<br>NOTE: Units need to be reported in 1-hour increments. |
| 65X | **Hospice Service.** Charges for hospice care services for a terminally ill patient. The patient would need to elect these services in lieu of other services for a terminal condition.<br>0    General Classification (HOSPICE)<br>1    Routine Home Care (HOSPICE/RTN HOME)<br>2    Continuous Home Care (HOSPICE/ CTNS HOME)<br>3    RESERVED<br>4    RESERVED<br>5    Inpatient Respite Care (HOSPICE/ IP RESPITE)<br>6    General Inpatient Care (Nonrespite) (HOSPICE/IP NONRESPITE)<br>7    Physician Services (HOSPICE/ PHYSICIAN)<br>9    Other Hospice (HOSPICE/OTHER)<br>NOTE: There must be a minimum of 8 hours of care (not necessarily continuous) during a 24-hour period to receive the Continuous Home Care rate from Medicare under code 652. If less than 8 hours of care are provided, code 651 should be used. Any portion of an hour counts as an hour.<br>    When billing Medicare under code 657, a physician procedure code must be entered in Item 44. Code 657 is used by the hospice to bill for physician's services furnished to hospice patients when the physician is employed by the hospice or receives payment from the hospice for services rendered. |

**Table 2–2** *(continued)*

| | |
|---|---|
| **66X** | **Respite Care.** Charges for hours of service under the Respite Care Benefit for homemaker or home health aide, personal care services, and nursing care provided by a licensed professional nurse.<br>0    General Classification (RESPITE CARE)<br>1    Hourly Charge/Skilled Nursing (RESPITE/SKILLED NURSE)<br>2    Hourly Charge/Home Health Aide/ Homemaker (RESPITE/HMEAID/ HMEMKR |
| **67X** | **Not Assigned.** |
| **68X** | **Not Assigned.** |
| **69X** | **Not Assigned.** |
| **70X** | **Cast Room.** Charges for services related to the application, maintenance, and removal of casts.<br>0    General Classification (CAST ROOM)<br>9    Other Cast Room (OTHER CAST ROOM) |
| **71X** | **Recovery Room.**<br>0    General Classification (RECOV RM)<br>9    Other Recovery Room (OTHER RECOV RM) |
| **72X** | **Labor Room/Delivery.** Charges for labor and delivery room services provided by specially trained nursing personnel to patients, including prenatal care during labor, assistance during delivery, postnatal care in the recovery room, and minor gynecological procedures if they are performed in the delivery suite.<br>0    General Classification (DELIVROOM/LABOR)<br>1    Labor (LABOR)<br>2    Delivery (DELIVERY ROOM)<br>3    Circumcision (CIRCUMCISION)<br>4    Birthing Center (BIRTHING CENTER)<br>9    Other Labor Room/Delivery (OTHER/DELIV-LABOR) |
| **73X** | **EKG/ECG (Electrocardiogram).** Charges for operation of specialized equipment to record electromotive variations in actions of the heart muscle on an electrocardiograph for diagnosis of heart ailments.<br>0    General Classification (EKG/ECG)<br>1    Holter Monitor (HOLTER MON)<br>2    Telemetry (TELEMETRY)<br>9    Other EKG/ECG (OTHER EKG/ECG) |
| **74X** | **EEG (Electroencephalogram).** Charges for operation of specialized equipment to measure impulse frequencies and differences in electrical potential in various areas of the brain to obtain data for use in diagnosing brain disorders.<br>0    General Classification (EEG)<br>9    Other EEG (OTHER EEG) |
| **75X** | **Gastrointestinal Services.**<br>0    General Classification (GASTR-INTS SVS)<br>9    Other Gastrointestinal (OTHER GASTROINTS)<br>      NOTE:  Use 759 with the procedure code for endoscopic procedure |
| **76X** | **Treatment/Observation Room.** Charges for the use of a treatment room, or observation room charges for outpatient observation services.<br>0    General Classification (TREATMT/OBSERVATION RM)<br>1    Treatment Room (TREATMT RM)<br>2    Observation Room (OBSERV RM)<br>9    Other Treatment/Observation Room (OTHER TREAT/OBSERV RM) |
| **77X** | **Not Assigned.** |
| **78X** | **Not Assigned.** |
| **79X** | **Lithotripsy.** Charges for using lithotripsy in the treatment of kidney stones.<br>0    General Classification (LITHOTRIPSY)<br>9    Other Lithotripsy (LITHOTRIPSY/ OTHER) |

**Table 2–2** (*continued*)

| 80X | **Inpatient Renal Dialysis.** A waste removal process that uses an artificial kidney when the body's own kidneys have failed. The waste may be removed directly from the blood (hemodialysis) or indirectly from the blood by flushing a special solution between the abdominal covering and the tissue (peritoneal dialysis). In-unit lab nonroutine tests are medically necessary tests in addition to or at greater frequency than routine tests that are performed in the dialysis unit.<br>0    General Classification (RENAL DIALY)<br>1    Inpatient Hemodialysis (DIALY/ INPT)<br>2    Inpatient Peritoneal (Non-CAPD) (DIALY/INPT/PER)<br>3    Inpatient Continuous Ambulatory Peritoneal Dialysis (DIALY/ INPT/CAPD)<br>4    Inpatient Continuous Cycling Peritoneal Dialysis (DIALY/ INPT/CCPD)<br>9    Other Inpatient Dialysis (DIALY/ INPT/OTHER) |
|---|---|
| 81X | **Organ Acquisition.** The acquisition of a kidney, liver, or heart for use in transplantation. Organs other than these are included in category 89X. Living donor is a living person from whom kidney is obtained for transplantation. Cadaver is an individual who has been pronounced dead according to medical and legal criteria from whom organs have been obtained for transplantation.<br>0    General Classification (ORGAN ACQUISIT)<br>1    Living Donor--Kidney (KIDNEY/ LIVE)<br>2    Cadaver Donor--Kidney (KIDNEY/ CADAVER)<br>3    Unknown Donor--Kidney (KIDNEY/UNKNOWN)<br>4    Other Kidney Acquisition (KIDNEY/OTHER)<br>5    Cadaver Donor--Heart (HEART/ CADAVER)<br>6    Other Heart Acquisition (HEART/ OTHER)<br>7    Donor--Liver (LIVER ACQUISIT)<br>9    Other Organ Acquisition (ORGAN/ OTHER) |
| 82X | **Hemodialysis--Outpatient or Home.** A program under which a patient performs hemodialysis away from the facility using his or her own equipment and supplies. Hemodialysis is the removal of waste directly from the blood.<br>0    General Classification (HEMO/OP OR HOME)<br>1    Hemodialysis/Composite or Other Rate (HEMO/COMPOSITE)<br>2    Home Supplies (HEMO/HOME/ SUPPL)<br>3    Home Equipment (HEMO/HOME/ EQUIP)<br>4    Maintenance 100% (HEMO/HOME/ 100%)<br>5    Support Services (HEMO/HOME/ SUPSERV)<br>9    Other Outpatient Hemodialysis (HEMO/HOME/OTHER) |
| 83X | **Peritoneal Dialysis--Outpatient or Home.** A program under which a patient performs peritoneal dialysis away from the facility using his or her own equipment and supplies. Waste is removed by flushing a special solution between the tissue and the abdominal covering.<br>0    General Classification (PERTNL/ OP OR HOME)<br>1    Peritoneal/Composite or Other Rate (PERTNL/COMPOSITE)<br>2    Home Supplies (PERTNL/HOME/ SUPPL)<br>3    Home Equipment (PERTNL/ HOME/EQUIP)<br>4    Maintenance 100% (PERTNL/ HOME/100%)<br>5    Support Services (PERTNL/HOME/ SUPSERV)<br>9    Other Outpatient Peritoneal (PERTNL/HOME/OTHER) |
| 84X | **Continuous Ambulatory Peritoneal Dialysis (CAPD)--Outpatient or Home.** A program under which a patient performs continual dialysis away from the facility using his or her own equipment and supplies. The patient's peritoneal membrane is used as a dialyzer.<br>0    General Classification (CAPD/OP OR HOME)<br>1    CAPD/Composite or Other Rate (CAPD/COMPOSITE)<br>2    Home Supplies (CAPD/HOME/ SUPPL)<br>3    Home Equipment (CAPD/HOME/ EQUIP)<br>4    Maintenance 100% (CAPD/HOME/ 100%)<br>5    Support Services (CAPD/HOME/ SUPSERV)<br>9    Other Outpatient CAPD (CAPD/ HOME/OTHER) |

**Table 2–2** *(continued)*

| | |
|---|---|
| 85X | **Continuous Cycling Peritoneal Dialysis (CCPD)--Outpatient or Home.** A program under which a patient performs continual dialysis away from the facility using his or her own equipment and supplies. A machine is used to make automatic exchanges at night.<br>0  General Classification (CCPD/OP OR HOME)<br>1  CCPD/Composite or Other Rate (CCPD/COMPOSITE)<br>2  Home Supplies (CCPD/HOME/ SUPPL)<br>3  Home Equipment (CCPD/HOME/ EQUIP)<br>4  Maintenance 100% (CCPD/HOME/ 100%)<br>5  Support Services (CCPD/HOME/ SUPSERV)<br>9  Other Outpatient CCPD (CCPD/ HOME/OTHER) |
| 86X | **Reserved for Dialysis (National Assignment).** |
| 87X | **Reserved for Dialysis (National Assignment).** |
| 88X | **Miscellaneous Dialysis.** Charges for dialysis services not identified elsewhere. *Rationale*: Ultrafiltration is the process of removing excess fluid from the blood of dialysis patients by using a dialysis machine but without the dialysis solution. The designation is only used when the procedure is not performed as a part of a normal dialysis session.<br>0  General Classification (DIALY/ MISC)<br>1  Ultrafiltration (DIALY/ ULTRAFILT)<br>2  Home Dialysis Aid Visit (HOME DIALY AID VISIT)<br>9  Miscellaneous Dialysis Other (DIALY/MISC/OTHER) |
| 89X | **Other Donor Bank.** Charges for the acquisition, storage, and preservation of all human organs (excluding kidneys).<br>0  General Classification (DONOR BANK)<br>1  Bone (DONOR BANK/BONE)<br>2  Organ (other than Kidney) (DONOR BANK/ORGN)<br>3  Skin (DONOR BANK/SKIN)<br>9  Other Donor Bank (OTHER DONOR BANK) |
| 90X | **Psychiatric/Psychological Treatments.** Charges for providing treatment for emotionally disturbed patients, including patients admitted for diagnosis and for treatment.<br>0  General Classification (PSYCH TREATMENT)<br>1  Electroshock Treatment (ELECTRO SHOCK)<br>2  Milieu Therapy (MILIEU THER)<br>3  Play Therapy (PLAY THERAPY)<br>9  Other (OTHER PSYCH RX) |
| 91X | **Psychiatric/Psychological Services.** Charges for providing nursing care and professional services for emotionally disturbed patients, including patients admitted for diagnosis and those admitted for treatment.<br>0  General Classification (PSYCH SVS)<br>1  Rehabilitation (PSYCH/REHAB)<br>2  Day Care (PSYCH/DAYCARE)<br>3  Night Care (PSYCH/NIGHTCARE)<br>4  Individual Therapy (PSYCH/INDIV RX)<br>5  Group Therapy (PSYCH/GROUP RX)<br>6  Family Therapy (PSYCH/FAMILY RX)<br>7  Biofeedback (PSYCH/BIOFEED)<br>8  Testing (PSYCH/TESTING)<br>9  Other (PSYCH/OTHER) |
| 92X | **Other Diagnostic Services.** Charges for other diagnostic services not otherwise categorized.<br>0  General Classification (OTHER DX SVS)<br>1  Peripheral Vascular Lab (PERI-VASCUL LAB)<br>2  Electromyogram (EMG)<br>3  Pap Smear (PAP SMEAR)<br>4  Allergy Test (ALLERGY TEST)<br>5  Pregnancy Test (PREG TEST)<br>9  Other Diagnostic Service (ADDL DX SVS) |
| 93X | **Not Assigned.** |

**Table 2–2**  *(continued)*

| | |
|---|---|
| 94X | **Other Therapeutic Services.** Charges for other therapeutic services not otherwise categorized.<br>0   General Classification (OTHER RX SVS)<br>1   Recreational Therapy (RECREA-TION RX)<br>2   Education/Training (EDUC/TRNG)<br>3   Cardiac Rehabilitation (CARDIAC REHAB)<br>4   Drug Rehabilitation (DRUG REHAB)<br>5   Alcohol Rehabilitation (ALCOHOL REHAB)<br>6   Complex Medical Equipment--Routine (CMPLX MED EQUIP-ROUT)<br>7   Complex Medical Equipment--Ancillary (CMPLX MED EQUIP-ANC)<br>9   Other Therapeutic Services (ADDITIONAL RX SVS)<br>    NOTE: Use 930 with a procedure code for plasmapheresis. Use 932 for dietary therapy and diabetes-related services, education, and training. |
| 95X | **Not Assigned.** |
| 96X | **Professional Fees.** Charges for medical professionals that the hospitals or third party payers require to be separately identified.<br>0   General Classification (PRO FEE)<br>1   Psychiatric (PRO FEE/PSYCH)<br>2   Ophthalmology (PRO FEE/EYE)<br>3   Anesthesiologist (MD) (PRO FEE/ ANES MD)<br>4   Anesthetist (CRNA) (PRO FEE/ ANES CRNA)<br>9   Other Professional Fees (OTHER PRO FEE) |
| 97X | **Professional Fees (continued).**<br>1   Laboratory (PRO FEE/LAB)<br>2   Radiology--Diagnostic (PRO FEE/RAD/DX)<br>3   Radiology--Therapeutic (PRO FEE/RAD/RX)<br>4   Radiology--Nuclear Medicine (PRO FEE/NUC MED)<br>5   Operating Room (PRO FEE/OR)<br>6   Respiratory Therapy (PRO FEE/ RESPIR)<br>7   Physical Therapy (PRO FEE/ PHYSI)<br>8   Occupational Therapy (PRO FEE/ OCUPA)<br>9   Speech Pathology (PRO FEE/ SPEECH) |
| 98X | **Professional Fees (continued).**<br>1   Emergency Room (PRO FEE/ER)<br>2   Outpatient Services (PRO FEE/ OUTPT)<br>3   Clinic (PRO FEE/CLINIC)<br>4   Medical Social Services (PRO FEE/ SOC SVC)<br>5   EKG (PRO FEE/EKG)<br>6   EEG (PRO FEE/EEG)<br>7   Hospital Visit (PRO FEE/HOS VIS)<br>8   Consultation (PRO FEE/CONSULT)<br>9   Private Duty Nurse (FEE/PVT NURSE) |
| 99X | **Patient Convenience Items.** Charges for items that are generally considered by the third party payors to be strictly convenience items and, as such, are not covered.<br>0   General Classification (PT CONV)<br>1   Cafeteria/Guest Tray (CAFETERIA)<br>2   Private Linen Service (LINEN)<br>3   Telephone/Telegraph (TELEPHN)<br>4   TV/Radio (TV/RADIO)<br>5   Nonpatient Room Rentals (NONPT ROOM RENT)<br>6   Late Discharge Charge (LATE DISCH)<br>7   Admission Kits (ADMIT KITS)<br>8   Beauty Shop/Barber (BARBER/BEAUTY)<br>9   Other Patient Convenience Items (PT CONVENCE/OTH) |

**Table 2–2** *(continued)*

# Type of Bill Codes
## (Form Locator 4)

| Code | 1st Digit: Type of Facility |
|------|------------------------------------------------------------|
| 1 | Hospital |
| 2 | Skilled nursing facility |
| 3 | Home health |
| 4 | Christian science (hospital) |
| 5 | Christian science (extended care) |
| 6 | Intermediate care |
| 7 | Clinic |
| 8 | Special Facility |
| **Code** | **2nd Digit: Bill Classifications (Clinics only)** |
| 1 | Rural Health |
| 2 | Clinic – Hospital Based or Independent Renal dialysis center |
| 3 | Free-standing |
| 4 | Other rehabilitation facility |
| 5 | Clinic – CORF |
| 6 | Clinic – CMHC |
| 9 | Other |
| **Code** | **2nd Digit – Bill Classifications (Except Clinics & Special Facilities)** |
| 1 | Inpatient (including Medicare Part A) |
| 2 | Inpatient (Medicare Part B only) |
| 3 | Outpatient |
| 4 | Other |
| 5 | Intermediate Care, Level I |
| 6 | Intermediate Care, Level II |
| 7 | SubAcute Inpatient |
| 8 | Swing Beds |
| **Code** | **2nd Digit – Bill Classifications (Special Facilities only)** |
| 1 | Hospice (Non Hospital Based) |
| 2 | Hospice (Hospital Based) |
| 3 | Ambulatory Surgical Center |
| 4 | Free Standing Birth Center |
| 5 | Critical Access Hospital |
| 6 | Residential Facility |
| 9 | Other |
| **Code** | **3rd Digit: Frequency** |
| 0 | Non-Payment/Zero |
| 1 | Admit through discharge claim |
| 2 | Interim: first claim |
| 3 | Interim: continuing claims |
| 4 | Interim: last claim |
| 5 | Late charge only |
| 6 | Reserved |
| 7 | Replacement of prior claim |
| 8 | Void/cancel of prior claim |
| 9 | Final Claim for a Home Health PPS Episode |

**Table 2–3** **Hospital Form Locator Codes**

*(continued on next page)*

# Sex Codes
## (Form Locator 15)

| Code | Definitions |
|------|-------------|
| M | Male |
| F | Female |
| U | Unknown |

# Marital Status Codes
## (Form Locator 16)

| Code | Definition |
|------|------------|
| S | Single |
| M | Married |
| X | Legally separated |
| D | Divorced |
| W | Widowed |
| U | Unknown |
| P | Life partner |

# Type of Admission Codes
## (Form Locator 19)

| Code | Definition |
|------|------------|
| 1 | Emergency |
| 2 | Urgent |
| 3 | Elective |
| 4 | Newborn |
| 5 | Trauma Center |
| 9 | Information not available |

# Source of Admission Codes Except Newborns
## (Form Locator 20)

| Code | Definition |
|------|------------|
| 1 | Physician referral |
| 2 | Clinical referral |
| 3 | HMO referral |
| 4 | Transfer from a hospital |
| 5 | Transfer from a skilled nursing facility |
| 6 | Transfer from another health facility |
| 7 | Emergency room |
| 8 | Court/law enforcement |
| 9 | Information not available |
| A | Transfer from a critical access hospital |
| B | Transfer from another HHA |
| C | Readmission to same HHA |

**Table 2–3** (continued)

## Additional Source of Admission Codes for Newborns
### (Form Locator 20)

| Code | Definition |
|------|------------|
| 1 | Normal delivery |
| 2 | Premature delivery |
| 3 | Sick baby |
| 4 | Extramural birth |
| 5 | Information not available |

## Patient Status
### (Form Locator 22)

| Code | Definition |
|------|------------|
| 01 | Discharged to home or self-care (routine discharge) |
| 02 | Discharged/transferred to another short-term general hospital |
| 03 | Discharged/transferred to a skilled nursing facility |
| 04 | Discharged/transferred to an intermediate care facility |
| 05 | Discharged/transferred to another type of institution (including distinct parts) or referred for outpatient services to another institution |
| 06 | Discharged/transferred to home under care of organized home health service organization |
| 07 | Left against medical advice or discontinued care |
| 08 | Discharged/transferred to home under care of home IV therapy provider |
| 09 | Admitted as an inpatient to this hospital |
| 20 | Expired (or did not recover – Christian Science patient) |
| 30 | Still a patient or expected to return for outpatient services |
| 31-39 | Reserved for National Assignment |
| 40 | Expired at home (for hospice care only) |
| 41 | Expired in a medical facility such as a hospital, SNF, ICF, or free-standing hospice (for hospice care only) |
| 42 | Expired, place unknown (for hospice care only) |
| 43 | Discharged/transferred to a Federal Hospital |
| 50 | Discharged to a hospice, Home |
| 51 | Discharged to hospice, Medical Facility |

**Table 2–3**  *(continued)*

# Condition Codes
## (Form Locator 24-30)

| Code | Definition |
|------|------------|
| 02 | Enter this code if the patient alleges that the medical condition causing this episode of care is due to environment/event from his/her employment. |
| 03 | Indicates that patient/patient representative has stated that coverage may exist beyond that reflected on this bill. |
| 04 | Indicates bill is submitted for informational purposes only. Examples would include a bill submitted as a utilization report, or a bill for a beneficiary who is enrolled in a risk-based managed care plan (such as Medicare+Choice) and the hospital expects to receive payment from the plan. |
| 05 | Enter this code if you have filed a legal claim for recovery of funds potentially due to a patient or on behalf of a patient. |

# Release of Information Indicator
## Codes (Form Locator 52)

| Code | Definitions |
|------|-------------|
| Y | Yes |
| R | Restricted or modified release |
| N | No release |

# Member's Relationship to the Insured Codes
## (Form Locator 59)
## (Date of Service is before October 16, 2003)

| Code | Definition |
|------|------------|
| 01 | Patient is the insured |
| 02 | Spouse |
| 03 | Natural child/insured has financial responsibility |
| 04 | Natural child/insured does not have financial responsibility |
| 05 | Stepchild |
| 06 | Foster child |
| 07 | Ward of the court |
| 08 | Employee |
| 09 | Unknown |
| 10 | Handicapped dependent |
| 11 | Organ donor |
| 12 | Cadaver donor |
| 13 | Grandchild |
| 14 | Niece/nephew |
| 15 | Injured plaintiff |
| 16 | Sponsored dependent |
| 17 | Minor dependent of a minor dependent |
| 18 | Parent |
| 19 | Grandparent |
| 20 | Life partner |

**Table 2–3** *(continued)*

## Member's Relationship to the Insured Codes

(Form Locator 59)

(Date of Service is after October 16, 2003)

| Code | Definitions |
|------|-------------|
| 01 | Spouse |
| 04 | Grandfather or Grandmother |
| 05 | Grandson or Granddaughter |
| 07 | Niece/nephew |
| 10 | Foster Child |
| 15 | Ward |
| 17 | Stepson or Stepdaughter |
| 18 | Self |
| 19 | Child |
| 20 | Employee |
| 21 | Unknown |
| 22 | Handicapped dependent |
| 23 | Sponsored dependent |
| 24 | Dependent of minor dependent |
| 29 | Significant other |
| 32 | Mother |
| 33 | Father |
| 36 | Emancipated minor |
| 39 | Organ donor |
| 40 | Cadaver donor |
| 41 | Injured plaintiff |
| 43 | Child where insured has no financial responsibility |
| 53 | Life partner |
| G8 | Other relationship |

## Valid Employment Status Codes

(Form Locator 64)

| Code | Definition |
|------|------------|
| 1 | Employed full-time |
| 2 | Employed part-time |
| 3 | Not employed |
| 4 | Self-employed |
| 5 | Retired |
| 6 | On active military duty |
| 9 | Unknown |

**Table 2–3** (continued)

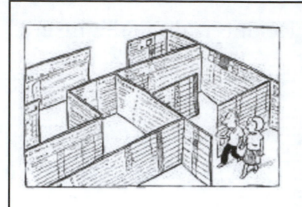

"It's not that hard to understand these forms.
Just follow my lead."

# On the Job Now

**Directions:** Look at the UB-92 form in **Figure 2–5**, and then answer the following questions.

1. What is the patient's name? _____

2. What is the name of the insured person on this claim? _____

3. What is the procedure code for the procedure performed? _____

4. What is the diagnosis code given? _____

5. What is the patient's marital status? _____

6. What insurance plan is the patient covered under? _____

7. Has the authorization to release information been signed? _____

8. Is this patient covered under more than one insurance policy? _____

9. Have benefits been assigned on this claim? _____

10. What is the name of the provider on this claim? _____

# CHAPTER REVIEW

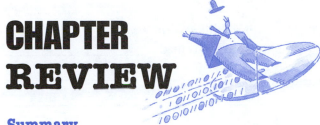

## Summary

- The *ICD-9-CM*, *CPT®*, *RVS*, *CDT*, HCPCS, *PDR*, medical dictionaries, and *Merck Manual* are the resource manuals most commonly used by health claims examining personnel.
- The *ICD-9-CM* is used to code diagnoses and conditions.
- The *CPT®* is used to code procedures and services rendered by providers.
- Use of the *PDR* assists in determining whether a drug is prescription or nonprescription, and lists some of the properties (i.e., manufacturer, chemical makeup, side effects, appearance) of a specific drug.
- Medical dictionaries list medical terms and their meanings, and the *Merck Manual* can assist in determining whether a service or *Red* and *Blue Book* procedure is appropriate for a given diagnosis or condition.
- Health claims examiners should familiarize themselves with the use of the reference books in this chapter. Without their proper utilization, delays and denials can result in claims submitted to payers.
- The CMS-1500 is the most accepted form for billing professional services.
- The UB-92 is the claim form used when billing for hospital services.
- The information in each field of these forms allows the claim to be processed quickly and accurately.
- While understanding the forms may seem simple, it takes practice to be able to accurately process these claims.
- You should familiarize yourself with these forms and know where to find the necessary information for claims processing.

## Assignments

Complete the Questions for Review.
Complete Exercises 2–1 through 2–2.

## Questions for Review

**Directions:** Answer the following questions without looking back at the material just covered. Write your answers in the space provided.

**1.** What is the CMS-1500 billing form used for? _____

_____

**2.** If the provider of service is an individual, what is shown in the block entitled Federal Tax ID Number? _____

_____

**3.** Which CMS-1500 block denotes that Workers' Compensation is involved in the claim? _____

**4.** What is the block at the top of the CMS-1500 form, labeled "Medicare, Medicaid, TRICARE, FECA, Black Lung, and Other" for? _____

_____

**5.** What does the term "Assignment of Benefits" mean? _____

_____

**6.** On the CMS-1500, what does block 24J "COB" stand for and what does the term mean? _____

_____

**7.** (True or False?) When a physician or provider of service signs a medical billing form, he/she is legally stating that the service(s) which they are seeking payment for have actually been performed. _____

**8.** What is a "Unit of Service?" _____

_____

**9.** What is the UB-92 billing form used for? _____

_____

**10.** What does form locator 17 on the UB-92 indicate? _____

_____

**11.** What are occurrence codes and occurrence span codes and what is the difference between them? _____

_____

_____

**12.** What would code 20 indicate in form locator 21 on the UB-92? _____

**13.** What would the code 03 indicate in form locator 22 on the UB-92? _____

**14.** On the UB-92, what is a value code used for? _____

_____

**15.** What do the following revenue codes indicate on a UB-92?

**a.** 722 _____

**b.** 351 _____

**c.** 559 _____

**d.** 207 _____

**e.** 450 _____

**f.** 622 _____

**g.** 815 _____

**h.** 657 _____

**i.** 490 _____

**j.** 341 _____

**16.** Which manual is used for coding diagnoses? _____

**17.** Name the two manuals that serve the same purpose and may be referred to interchangeably.

**1.** _____

**2.** _____

**18.** The full name of the *PDR* is _____

**19.** If you needed to verify a diagnosis, affected body area, or spelling of terms and definitions, you would probably refer to the _____

**20.** The _____ is useful in determining the appropriateness of services for a reported diagnosis.

If you were unable to answer any of these questions, refer back to that section and then fill in the answers.

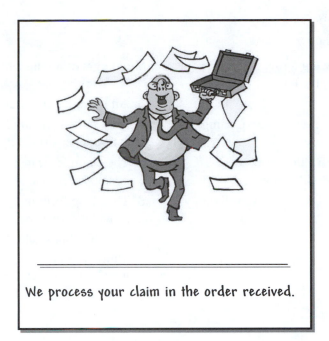

We process your claim in the order received.

# Exercise **2-1**

**Directions:** Find and circle the words listed below. Words can appear horizontally, vertically, diagonally, forward, or backward.

```
P H J C P U L H A C C V E E M P S T G B G M P Z A
M Y V L H C R J L J Z E S C P Q N K F X O N G W G
T E X C I J P U O I E S T N A K O M L B C A I M E
C E D V Q M B A Q C T Y G E H O E R C V O T K Q K
T E C I W E X L N J D N D R B B P T X U L F T V T
F B E I C A L X Q R E W L E I R H W P W A A I I V
D N I Z G A Q B B M U F U F A U T X M Y S W M W O
R B B I R O L L V O V L G E U R U N U M I K X Z I
A K U C K Q G D S X B F R R E N O F F W N O S A K
E H W B T F Q M I D P I O K L W J Z K L U S S K H
G F T B W T D C N C L G D S S U W Q L D M L J C X
G X B T W S V A V L T R B E H F O I Y Z E B R O H
V E U Q Z Q K Y R O W I P D F R S T Y J R A W V G
C Q K Y C O R N D C K L O S N V L T N M C D C M S
F T Z B O Y P S L G G Y D N K T F P O X K C A Z N
N W G B P A P S P J W G G A A P S L Q Y M J P E M
T O D C O Y D L U C J N C I K R T Q I R A R B O L
G E E H J F B L V K X S R C D L Y J H X N O Y Z O
R I O Q N F E I D L H P S I W W R I S K U C F Y J
N E P V U L R J J Q V D R S A T I G B Q A V N F T
C G V N D G O Q G X T O H Y Q G F V V O L Y D S U
S Q C M O N I H T U S K Z H L Y K D P V D A Y X N
D C K O V X K L U M M B P P E J U P Y A D W X R V
D L I H X W C A U E P N K J I Q C A C J G B S M J
R E L A T I V E V A L U E S T U D Y U Z X S Z V B
```

1. Medical Dictionary
2. *Merck Manual*
3. *Physicians Desk Reference*
4. *Red Book* and *Blue Book*
5. Relative Value Study

# Exercise 2-2

**Directions:** Match the following terms with the proper definition by writing the letter of the correct definition in the space next to the term.

1. _____ CMS-1500

2. _____ Health Care Common Procedure Coding System

3. _____ International Classification of Disease-9th Revision Clinical Modification

4. _____ Physicians' Current Procedure Terminology

5. _____ UB-92

a. An indexing of conditions.

b. A systematic listing for coding the procedures or services performed by a physician.

c. The claim form most commonly used to bill for hospital services.

d. The claim form most commonly used to bill for provider's services.

e. A coding book which came about because of the limitations in the *CPT*® and RVS for billing injections, medication, supplies, and durable medical equipment.

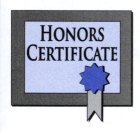

## Honors Certification™

The Honors Certification™ challenge for this chapter consists of a written test. You will be given several claim forms and asked to pull information from them, similar to that found in the Exercises. Any errors will result in a deduction of up to 5% from your grade. You must achieve a score of 85% or higher to pass this test. If you fail the test on your first attempt, you may retake the test one additional time. The items included in the second test may be different from those in the first test.

# 3
# Medical
## Plan Provisions

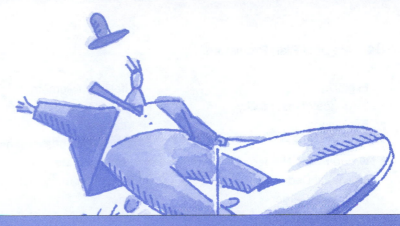

## After completion of this chapter
**you will be able to:**

- List the items that are necessary for a contract to be valid and enforceable.
- Define the provisions for coverage (i.e., eligibility, effective date, termination of coverage).
- List and explain common basic benefits.
- List and explain common major medical benefits.
- List and define common stipulations or items which can affect major medical payments (i.e., deductible, stoploss, etc.).
- Determine the order of benefit payments.
- Define eligibility and termination of coverage and explain their purposes.
- List eligibility guidelines for employees and dependents.
- List those people who are commonly considered to be dependents on an insurance policy.

- Determine a patient's eligibility status in a given scenario.
- Explain what COBRA is and how it functions.
- List conditions that may affect a person's ability to obtain continuation of coverage.
- Explain how HIPAA has affected eligibility for coverage.
- Identify possible third party liability and preexisting claims.
- Investigate possible third party liability and preexisting claims.
- Track payments which may be affected by third party liability.
- Identify the mandates that affect payment in their state.

## Keywords and concepts
**you will learn in this chapter:**

- Accident
- Active Work (Actively at Work)
- Actively-at-Work
- Acts of Third Parties (ATP)
- Aggregate
- Basic Benefit
- Beneficiary
- Carryover Deductible
- Coinsurance
- Coinsurance Limit
- Consideration
- Consolidated Omnibus Budget Reconciliation Act of 1985 (COBRA)
- Contract
- Contributory Plan
- Conversion
- Copayment
- Credible Coverage
- Deductible
- Dependent
- Effective Date

- Eligibility
- Evidence of Insurability
- Exclusions
- Group Contract
- Group Policy Holder
- Individual Deductible
- Insurance Carrier
- Insurance Company
- Insurance Premium
- Insured or Member

- Lifetime Maximum
- Major Medical Benefits
- Mandates
- Mental/Nervous Expenses
- Nonaggregate
- Noncontributory Plan
- Offer
- Open Enrollment
- Out-of-Pocket
- Policy

- Preadmission Testing
- Preexisting Conditions
- Qualified Beneficiary
- Qualifying Event
- Second Surgical Opinion
- Subrogation
- Summary Plan Description
- Termination of Coverage
- Third Party Liability (TPL)
- Treatment-Free Period

A **contract** is a legal and binding written document that exists between two or more parties. Written contracts are present in every aspect of society. Essentially, any agreement between two or more persons that is enforceable by law is considered a contract. However, written contracts have several advantages over non-written (oral) contracts: the existence of a written contract cannot be denied, and the terms of a written contract can be enforced more easily in the event of death or incapacity (i.e., insanity, coma) of one of the parties of the contract.

In health insurance, the contract is used to determine eligibility requirements and covered services and to determine how those covered services are to be paid. The contract also indicates services that are excluded and services that have limitations. Therefore, the health claims examiner must learn to read and interpret the contract in order to pay the proper benefits.

## Contract Validity

For a contract to be valid, the persons signing the contract must agree on the terms. For the parties to agree there must be some form of offer and acceptance. To **offer** means to propose or undertake to do or give something in exchange for a return promise from the person to whom the act or gift is being offered. An offer must be communicated in one form or another before it can be accepted. However, acceptance need not always be communicated to create a contract.

For example, banks often send out a letter to their patrons informing them of a change in interest rates or other terms regarding their accounts. These letters often state that if the bank is not contacted within a specified period of time, it will be assumed that the patron has agreed to and accepted the new terms or rates.

For a contract to be valid and enforceable, the following principles must be met:

1. The contract must be based on a mutual agreement by the parties to do or not to do a specific thing or things.

2. The contract must be made by parties who are able and competent to enter into the contract and to enforce the terms of the contract. In some states, this may mean that minors may not enter into certain types of contracts.

3. The contract must include consideration to pay money, deliver services, or promise to do or refrain from doing some lawful act that has not yet occurred (i.e., a contract cannot be made to enforce an event that has already occurred).

4. The purpose of the contract must be lawful. Contracts for unlawful acts are unenforceable.

5. If the contract falls into a class of contracts required by law to be in a special form, the format of the contract must meet those laws or requirements.

## Group Contracts

Every health benefit plan, whether it is insured or not, is required by law to have a written document describing the plan benefits. This written legal document is used both by the plan members and by the administrator in determining how claims are to be paid. If any settlement disputes develop, the document is entered as evidence of what is and is not covered, what allowances are provided towards specific services, what books are used for reference in calculating benefits, and what the appeal procedures are.

Insured plans call this written document a **contract** or **policy**. Noninsured plans usually refer to it as a **summary plan description**. For our purposes, we will refer to the documents generically as contracts without implying whether or not a plan is insured.

The **group contract** is an instrument through which an insurance company can meet the financial security needs of a group of persons. In essence, it is an agreement between the insurance company and the policyholder to insure the lives and health of the members of a defined group of persons and to pay the insurance benefits to the insured person or their beneficiaries. An **insured** (also called **member**) is the person who obtains or is otherwise covered by insurance on his health, life, or property. The specific terms and conditions of the contract are determined by negotiation between the insurance company and the policyholder. With the exception of benefit provisions, they are largely determined by standard provisions, generally accepted throughout the industry.

The group contract must consist of the following three parts:

1. The group master policy.
2. The application of the group policyholder.
3. The individual applications, if any, of the persons insured.

The term **insurance company** is often used to refer to companies that sell policies offered by insurance carriers. The parties to a group contract are the insurance company and the **group policy holder**. In most cases, this is an employer. However, the policyholder may be a union or the trustee of a fund established by employers, unions, or both. For a group contract to be valid, a written application must be made. For it to remain valid, premiums must continue to be paid.

A basic principle of the law of contracts is consideration. Consideration can be a very broad term. For our purposes, **consideration** will be defined as anything that is given, done, promised, forbidden, or suffered by one party as an inducement for the agreement. The most common form of consideration is the payment of money in exchange for a promise. For insurance, consideration is the premium paid by the group policyholder. The individual insured may contribute toward these premiums or provide the entire amount. In most cases, however, the premium is paid by the policyholder to the insurer, even though the individual insured may contribute part or all of the monies.

Interpreting and understanding contracts is one of the most important aspects of being a health claims examiner. The healthcare contract is the one document which is used to determine the benefits which the insurance carrier will pay for services rendered. The **insurance carrier** is the company which offers the health insurance policy; a corporation or association whose business is to make contracts of insurance.

The wording and terminology of health insurance contracts can often be confusing to someone who is not well versed in the insurance field. For this reason, health claims examiners will often be called upon to interpret the provisions of a contract for billing purposes or to explain benefits to a patient.

# Contract Provisions

In the following sections, we will briefly look at each of the items in a contract. These items, and how to calculate them, will be discussed in more detail in subsequent chapters. For now, just familiarize yourself with where to find items in a contract.

## Eligibility

The first item that is considered on the contract is **eligibility**, or the qualifications which make the person eligible for coverage. Usually, this includes items such as working full-time for a company and the description of what is considered full time. For example, in the Winter contract, an employee must work a minimum of 30 hours per week to be eligible for coverage. The contract also discloses who is considered a dependent of the employee.

If a person has purchased individual coverage and is not covered by their place of work, there would be no minimum work requirements. However, there would still be qualifications to have coverage under the plan.

Dependent eligibility is usually defined by the relationship to the employee and the age (if the dependent is a child). For example, in the Winter contract a child is covered until age 19 or to age 23 if they are a full-time student. If an eligible dependent becomes disabled before age 19, or if a student and the eligible dependent becomes disabled before age 23, dependent coverage would continue until age 23. Children include unmarried natural children, legally adopted children, foster children, and those for whom the employee is considered the legal guardian.

On some contracts there are provisions which state that if a husband and wife (or parent and child) work for the same employer and are covered under the same contract, the spouse or child cannot be covered as a dependent on the employee's policy. Also, some contracts state that if both spouses are working at the same company and are covered under the same contract, the children may be covered by one parent or the other, but not both. This prevents the insurance carrier from having to pay twice for the same patient and services rendered.

## Effective Date

The next item to be considered is whether or not the contract was in force at the time the services were rendered. This is often dependent on a minimum length of time an employee must have worked for a company in order for the contract to be in force. An **effective date** is the date a contract began to be in force.

There is also an **"actively-at-work"** stipulation that is included in many contracts. This clause states that a person must be at-work (or actively engaged in their normal activities if a dependent) on the date coverage becomes effective. If he or she is not at work or actively engaged in their normal activities, the contract does not become effective until the employee or dependent returns to work or their normal activities.

It should be noted that the employee does not have to be actively-at-work if the effective date of coverage falls on a date the employee would not normally be scheduled to work (i.e., an employee who works Monday through Friday, but his effective date falls on Saturday). In this instance the employee's coverage would become effective on Saturday. For an eligible dependent, if the dependent is hospital-confined on the date coverage was to become effective, the coverage will not become effective until after release from the hospital.

As a claims examiner, it is important that you ensure that a patient is eligible and is covered under an insurance policy in order to receive benefits. Many providers contact the insurance company prior to performing a procedure to be sure that the patient is covered. This is especially important when a patient is covered under an individual policy and pays a monthly premium for coverage.

## Termination of Coverage

This section provides information regarding when coverage will terminate for the employee and their dependents. It is important to note when coverage ceases, as the insurance carrier should not pay benefits after this date. **Termination of coverage** means a cessation of eligibility under the plan. Coverage will often continue until the end of the month in which an employee terminates.

# On the Job Now

**Directions:** Answer the following questions without looking back at the material just covered. Write your answers in the space provided.

1. For a contract to be valid and enforceable, what five principles must be met?

1. _____

   _____

2. _____

   _____

3. _____

   _____

4. _____

   _____

5. _____

   _____

**2.** The group contract must consist of what three parts?

**1.** _____

**2.** _____

**3.** _____

# Contract Benefits

The next section usually details the benefits that the contract covers. These can include basic and major medical benefits. Premiums are based on the number and amount of benefits which a contract covers. The greater the coverage is, the higher the cost of the premiums. For example, a contract which covers charges at 90% of the allowed amount and has a $100 deductible will usually cost more than a similar contract which covers charges at 70% of the allowed amount and has a $250 deductible.

## Basic Benefits

A **Basic Benefit** provides a specified allowance for a certain type of service, is usually paid at 100% of covered expenses, and is paid before major medical benefits are paid. Therefore, it is possible for the insurance plan to pay basic benefits even when the patient has not yet met their deductible. Not all contracts will have basic benefits. Most basic benefit plans have been replaced with managed care plans.

Some contracts have a basic benefit which is based upon the unit value (a number based upon the difficulty of a procedure and the overhead needed) being multiplied by a basic conversion factor (see Ball contract). This allows a small portion of most services to be paid at 100% with the remaining portion paid at the normal coinsurance percentage. Often these types of basic benefits do not cover all procedures.

## Accident Benefits

One of the most common basic benefits is an accident benefit. An **accident** is defined as an unintentional injury which has a specific time, date, and place. Under the Winter contract, the first $300 of services that are due to an accident are paid at 100%. The remaining charges are then paid at 90%. This benefit is for the first $300 of charges that are incurred within 120 days of the date of the accident.

On the CMS-1500 form, blocks 10b & 10c indicate services due to an accident with the date of the accident indicated in block 14.

## Preadmission Testing

In the past, a patient would enter the hospital the day before surgery for routine tests such as a chest x-ray and blood tests. The hospital would then admit the patient and watch over them to ensure that they had nothing to eat or drink in the 24 hours prior to surgery. Insurance carriers realized there would be a great cost savings if the patient were to visit the hospital for the tests, return home, and return the next day for the surgery. This eliminated the charges for an overnight hospital stay.

To encourage this practice, some insurance carriers offer an extra incentive for **preadmission testing**. Preadmission testing consists of routine laboratory and x-ray tests performed on an outpatient basis before a scheduled inpatient admission. Some insurance carriers now cover these charges at 100% rather than at their normal coinsurance percentage. Only tests done at the facility where the patient will be admitted and done within 24 hours of admittance are usually allowed under this benefit.

## Second Surgical Opinions

A **second surgical opinion** is an opinion provided by a second physician when one physician recommends surgery to an individual. This provision is designed to insure that the diagnosis of diseases and recommendation of treatments are accurate, or to investigate alternative and less invasive treatment.

Some insurance carriers pay 100% of allowable charges for a second surgical opinion. This originally started out as a cost containment measure. The hope was that only those surgeries that were necessary would be confirmed, with some patients receiving alternative and less expensive treatments, or with treatment being considered unnecessary.

Second surgical opinions have become less popular among insurance carriers since the cost savings seems to be minimal, if any. Many doctors are reluctant to go against the word or prescribed treatments of another physician. They do not want to contradict their peers, and also do not want to open themselves up to a lawsuit by suggesting a less radical treatment which may eventually prove less effective. Therefore, they will often simply confirm the diagnosis and prescribed treatment of the original physician.

## Outpatient Facility Charges

Some surgeries are simple or routine enough to be performed on an outpatient basis. This means the patient enters the facility in the morning, has surgery, and, after a brief recovery period, returns home the same day. There are no overnight or room and board charges. To encourage outpatient surgery when and where possible, some insurance carriers will cover such charges at 100%.

## Major Medical Benefits

**Major Medical Benefits** are those benefits paid after Basic benefits, and which are usually subject to a deductible and coinsurance. Major medical plans usually cover a broad list of medical expenditures. This section lists the particular benefits and stipulations which a Major Medical contract generally provides.

### Individual Deductible

The first item usually listed is the amount of the **deductible**. This is the amount which the member must pay prior to the insurance paying benefits. An **individual deductible** is the amount of covered expense that must be paid by the individual family member before benefits become payable by the plan. Deductibles are usually accumulated according to a calendar year. Thus, each January 1st, the amount the patient has paid toward their deductible returns to zero and the patient must start paying again.

The exception to this is in contracts which have a "carryover deductible provision." A **carryover deductible** means that any amounts which the patient pays toward their deductible in the last three months of the year will carry over and will be applied toward the next year's deductible. Remember, the member pays their deductible before the insurance is required to pay any benefits. Therefore, if the patient is still paying a deductible in the last three months of the year, the insurance carrier has not had to pay any major medical benefits on this patient up to that time.

### Family Deductible

Family deductibles work the same way individual deductibles do in that once a certain limit is reached, no more deductible is taken. There are two ways to accumulate family deductible amounts: aggregate and nonaggregate.

**Aggregate** means that any amounts paid toward the deductible by any member of the family will be added up to reach the deductible.

**Nonaggregate** means a specified number of individual deductibles must be satisfied before the family limit is met.

### Out-of-Pocket Limit

A member's **"out-of-pocket"** costs include the deductible, cost-sharing arising from the operation of the coinsurance clause, and medical expenditures that are deemed by the plan to be in excess of reasonable and customary charges.

### Copayment

A **copayment** is when the member is required to pay a set or fixed dollar amount (i.e., $15, $20, or $25) each time a particular medical service is provided. Copayment provisions are frequently found in PPO and HMO plans.

### Coinsurance

**Coinsurance** is the portion of covered expenses the member pays, and the portion the plan pays after any deductible amounts are met. This is usually expressed in percentages (i.e., the insurance covers 80% of the approved amount of a bill, and the member covers 20%).

### Coinsurance Limit

Many insurance companies are aware that the costs of a catastrophic illness can ruin a family financially. Since insurance carriers want to keep people on the member rolls, they must leave them with enough resources to consistently pay premiums. For this reason many insurance carriers have a **coinsurance limit**. This limit stipulates that if the coinsurance portion of a patient's bills reaches a certain amount, all subsequent claims will be paid at 100% of the allowed amount.

### Mental/Nervous Expenses

**Mental and nervous expenses** include claims submitted for psychiatric services, marriage and family counseling services, and drug and alcohol treatment. A lower coinsurance percentage (i.e., 50%) and a higher copayment may apply. Also, the coverage may depend on whether treatment is provided on an inpatient or outpatient basis.

Many contracts have a calendar year maximum or a maximum number of visits for these types of services.

## Practice
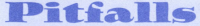
**Pitfalls**

The Ball Insurance Carriers contract has a coinsurance limit of $400. Since the coinsurance amount is based upon 20% of the allowed amount (with the insurance covering 80% of the allowed amount), the patient must have bills with approved amounts totaling over $2,125 in a calendar year ($125 is applied toward the deductible, $2,000 multiplied by 20% equals the $400 limit).

## Lifetime Maximum

There is a lifetime maximum payment amount placed on most contracts. Once the patient reaches the **lifetime maximum** amount, the insurance carrier will not cover any additional expenses. Essentially this amount is the total dollar payments the insurance carrier will make toward the care of this member. However, this amount is so high that it is seldom reached, except in extreme cases.

## Preexisting Limitations

Many contracts will not cover conditions which existed prior to a patient becoming covered under a contract (called **preexisting conditions**). This prevents a patient from not paying for insurance coverage, then suddenly discovering they have a serious illness and seeking insurance to cover that illness.

By law, preexisting limitations must be included in the contract. The term *preexisting* is different for each contract. Most often it is defined as a condition for which the patient has sought treatment within a given time period before insurance coverage has begun. If the patient has sought treatment for such a condition within this time period, benefits for treatment may not

be covered, or may be limited to a certain dollar amount. Usually, the restraints for benefits will cease once the patient has been covered under a contract for six months or longer.

Some contracts also have a **"treatment-free"** period. With this provision, if the patient can go without treatment for a specified period of time (often 90 days), then the insurance carrier will no longer consider the condition to be preexisting and will cover the illness or condition under the normal terms of the contract.

Remember that treatment includes any kind of contact in relationship with the illness, including the office visit or testing which was used to diagnose the illness. It also includes treatment of the condition, tests or office visits to monitor the condition, and filling of prescriptions relating to the condition.

## Exclusions

Every contract will have a list of **exclusions**; which are conditions or expenses for which no coverage is provided. It is important to check the list of exclusions before verifying benefits for services. If the procedures or treatments are not covered, the member will be responsible for the entire amount of the bill.

# On the Job Now

**Directions:** Answer the following questions without looking back at the material just covered. Write your answers in the space provided.

1. Basic benefits are usually paid at 100% and are _____

2. Define accident. _____

3. What is preadmission testing? _____

4. What is outpatient surgery? _____

_____

5. What is a deductible? _____

_____

**6.** What is coinsurance? _____

_____

**7.** What are mental/nervous expenses? _____

_____

**8.** What happens when a patient reaches their lifetime maximum? _____

**9.** What is a preexisting condition? _____

_____

# On the Job Now

**Directions:**   Read through the Ninja Enterprises (Rover Insurers) contract and possible preexisting conditions (see Appendix A), then list the amounts for the following provisions in the space provided.

**1.** What is the individual deductible amount?   _____

**2.** What is the dependent eligibility age limit? _____

**3.** What is the family calendar year deductible? _____

**4.** What is the individual coinsurance limit?   _____

**5.** What is the coinsurance percentage?   _____

**6.** What is the lifetime maximum amount? _____

**7.** How many hours must the employee work to be eligible? _____

**8.** Does the contract include dental coverage?   _____

**9.** What is the family coinsurance limit?   _____

**10.** Is the family coinsurance aggregate or nonaggregate? _____

**11.** Is there a carryover provision on the individual deductible? _____

**12.** How many months must the employee work before coverage becomes effective? _____

**13.** What is the amount of the basic accident benefit? _____

**14.** What basic benefits does the contract have?   _____

_____

**15.** What are the terms of the accident benefit? _____

_____

_____

# On the Job Now

**Directions:** Read the dental portion for the contracts (see Appendix A) and list the amounts for the following dental provisions in the spaces provided.

|  | ABC | XYZ | Ninja |
|---|---|---|---|
| 1. What is the individual deductible amount? | _____ | _____ | _____ |
| 2. What is the dependent eligibility age limit? | _____ | _____ | _____ |
| 3. What is the family calendar year deductible? | _____ | _____ | _____ |
| 4. What is the calendar year maximum? | _____ | _____ | _____ |
| 5. What is the coinsurance percentage? | _____ | _____ | _____ |
| 6. How many hours must the employee work to be eligible? | _____ | _____ | _____ |
| 7. Are orthodontics covered? | _____ | _____ | _____ |
| 8. Is oral surgery covered? | _____ | _____ | _____ |
| 9. Are fluoride treatments covered for a 20-year-old? | _____ | _____ | _____ |
| 10. Does the missing and unreplaced rule apply? | _____ | _____ | _____ |

## Eligibility

**Eligibility** is defined as the quality or qualities that make someone eligible. Eligible is defined as fit to be chosen or legally or morally qualified. Therefore, as far as insurance is concerned, eligibility means those qualities or requirements that a person must meet to be covered by the plan. Do not confuse "eligible" with "effective." In insurance, these are two very different concepts. A person can be eligible for coverage without the coverage ever becoming effective. (The concept of coverage becoming effective will be covered later in this chapter).

The definition of an eligible person varies from plan to plan. However, most plans have separate definitions for eligible employees or subscribers compared with eligible dependents. The requirements for the insured can include such things as the number of hours worked for the policyholder and a minimum of months that the employee has been employed by the policyholder. The requirements for the dependents of the insured can include such things as being a lawful spouse, domestic partner, or dependent child of the insured, being under a certain age limit, or attending school full-time. The eligibility of these relationships varies by plan as well as by insurance company. Before verifying eligibility and benefits, be sure to review the plan definition of an eligible dependent and the company policy for covering domestic partners.

It is important for the health claims examiner to understand the concept of eligibility and the eligibility requirements under each contract in order to process claims correctly.

## Employee Eligibility

Most contracts define participants (also called employees, subscribers, members, or insureds) according to the minimum number of hours that the employee or subscriber must work per specified period of time, which is

# On the Job Now

**Directions:** Read the following list of exclusions and place an E in the space provided if the service is excluded under the applicable contract (see Appendix A). Place an N/E in the space provided if the service is not excluded under the contract.

|  | ABC | XYZ | Ninja |
|---|---|---|---|
| 1. Gender-altering treatments or surgeries or related studies. | | | |
| 2. Work-related injuries or illnesses. | | | |
| 3. Changes or services in excess of UCR. | | | |
| 4. Charge made for failure to keep an appointment. | | | |
| 5. Routine, preventative, or experimental services. | | | |
| 6. Mental/Nervous expenses above $15,000. | | | |
| 7. Orthopedic shoes (medically necessary) following foot surgery. | | | |
| 8. Radial keratotomy. | | | |
| 9. Cosmetic surgery for breast following mastectomy. | | | |
| 10. Services for which there is no charge in the absence of insurance. | | | |
| 11. Surgical correction of cleft palate. | | | |
| 12. Custodial care. | | | |
| 13. Reversal of voluntary sterilization. | | | |
| 14. Contraceptive materials or devices. | | | |
| 15. Expenses resulting from self-inflicted injuries. | | | |
| 16. Elective abortions. | | | |
| 17. Expenses for weight reduction for someone 90 lbs. overweight. | | | |
| 18. Charges for services not medically necessary. | | | |
| 19. Vitamins, food supplements, or protein supplements. | | | |
| 20. Experimental transplants. | | | |

usually per week. Generally, part-time employees and full-time employees working fewer than 30 hours per week are not considered eligible for coverage.

Other contracts define the subscriber in terms of membership in an organization, such as the CPA Society or real estate societies. A minimum number of hours worked may also apply in these circumstances. Partners and proprietors are also considered participants as long as they engage in the conduct of business on a full-time basis or a minimum number of hours per week.

For example, refer to the XYZ Corporation contract (see Appendix A). As indicated therein, the employee must:

- Routinely work a minimum of 30 hours per week,

- Be considered a full-time employee. (Even though the contract does not specifically indicate this, it is an industry standard.) Therefore, unless the booklet or contract says otherwise, this is to be assumed, and

- Work three consecutive months to be eligible. Coverage may become effective the first of the month following the completion of three months of work (application must still be made).

## Practice Pitfalls

Suppose an employee is hired on 3/2/CCYY and works 40 hours per week, and is covered under the XYZ Corporation contract. This contract states that an employee is eligible for coverage the first of the month following three consecutive months of continuous employment. Three months would end on 6/2/CCYY. However, since 6/2/CCYY is past the first of the month, coverage will become effective the first of the month following the completion of the three-month waiting period. Therefore, coverage would become effective on 7/1/CCYY.

Under many union contracts, eligibility depends on the number of hours the member worked during the previous year or the previous month. With unions, a member may work for multiple employers during a month or week. As long as both the employer and the employee are members of the union, hours are accumulated toward the satisfaction of the hourly requirement.

For example, a common type of wording for union contracts is: If you are a bargaining unit employee, you will become eligible for benefits on the first day of the second month following any three consecutive months during which you worked for one or more contributing employers a minimum total of 300 hours. Once eligibility has been established, you and your dependents will be covered for a minimum of three consecutive months.

For example, if you worked:

| | |
|---|---|
| January | 110 hr |
| February | 0 hr |
| March | 190 hr |
| Total | 300 hr |

Your coverage will begin May 1.
In this example, the requirements are:

- 300 hours in any consecutive three-month period,
- Eligibility begins on the first day of the second month following the three consecutive months, and
- Coverage will be for a minimum of three consecutive months.

It is not unusual for a plan to have different eligibility provisions for different classifications of employees. For example, separate provisions may be given for employees classified as Active Officers, Board Members, Management Employees, or Retired Employees. Special provisions may also be applicable to employees who are laid off or on leave. Therefore, it is very important to check the plan provisions to determine whether there are a variety of classifications and, if so, to know how to verify the specific classifications of the claimants whose claims you are handling.

## Dependent Eligibility

The first step in determining whether a dependent is eligible is to verify whether the dependent fits the definition of an eligible dependent (ED). Defining a dependent is much more difficult than defining an employee because of the complex family and social dynamics in our society. A plan must try as much as possible to define all the dependents that can exist and to place those definitions into either covered or noncovered categories.

In general, "**dependent**" means:

1. The employee's legal spouse (either through marriage or through common-law status if recognized by the state in which they are residing). The employee and spouse cannot be divorced or legally separated, even if there is a court decree stating that the employee is responsible for providing medical coverage.

2. Dependent, unmarried children within the age limitations specified by the plan. The term "dependent" means that the child must rely on the employee for daily maintenance and care. The term "children" always includes one's natural children and may include:

   a. Adopted children for whom the final court order has been issued or for whom it is specified by the adoption agreement during any state-mandated waiting period that the adoptive parents provide for all medical care.

   b. Stepchildren residing with the employee.

   c. Grandchildren residing with the employee, who depend on the employee for more than 50% of their support.

   d. Foster children whose foster child agreement specifies that the state is not responsible for their health care and that the foster parents are responsible. (The state usually maintains responsibility for the foster children's health care).

**e.** Any other children related to the employee by blood or marriage, provided that they are living in a regular parent-child relationship and dependent on the employee for support and maintenance. In the case of grandchildren, a regular parent-child relationship does not exist if either of the child's parents also reside with the employee.

Plans will further specify that to be eligible, children must be under a certain age, usually 18 or 19 years. Unmarried children of a specified age limitation, usually 23 through 25 years of age, who attend a licensed or accredited school on a full-time basis, are generally also eligible. For coverage to continue during vacation periods, the child must be scheduled and registered to enter school on the next enrollment date.

In conjunction with this requirement, plans must define what is considered a "licensed" or "accredited" school. Many plans cover only colleges or universities. Other plans allow vocational schools and rehabilitation schools. The plan must specify what is considered to be full-time. Most schools define what constitutes a full-time student, and most plans accept the school-specific definition. However, this must be verified by reading the contract provisions.

Many states have enacted legislation concerning coverage for dependent children from birth. Although specific wording and intent are determined by individual state legislation, the laws generally provide that newborn children can be afforded the same eligibility for accident and health coverage as any other dependent and are covered from birth for treatment of a disease or injury. Preexisting limitations by definition cannot be applied to newborn children. This automatic coverage is generally for an initial 31-day period from date of birth. For such coverage to continue past the 31-day period, the employee must:

- Complete any required enrollment form,
- Make any required contributions, effective from the date of birth.

The law does not usually create an obligation for plans to pay for well-baby or custodial care. However, a few states require insured plans to have well-child care provisions. (Refer to the mandates listed later in this chapter.)

Many plans also specify that a person who is eligible as an employee cannot be enrolled as a dependent on the same plan. And, if both husband and wife are covered under the same plan as employees, one or the other, not both, may elect to cover their dependents. This prevents a particular child from being covered as a dependent under both parents. Some self-funded plans do permit dual coverage under the same plan, for husbands, wives, and dependent children. Unless specifically excluded from being covered as both employees and dependents or as a dependent under both parents, dual coverage is permitted. Be sure to review the contract for the definition of dependent coverage.

# Employee Effective Date of Coverage

For an eligible employee's coverage or a dependent's coverage to become effective, the person is usually required to complete the necessary enrollment papers prior to the date of eligibility.

The rules defining the effective date of coverage vary, depending on whether the plan is considered a contributory or noncontributory plan.

In a **contributory plan**, the employees contribute to the cost of the coverage, usually through payroll deductions. In a **noncontributory plan**, the employer bears the complete cost of the coverage and the employee does not contribute.

In a contributory plan:

- The employee must complete the enrollment card listing himself or herself and the dependents he or she wants to be covered; usually, all eligible dependents must be listed,
- Such application must be received by the employer or by the plan administrator on or before the eligibility date of the coverage for coverage to become effective on that date, and
- The employee must also authorize the applicable payroll deductions or make the necessary premium payments.

**Example:** Sammy Subscriber begins working for White Corporation on 1/15/CCYY. The Winter contract states he will become eligible on the first of the month after 90 days of employment. Therefore, he will become eligible on 5/1/CCYY. If he has not completed the enrollment card, turned it in to the employer, and made arrangements for payment before 5/1/CCYY, his insurance will not become effective. Thus, he will not be insured.

If the enrollment card is not received on or before the eligibility date of coverage, but is received within one month (or 30 or 31 days) after the date of eligibility, the employee is considered to be a "late applicant" and coverage will begin either on the date of application or the first or fifteenth of the month following the date of application (the plan provisions must specify which of the time limitations are to be applied).

If the enrollment application is not submitted within one month (or 30 or 31 days) after the date of eligibility, the employee may be required to submit proof of good health. Also known as **evidence of insurability**, this is often a health questionnaire required for the policy holder and all eligible dependents seeking coverage. The questionnaire will be submitted to the medical consultants of the insurer or plan administrator for review. If the participant appears to be a good "risk," that is, he or she does not appear to have any active illness or conditions, coverage may be approved. If the participant appears to be a poor risk because of active illnesses, coverage may not be approved and the employee and dependents may not be able to obtain coverage under the plan at that time (some plans provide for open enrollment periods, which will be discussed later.) Dependents cannot be covered unless the employee is covered. Therefore, if the dependents are healthy but the employee is not, the employee's eligibility is denied. Thus, even though the dependents may be a good risk, they will not be covered under the plan.

In a noncontributory plan in which the employer pays the full cost, a request for coverage is not necessary except for record purposes and beneficiary designations. A **beneficiary** is the person who receives payment on a claim, often the person who receives the benefit in the case of a deceased member. Coverage for employees and, in some instances, their dependents begins automatically on the employee's eligi-

bility date, regardless of when the enrollment application is completed and submitted. If the insurer or administrator is not informed of an employee's eligibility on the appropriate date and a claim or an enrollment card is subsequently submitted, the insurer/administrator will automatically add the member and bill the employer for all back premiums due. After the back premiums are paid, the claim(s) will be paid. Evidence of insurability is not required in these cases and there are not considered to be any "late applicants" on the plan.

Be aware that a plan can be noncontributory for the employee and contributory for the dependents. Therefore, a combination of the above rules may apply. For example, a company provides free health insurance for their employees (noncontributory), but any employees who also want coverage for their spouse and children must pay for it (contributory).

Whether the group is contributory or noncontributory, the usual effective date of coverage is deferred if on the effective date the employee is absent from work because of illness or injury. Most plans stipulate that for coverage to become effective, the employee must have completed either a full day of active work on that date or a full day of active work on the last regularly scheduled work day and be able to work on the date of eligibility. If the employee does not meet these requirements, the coverage will become effective on the date he or she returns to active work.

**Active work** and **actively-at-work** usually means performing the regular duties of a full workday for the employer.

**Practice**

# Pitfall

Susan Subscriber's insurance was to become effective on 5/1/CCYY. However, on 4/30/CCYY she came down with a bad cold and was absent from work for a week. She returned on 5/7/CCYY. Therefore, her insurance coverage will not begin until 5/7/CCYY.

## Dependent Effective Date of Coverage

The rules regarding the effective date of dependents are similar to the rules for employees, since the rules depend on whether the plan is contributory or noncontributory.

In the case of an employee, the plan usually makes a stipulation regarding being actively at work. A similar provision is also made for dependents. However, since a dependent often does not work, policies usually state that if a dependent is in the hospital, the coverage for that dependent becomes effective on the day after the date of discharge, or the date on which the dependent is able to perform all the duties he or she usually performs. In other words, if the dependent is of school age, coverage might begin when the child returns to school. An exception would be that of a newborn child, who is usually born in a hospital. In such a case, coverage begins immediately.

In a contributory plan, dependents are handled in the same way as with employees regarding late enrollment. However, many contributory plans require that for dependent coverage, all eligible dependents must be enrolled in the plan. This requirement prevents an employee from selectively putting sick dependents on one plan and healthy dependents on another plan.

# On the Job Now

**Directions:** Indicate whether the person listed would be considered an eligible dependent (ED) or a noneligible dependent (NED) under the general provisions. Assume that the first person is covered under the general provisions, and the second person is applying as his or her dependent.

**1.** Natalie's legally married spouse. _____

**2.** Nathaniel's dependent child, age four. _____

**3.** Bryant's cousin Terrell. _____

**4.** Tabari's divorced ex-spouse. _____

**5.** Tiron's son, age 45, fully functional. _____

**6.** Kyra's dependent child, age 19, who is a full-time student. _____

**7.** Kayla's brother Kenneth. _____

**8.** Ann's dog Pepper. _____

**9.** Aaron's adopted daughter. _____

**10.** Brittany's mother-in-law. _____

## Open Enrollment

**Open enrollment** is a process that allows late applicants to enroll in a plan without having to complete evidence of insurability. This enrollment process usually occurs on the anniversary date of the plan, and when an employer has multiple plan options. For example, larger employers are required by law to offer their employees an HMO option. These employers often offer an HMO plan, a low-indemnity plan (i.e., higher deductibles, lower coinsurance payable by the plan), and perhaps a high-indemnity plan (lower deductible, higher coinsurance payable by the plan). By having an open enrollment period, employees may switch from one plan to another without penalties or a gap in coverage and without having to complete a health statement.

## Termination of Coverage

The provisions for terminating an individual's coverage vary according to the type of group and how the employer wants the plan administered. In a union or association group, for example, coverage terminates when the employer terminates the group's membership in the union or association. The most common termination provisions are those based on conditions pertaining to employment. Coverage is usually terminated under one of these conditions:

- The group policy terminates (i.e., a company terminates the policy).
- The policy is amended to terminate the eligibility of the class of employees to which the individual belongs (i.e., the employer decides they will no longer cover commissioned sales people).
- The employee transfers out of a class covered by the policy (i.e., an employee goes from full-time to part-time).
- Active employment ceases (i.e., the employee quits).
- The employee ceases to pay the required contributions for the coverage.

When coverage ceases, regardless of the reason, some form of continuation of coverage may be available.

## Continuation of Coverage

Many plans allow benefits to extend beyond the normal date or terms of eligibility. These extensions can be of several types, depending on the reason for the continuation (i.e., disability, COBRA). We will discuss the main situations in which benefits are extended beyond normal eligibility and the requirements for continuing such coverage.

An employee or dependent losing coverage may qualify for continuation of benefits under more than one provision. It should be noted that the order in which these provisions apply is important. Continuation is first considered under COBRA (see heading COBRA) because it is premium-based and covers all conditions. The extension of benefits for disability is second because the only person eligible for coverage under this provision is the person, and only the disabling condition is covered. The coverage is usually for 12 months and the premium contributions are waived. The conversion privilege is the last coverage option to be exercised.

# On the Job Now

**Directions:** Answer the following question without looking back at the material just covered. Write your answers in the space provided.

List the five conditions under which coverage is usually terminated.

1. _____

2. _____

3. _____

4. _____

5. _____

## Extension of Benefits

Because extension of benefits for disability and conversion are more easily explained, we will cover those first. Most plans contain an extended benefits provision for totally disabled members. This type of provision requires that:

- The person was eligible and covered under the plan when his or her coverage terminated.

- As of the termination date, the person was totally disabled due to an injury or illness.

- Only covered expenses (as defined by the plan provisions) incurred for the illness or injury causing the disability will be considered eligible for benefit consideration.

- Coverage will last only for the length of time specified in the policy.

The latter requirements indicate that first there must be documented proof that the person was totally disabled with an injury or illness when he or she terminated. Second, only eligible expenses incurred for the injury or illness causing the disability are considered for benefits after the termination date.

Refer to the three contracts in Appendix A. As indicated, ABC and XYZ contracts both have a standard extension of benefits provision. Coverage will continue for 12 months from the date of termination under the plan or until the person is no longer totally disabled, whichever interval is less. Ninja Enterprises does not have an extension of benefits provision.

Therefore, in determining whether an extension of benefits provision is applicable, the following steps must be followed:

1. Was the member eligible and effective under the plan when coverage terminated? If no, the investigation would end, since the member could not continue coverage if he or she was not eligible and effective on the plan when the coverage terminated. If yes, then:

2. Was the member totally disabled at the time the coverage terminated? If no, extension of benefits would not apply. If yes, then:

3. A letter from the attending physician must be obtained stating the condition or conditions causing the disability, the date the member became totally disabled, and the anticipated end of the total disability.

4. Also, if the employee is claiming disability, try to find out if he or she is employed anywhere. Sometimes, members apply for this type of extension because premiums are not required (continuation is provided for the maximum 12 months free of charge to the employee but only for the person totally disabled) and the member wants coverage between jobs.

## Conversion Policies

Most states have legislatively mandated that insurance policies contain a continuation of coverage provision known as conversion. **Conversion** permits employees and dependents to continue their insurance protection on an individual basis when their coverage under a group plan ceases because:

- The employee's employment in the class of employees insured under the group policy terminates.

- The policy is amended to terminate coverage for the class to which the employee belongs.

- The employee terminates employment with the employer.

- A dependent child reaches the plan limiting age.

- The employee and spouse are divorced or legally separated so that the spouse is no longer considered eligible under the provisions of the plan.

Evidence of insurability is not required, but the person must apply in writing and pay the required premiums within a specified time period of the date of termination of coverage under the group plan (usually 31 days). Those who voluntarily discontinue their insurance coverage while still employed are not eligible to convert, nor is the conversion privilege available when the employer's complete policy is terminated.

As a rule, conversion policies are extremely expensive. The reason for the high cost is that usually only those employees who are disabled and extremely ill convert their policy. Because of the high expenses on the conversion policy, the resulting premiums are also very high.

Unfortunately, if an individual is so ill that he or she must cease working, it is extremely difficult to afford the high premiums. Nevertheless, it is an available option.

# On the Job Now

**Directions:** Place a "yes" or "no" next to each of the following to show whether coverage would be terminated under the circumstances given. Assume that each person listed is the member on the plan. Do not be concerned about whether the person is entitled to continuation of coverage.

1. Nancy goes from full-time to 20 hours per week.  _____

2. Alonzo is terminated by the company.  _____

3. Kerri's company terminates the policy.  _____

4. Sydney becomes self-employed but works on a contract basis for the same company.  _____

5. Sean stops paying the premium for his insurance.  _____

6. Thomas goes on vacation for two weeks.  _____

7. Floree forgets to enroll during her company's open enrollment period.  _____

8. Mia is transferred out of a class covered by the policy.  _____

9. Mayra goes on maternity leave.  _____

10. Carol gets married.  _____

## COBRA

In 1986, President Ronald Reagan signed into law HR3128, the **Consolidated Omnibus Budget Reconciliation Act of 1985 (COBRA)**, also referred to hereafter as **continuation of coverage**. Within this act, there is a very significant provision, Title X, which has had profound effects on employee welfare benefits plans.

Previous to COBRA, employers were generally not required to provide continuation of group insurance coverage for individuals who ceased to be eligible for such coverage. The objective of Congress through Title X was to require employers to permit employees and their dependents to purchase transitional health care coverage at favorable group rates until replacement coverage could be obtained. The intended result was to reduce the number of people without health care coverage.

Title X is composed of the following amendments:

Section 10001  Amendments to the Internal Revenue Code (IRC).

Section 10002  Amendments to the Employee Retirement Income Security Act (ERISA).

Section 10003  Amendments to the Public Health Service Act (PHSA).

The effect of these amendments is to require virtually every type of group health plan, insured or self-funded, to provide the option of self-payment for continuation of coverage. And, since the penalties for nonconformance will be administered by the IRS, noncompliance will be costly.

### COBRA Applicability

COBRA applies to all private employers who regularly employ 20 or more employees (including both full-time and part-time) on a typical working day. It applies to single employer health plans, multiple employer trust plans, collectively bargained plans, insured plans, and self-funded plans.

Under the amendment to the Public Health Service Act (PHSA) (Section 10003), certain state and local governmental employers of 20 or more employees are required to offer continuation of coverage even though these employers are exempt from both taxes and ERISA. The applicability of COBRA to state and local governmental employers is based on the receipt of funds under PHSA. If the state or local governmental employer received funds under PHSA, compliance is required.

In sum, all employee group health benefit plans are required to comply in offering continuation of coverage, with the exception of the following:

- Any group health plan for any calendar year if the employer normally maintained fewer than 20 employees on a typical business day during the preceding calendar year.
- Certain church plans.
- Group health plans maintained by state or local governmental employers who do not receive funds under PHSA.
- Group health plans maintained for employees by the government of the District of Columbia or any territory or possession of the United States.

Governmental and nongovernmental group health plans that are not collectively bargained were subject to the COBRA requirements as of the first of the plan year, beginning subsequent to June 30, 1986.

## Qualified Beneficiaries

The option of self-payment continuation of coverage must be offered by the affected employers to certain individuals referred to as qualified beneficiaries. A **qualified beneficiary** is defined as anyone who, on the day before the Qualifying Event, is covered under the health coverage plan as an employee, a dependent spouse, or a dependent child.

## Qualifying Event

The term **qualifying event** refers to one of the following events which results in the loss of eligibility under the employer sponsored health plan:

- Voluntary or involuntary termination of employment, with the exception of termination for gross misconduct.
- Reduction in work hours.
- Eligibility of the employee only for Medicare.
- Death of the employee.
- Divorce or legal separation.
- Disqualification of a dependent child as an eligible dependent.

Employers are required to offer the self-pay continuation of coverage option to the following:

- Terminated or laid-off employees (except those terminated for gross misconduct); employees for whom a reduction in work hours would result in

the loss of coverage; retired employees who are not eligible for Medicare.
- The surviving spouse and dependent children of a deceased employee.
- Divorced spouses and their dependent children.
- Spouses and dependent children of employees who are eligible for Medicare.
- Dependent children who cease to meet the plan definition of a "dependent child".

There are no "length of service" requirements connected to COBRA. As long as the employee was covered under the employer-sponsored health plan prior to the qualifying event, he or she has the right to elect continuation. This right also applies to the employee's spouse and dependent children, provided they were covered under the plan the day before the event.

The covered employee or spouse (when spouse is the elector) may act as the agent for the entire family. It is not necessary for each family member to make an individual election.

## Duration of Coverage

COBRA requires that affected employers permit employees and covered dependents, at the time their coverage would cease because of a qualifying event, to elect continuation of their insurance coverage for up to 18, 29, or 36 months, depending on the circumstances.

For employees and their dependents, a maximum of 18 months is allowed after one of the following events:

- Voluntary or involuntary termination of employment other than for gross misconduct.
- Reduction of work hours below the plan eligibility requirements.

For employees or dependents who are permanently disabled at the time of the event, coverage may be continued for up to 29 months rather than 18 months. The plan may use the Social Security standard of permanent disability as a qualifying condition of the extended coverage.

For covered dependents only, a maximum of 36 months of continued coverage is allowed after one of the following events:

- Death of the employee.
- Divorce or legal separation from the employee.
- The employee becomes eligible for Medicare.
- A child ceases to be an eligible dependent as defined by the plan provisions.

If a second qualifying event occurs during the time of the continuation of coverage for dependents, the maximum time allowed can be increased from 18 to 36 months if a qualifying event occurs as indicated above. For example, an employee terminates (allows 18 months of coverage). During these 18 months, the child ceases to be an eligible dependent. That dependent may continue coverage but other family members may not. Also, it may be possible to extend coverage from 18 to 29 months if an employee becomes totally disabled while covered. However, coverage cannot be extended beyond 29 months for employees.

## Notification of Eligibility

One of the most important aspects of the COBRA Act is the requirement that eligible members be informed of their eligibility for COBRA. Many employers have interpreted this to mean that when an employee terminates coverage, usually in the form of employment termination, he or she will be informed of the COBRA rights. However, this procedure addresses only a portion of those actually eligible for continuation of coverage.

Few personnel departments of large employers can maintain adequate monitoring of the mobility of all employees, much less of dependents. Yet this segment of the eligible member base may represent a significant portion of continuation eligibility.

**Figure 3–1** is an example of a document that may be used to enroll the applicant for continuation of coverage. In addition, the employer must provide notification of the availability of COBRA to all employees and their dependents. By early distribution of reference materials, liability for failure to notify affected employees/dependents can be avoided, and the responsibility for timely application would be shifted entirely to the affected employee if (1) dependents become overage, (2) a divorce or separation occurs, or (3) the employee abandons or terminates employment without advance notification. The applicant has 60 days from the date that such coverage is terminated due to a qualifying event in which to submit the application for continuation to the administrator or insurance company, or 60 days from the date the notice of the right to elect COBRA continuation is sent to the employee. Therefore, if the employer/plan fails to send out notification of the election right for two years after the actual event date, the employee would have to be given 60 days from the two year date in which to elect coverage. Mistakes like this can prove to be very costly to a plan.

## Premium Payments

After COBRA has been elected, 45 days are allowed in which to pay the initial premium including all retroactive premiums due since the termination of coverage as a regular employee. If the initial premium and all back premiums are not paid within this time, coverage will remain terminated and COBRA coverage will not become effective.

Normally, a monthly COBRA statement is provided to the employee, which reflects the premium due date for each month and the amount of the monthly premium based on the coverage elected by the applicant. However, the law permits a 30-day grace period from the premium due date. This allows the applicant 30 additional days in which to pay the required premium amount. If the premium is not mailed within the 30-day grace period, coverage will automatically lapse back to the last premium paid date. The amount of the premium can be up to 102% of the premium costs for employees. The 2% is to cover administrative costs. For employees who are eligible for the 29-month extension, the premium can be up to 150% of the employee premium cost for months 19 through 29.

Normally, claims are not paid until the member has paid the premium for the month in which the services were incurred or until the grace period has lapsed. Consequently, if the member consistently pays at the end of the grace period, claim payments may be consistently delayed (again, the incurred date of services will be compared with the paid through date. If the premium for the month in which services were incurred has not been paid, processing will be delayed until the end of the grace period).

Bounced checks or any type of non-paid check may result in lapse of coverage if the check is returned from the bank after the premium due date and a replacement check is not received prior to the end of the grace period. The mailing date of premiums should be strictly monitored with no exceptions. The date of receipt is not important. Judgment of whether or not a payment was received timely is based on the postmark on the envelope. By law, if the payment was mailed within the specified time, it must be accepted as being paid timely.

It is very important that all applicants/members be treated equitably regarding the premium payment policy since deviations may set precedents and extend plan liabilities above acceptable limits.

**ABC Company**
**333 Whata Way**
**Hollywood, CA  91731**

# Continuation of Coverage Request

If you were eligible under your employer's group health insurance plan, you may be eligible to continue your coverage.  In order to apply, this form must be completed and returned to the Administrator's office indicated above within 60 days of the date your eligibility under the group plan terminates.  Within 14 days of our receipt of this request, you will be sent a copy of your Election Rights under the Consolidation Omnibus Reconciliation Act of 1985 (COBRA), Public Act 99-272, Title X.

| EMPLOYEE NAME – LAST | FIRST | FACILITY | ID NO. |
|---|---|---|---|
| | | | |

| COMPLETE HOME ADDRESS | CITY | STATE | ZIP |
|---|---|---|---|
| | | | |

Qualifying Event:  Check off the event and give the event date.
□ Reduction in Work Hours.  Effective: _____
□ Employment Termination (Except due to "gross misconduct"). Last Work Day: _____
□ Dependent Child Attained Maximum Age Defined by Plan. _____
□ Legal Separation and/or Divorce. Date: _____
□ Death of Covered Employee. Date: _____

CONTINUATION OF COVERAGE REQUESTED FOR: (Coverage(s) cannot be added. May be dropped only.)

| □ Employee Only | □ Employee & Dependent(s) | □ Dependent(s) Only |
|---|---|---|
| □ Medical Only | □ Medical Only | □ Medical Only |
| □ Dental + Vision Only | □ Dental + Vision Only | □ Dental + Vision Only |
| □ Medical + Dental + Vision | □ Medical + Dental + Vision | □ Medical + Dental + Vision |

ALL DEPENDENTS MUST BE LISTED BELOW.  LIST THE SOCIAL SECURITY NUMBER OF THE EMPLOYEE'S SPOUSE AND OVER AGE DEPENDENT CHILDREN.

| NAME | ID NO. | BIRTHDATE | RELATIONSHIP |
|---|---|---|---|
| | | | |
| | | | |
| | | | |
| | | | |
| | | | |

Signature of Applicant/Date Signed

■ **Figure 3–1**  Continuation of Coverage Request

## Termination of Coverage

An individual may terminate the continuation of coverage before the completion of the 18-, 29-, or 36-month period. However, if coverage is terminated before the completion of the maximum period, the employer is not required to offer a second election of extension. In other words, once continuation is discontinued, coverage will not be reinstated or restarted.

If any of the following events occurs before the end of the 18-, 29-, or 36-month continuation period, coverage will cease at the end of the month following the date of the occurrence:

- Termination of all of the employer's sponsored group health plans.

- Failure to pay required premium contributions within 30 days of premium due date.

- Becoming covered under another group sponsored health plan, unless the replacement plan exempts coverage for a preexisting condition affecting the member. Under this circumstance, the member may continue COBRA with the COBRA plan covering only those expenses incurred as a result of the preexisting condition. The replacement plan would cover all other expenses.

- Becoming entitled to Medicare coverage.

# On the Job Now

**Directions:** Answer the following questions without looking back at the material just covered. Write your answers in the space provided.

1. To whom does the COBRA Act apply? _____

_____

2. What is a qualified beneficiary? _____

_____

3. What is a qualifying event? _____

_____

4. What is the maximum time in which a dependent can continue COBRA? _____

5. What is the maximum time in which an employee can continue COBRA? _____

6. How long does a member have to apply for COBRA after termination of coverage? _____

_____

# On the Job Now

**Directions:** Read through the XYZ Corporation (Ball Insurance Carriers) contract and possible preexisting conditions (see Appendix A) and list the amounts for the following provisions in the space provided.

1. What is the individual deductible amount? _____

2. What is the dependent eligibility age limit? _____

3. What is the family calendar year deductible? _____

4. What is the individual coinsurance limit? _____

5. What is the coinsurance percentage? _____

6. What is the lifetime maximum amount? _____

7. How many hours must the employee work to be eligible? _____

8. Does the contract include dental coverage? _____

9. What is the family coinsurance limit? _____

10. Is the family coinsurance aggregate or nonaggregate? _____

11. Is there a carryover provision on the individual deductible? _____

12. How many months must the employee work before coverage becomes effective? _____

13. What is the amount of the basic accident benefit? _____

14. What basic benefits does it have? _____

_____

_____

15. What are the terms of the accident benefit? _____

_____

## General Plans and Provisions

There are several provisions which affect most, if not all, insurance plans. These provisions include:

**Acts of third parties and subrogation**—These provisions allow a plan to be reimbursed for medical expenses they have covered that should have been covered by another party.

**Preexisting conditions**—This is how insurance carriers attempt to limit amounts paid on behalf of people who were ill or injured before they obtained insurance. This prevents someone from only getting insurance coverage when they need it to cover a serious illness or injury.

**Mandates**—Some states mandate that certain items, situations, or patients be covered or eligible for coverage within their state.

These common provisions can affect payment on certain claims. It is important that the health claims examiner be aware of these provisions and is able to apply them properly. Without proper application of these provisions, an insurance carrier could have thousands of dollars of benefit payments made on claims that they are not responsible for.

## Practice

# Pitfalls

A claimant is injured while on the premises of a grocery store. The claims for the injuries are submitted to the benefit plan for payment. Subsequently, the claimant seeks recovery from the store. When recovery is successful, the claimant is required to reimburse the benefit plan for its losses.

# Acts of Third Parties

**Acts of Third Parties (ATP)** and **Subrogation** are provisions that are included in many benefit plans to allow for recovery of money paid on claims incurred as a result of a third party's act or acts for which that party is financially responsible.

Subrogation and Acts of Third Parties (ATP) (also known as Third Party Liability [TPL]) have some similarities but are actually different. Many older plans had Subrogation, whereas many new plans have TPL.

State laws affect general plan provisions. Although a plan may contain one of these provisions, it may not always be allowed to function if prohibited by a specific state statute or statutes.

Under **Third Party Liability**, the plan advances money to the injured person with the understanding that, if the claimant is successful in obtaining reimbursement from a third party, the plan will be reimbursed for its losses. The plan's interests lie with the claimant, not with the third party. An example of a third party provision is as follows:

A special provision applies when you or your dependent covered under the plan is injured through the act or omission of another person. When this happens, the plan will advance the benefits under the policy only under the condition that you or your dependents agree in writing to the following:

1. To repay the plan in full for any sums advanced to cover such claims paid by the plan, from the judgment or settlement you or a dependent receives.

2. To provide the plan with a lien to repay the plan to the extent of benefits advanced by the plan. The lien may be filed with the person whose act caused the injuries, his or her agent, the court, or the attorney of the person covered under the plan.

Thus, when such a claim is received, a repayment agreement must be sent to the claimant. This agreement requires the member to provide the in-formation necessary to investigate the claim and subsequently, if appropriate, to file a lien with the member's attorney for reimbursement against any settlement procured by the member. Usually, payment of losses is not made until the claimant has signed the repayment agreement and returned it to the administrator.

A demand by the plan for reimbursement cannot be made until the insured has been compensated for the loss by the third party. Filing a lien against such compensation protects the plan by making it mandatory that the plan be reimbursed before the claimant receives such compensation. Although the loss claimed by the claimant may include medical expenses, property damage, loss of earnings, pain and suffering, and even future medical expenses, the plan is permitted to recover only the amount actually paid out as a result of the injury. A sample of a payment demand is shown in **Figure 3–2**. When any payments are received, they should be noted on a Right of Reimbursement Claims Ledger Sheet. A sample copy of such a ledger sheet is shown in **Figure 3–3**.

When a claim is received for expenses incurred as a result of an injury, determine how, when, and where the injury occurred. If this information is not indicated on the forms submitted, write to the member and request details. Samples of a letter and questionnaire are shown in **Figures 3–4** and **3–5**.

If the injury occurred as the result of another party's acts and the plan has a TPL or subrogation provision, a letter informing the claimant regarding the appropriate provision should be sent along with an agreement. A sample copy of such letter is shown in **Figure 3–6**. The claimant must sign the agreement indicating that if monies are received from another source to cover these expenses, he or she is legally obligated to reimburse the plan. A sample copy of the agreement is shown in **Figure 3–7**. This signed agreement is then kept on file with occasional follow-ups to track recovery; some payers file a lien against monies that the claimant might be entitled to. If the plan does not have either of these types of provisions, reimbursement from a third source cannot be sought.

As a rule, these provisions cannot be used to recover against the member's own auto liability carrier or homeowner's insurance carrier.

Administration of this provision tends to be long-term and time-intensive. Therefore, many plans retain special agencies to help track and recover TPL monies. In exchange, the agency is paid from the proceeds that they recover.

**ANY INSURANCE CARRIER, INC.**
123 Any Drive, Anywhere, USA 12345 ● (800) 555-1234

Date:

Policyholder: _____

Control: _____

Employee: _____

Dependent: _____

Dear

This is to advise you that benefits totaling _____ have been paid to date to

_____ as a result of the accident on

_____.

Under the terms of _____ group health coverage, the insurance carrier is entitled to claim reimbursement from any third party liability coverage applicable to the same accident. Therefore, subrogation rights are claimed. Please advise as soon as possible when we might expect payment.

Sincerely,

Any Insurance Carrier

■ **Figure 3–2** Sample of a Payment Demand Letter

**ANY INSURANCE CARRIER, INC.**
**123 Any Drive, Anywhere, USA 12345 ● (800) 555-1234**

## For Right of Reimbursement Claims

Claimant: _____    Policyholder: _____

Attorney: _____

Date of Accident: _____    Control No.: _____

Description of Condition/Diagnosis: _____

| Type of Transaction | Payee/Receiver | Date | By | Amount of Payment | Total Paid to Date |
|---|---|---|---|---|---|
| | | | | | |
| | | | | | |
| | | | | | |
| | | | | | |
| | | | | | |
| | | | | | |
| | | | | | |
| | | | | | |
| | | | | | |
| | | | | | |
| | | | | | |
| | | | | | |
| | | | | | |
| | | | | | |
| | | | | | |
| | | | | | |
| | | | | | |
| | | | | | |
| | | | | | |
| | | | | | |
| | | | | | |
| | | | | | |
| | | | | | |
| | | | | | |
| | | | | | |
| | | | | | |

■ **Figure 3–3** Right of Reimbursement Claims Ledger Sheet

**ANY INSURANCE CARRIER, INC.**
123 Any Drive, Anywhere, USA 12345 • (800) 555-1234

Insured's I.D. No. _____

Re: _____

Dear _____

The claim that you recently submitted for accidental bodily injuries expenses is under review. Circumstances of the accident indicate that a third party may be liable for the payment of your medical or dental bills.

Accordingly, the policy in force between _____ and _____ contains a Third Party Liability exclusion, which provides that no medical or dental benefits are payable for injuries or illness caused by a third party if payment for such expenses has been or will be received from the third party or insurer. A copy of the entire provision is attached.

To assist us in evaluating the claim, please complete the enclosed questionnaire detailing particulars regarding the accident and parties involved. Any additional information would be greatly appreciated.

Additionally, if a third party is liable for your expenses, we have enclosed a Third Party Liability Reimbursement Agreement, to be signed, witnessed, and returned to us before benefits can be released.

If you have any questions regarding this matter, please do not hesitate to contact me.

Sincerely,

**■ Figure 3–4** Sample of a letter requesting further information on a possible TPL claim

---

**ANY INSURANCE CARRIER, INC.**
123 Any Drive, Anywhere, USA 12345 • (800) 555-1234

**TPL INVESTIGATION QUESTIONNAIRE**

1. Name and address of responsible third party.

   _____

   _____

   City _____ State _____ Zip Code _____

2. Name and address of responsible third party's insurance company and policy number.

   _____

   _____

   City _____ State _____ Zip Code _____

3. If an accident, what were the circumstances?

   _____

   _____

   _____

   _____

4. If Any Insurance Carrier, Inc. is to pay medical benefits under the terms of the contract, when is settlement expected or how often may we expect status reports?

   _____

   _____

   _____

5. Is legal counsel involved? If yes, please give name and address.

   _____

   _____

   City _____ State _____ Zip Code _____

**■ Figure 3–5** Sample of a TPL questionnaire

**ANY INSURANCE CARRIER, INC.**
123 Any Drive, Anywhere, USA 12345 • (800) 555-1234

Third Party Liability Exclusion Rider Effective
Attached to and made part of Group Insurance Policy No. _____
Issued by _____

to _____

No benefits will be paid under this policy to or on behalf of an insured individual who has:

1.  medical or dental charges, or
2.  loss of earnings

if the insured individual has received payment, in whole or in part, from a third party, or its insurer, for past or future medical or dental charges or loss of earnings as the result of negligence or intentional acts of a third party.

If an insured party makes a claim to Any Insurance Carrier for medical, dental, or loss of earnings benefits under this policy prior to receiving payment from a third party, or its insurer, the insured individual (or legal representative of a minor or incompetent) must agree in writing to repay Any Insurance Carrier from any amount of money received by the insured individual from the third party, or its insurer. The repayment will be to the extent of the benefits paid by Any Insurance Carrier. However, the reasonable pro rata expenses, such as lawyer's fees and court costs, incurred in affecting the third party payment may be deducted from the repayment to Any Insurance Carrier.

The repayment agreement will be binding upon the insured individual (or legal representative of a minor or incompetent) whether:

1.  The payment received from the third party, or its insurer, is the result of:
    a.  a legal judgment, or
    b.  an arbitration award, or
    c.  a compromise settlement, or
    d.  any other arrangement, or
2.  The third party, or its insurer, has admitted liability for the payment, or
3.  The medical or dental charges or loss of earnings are itemized in the third party payment.

**Figure 3–6** Sample of a Third Party Liability Exclusion Rider

**ANY INSURANCE CARRIER, INC.**
123 Any Drive, Anywhere, USA 12345 • (800) 555-1234

**Third Party Liability Reimbursement Agreement**

I, _____, an insured individual (or his or her legal representative) under group insurance policy number _____ issued by Any Insurance Carrier, Inc. to _____, the policyholder, pursuant to the terms of the group insurance policy, do hereby agree to reimburse Any Insurance Carrier for any medical or dental expenses or loss of earnings benefits which are paid by Any Insurance Carrier or will be paid by it, which expenses or benefits arise out of the accident or sickness commencing _____, 20___, if payment is received from a third party, or its insurer.

I understand that this agreement to reimburse shall be binding on me regardless of whether:

1.  the payment received from the third party, or its insurer, is the result of a legal judgment, arbitration award, compromise settlement or otherwise; or,
2.  such third party, or its insurer, has admitted liability in connection with such payment; or,
3.  such medical or dental expenses actually incurred or loss of earnings realized are itemized in such third party payment.

I further understand that the reasonable pro rata costs, including attorney fees, actually incurred by me in effecting the third party payment for such medical or dental expenses or loss of earnings may be deducted from any such reimbursement.

_____
(Witness)

_____
(Insured Individual or his or her Legal Representative)

**Figure 3–7** Third Party Liability Reimbursement Agreement

# Completion of the Right of Reimbursement Claims Ledger Sheet

The information on this sheet must be written or typed in a legible manner. This sheet is used to track all payments made on this case, and all correspondence sent or received regarding the case.

This form is often created on letterhead so that a copy of this form may be attached to any liens filed with the claimant's attorney. This ledger then becomes a statement of the amount due on the case, as of the date it is sent.

The fields on the Right of Reimbursement Claims Ledger Sheet are to be filled in as follows:

**Claimant:** Enter the name of the claimant (patient).

**Policyholder:** Enter the name of the policyholder or insured.

**Attorney:** Enter the name, address, and phone number of the attorney who is representing the claimant.

**Date of Accident:** Enter the date of the accident. If this claim is pertaining to an illness (i.e., an illness which may be covered under worker's compensation), enter the date the patient was diagnosed with this condition.

**Control No.:** Enter the control number assigned to this case. Each case will be assigned a control number to aid in tracking the case and all claims payments associated with it.

**Description of Condition/Diagnosis:** Enter the conditions or diagnoses associated with this situation. All conditions and diagnoses related to the accident or illness should be entered together on one sheet.

**Type of Transaction:** Enter the type of the transactions which occurred. This could be a claim which was processed, an agreement letter sent, a lien notice sent, correspondence sent, or any other transaction that occurred for this case.

**Payee/Receiver:** Enter the name of the person or facility that received payment on the claim. If the transaction was a letter or other item sent through the mail, enter the name of the person the item was sent to.

**Date:** Enter the date the item (check or other item) was sent out.

**By:** Enter the name of the person who sent the item or who processed the claim.

**Amount of Payment:** Enter the amount of the payment that was made on this claim. If the item is not a claim and no value is assessed (i.e., a lien notice sent or agreement sent), enter N/A for Not Applicable.

**Total Paid to Date:** Add the amount paid with this transaction to the remaining balance (prior line of this column). This amount will show the total amount that the carrier should be reimbursed for claims paid out on this TPL case.

**Payments Received**

If a payment is received by the insurance carrier for repayment of part or all of the case, this should also be recorded on the ledger sheet. In this case the following information would be entered:

**Type of Transaction:** Enter "Payment Received."

**Payee/Receiver:** Enter the name of the insurance carrier, and the name of the party the payment is from (i.e., Any Ins. Car. from Client's Attorney).

**Date:** Enter the date the payment was received.

**By:** Enter the name of the contact person or the person who sent the payment.

**Amount of payment:** Enter the amount of the payment.

**Total Paid to Date:** Subtract any payment amounts from the total amount shown on the previous line. This will allow you to always see the total amount due for this case on the last line.

# Subrogation

Under **subrogation**, the insurance carrier has an obligation to pay a benefit under the contract, but has a subrogated right for a portion of the recovery that the claimant may obtain from a third party. The insurance carrier has a direct interest with the third party. An example of a subrogation provision is as follows:

When benefits are paid to or for you or a dependent under the terms of the plan, the plan shall be subrogate, unless otherwise prohibited by law, to your right of recovery or the rights of recovery of a dependent against any person who might acknowledge to be liable or might be found legally liable by a court of competent jurisdiction for the injury that necessitated the hospitalization or the medical or surgical treatment for which the benefits were paid.

Such subrogation rights shall extend only to the recovery by the insurance carrier of the benefits it has paid for such treatment, and the insurance carrier shall pay fees and costs associated with such recovery.

When a claim is received for expenses incurred as a result of any injury involving another party, a subrogation letter along with a subrogation statement should be sent to the claimant.

The subrogation statement requires the member to provide information necessary to investigate the claim. The form also requires the member to agree to allow the plan to file a lien against any settlement made by another party.

Although technically these two provisions are not the same, from the health claims examiner's standpoint, the differences are moot. Do not be concerned with what the differences are at this point. Be concerned with the concepts behind them, what the objective is, and how to obtain that objective.

# On the Job Now

**Directions:** Answer the following questions without looking back at the material just covered. Write your answers in the space provided.

1. Why are Acts of Third Parties and Subrogation provisions included in many benefit plans? _____

_____

2. Under _____, the plan advances money to the injured person with the understanding that if the claimant is successful in obtaining reimbursement monies from a third party, the plan will be reimbursed.

3. Under _____, the plan has an obligation to pay a benefit under the contract, but a subrogated right for a portion of the recovery that the claimant may obtain from a third party.

## Preexisting Conditions

A **preexisting condition** is a condition that the claimant was treated for within a specified time period before the claimant became covered under the plan. This provision must be reviewed carefully because there are many variations. For example, it may apply to dependents only; time limits may be different for members versus dependents; or, the provision may be waived for all individuals who are covered on the effective date of the plan. See **Appendix C** for a list of possible preexisting conditions.

Whether the expense or expenses incurred are excluded completely or limited to a specific dollar benefit, most clauses provide that benefits will become payable after the member has been covered under the plan for a specific period of time and has not received any treatment for the preexisting condition.

### Handling Procedures

Improperly handled claims for preexisting conditions are a frequent source of complaints and lawsuits. An examiner has an obligation to:

1. Investigate thoroughly, at the earliest appropriate time, preferably on the very first claim receipt. If the expenses result from an injury incurred after the effective date of the plan or are not chronic, such as a cold or flu, an inquiry should not be made. Always consider the specific plan provisions.

2. Notify the member and the provider, if appropriate, of the delay, in writing.

3. Bring the investigation to a conclusion as rapidly as possible with either a decision to pay or a fully documented denial.

### Treatment-Free Provisions

To qualify for payment on the basis of having satisfied the treatment-free provision and the total limitation (no payment of preexisting conditions for 12 months), it must be determined that the patient did not receive any treatment for the preexisting condition from a doctor, hospital, clinic, or other medical practitioner. Advice from a practitioner without treatment may be considered "treatment" in the case of a preexisting condition. To determine whether a given condition is preexisting, the following procedures should be followed:

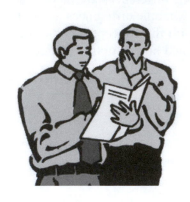

Examiner:    I'm trying to process this claim, but the doctor abbreviated the patient's condition and I can't figure out what FDSTW means.

Boss:    Found dead, stayed that way.

1. Identify all potential preexisting conditions by noting the diagnosis and the length of time between the effective date of the plan and the first treatment documented on the claim form or in the claim file. Special attention should be paid to claims for chronic conditions or for major surgery with little or no preliminary diagnostic work or medical treatment.

2. Initiate the investigation as soon as appropriate by writing to the attending physician and all other consulting or referring physicians whose names can be determined. **Figure 3–8** Shows an example of a letter used to obtain additional information regarding a possible preexisting condition. Write to the following sources as well:

- All hospitals involved and request a copy of hospital records including the admitting history and physical, discharge summary, consultation, and operative reports.
- Pharmacies to obtain drug names, dates filled, and names and phone numbers of prescribing physicians.

- Attending physicians to request copies of treatment histories that should detail the onset of the condition, referring physicians, and other pertinent information.
- Claimants to request the names, addresses, and phone numbers of all doctors seen and all medications taken during the appropriate time period stipulated in the plan.

Many insurance carriers have a standard form letter for requesting information regarding a pre-existing condition.

3. Act immediately on leads or additional information supplied in response to the initial requests for information.

4. Bear in mind that the burden of proof lies with the plan to prove that a condition is preexisting. No matter how certain you may be that a condition is preexisting, a claim cannot be denied as such unless there is adequate documentation in the claim file.

5. If answers to the inquiries are not received, follow the administrator's guidelines for denying the claim. Do not deny the claim as preexisting. Instead, deny pending receipt of previously requested information.

6. Determining whether a condition is a chronic illness or a new illness is essential in deciding whether the preexisting exclusion would apply. For example, infectious conditions such as upper respiratory infection, otitis media, bronchitis, and urinary tract infection may occur repeatedly with resolution between episodes. If a period elapses between treatments, a new episode (and therefore, a new illness) may exist, in which the preexisting exclusion would not apply.

7. Related conditions and complications of existing conditions may pose problems in determining whether an illness is preexisting. Certain diseases are progressive, and a different diagnosis may be assigned to the successive stages of the disease. *The Merck Manual* may be helpful in researching such conditions, but any questionable case should be referred to the supervisor, medical review department, or a consultant for review.

Refer to the ABC contract in Appendix A. According to this plan, if the claimant was effective when the plan became effective 06/01/2002, the preexisting exclusion will not apply to that person. If the claimant was not effective on the plan effective date of 06/01/2002, the exclusion would apply.

**Any Insurance Carrier, INC.**
**123 Any Drive**
**Anywhere, USA 12345**
**(800) 555-1234**

Re:

Control: _____

Insured: _____

Dear

We are presently processing a claim for the above patient. In order to give it full consideration, we need additional information. Please answer the questions outlined below. A pre-addressed envelope is provided for your convenience. Your cooperation will be appreciated and will help expedite the matter for your patient. (Authorization to release information is attached.)

Sincerely yours,

Claims Representative

Condition(s) described on claim form as: _____

_____

_____

1. Did you prescribe medication for, or treat the above condition or related symptoms from _____ through _____ ? ☐ Yes ☐ No  If so, specify below:

| Condition | Date Treated |
|-----------|--------------|
| _____ | _____ |
| _____ | _____ |
| _____ | _____ |

2. Drug                    Date Prescribed        Drug                    Date Prescribed

| | | | |
|---|---|---|---|
| _____ | | _____ | |
| _____ | | _____ | |
| _____ | | _____ | |

3. Was the patient referred to you by another physician? ☐ Yes ☐ No If so, please provide name and address of referring doctor. _____

Dated _____    Signed _____

■ **Figure 3–8** Preexisting Condition Form

Once the claimant has been covered under the plan for 12 consecutive months, the preexisting exclusion no longer applies whether or not the condition was preexisting.

On a plan that includes a specific money limit for preexisting conditions, it is not necessary to pend the claims and request information. However, the allowable amounts that have been paid under the plan must be tracked so that once the specified limit has been reached for each condition, the preexisting inquiry can be initiated.

Properly applying preexisting limitations takes experience. Remember what is being investigated and what the plan provisions allow or do not allow. Also, request assistance at the beginning of the process until you are familiar with the application of the various provisions. In doing so, you will not delay the claim unnecessarily.

# Practice Pitfalls

Claimant is covered under the ABC Corporation contract, and is effective 07/01/CCYY. A claim is received for a diagnosis of diabetes for the date of service 08/01/CCYY. Diabetes is a chronic condition; therefore, it may be preexisting. An investigation must be pursued in a manner previously indicated so that the claim file can be properly documented to substantiate the claims decision. Let's examine the claim form. Does it list the following: The date of the first treatment of the condition? Was the treatment before the effective date? If so, the condition is possibly preexisting because persons with some diabetic conditions require insulin injections or pills on a daily basis.

If not, is there a name of a referring physician? If so, write to that physician and request treatment information. If the first treatment date is not indicated, write to the physician who submitted the claim and to the claimant, requesting the following information:

- The names of all physicians seen between 04/01/CCYY and 08/01/CCYY (this covers the 90-day period prior to the effective date of coverage, up to and including the current treatment date).

- The names and dates of all prescriptions written during this same period of time.

- The names of all other medical providers referred to or from and the dates of treatments during this period of time.

The objective of this questioning is two-fold as follows:

1. To determine whether treatment commenced during the 90-day period of time before the effective date.

2. To determine whether a three-month period of time has occurred in which the claimant did not receive treatment (determine whether the three-month treatment-free period provision applies).

## HIPAA and Health Insurance Portability

In 1996, a new law regarding health insurance was signed by President William Clinton. This law is called the Health Insurance Portability and Accounting Act of 1996 (HIPAA). The most important changes include preexisting limitations, prior coverage certification, and privacy issues. Here we will discuss preexisting limitations and prior coverage certification.

This law has a direct impact on insurers, unlike other health care legislation which primarily impacts the employer.

HIPAA restricts the circumstances and the period for which a group health plan may exclude coverage for a preexisting condition. The restriction has five parts:

1. A group health plan may not impose a preexisting condition limit unless the plan provides prior notice to the member of the existence and terms of the preexisting condition exclusion.

2. A group health plan may not impose a preexisting condition exclusion unless the member received treatment or advice from a state-licensed medical practitioner for the condition within the six-month period preceding the date of enrollment under the group health plan.

3. The group health plan must credit an individual's prior health coverage toward satisfaction of the preexisting condition limit unless that coverage was solely for excepted benefits, commonly called riders or waivers.

4. The maximum period allowed for a preexisting condition exclusion is generally 12 months (18 months in the case of an individual who does not enroll when first eligible).

5. The group health plan may not impose any preexisting condition exclusions for pregnancy or for a newborn or newly adopted child enrolled within 30 days.

## Prior Notification

Unless the insurer gives the insured prior information regarding preexisting limitations, they may not impose them. Most insurance carriers include preexisting clauses in their contracts. Placing the information within the contract satisfies the requirement of prior notification.

## Preexisting Requirements

HIPAA limits the preexisting period (also called the look back time) in determining whether a condition is preexisting to six months. A preexisting provision generally applies to medical advice, diagnosis, care, or treatment that is either recommended or received for a condition. The look back period is the six-month period prior to the enrollment date in any new health plan. Some states use the prudent person standard in determining a preexisting condition. This means that a condition is preexisting if a prudent person would have sought care or treatment. HIPAA rejects this standard. Therefore, a condition is only preexisting if advice or care is actually sought.

# On the Job Now

**Directions:** Indicate whether or not the following situations would warrant a preexisting investigation and why.

1. Thomas is covered under the ABC Corporation plan. His effective date of coverage is 1/1/CCYY. He received treatment for chronic allergies on 12/15/CCPY, and a claim was received for services rendered on 1/25/CCYY.

   _____

2. Gerald is covered under the Ninja Enterprises plan. His effective date of coverage is 7/4/CCPY. He received treatment for a finger laceration on 4/23/CCYY.

   _____

3. Adam is covered under the XYZ Corporation plan. His effective date of coverage is 4/14/CCYY. He received treatment for leukemia on 3/15/CCYY, and a claim was received for this same diagnosis for services rendered on 5/15/CCYY.

   _____

4. Alyse is covered under the Ninja Enterprises plan. Her effective date of coverage is 11/1/CCYY. She received treatment for diabetes on 12/1/CCYY, and a claim was received for these services.

   _____

5. Sebastian is covered under the ABC Corporation plan. His effective date of coverage is 2/15/CCYY. A claim with a diagnosis of hypertension is received with a date of service of 2/20/CCYY.

   _____

## Credit for Prior Coverage

HIPAA also states that an employee may be given credit for the period of time he was covered by his former employer, provided the coverage is considered "credible." Therefore, if an employee only had medical coverage with his former employer, the employee would be given credit for prior medical coverage, but preexisting exclusions could be applied to dental, vision, and other services.

**Credible coverage** does not take into consideration the benefits of the old and new plan, but only that the former plan was medical and the new plan is medical coverage. A new insurance carrier may choose to enact the preexisting limitations on certain items that were not included in previous medical coverage. This allowance is limited to coverage for mental health, substance abuse treatment, prescriptions, dental care, and vision care. For example, if a participant's old plan did not include coverage for mental health benefits, then the new plan may elect to enact a preexisting limit on the mental health benefits that it normally offers in the plan.

Under the new law, preexisting exclusions are limited to a six-month look back period, and credit must be given for prior coverage. Therefore, if a person is covered by insurance, and transfers insurance coverage to a new company prior to 63 days of ceasing coverage at the old company, the new insurance carrier may not apply preexisting limitations to treatment. If there was a break of 63 days or more between termination of the old coverage and the available date of new coverage, preexisting exclusions are limited to six months.

If a person declines coverage under a new plan because they are covered under a previously existing plan, and then they lose their benefits under the old plan, they can enroll under a new plan without preexisting limitations. No preexisting limitation may be applied to those who transfer from one plan to another during a company's open-enrollment period.

Employees are no longer allowed to continue COBRA coverage on a policy if they are covered under a new policy. In the past, many employees would continue coverage on an old policy until the preexisting limitation had been satisfied on the new insurance. Since the new insurance is no longer allowed to apply preexisting limitations, the need for this coverage has been eliminated. Many people may still elect to continue coverage on the old policy until they have satisfied any length of employment (i.e., must be employed for 90 days) requirements. However, the waiting period is not considered a break in coverage for purposes of the 63-day break in coverage. Therefore, if an employee terminates at one company (and ceases coverage), and

is hired at a second company within 63 days, they are considered continuously covered even if they must satisfy a 90-day waiting period before coverage begins with their new employer.

Employers are not allowed to discriminate against those with higher medical costs in their hiring practices. This is true even though the higher costs will eventually show an increase in the company's insurance premiums. An **insurance premium** is the amount of money required for coverage under a specific insurance policy for a given period of time. Depending on the policy agreement, the premium may be paid monthly, quarterly, semiannually, or annually.

An employee leaving his employer should obtain a certificate of credible coverage which states that the employee was covered, what type of plan it was (dental only, medical etc.), and for how long. This certificate of credible coverage is then applied to the new carrier's preexisting conditions clause.

Companies are also now required to provide written certification of all prior coverage. They must provide this information upon termination of coverage, and for up to 24 months after termination if the employee requests it. Certificates must include:

- The date the certificate is issued.
- The name of the group health plan that provided the coverage described in the certificate.
- The name of the participant or dependent covered and identifying information on them (i.e., social security number, identification number, etc.).
- A telephone number to call for further information regarding the certificate.
- Either:
  a. A statement that the individual has had at least 18 months of creditable coverage, or
  b. The beginning date for any creditable coverage (and any waiting period).
- The ending date of coverage, or (in cases of COBRA) a statement that the participant or dependent is continuing coverage as of the date the certificate was issued.

If the information for a participant and their dependents is identical, one certificate may be issued, provided all persons are properly named and identified on the certificate. If information is different for each individual (i.e., beginning and ending dates of coverage), then a plan administrator may either issue a separate certificate for each person, or the information for each person may be detailed on one certificate.

## Practice
# Pitfalls

A new employee with ABC Company was hired on 2/1/CCYY and has a three-month waiting period. The employee signs up in a timely manner and is covered effective 5/1/CCYY. He has been continuously taking medication for hypertension for the past two years. The employee was covered by his prior medical plan for a period of six months; from 8/1/CCPY through 1/31/CCYY. He has a certificate of credible coverage from the prior carrier. His diagnosis of hypertension is considered preexisting by the new carrier. The 12-month exclusion period under the ABC Company plan, begins on 2/1/CCYY. Because the employee has credible coverage, the new carrier must give the employee credit for the six months he was covered under the prior plan. Therefore, the hypertension is only excluded for a period of six months; or until 8/1/CCYY.

## Practice
# Pitfalls

A new employee with ABC Company was hired on 2/1/CCYY and has a three-month waiting period. The employee signs up in a timely manner and is covered effective 5/1/CCYY. He has been continuously taking medication for hypertension for the past two years. The employee was covered by his prior medical plan for a period of 36 months. He has a certificate of credible coverage from the prior carrier. His diagnosis of hypertension is considered preexisting by the new carrier. The 12-month exclusion period under the ABC Company plan begins on 2/1/CCYY. The employee was covered by his prior medical plan for a period of 36 months and has a certificate of credible coverage. Because there is a certificate of credible coverage for 36 months, the preexisting exclusion period does not apply.

### Maximum Periods

For those who do not satisfy the continuous coverage requirements, preexisting exclusions are limited to conditions for which treatment was received within six months prior to coverage. Exclusions are only allowed to remain in effect for 12 months. Therefore, after 12 months the carrier must cover the condition, whether it was preexisting or not. If a person did not enroll when they first became eligible, then preexisting exclusions are allowed to continue for 18 months. This is because some people will not apply for coverage until they have a condition that they know is going to require extensive treatment. They will then attempt to get coverage for that condition.

HIPAA also states that if a preexisting condition exists, the 12-month period for imposing the preexisting exclusion is measured from the employee's enrollment date. The enrollment date is defined as the earlier of; 1) the date of coverage in the plan, or 2) the first day of the waiting period before the coverage begins (usually the employment date). The waiting period rule does not apply when the enrollee is a late enrollee.

## Practice
# Pitfalls

A new employee with ABC Company, was hired on 2/1/CCYY, and has a three-month waiting period before signing up for coverage. The employee signs up in a timely manner and is covered for benefits on 5/1/CCYY. The employee takes medication for hypertension, which is considered a preexisting condition. The plan's 12-month coverage exclusion for a preexisting condition begins on 2/1/CCYY because that is the earliest date of enrollment under HIPAA.

## Practice
# Pitfalls

A new employee with ABC Company, hired on 2/1/CCYY, has a three-month waiting period before signing up for coverage. The employee does not sign up right away and so does not become covered until 7/15/CCYY. The employee takes medication for hypertension, which is considered a preexisting condition. HIPAA states that the late enrollee does not get the benefit of his waiting period; therefore, the 12-month preexisting exclusion period begins on the actual effective date of coverage, in this case 7/15/CCYY.

Note should be taken if an employer requires a physical examination as a condition of employment and that examination is done **after** the date of employment. Any condition first identified during that examination cannot be applied to the preexisting condition exclusion clause. However, if the physical examination takes place **prior** to the employment date and the condition is first identified at that time, the preexisting condition exclusion clause can apply.

### Pregnancies, Newborns, and Adopted Children Under 18 Excluded

Preexisting limits are not allowed for pregnancy, newborns, or adopted children under 18 years of age. Therefore, if a woman transfers coverage while she is pregnant, the new insurance carrier must cover the costs associated with the pregnancy. Also, a preexisting condition exclusion cannot be applied to a newborn or adopted child under age 18 as long as the child became covered under the health plan within 30 days of birth or adoption.

HIPAA does much to reduce the burden placed on employees due to a preexisting condition. It does not eliminate the right of a carrier to investigate and impose the preexisting clause when applicable. This legislation is complex and all questions should be directed to your supervisor.

A good understanding of the preexisting condition clause in a plan is essential for applying the rules under HIPAA.

# On the Job Now

**Directions:**  Read each scenario below and determine whether or not the certificate of prior insurance should be checked and why or why not.

1. Jennifer received treatment for a chronic ulcer on 7/1/CCYY and again on 8/1/CCYY. On 10/01/CCYY she quit her old job and began working for a new employer two weeks later, on 10/15/CCYY. She immediately signed up for insurance and her coverage became effective after a 30-day waiting period, on 11/15/CCYY. On 1/15/CCNY, she was seen by the doctor for additional treatment for chronic ulcer. Do you need a copy of her coverage certificate with the 1/15/CCNY claim?

   _____

   _____

2. Mary received treatment for diabetes on 7/1/CCYY and again on 8/1/CCYY. On 10/1/CCYY she quit her old job and began working for a new employer two weeks later, on 10/15/CCYY. She immediately signed up for insurance and her coverage became effective after a 90-day waiting period, on 1/15/CCNY. On 10/15/CCNY, she was seen by the doctor for additional diabetes treatment. Do you need a copy of her coverage certificate with the 10/15/CCNY claim?

   _____

   _____

3. Tom received treatment for kidney disease on 2/1/CCYY and again on 3/1/CCYY. On 10/1/CCYY he quit his old job and began working for a new employer two weeks later, on 10/15/CCYY. He immediately signed up for insurance and his coverage became effective after a 30-day waiting period, on 11/15/CCYY. On 12/15/CCYY, he was seen by the doctor for additional treatment for kidney disease. Do you need a copy of his coverage certificate with the 12/15/CCYY claim?

   _____

   _____

4. Betty received a routine visit for pregnancy on 7/1/CCYY and again on 8/1/CCYY. On 10/1/CCYY she began working for a new employer. She immediately signed up for insurance and her coverage became effective after a 30-day waiting period, on 11/1/CCYY. She did not have prior coverage. On 1/15/CCNY, she was seen by the doctor for an additional routine visit. Do you need a copy of her coverage certificate for the 1/15/CCNY claim?

_____

_____

5. Jesse received treatment for anorexia on 7/1/CCYY and again on 8/1/CCYY. On 10/16/CCYY she quit her old job and chose not to continue coverage under COBRA rules. On 12/15/CCYY she began working for a new employer. She immediately signed up for insurance and her coverage became effective after a 30-day waiting period, on 1/15/CCNY. On 1/25/CCNY, she was seen by the doctor for treatment of diabetes. Do you need a copy of her coverage certificate with the 1/25/CCNY claim?

_____

_____

# Mental Health Parity Act

In 1996 the Federal Government passed the Mental Health Parity Act. This act states that group insurance plans for employers with more than 50 employees must provide parity (an equal amount of coverage) between the benefits for mental health treatments and for medical/surgical treatments. Thus, if the lifetime maximum for medical/surgical benefits is $1,000,000, then the lifetime maximum for mental health benefits must also be $1,000,000.

The law also states that plans that do not have a calendar year maximum on medical/surgical benefits may not impose such a maximum on mental health benefits.

However, plans are allowed to increase the amount of coinsurance required for mental health benefits, increase the copayment amounts for mental health benefits, or to limit the number of visits allowed per year.

Some states have increased provisions to these laws (i.e., requiring mental health parity by employers with 20 or more employees).

# Mandates

**Mandates** are laws enacted by states that require insurance carriers to cover certain services or dependents, or services provided by certain providers.

Mandates generally take one of two forms:

1. The insurance carrier is required to provide the coverage as part of all plans offered by the carrier, or

2. The insurance carrier within the state must offer the benefit. However, it is not required to be part of a standard policy.

The second requirement is satisfied if the insurance carrier offers a second policy (often with a higher premium) which includes the benefit. Employers are not required to purchase them for employees. Since most insurance coverage is offered as a benefit of employment, most employers will opt for the lower priced coverage that does not include the benefit. For that reason, many people with health insurance coverage provided through their employer often are not covered by the benefit. Individuals who buy an individual insurance plan may choose to have these options included or not.

There are over 1,000 mandates on the books as of this writing. However, special interest groups are constantly submitting bills to state legislatures requesting additional coverage. Each insurance carrier is required to obtain a copy of the mandates in any states they sell coverage in. Regardless of where the insurance carrier is located, if the policy is sold and coverage is offered in a state, then that state's mandates apply to the coverage offered in that state.

Some limitations may apply to these benefits (i.e., they apply to group insurance only). For more complete and current information for a state, contact that state's Department of Insurance.

## Benefits

1. Required Benefits. These benefits must automatically be included in the contract.

2. Benefits required to be offered.

**Figure 3–9** is an example of a list of state mandates regarding health insurance benefits.

**Alcoholism treatment: (1)** AK, CT, DC, HI, IL, KS, MD, MA, MI, MN, MS, MO, MT, NE, NV, NJ, NY, ND, OH, OR, PA, RI, TX, VT, WA, WV, WI. **(2)** AL, AR, CA, CO, FL, GA, KY, LA, ME, NM, NC, SC, SD, TN, UT, VA, WY.

**Alzheimer's treatment: (2)** MD.

**Ambulance transportation: (1)** CT, FL, LA, MS, OK.

**Ambulatory care: (2)** NY.

**Ambulatory surgery: (1)** AZ, AR, FL, HI, KY, MN, OK.

**Autism: (1)** IN.

**Blood lead screening: (1)** MA, NJ, RI. **(2)** CA

**Bone mass measurement: (1)** KS, MD, NC, OK, TN, TX. **(2)** GA, KY.

**Bone marrow transplants: (1)** FL, KY, MA, MN, NH. **(2)** GA, NJ, TN, VA.

**Blood products: (1)** MD.

**Breast reconstruction: (1)** AL, AK, AZ, AR, CA, CO, CT, DC, GA, HI, ID, IL, IN, IA, KS, KY, LA, ME, MD, MO, MI, MN, MS, MT, NE, NV, NH, NJ, NM, NY, NC, ND, OH, OK, OR, PA, RI, SC, SD, TN, TX, UT, VT, VA, WA, WV, WI, WY. **(2)** FL.

**Cancer hormone treatment: (1)** PA.

**Cancer pain drugs: (1)** VA.

**Cardiac rehabilitation: (1)** ME, MA.

**Cervical cancer screening (Pap smear): (1)** AK, CA, CT, DE, DC, GA, IL, LA, ME, MA, MN, MO, NM, NV, NJ, NY, NC, OH, OR, RI, PA, SC, VT, VA, WY. **(2)** TN.

**Chemotherapy: (1)** PA, TN. **(2)** MO.

**Childhood immunizations: (1)** DE, MO, NJ, OK, PA, TX, WI.

**Chiropractic care: (1)** ME, NY, ND, VT. **(2)** SC.

**Chlamydia screening: (1)** MD. **(2)** TN.

**Cleft palate: (1)** CO, FL, ID, IN, LA, MD, MN, NC, SC.

**Clinical trials: (1)** CA, CT, DE, GA, LA, MD, NH, NC, RI, VT, VA. **(2)** IL.

**Colorectal cancer screening: (1)** CT, DE, MD, MO, NC, OK, WY.

**Complications of pregnancy: (1)** CA, CO, NV, NC, ND.

**Congenital bleeding disorders: (1)** NJ, VA.

**Contraceptives: (1)** AZ, CA, CT, DE, GA, HI, IA, ME, MD, MO, NV, NH, NM, NC, TX, VT, VA, WA.

**Dental anesthesia: (1)** CA, CO, ST, FL, GA, IN, KS, LA, MD, MN, MO, NE, NH, NJ, NC, ND, OK, SD, WI.

**Dental, vision, hearing: (2)** AK.

**Dermatological care: (1)** SC.

**Diabetic supplies and education: (1)** AK, AZ, AR, CA, CO, CT, DE, FL, HI, IL, IA, IN, KS, KY, LA, ME, MD, MI, MN, NV, NE, NH, NJ, NM, NY, NC, OK, OR, PA, RI, SC, SD, TN, TX, UT, VT, WV, WI, WY. **(2)** GA, MS, MO.

**Drug abuse treatment: (1)** AL, AK, CT, DC, HI, KS, ME, MD, MI, MN, MT, NV, NY, ND, OR, PA, RI, TX, VT, WA, WI. **(2)** AR, CA, FL, GA, LA, MO, NC, SC, TN, UT, VA.

**Elimination of port-wine stains: (1)** MN.

**Emergency services: (1)** AZ, AR, CA, CO, CT, DE, DC, FL, GA, HI, ID, IN, IA, KS, KY, LA, MD, MI, NE, NV, NH, NJ, NM, NY, NC, ND, OH, OK, OR, PA, SC, TN, TX, UT, VT, VA, WA, WV, WI.

**Enteral formulas: (1)** MA, NY.

■ **Figure 3–9** State Mandated Health Insurance Benefits

| | |
|---|---|
| **Gynecological exams:** (1) DE, KS, PA, SC. | **Metabolic formula:** (1) ME. |
| **Hair prosthesis:** (1) MD, MA, MN, NH, OK. | **Midwife services:** (1) DE. |
| **Hearing aids:** (1) CT, MD, OK, PA. | **Minimum mastectomy stays:** (1) AR, CA, CT, FL, GA, IL, KY, ME, MD, MT, NJ, NM, NY, NC, OK, PA, RI, SC, TX, VA. |
| **Hearing screening for children:** (1) MA, MO, NE, NC, TX, VA. | |
| **Hemophilia:** (1) NJ. | **Minimum hysterectomy stays:** (1): VA. |
| **Home health care:** (1) AZ, CT, FL, MD, MA, NJ, NY, VT, WI. (2) CA, CO, KY, ME, MT, NM, RI, SC, TX, WA. | **Minimum maternity stays:** (1) All states. |
| | **Minimum testicular cancer stays:** (1) MD. |
| **Hospice care:** (1) MA, NV, VA. (2) AR, CO, MD, MI, NY, WA. | **Morbid obesity treatment:** (1) IN, MD. (2) GA, VA. |
| | **Neurodevelopment therapy:** (1) WA. |
| **Human leukocyte antigen testing:** (1) MA. | **Newborn care:** (1) DC, DE, ME, WI. |
| **Infertility services and/or in vitro fertilization:** (1) AR, HI, IL, MD, MA, MT, NJ, RI, WV. (2) CA, CT, NY, TX. | **Newborn sickle cell testing:** (1) PA, RI. |
| | **Nursing home care:** (1) NY. |
| **Kidney disease:** (1) WI. | **Off-label drug use:** (1) AL, AR, CA, FL, GA, IL, IN, KS, KY, LA, ME, MD, MA, MN, MS, NE, NV, NH, NJ, NY, NC, OH, OK, RI, TN, TX, VA. |
| **Lead poisoning screening:** (1) DE. | |
| **Long term care:** (1) KY, WV. | |
| **Lyme disease:** (1) CT, MN. | **Orthotics/prosthetics:** (1) CT, MD. (2) CA, FL, MI. |
| **Mammography screening:** (1) All states except (2) AR, IN, MI, MS. | **Osteoporosis:** (1) GA |
| | **Ovarian cancer monitoring:** (1) DE. |
| **Maternity care:** (1) CO, GA, HI, ME, MD, MA, MN, MO, NY, OR, PA. (2) CA, KS, TN. | **PKU Formula:** (1) AK, AR, CA, CT, FL, HI, ME, MD, MA, MN, MO, MT, NV, NH, NJ, ND, PA, TN, TX, UT, VT, WA. (2) SD. |
| **Mental health, general:** (1) CA, DC, HI, IL, KS, ME, MD, MN, MS, MO, MT, NH, ND, OR, VA, WV, WI. (2) AR, FL, GA, KY, LA, NY, NH, TN, VT, WA. | |
| | **Prescription drugs (medically necessary):** (1) DE, ME, NC, ND. (2) CA. |
| **Mental health, parity:** (1) AR, CA, CO, DE, DC, GA, HI, IN, KS, LA, ME, MD, MA, MN, MT, NE, NH, NJ, OK, PA, RI, SC, SD, TN, TX, VT, VA. | **Prostate cancer screening:** (1) AK, CA, CO, CT, GA, IL, IN, KS, LA, MD, MO, NJ, NY, NC, ND, OK, SC, SD, TN, TX, VT, VA, WY. (2) ME. |
| | **Referrals:** (1) DE. |
| **Mental illness (serious):** (1) DE, DC, NY, SC, TX, UT. | |
| **Mentally retarded children care:** (1) PA. | **Rehabilitation services:** (1) MD, MA, WV. (2) CT, LA. |

■ **Figure 3–9** (continued)

| Second medical and surgical opinion: (1) CA, MD, NY, WA, WI. (2) NJ, RI. |
| Speech, language and hearing disorders: (1) MA. (2) MO. |
| TMJ disorders: (1) CA, FL, GA, KY, MN, NV, NM, NC, ND, TX, VT, VA, WI. (2) IL, MS, NE, WA, WV. |
| Well-child care: (1) CA, CO, CT, DC, FL, GA, HI, IN, IA, KS, LA, MD, MA, MN, MO, MT, NE, NM, NY, PA, RI, TS, UT, WV, WI. (2) MS, OK, VA. |
| Wellness care: (1) NJ. |
| Wilm's tumor: (1) NJ. |

■ **Figure 3–9** *(continued)*

## Persons Who Must Be Covered

Some states require health plans to cover specific groups of people to ensure that they are not excluded from coverage.

**Figure 3–10** is an example of a list of state mandates regarding people who must be covered.

| Adopted Children: AK, AR, AZ, CO, CT, FL, GA, HI, IL, IN, IA, KS, MD, MA, MN, MT, NE, NV, NM, NY, NC, ND, OH, OK, OG, RI, SC, SD, TX, UT, VA, WA, WY. |
| Civil union same sex partners: VT. |
| Children of dependents: MA. |
| Continuation – dependents: AR, CA, CO, ST, FL, GA, IL, IA, KS, KY, LA, ME, MD, MI, MN, MS, MD, NE, NV, NH, NM, NY, NC, ND, OK, OR, RI, SC, SD, TN, TX, UT, VT, VA, WA, WV, WI. |
| Continuation – spouses: CA, IL. |

■ **Figure 3–10** State Mandated Member Coverages

| Continuation – employees: AR, CA, CO, CT, FL, GA, HI, ID, KS, KY, LA, ME, MD, MA, MN, MS, MO, MT, NE, NV, NH, NY, ND, OK, OR, SC, TN, TX, UT, VT, VA, WA, WV, WI, WY. |
| Conversion to non-group: AZ, AR, CA, CO, FL, GA, ID, IL, IN, IA, KS, KY, LA, MD, MN, MO, MT, NV, NM, NY, NC, ND, OH, OR, PA, RI, SD, TN, TX, UT, VT, VA, WA, WI, WY. |
| Dependent students: CT, FL, GA, LA, MN, NE, ND, TX. |
| Foster children: NC. |
| Grandchildren: WI. |
| Handicapped dependents: AZ, AR, CA, CT, FL, GA, HI, ID, IL, IN, LA, MD, MA, MI, MN, MS, MT, NH, NJ, NM, NY, NC, ND, OH, PA, SC, SD, TN, TX, UT, VT, VA, WA, WI, WY. |
| Handicapped employees: NJ. |
| Newborns: All States. |
| Non-custodial children: CT, MN, MT, ND, OR, TX, UT, WY. |
| Spouses: AK. |
| Unmarried children to age 26: UT. |

## Preexisting

HIPAA mandates that the look back period is six months, preexisting conditions can be excluded for only 12 months, and credit from any previous eligible group health plan must be applied to the 12-month waiting period. Some state laws shorten that waiting period for plans. If a state shortens the HIPAA requirement, it is listed under the correct time limit (**Figure 3–11**). In this listing, the first number indicates the amount of time health plans can review your medical records. The second number indicates the time insurers can exclude coverage of preexisting conditions after the purchase date of the policy. States which do not shorten the HIPAA requirements are listed under the word NO. Some states allow health plans to utilize exclusionary riders or endorsements to exclude certain conditions indefinitely.

| |
|---|
| **Three months/nine months:** NH. |
| **Six months/six months:** NM, MA (prior coverage credited) OR. |
| **Six months/nine months:** WA. |
| **Six months/12 months:** CA, CO, CT, DE. |
| **NO:** AL, AK, AZ, AR, FL, IL (non-HMO), IA, GA, KS, MO, MT, NB, NV, NC, OK, SC, TN, TX, WV, WI. |

■ **Figure 3–11** State Mandates for Special Preexisting Conditions

The following states (**see Figure 3–12**) have provisions which did not fit in the above categories.

| |
|---|
| **IL** – HMOs may not deny coverage for preexisting conditions. However, they may apply a copayment for the first 12 months of coverage of up to 50 percent for those conditions present in the 12 months prior to the effective date of coverage. |
| **PA** – HIPAA rules for most plans, however Blue Cross & Blue Shield plans must "take all comers," regardless of preexisting conditions. |
| **RI** – No preexisting exclusion periods are allowed. |

■ **Figure 3–12** State Mandates for Special Preexisting Conditions

## Prompt-pay Laws

Prompt-pay laws require health plans to pay health insurance claims within a specified time period, or face fines, added interest payments, and other penalties. Note that prompt-pay laws apply only to "clean claims" (meaning claims without defect and with full information provided). If a state requires clean claims to be paid within a certain time, the state is listed under the appropriate time limit (**see Figure 3–13**). (e) = Electronic claims. (ne) = Non-electronic claims.

| |
|---|
| **15 Working Days:** GA, ND. |
| **25 Working Days:** AL (provider claims). |
| **25 Calendar Days:** LA(e). |
| **30 Working Days:** CA (insurers). |
| **30 Calendar Days:** AK, AZ, CO(e), HI, IL, IN(e), IA, KS, KY(Non-organ transplants), ME, MD, MN, NH, NJ(e), NC, OH, OR, RI(e), TN, UT, WV(e), WI. |
| **35 Calendar Days:** FL (HMOs). |
| **40 Calendar Days:** NJ(ne), RI(ne), VA, WV(ne). |
| **45 Working Days:** AL (consumers), CA (HMOs). |
| **45 Calendar Days:** CO(ne), CT, DE, FL(insurers), IN(ne), LA(ne), MA, MI, MS, MO, NM, NY (undisputed), PA, SD, TX, VT, WY. |
| **60 Calendar Days:** KY (organ transplant claims), NV, OK, WA. |
| **90 Calendar Days:** CO (disputed claims). |
| **No prompt payment requirement:** AR, DC, ID, MT, NE, SC. |

■ **Figure 3–13** State Mandates for Prompt-pay Laws

## External or Independent Grievance Systems

External grievance systems allow claimants to take a dispute with their health plan to a doctor or review board unaffiliated with their health plan. Thus, both the claimant and their health plan receive an impartial ruling on its decision to deny coverage of services or treatment. Additionally, claimants can file a complaint against their health insurer with their state's department of insurance.

The following information (**Figure 3–14**) identifies the grounds of the original denial where a claimant may appeal a health plan's unfavorable decisions, and whether the panel's decision is binding or advisory. Information given applies to all health plans unless otherwise stated.

**There is no external grievance procedure in:** AL, AR, ID, MS, NE, NV, ND, SD, WY.

**AK** – For experimental, investigative, medical judgment, or medical necessity. Binding, unless appealed to state superior court within six months.

**AZ** – For any denial. Binding.

**CA** – For investigational treatment appeals and medical necessity. Binding.

**CO** – For medical necessity. Binding.

**CT** – For investigational treatment appeals and medical necessity. Binding on both parties.

**DE** – For managed care plans only, on grounds of investigational treatment appeals and medical necessity. Advisory.

**DC** – For any denial. Advisory.

**FL** – For HMOs, on grounds of any denial. Advisory.

**GA** – For HMO and PPO plans, on grounds of investigational treatment appeals and medical necessity. Binding.

**HI** – For any except medical malpractice. Appealable to state court.

**IL** – Only for HMOs, on grounds of denial of medical necessity, and disputes over length of stay or referrals. Binding.

**IN** – For HMOs, on grounds of investigational treatment appeals, medical necessity, violation of prompt-pay laws. Binding.

**IA** – For medical necessity. Binding on both parties.

**KS** – For investigational treatment appeals and medical necessity. Advisory.

**KY** – For any denial. Binding.

**LA** – For medical necessity. Binding on both parties.

**ME** – For investigational/experimental treatment, medical necessity, preexisting conditions. Binding only on carrier.

**MD** – Through the Maryland Insurance Administration, on grounds of medical necessity. Binding.

**MA** – After all internal plan appeals are exhausted. Binding.

**MI** – For any denial. Advisory.

**MN** – For any denial. Binding.

**MO** – For investigational treatment appeal, medical necessity. Binding on both parties.

**MT** – For medical necessity. Binding.

**NH** – For investigational treatment appeals and medical necessity. Binding.

**NJ** – For investigational treatment appeal, medical necessity. Binding.

**NM** – For any denial. Advisory.

**NY** – For medical necessity, investigational treatment, experimental treatment, clinical trials. Binding.

**NC** – For medical necessity. Binding.

**OH** – For investigational treatment appeal, medical necessity. Binding.

**OK** – For medical necessity. Advisory.

**OR** – Grounds unspecified. Binding for both sides.

**PA** – For medical necessity, coverage disputes, and exclusions. Binding.

■ **Figure 3–14** State Mandates for Grievance Systems

| |
|---|
| **RI** – For medical necessity and appropriateness of medical treatment. Binding. |
| **SC** – For emergencies, experimental or investigational treatment, medical necessity, untimely internal appeal delay, waiver of internal appeal by carrier. Binding for both sides. |
| **TN** – For HMOs only, on grounds of medical necessity. Binding. |
| **TX** – For medical necessity. Binding. |
| **UT** – For denial, modification, or reduction of claims payments or termination of coverage. Binding. |
| **VT** – For investigational treatment appeal, medical necessity. Binding. |
| **VI** – For medical necessity. Binding on both parties. |
| **WA** – For denial, modification, or reduction of claims payments, or termination of coverage. Binding for the insurer. |
| **WV** – For experimental treatment, medical necessity. Binding. |
| **WI** – For medical necessity. Binding. |

■ **Figure 3–14** *(continued)*

# On the Job Now

**Directions:** Go through the mandates on the above pages. Highlight each mandate that applies to your state. Then obtain a copy of the mandated insurance coverage in your state (usually available through the State Department of Insurance).

# CHAPTER REVIEW

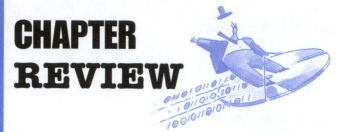

## Summary

- The term "contract," in general, is an agreement among two or more persons that is enforceable by law. For a contract to be valid, the parties must agree on its terms. There must also be some form of offer and acceptance.

- When an offer has been properly communicated and accepted, a binding contract is formed.

- A group contract allows an insurance company to meet the financial security needs of a group of persons.

- It is vital that health claims examiners understand how to interpret contracts. It will take practice to accurately understand the coverages provided under contracts and to pay benefits properly.

- Basic and Major Medical plans are generally classified as indemnity contracts.

- These plans indemnify or reimburse the insured for medical expenses incurred and typically require the completion and filing of claims.

- These plans often also contain deductible and coinsurance provisions and may restrict coverage for certain types of medical care expenditures.

- Indemnity plans, in contrast to HMO and PPO plans, provide the member with substantial freedom regarding the choice of physicians or specialists seen.

- HMO and PPO plan coverage emphasizes comprehensive (including preventive) care and typically contains fewer exclusions, small or no deductibles, and nominal copayments. However, there is much less freedom in choosing a physician.

- The three contracts found on the following pages will be used throughout the course to calculate benefits on sample claims and to add clarification to examples used to demonstrate the application of plan provisions.

- These sample contracts are based on actual plans and should be used as examples of what is possible within the industry. There is no such thing as a definitive plan. As you will discover, there are a multitude of possible contract provisions. Therefore, use these samples as learning tools only.

- Eligibility and effective dates of coverage are probably the greatest factors to be considered when processing a claim.

- Thus, eligibility and effective date is the first thing that should be checked when a claim is received for payment. If the patient is not eligible, no further action need be taken on the claim.

- Acts of Third Parties and Subrogation can drastically alter the way a claim is paid and who is responsible for the claim payment.

- Preexisting conditions account for one of the highest dollar amounts of claims paid incorrectly, costing insurance companies thousands of dollars.

- The health claims examiner must understand these concepts and when they come into play.

## Assignments

Complete the Questions for Review.
Complete Exercises 3–1 through 3–5.

## Questions for Review

**Directions:** Answer the following questions without looking back at the material just covered. Write your answers in the space provided.

1. (True or False?) Every health benefit plan, whether it is insured or not, is required by law to have a written document describing the plan benefits. _____

2. Define offer. _____

_____

**3.** Define eligibility. _____

_____

**4.** What is an exclusion? _____

**5.** _____ refers to the requirements that must be fulfilled for a person to be covered by the plan.

**6.** Most contracts define employees in terms of _____

_____

**7.** What is a qualified beneficiary? _____

_____

**8.** What is a qualifying event? _____

_____

**9.** (True or False?) Improperly handled claims for preexisting conditions are a common source of complaints and lawsuits. _____

**10.** (True or False?) An examiner should not notify the member and the provider of the delay of a claim. _____

If you were unable to answer any of these questions, refer back to that section and then fill in the answers.

# Exercise 3-1

**Directions:**  Read through the ABC Corporation (Winter Insurance) contract and possible preexisting conditions (see Appendix A) and list the amounts for the following provisions in the space provided. Do not concern yourself with the definitions of terms or how to calculate the amounts, since these subjects will be covered in another chapter.

**1.** What is the individual deductible amount? _____

**2.** What is the dependent eligibility age limit? _____

**3.** What is the family calendar year deductible? _____

**4.** What is the individual coinsurance limit? _____

**5.** What is the coinsurance percentage? _____

**6.** What is the lifetime maximum amount? _____

**7.** How many hours must the employee work to be eligible? _____

**8.** Does the contract include dental coverage? _____

9. What is the family coinsurance limit? _____

10. Is the family coinsurance aggregate or nonaggregate? _____

11. Is there a carryover provision on the individual deductible? _____

12. How many months must the employee work before coverage becomes effective? _____

13. What is the amount of the basic accident benefit? _____

14. What basic benefits does it have? _____

15. What are the terms of the accident benefit? _____

_____

# Exercise 3-2

**Directions:** Place a "yes" or "no" next to each of the following people to show which would be eligible for coverage under the Ninja contract.

1. Mother, Kanika, works 35 hours per week for Ninja. _____

2. Father, Kenneth, is self-employed. He is Kanika's second husband. _____

3. Ryan, 20-year-old son of Kanika and her first husband, is currently unemployed and is not a full-time student. _____

4. Ravyn, 20-year-old daughter (Ryan's twin) is going to the local university full-time. _____

5. Jordan, 16-year-old daughter, a high school dropout. _____

6. Sheila, a 13-year-old foster child who lives with the family. _____

7. Sharon, a 10-year-old legally adopted child. _____

8. Paris, the three-year-old daughter of Ravyn. _____

9. Kytrena, Kanika's mother. She has Alzheimer's Disease and is listed as a dependent on Kanika's income tax form. _____

10. Caitlind, Kanika's mentally retarded sister. Kanika is not her legal guardian. _____

# Exercise **3-3**

**Directions:** Find and circle the words listed below. Words can appear horizontally, vertically, diagonally, forward, or backward.

```
Q E K Z S Q L Z B B X N I C X Q T S N O
C X Y H X U P T L D D O N C L C K G A Q
Y Y T Y Y A Q B D B H N F M A Q U E L N
G I Y I L L V F K A X C V R J E R T P X
S C F E A I G S R V K O T V U B B C Y F
Q U A L I F I E D B E N E F I C I A R Y
A O B K Y Y Q Q L A O T E E W D A R O C
T F K R U I K H P C I R S T J S S T T O
L N G D O N L Q T Z E I Y T H K A N U N
O D E N Z G E L I G I B I L I T Y O B V
U J M D K E A T S R L U F Z D N E C I E
W S C H N V U T Q Q Y T L B N E Z P R R
L X P F K E F E I D Y O B R U D X U T S
M O X G R N P T I O M R R T O I D O N I
Y R U S O T Z E Y P N Y H S A C S R O O
I E L B I T C U D E D P B X M C W G C N
Y M A N D A T E S C N L E B Y A V Y Y Z
V R P T I M I L E C N A R U S N I O C Q
L O B Z H L S T I F E N E B C I S A B L
L I F E T I M E M A X I M U M C K A C F
```

1. Accident
2. Basic Benefits
3. Coinsurance Limit
4. Contract
5. Contributory Plan
6. Conversion
7. Deductible
8. Dependent

9. Eligibility
10. Group Contract
11. Lifetime Maximum
12. Mandates
13. Noncontributory Plan
14. Qualified Beneficiary
15. Qualifying Event
16. Subrogation

# Exercise 3-4

**Directions:** Complete the crossword puzzle by filling in a word from the keywords that fits each clue.

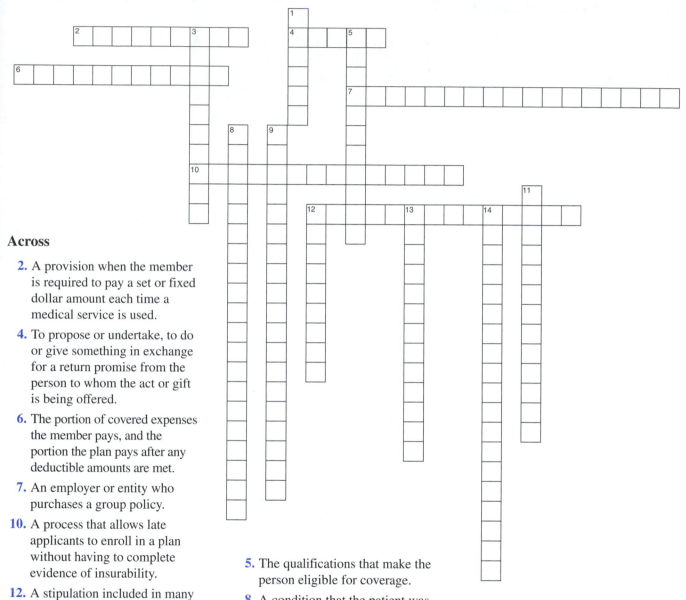

### Across

**2.** A provision when the member is required to pay a set or fixed dollar amount each time a medical service is used.

**4.** To propose or undertake, to do or give something in exchange for a return promise from the person to whom the act or gift is being offered.

**6.** The portion of covered expenses the member pays, and the portion the plan pays after any deductible amounts are met.

**7.** An employer or entity who purchases a group policy.

**10.** A process that allows late applicants to enroll in a plan without having to complete evidence of insurability.

**12.** A stipulation included in many contracts that states that a person must be at work (or actively engaged in their normal activities if a dependent) on the date coverage becomes effective.

### Down

**1.** A legal and binding written document that exists between two or more parties.

**3.** Any condition or expense for which, under the terms of the policy, no coverage is provided.

**5.** The qualifications that make the person eligible for coverage.

**8.** A condition that the patient was treated for within a specified time period before becoming effective under the plan.

**9.** With this provision, if the patient can go without treatment for a specified period of time, then the insurance carrier will no longer consider the condition to be preexisting and will cover the illness or condition under the normal terms of the contract.

**11.** Anything that is given, done, promised, forbidden, or suffered by one party as an inducement for the agreement.

**12.** Any amounts paid toward the deductible by any member of the family will be added up to reach this deductible.

**13.** The date a contract began to be in force.

**14.** A provision that allows the insurance carrier to recoup medical expenses paid if it is found that a third party is liable for damages.

# Exercise 3-5

**Directions:** Match the following terms with the proper definition by writing the letter of the correct definition in the space next to the term.

1. _____ Active Work

2. _____ Acts of Third Parties

3. _____ Carryover Deductible

4. _____ Coinsurance Limit

5. _____ COBRA

6. _____ Credible Coverage

7. _____ Evidence of Insurability

8. _____ Major Medical Benefits

9. _____ Nonaggregate Family Deductible Limits

10. _____ Out-of-Pocket

11. _____ Preadmission Testing

12. _____ Preexisting Condition

13. _____ Second Surgical Opinion

a. Like or similar coverage. For example if the former coverage was medical only, and the new coverage is medical, dental, and vision, only the medical portion would be considered. Therefore, the employee would be given credit for prior medical coverage, but preexisting exclusions could be applied to dental and vision services.

b. Cessation of eligibility for benefits under the plan.

c. A legal and binding written document that exists between two or more parties.

d. Consists of routine laboratory and x-ray tests performed on an outpatient basis before a scheduled inpatient admission.

e. A member's costs, which include the deductible, cost-sharing arising from the operation of the coinsurance clause, and medical expenditures that are deemed by the plan to be in excess of reasonable and customary charges.

f. A specified number of individuals in the family must meet their individual deductible limit in order for the family limit to be met.

g. Those benefits paid after basic benefits and which are usually subject to a deductible and coinsurance

h. An opinion provided by a second physician when one physician recommends surgery to an individual.

i. The employee will be required to submit proof of good health, usually by filling out a health questionnaire.

j. Usually means performing the regular duties for a full workday for the employer.

k. Any amounts which the patient pays toward their deductible in the last three months of the year will carry over and will be applied toward the next year's deductible.

l. This limit stipulates that if the coinsurance amount reaches a certain level, all subsequent claims will be paid at 100% of the allowed amount.

m. A medical condition that existed before an insurance policy was purchased. Depending on the policy, this condition may be defined based on when it originated, when symptoms first appeared, or when treatment was first sought.

14. _____ Summary Plan Description

n. The law requires employers to permit employees and their dependents to purchase transitional healthcare coverage at favorable group rates until replacement coverage could be obtained. The intended result was to reduce the number of people without healthcare coverage.

15. _____ Termination of Coverage

o. A provision that allows the insurance carrier to recoup medical expenses paid, if it is found that a third party is liable for damages.

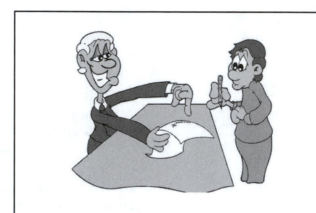

"Just sign right here and we'll cover 80% of everything we think the doctor should charge."

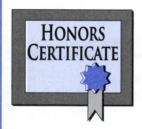

### Honors Certification™

The Honors Certification™ challenge for this chapter comprises a written test. You will be given questions pertaining to the information covered in this chapter. In addition, you will be given a number of questions dealing with the three contracts presented. Any incorrect answers will result in a deduction of up to 5% from your grade. You must achieve a score of 80% to pass this test. If you fail the test on your first attempt, you may retake the test one additional time. The information included in the second test may be different from that included in the first test.

# 4

# Medical Benefit
## Structures

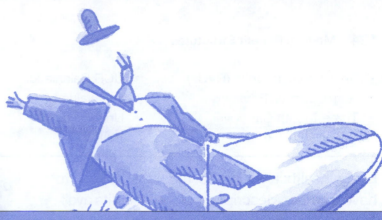

## After completion of this chapter
### you will be able to:

- Identify three major types of coverages available under indemnity contracts.
- Define and explain basic benefit terms.
- Accurately interpret contract provisions.
- Accurately calculate deductible amounts given a contract and scenario.
- Accurately calculate benefit amounts when given a contract and specific scenarios.
- List and explain situations that may be considered accident situations.

- Determine the correct unit value of a given procedure code.
- Determine the appropriate conversion factor as indicated by geographic region and status of a given provider.
- Accurately calculate customary and reasonable allowances.
- Identify cost-containment programs and describe their implementation.

## Keywords and concepts
### you will learn in this chapter:

- Accidental Injury
- Accumulation Period
- Allowed Amount
- Automatic Annual Reinstatement (AAR)
- Common Accident Provision
- Concurrent Review
- Conversion Factor
- Covered Expense
- Cumulative Benefit
- Exclusive Provider Organization (EPO)
- Extended Benefits

- Fee Schedule
- Gatekeeper PPO
- Health Maintenance Organization (HMO)
- In-Network
- Loss Date
- Managed Care
- Management Service Organization (MSO)
- Mandatory Program
- Maximum
- Medical Case Management (MCM)

- Nondisabling or Per Visit Benefit
- Out-of-Network
- Out-of-Pocket (OOP)
- Out-of-Pocket Maximum
- Per Period of Disability
- Physician Hospital Organization (PHO)
- Preauthorization
- Precertification
- Predetermination
- Preferred Provider Organization (PPO)
- Region

- Relative Value Units (RVUs)
- Retrospective Review
- Three-Month Carryover Provision (C/O)
- UCR Calculation
- Unit Value
- Unnecessary Surgery
- Usual, Customary, and Reasonable (UCR)
- Utilization Review (UR)
- Voluntary Program

Every healthcare plan is required by law to have a written description of the benefits available to the members of that plan. This plan document must indicate, in detail, and in layman's terms, the provisions of the coverage.

Three major types of indemnity coverage are currently available:

- Basic only.
- Basic-Major Medical.
- Comprehensive Major Medical.

Within these types there may be numerous variations. Additionally, under managed care provisions there can be PPO and HMO contracts.

Since the benefit payments calculated under each type of coverage can be identical, do not let the names confuse you. It is the concept that is important. Be sure you understand the types of benefit payments before processing any claims, since accurate benefit payment calculation is essential to being a good claims examiner. Inaccurate payments can cost an insurance carrier thousands of dollars.

## Benefit Definitions

Following are some common terms that are used when dealing with benefits. These definitions may not have calculations associated with them, so they are covered here. Benefit definitions that require you to calculate items will be discussed in the Benefit Calculations section.

**Accumulation Period**—Period of time (normally January 1 through December 31) in which to satisfy the deductible, accumulate COB credit reserves, reach maximums, and so on.

**Covered Expense**—Those expenses that are allowable under the plan. Services specifically excluded by the plan or in excess of UCR (usual, customary, and reasonable fees) are not considered to be covered expenses (also called Allowed Amount).

### Practice Pitfalls

**Example:** Surgery is billed at $500. The plan's UCR amount is $350; therefore, the covered expense would be $350. Therefore, any applicable deductible would be taken from the $350 allowance, and any remaining amount would be paid at the Major Medical coinsurance percentage. The difference between the submitted amount of $500 and the covered/allowable amount of $350 ($150) would be the member's responsibility, for a non-PPO provider.

**Extended Benefits**—The continued entitlement of a member, under certain circumstances, to receive benefits after the coverage has terminated. A doctor's certification of total disability is required before benefits can be extended. Usually, such coverage will continue only for expenses incurred from the condition that caused the disability and for a maximum of 12 months following the date of disability or the date that the member is no longer totally disabled, whichever is less.

**Loss Date**—The loss date is always the date of the accident. Regardless of the date of service, the loss date remains the same.

**Maximum(s)**—The maximum amount payable by the plan. The maximum may be a calendar year or lifetime maximum. In addition, it may apply only toward expenses paid under Basic or only toward expenses paid under Major Medical or a combination of all payments, Basic and Major Medical. The policy must specify the type.

**Out-of-Pocket (OOP) Maximum**—A yearly limit on the OOP that the insured is responsible for paying. When this limit or maximum is reached, the plan pays subsequent covered expenses at 100% (or other specified percentage) instead of the usual percentage for the remainder of the calendar year.

**Per Period of Disability**—Basic Benefit waiting periods and deductibles; may be based on a per illness basis or a waiting period basis. With a per illness waiting period, for each new illness or injury a new benefit amount may be applicable or a new waiting period may apply. If there is a time period basis for renewal of the benefit, the patient must go for a specified time period without treatment of the specific illness or any illnesses. This most often applies to medical treatment while hospitalized or office visit benefits.

**Unit Value**—A numerical value assigned by a relative value study to a procedure code. The unit value is multiplied by the conversion factor to determine the UCR allowance or a basic allowance.

# Benefit Calculations

The following items may need to be calculated in order to determine the proper benefit. This section will cover the calculation of each of these items. Since not all items are needed on every claim, we will look at each item separately. This way you can check back in this section when you are unsure of a calculation.

When you reach the Medical Claims Administration chapter and the chapters which discuss the various types of claims, these calculations will be used to complete the Payment Worksheet.

**Automatic Annual Reinstatement (AAR)** A contractually specified amount of money (credit) that may be added to the balance of available lifetime benefits. Usually, this applies to Major Medical benefits and is important only when a member has a catastrophic illness or injury and is calculated only when lifetime benefits have been exhausted.

**Example:** This Plan has a lifetime maximum amount of $300,000, with a $1,000 yearly reinstatement (AAR). The Plan has been in effect since 2003.

**Expenses Submitted to Plan   Lifetime Maximum**
**Year 2004**

| | |
|---|---|
| $150,000 Covered Expenses | $300,000 Lifetime Maximum |
| | −$150,000 Payments Made |
| | $150,000 Lifetime Maximum Remaining |

**Year 2005**

| | |
|---|---|
| $175,000 Covered Expenses | $150,000 Remaining Lifetime Maximum |
| | +1,000 2003 AAR |
| | +1,000 2004 AAR |
| | $152,000 Remaining and Payable |
| | $175,000 Covered Expenses Submitted |
| | −152,000 Benefits Paid |
| | $23,000 Unpaid/Amount Exceeds the Lifetime Maximum. |

Although the member has submitted $175,000 in covered expenses the plan will only pay $152,000, because this is the remainder of the lifetime maximum after crediting the AAR amounts for 2003 and 2004. Therefore, $23,000 remains unpaid because it is over the lifetime maximum.

The maximum amount that can be reinstated in one year can be either a specific dollar amount, or the total amount paid out in that year; or the plan language may indicate that the reinstated amount is the lesser of these two amounts. For example, if $800 had been paid out in 2004, only $800 could be reinstated. Usually, reinstatement is allowed for every year that the member is covered up to either the specified dollar amount stated in the contract, or the amount paid out; or whichever is less. In essence, any amount not used will not be carried over to succeeding years.

**Coinsurance** To calculate this amount, simply multiply the amount subject to Major Medical (after all Basic amounts, deductible and other benefits have been deducted) by the coinsurance amount the plan provides. For example, if the amount subject to Major Medical is $120 and the plan pays 80%, the plan's Major Medical payment would be $96.

**Out-of-Pocket (OOP)** The calculation of this amount is the reverse of the coinsurance amount. Thus, if the insurance carrier pays 80% of the amount subject to Major Medical, then the out-of-pocket amount would be 20% of the amount subject to Major Medical.

**Copayment** This amount will be a fixed dollar amount (i.e., $20, $25, etc.) which is paid or deducted each time a particular medical service is provided.

# Calculating the Deductible

A deductible must be paid by the member before benefits become payable by the plan under the Major Medical portion of the contract. Usually, this is a calendar year deductible (taken once each calendar year), but not always. The deductible is always taken out of the first eligible expense(s) submitted each year. The three common types of deductibles are:

**1.** Individual Deductible.

## Practice
# Pitfalls

Billy Barton is covered under the Winter Insurance Company contract. The individual deductible amount is $100; of which Billy has satisfied $0. Billy submits a claim for $25; of which $25 is considered covered expenses. Because Billy has not satisfied any portion of his individual deductible, the $25 would be applied toward his deductible.

**2.** Aggregate Deductible.

# Practice
# Pitfalls

If the Barton Family is covered under the Winter Insurance Company contract, their family deductible would be $200, aggregate. Therefore:

| Family Member | Deductible Satisfied |
|---|---|
| Billy | $25 |
| Barry | $45 |
| Bobby | $85 |
| Betty | $0 |

Betty now submits a claim for $500 in covered expenses. She only needs to satisfy $45 toward her deductible, because the family will have reached the $200 family deductible limit. Even though none of the family members have met their individual limit, the family limit has been satisfied. Therefore, no more deductible will be taken on any family members for this deductible period.

**3.** Nonaggregate Deductible.

# Practice
# Pitfalls

Nonaggregate family limits often require that the family pay more money toward the deductible. For example, if the Barton family were covered under the Ball Insurance Carriers contract, the family deductible limit would be two family members satisfying their $125 individual deductible.

| Family Member | Deductible Satisfied |
|---|---|
| Billy | $25 |
| Barry | $45 |
| Bobby | $85 |
| Betty | $0 |

Betty now submits a claim for $500 in services. She must pay the full $125 toward her deductible. Even so, the family deductible has still not been satisfied for this deductible period.

If the next claim is for Billy for $75, the full $75 amount would be considered part of the deductible, thus bringing the amount Billy has paid toward his deductible to $100. However, the family deductible for

this period would still not have been met since only one family member (Betty), not two, have reached their individual limit.

Only when either Billy, Barry, or Bobby has paid $125 toward their individual deductible during this deductible period will the family deductible be met. After the family deductible limit has been met, no more deductible would be taken on any member of the family for this deductible period.

## Three-Month Carryover Provision (C/O)

A **three-month carryover provision** states that eligible charges incurred in the last quarter of the calendar year (October, November, December) and applied toward the member's deductible will also carry over toward satisfying the following year's deductible. However, if the plan year is different from the calendar year, the last three months of the plan year will constitute the carryover deductible period. These monies may or may not be applied toward the family limit (see the terms of the contract).

# Practice
# Pitfalls

The deductible for John is $100 per year. The first claim submitted is for services in June, CCYY. Thirty five dollars were applied toward his CCYY deductible. The second claim submitted for John is for services dated November, CCYY. A $65 deductible was taken on this claim, thus satisfying the CCYY deductible. In addition, since $65 of the deductible was satisfied during the last three months of CCYY, $65 of CCNY's deductible will also be considered satisfied.

Carryover deductibles reward a patient who has been treatment-free for most of the year. If the patient is still paying their deductible during the last three months of the year, they have remained treatment-free for most of the year. Since deductibles are paid before the insurance carrier pays out any benefits, this means that the insurance carrier has not had to pay out any benefits during the year.

## Common Accident Provision

A **common accident provision** states that only one deductible, under Major Medical, will be taken for all members of a family involved in the same accident. After the one deductible, remaining deductibles will be waived on all other members for expenses incurred for that accident only.

As a claims examiner, try to be aware of where each member of a family stands in relation to their deductible payments. The patient with the most charges during the year has probably gone the farthest toward meeting their deductible. Also, if the insurance carrier has previously made several payments, the deductible has usually (though not always) been satisfied.

If more than one member of a family is being treated, many insurance carriers will take the single deductible from the claim that comes in first. If several claims for the family come in at the same time, often the deductible is taken from the patient who owes the most on their deductible.

## Practice
# Pitfalls

The entire Barton family was involved in an accident and they all visited the doctor on the same day. All claims were received by the insurance carrier at the same time. Their policy has a common accident provision, a $125 deductible, and the following family deductible accumulations:

| Family Member | Deductible Satisfied |
|---|---|
| Billy | $25 |
| Barry | $45 |
| Bobby | $85 |
| Betty | $0 |

Most insurance carriers would take the full deductible amount from Betty, and would then waive the deductible for the other family members.

# On the Job Now

**Directions:** Calculate the amount of deductible which will be taken and answer the following questions.

The Bear family is covered under the Rover Insurers Inc. contract. Their previous deductible payments are as follows:

|  | Brad | Bonnie | Barbra | Brian |
|---|---|---|---|---|
| C/O paid | 0.00 | 5.00 | 10.00 | 55.00 |
| Deductible paid | 10.00 | 0.00 | 5.00 | 5.00 |

**1.** What is the individual deductible limit on this contract? _____

**2.** What is the family deductible limit on this contract? _____

**3.** Is the family limit aggregate or nonaggregate? _____

**4.** How many people are needed to meet the family deductible for this year? _____

**5.** Bonnie incurs allowed charges of $55. How much will be applied to the deductible? _____

**6.** How much has Bonnie now met on her deductible? _____

**7.** How many people are now needed to meet the family deductible? _____

**8.** Brian incurs allowed charges of $85. How much will be applied to the deductible? _____

**9.** How much has Brian now met on his deductible? _____

**10.** How many people are now needed to meet the family deductible? _____

**11.** Barbra incurs allowed charges of $105. How much will be applied to the deductible? _____

**12.** How much has Barbra now met on her deductible? _____

**13.** How many people are now needed to meet the family deductible? _____

**14.** Brad incurs allowed charges of $60. How much will be applied to the deductible? _____

**15.** How much has Brad now met on his deductible? _____

**16.** How many people are now needed to meet the family deductible? _____

**17.** Bonnie incurs allowed charges of $35. How much will be applied to the deductible? _____

**18.** How much has Bonnie now met on her deductible? _____

**19.** How many people are now needed to meet the family deductible? _____

**20.** Brian incurs allowed charges of $35. How much will be applied to the deductible? _____

**21.** How much has Brian now met on his deductible? _____

**22.** How many people are now needed to meet the family deductible? _____

**23.** Barbra incurs allowed charges of $55. How much will be applied to the deductible? _____

**24.** How much has Barbra now met on her deductible? _____

**25.** How many people are now needed to meet the family deductible? _____

**26.** Brad incurs allowed charges of $60. How much will be applied to the deductible? _____

**27.** How much has Brad now met on his deductible? _____

**28.** How many people are now needed to meet the family deductible? _____

# On the Job Now

**Directions:**  Calculate the amount of deductible which will be taken and answer the following questions.
The Carpenter family is covered under the Ball Insurance Carriers contract. Their previous deductible payments are as follows:

|                 | Carrie | Connie | Cathy | Chris |
|-----------------|--------|--------|-------|-------|
| C/O paid        | 0.00   | 5.00   | 10.00 | 55.00 |
| Deductible paid | 10.00  | 0.00   | 5.00  | 5.00  |

1. What is the individual deductible limit on this contract? _____

2. What is the family deductible limit on this contract? _____

3. Is the family limit aggregate or nonaggregate? _____

4. How many people are needed to meet the family deductible? _____

5. Connie incurs allowed charges of $35. How much will be applied to the deductible? _____

6. How much has Connie now met on her deductible? _____

7. How many people are now needed to meet the family deductible? _____

8. Carrie incurs allowed charges of $55. How much will be applied to the deductible? _____

9. How much has Carrie now met on her deductible? _____

10. How many people are now needed to meet the family deductible? _____

11. Chris incurs allowed charges of $60. How much will be applied to the deductible? _____

12. How much has Chris now met on his deductible? _____

13. How many people are now needed to meet the family deductible? _____

14. Chris incurs allowed charges of $35. How much will be applied to the deductible? _____

15. How much has Chris now met on his deductible? _____

16. How many people are now needed to meet the family deductible? _____

17. Connie incurs allowed charges of $95. How much will be applied to the deductible? _____

18. How much has Connie now met on her deductible? _____

19. How many people are now needed to meet the family deductible? _____

**20.** Carrie incurs allowed charges of $45. How much will be applied to the deductible? _____

**21.** How much has Carrie now met on her deductible? _____

**22.** How many people are now needed to meet the family deductible? _____

**23.** Cathy incurs allowed charges of $105. How much will be applied to the deductible? _____

**24.** How much has Cathy now met on her deductible? _____

**25.** How many people are now needed to meet the family deductible? _____

**26.** Carrie incurs allowed charges of $85. How much will be applied to the deductible? _____

**27.** How much has Carrie now met on her deductible? _____

**28.** How many people are now needed to meet the family deductible? _____

**29.** Chris incurs allowed charges of $85. How much will be applied to the deductible? _____

**30.** How much has Chris now met on his deductible? _____

**31.** How many people are now needed to meet the family deductible? _____

**32.** Cathy incurs allowed charges of $90. How much will be applied to the deductible? _____

**33.** How much has Cathy now met on her deductible? _____

**34.** How many people are now needed to meet the family deductible? _____

# On the Job Now

**Directions:** Calculate the amount of deductible which will be taken and answer the following questions.

The Apple family is covered under the Winter Insurance Company contract. Their previous deductible payments are as follows:

|                | Annie | Adam | April | August | Ashley |
|----------------|-------|------|-------|--------|--------|
| C/O paid       | 0.00  | 5.00 | 10.00 | 55.00  | 0.00   |
| Deductible paid| 10.00 | 0.00 | 5.00  | 5.00   | 0.00   |

**1.** What is the individual deductible limit on this contract? _____

**2.** What is the family deductible limit on this contract? _____

**3.** Is the family limit aggregate or nonaggregate? _____

**4.** How much has been paid toward the family deductible? _____

**5.** Annie incurs allowed charges of $35. How much will be applied to the deductible? _____

**6.** How much has Annie now met on her deductible? _____

**7.** How much has now been paid toward the family deductible? _____

**8.** August incurs allowed charges of $55. How much will be applied to the deductible? _____

**9.** How much has August now met on his deductible? _____

**10.** How much has now been paid toward the family deductible? _____

**11.** April incurs allowed charges of $55. How much will be applied to the deductible? _____

**12.** How much has April now met on her deductible? _____

**13.** How much has now been paid toward the family deductible? _____

**14.** Adam incurs allowed charges of $60. How much will be applied to the deductible? _____

**15.** How much has Adam now met on his deductible? _____

**16.** How much has now been paid toward the family deductible? _____

**17.** Annie incurs allowed charges of $35. How much will be applied to the deductible? _____

**18.** How much has Annie now met on her deductible? _____

**19.** How much has now been paid toward the family deductible? _____

# Basic Benefits

A Basic Benefit provides a specified allowance for a certain type of service. Usually, the allowance is 100% of either UCR (as defined by the plan) or some other amount based on the relative value study (RVS) and conversion factors.

A Basic Benefit usually has a stated calendar year dollar maximum, or number of visits or treatments, or a combination of both.

For example, refer to the XYZ contract under "Surgical" benefits. As indicated, this Basic Benefit pays 100% of the allowable using an $8.50 conversion factor. A maximum of $1,600 is payable under the Basic Benefits only per surgery or operative session. Any money charged in excess of either the $1,600 or the allowable amount up to the UCR amount would be covered under Major Medical subject to any limitations specified by that provision. Basic Benefits are al-ways paid first. It is possible for a single expense to be covered under multiple Basic Benefits. In this case, the first Basic Benefit would be computed, then any excess would be allowed under any other applicable Basic Benefit, and finally any remaining amount would be considered under Major Medical.

Following are some guidelines for calculating Basic Benefits:

1. Basic Benefits are always paid first before applicable Major Medical benefits are calculated.
2. Basic Benefits are usually paid at 100% of the stated amount. Any other applicable percentage must be specifically stated in the policy.
3. Basic Benefits usually have a dollar or number limit.

Under a basic only plan, any amount not paid by the Basic Benefit would not be covered at all. These charges would be the patient's responsibility.

# Common Basic Benefits

There are several different types of Basic Benefits. The most common are listed below.

## Accident Benefits

An **accidental injury** is a sudden and unforeseen event, definite as to time and place. This includes trauma happening involuntarily or as a result of a voluntary act entailing unforeseen consequences. The following is terminology related to accidental injuries:

1. **Aggravated physiologic weakness** Injury caused when an individual has a physical weakness that is aggravated by some voluntary activity. Overexertion or unusual physical exertion is also considered an accident if there is a specific time and circumstance involved. Do not consider routine bodily movements to be an injury if there is a history of related illness, such as arthritis and chronic strain of the affected area. Strains or sprains resulting from an unknown cause would not be considered an accident.

2. **Aggressor acts while intoxicated** The aggressor may not be considered responsible for his or her actions. Therefore, resulting injuries may be covered under this provision. However, this rule is changing due to tougher intoxication laws and the push toward encouraging responsible drinking.

3. **Aggressor claims** If someone is the victim of an aggressor, his or her injuries are usually considered accidental. When an investigation does not clearly show who the aggressor was, the determination is usually made in the claimant's favor. As a rule, a person who is the aggressor or who is injured in the commission of a crime is not usually covered under an accident benefit.

4. **Family altercations** If an employee unintentionally injures a member of his or her family without provocation, the injuries would be considered accidental. Cases of this sort need to be investigated to ascertain the facts.

5. **Internal reaction with external trauma** Injury incurred as the result of an internal condition (i.e., by falling after fainting) is considered accidental. There must be an external impact involved in the injury.

6. **Reactions to external stimulus** Unforeseen consequences of voluntary acts, such as insect bites, allergic reactions to poison ivy or other foliage, food poisoning, and animal bites.

Benefits under this provision usually pay the first charges submitted up to a specified limit at 100% for all expenses incurred within a specified time period of the date of the accident. Amounts over the dollar limit or after the time limit are covered under other plan provisions.

**Note:** Any complication involved in the treatment of what was originally deemed an "accident" would continue to be part of that accident. This includes reactions to drugs given as a result of the accident.

## Nonaccidental Injuries

Injuries received as a result of any of the following are usually not considered accidental. These include:

- Injuries resulting from willful or reckless actions which are known to result in serious bodily injury, including extremes such as playing Russian roulette, parachute jumping, high-speed auto racing on city streets, and injuries sustained in the commission of a crime.
- Intentionally self-inflicted injuries, such as those sustained during an attempted suicide.

## Practice
# Pitfalls

Holly Hiker (covered under the XYZ contract) was hiking along a mountain trail when a snake jumped out and bit her. She ended up incurring allowable charges of $150 for the ambulance, $125 for the emergency room doctor, $225 for the second doctor, $1,100 in hospital fees, and $250 in lab fees. The total allowable amount is $1,850. Under the XYZ contract the first $300 is covered at 100%. Therefore, if the bills were submitted in the order shown above, the ambulance charge ($150), the emergency room doctor's charge ($125), and $25 of the second doctor's charge would be paid at 100%. Thus, $200 for the second doctor, $1,100 for the hospital fees and $250 for the lab fees would be paid under Major Medical.

It is important to note that accident benefits usually have a date provision attached. Benefits may be limited to charges incurred within the first 90 days of the accident. Therefore, any treatments that occurred after the 90 day limit would not be allowed under Basic Benefits. They would only be paid under Major Medical benefits.

- Injury sustained as a result of a family quarrel, unless the injured party takes legal action and receives a favorable court decision and it is the injured party who is the insured.

- Sunburn for any person over the age of 16. However, severe sunburn resulting from being stranded (i.e., in a desert) is covered as an accident for a person of any age.

- Any trauma resulting from the normal risks a person takes when undergoing surgical or medical treatment for an illness. Included in this category would be circumstances similar to the following: the unintentional severing of a ureter during a hysterectomy, leaving a clamp or surgical instrument in the operative field, and allergic reactions to prescribed medications.

- Injuries sustained in a fight or brawl, if it is determined that the member was the aggressor.

- A "bad trip" as the result of voluntary injection, ingestion or inhalation of illegal drugs in anyone over 16 years of age. In a person under 16 years of age, the first such experience may be considered "accidental".

- Any injury in which the patient cannot recall how it happened, with the exception of anything as obvious as a fracture, burn, or laceration, and except in a small child who cannot be expected to remember.

## Attempted Suicide

Most plans will not cover attempted suicides as an accident. Some plans specifically exclude expenses incurred as a result of an attempted suicide or self-inflicted injury. Thus, the policy should be checked to determine whether such exclusion is applicable.

## Diagnostic X-Ray and Laboratory (DXL)

Benefits for x-rays and labs can be handled in a variety of ways. In the past, it was not uncommon to have what was called a "scheduled benefit." This type of benefit specified that a set dollar amount was allowed for each test. Today, most basic plans provide an alternative type of benefit called an "unscheduled" Basic Benefit, which limits payment under the Basic Benefit to a specified dollar amount per calendar year based on UCR or based on a conversion factor and RVS units. Once the calendar year maximum has been paid, subsequent expenses

would be paid under the Major Medical benefit. If a Basic DXL benefit is provided by the plan, inpatient charges are usually excluded. That is, inpatient expenses would be covered only under Major Medical. However, outpatient hospital claims would allow a Basic Benefit for DXL charges. Therefore, it is important to read the benefit plan before determining benefits.

### Practice Pitfalls

Gen Gym is covered under the ABC contract. He had lab tests performed by his doctor and the billed and allowed amount is $25. The unit value for the lab tests is .96. The contract pays a basic benefit for laboratory charges; at a $7 conversion factor. Thus, the .96 unit value would be multiplied by $7 totaling $6.72. This $6.72 would be paid at the basic benefit rate of 100%, and the remaining $18.28 would be paid under Major Medical benefits.

## Hospital Benefits

This Basic Benefit may provide a per admission deductible that does not usually carry over to the Major Medical plan. This benefit usually applies not only to hospital expenses but also to outpatient surgery expenses and charges incurred as a result of an accident within a specified time period (generally 24 hours).

This type of benefit usually has a dollar limit that is allowed per day for room and board and a separate allowance limit for ancillary expenses. As with other Basic Benefits, the provisions of this type of benefit vary widely from plan to plan.

## Medical While Hospitalized (MWH)

Inpatient hospital care is often known as medical while hospitalized. The patient is admitted into a facility, and the physician visits him or her in the hospital.

### Cumulative Benefit

Many types of MWH benefits are available. One of the more common types is called a **cumulative benefit**. To calculate benefits under this provision, the number of days hospitalized is multiplied by the benefit amount.

This is the maximum amount of Basic Benefit that can be paid out for this admission, regardless of how many doctors see the patient on a single day or the actual number of visits during the period. Some provisions allow multiple doctors to receive the benefit, but most

## Practice
## Pitfalls

The XYZ contract allows for an inpatient hospital Basic Benefit of room and board up to the semi-private room charge (ICU is limited to $600 per day). Miscellaneous fees (all other hospital fees) are unlimited, but the Basic Benefit only allows 10 days per period of disability. This amount is also subject to a $50 deductible.

Therefore, if Emily Emerson was admitted to the hospital for 14 days, the Basic Benefit would pay the cost of the room and board up to the semi-private room rate for the first 10 days. The additional four days would be paid under Major Medical. Likewise, the miscellaneous fees would be covered for the first 10 days under Basic benefits and the remaining four days under Major Medical benefits. Basic benefits are paid at 100%, and Major Medical benefits are covered at 80%.

The $50 hospital deductible would apply to the hospital charges. However, the patient would also have to pay the full $125 Major Medical deductible on any Major Medical charges, since the hospital deductible is separate from the Major Medical deductible. Additionally, if Emily Emerson was hospitalized again at a later date, she would owe another $50 basic hospital deductible for the hospital charges since the benefits (and deductible) in this case is per occurrence.

plans limit the benefit to one, which may be split up and paid to multiple providers as long as it does not exceed the maximum as calculated above. For an example of this benefit type, see the XYZ Corporation contract.

## Practice
## Pitfalls

Bobby Brainerd was hospitalized from 3/1/CCYY through 3/14/CCYY. His contract allows a $21 basic benefit for the first day of hospitalization and $7 per day thereafter.

The day of admission and the day of discharge are counted to determine the maximum allowance. To determine the cumulative basic benefit; $7 is multiplied by 13 days, which totals $91. Ninety one dollars is added to the first day benefit of $21; for a total basic benefit payment of $112.

### Per Visit Benefit

A second type of benefit has multiple names, which may include the terms **nondisabling** or **per visit benefit**. For this type of benefit, there is a waiting period, a daily maximum, and a calendar year maximum. For example, the provision may indicate, "$10 per day payable after seven days and $200 per calendar year."

Using the same hospitalization as above, this benefit is substantially different from the prior example. The day of admission and the day of discharge are counted to determine the maximum allowance. The seven-day waiting period is subtracted from the 14 days, and the remaining number of days (seven) is multiplied by the daily benefit amount of $10 for a total of $70. Usually, this provision allows for the circumstance in which a patient is discharged and then readmitted within a specified period of time, and another seven-day waiting period is not required. The plan provisions must be checked for this and any other exceptions.

### Surgery While Hospitalized

If surgery is performed during the hospitalization, there are many ways to apply an inpatient visit provision, depending on the wording of the benefit and how the services are provided. The following is a summary of some of the more common circumstances. These rules apply to visits performed by the operating surgeon.

1. If surgery is performed, there should not be a charge for a visit on the same day as surgery, excluding diagnostic procedures such as proctosigmoidoscopy and other procedures with no follow-up days.

2. If the surgery has follow-up days listed but the surgery is not performed on the day of admission:
   - Visits billed before the date of surgery are allowed. Calculate as indicated in the examples above, counting the date of admission and every day up to but not including the day of surgery.
   - Visits billed on the day of surgery are combined with the surgery charge. There should not be a separate charge for a visit on the same day of surgery. Allow up to the plan maximum for the surgery.
   - Visits billed on the days following surgery within the follow-up days listed are to be combined with the surgery charge. Visits billed after the follow-up days can be paid separately.
   - If surgery is performed on the first day of admission, all visits occurring within the follow-up days should be combined with the

surgery charge. An emergency consultation on the same day as surgery may be an exception to combining the visits with the surgery charge. The regular surgery benefit will be calculated in accordance with the plan provisions.

**Example:** Araceli Alejandro enters the hospital for treatment of a bone cyst (code 20615) on 3/1. Surgery is performed on 3/2 and she is discharged on 3/12. The RVS lists 10 follow-up days for this procedure. Therefore, a physician visit benefit would be allowed on the first day, since surgery was not performed on that day. The visits for the next 10 days would be covered under the surgical charge. The visit for the last day would be paid since it occurred after the 10 follow-up days.

## Office Visits

Like the MWH benefit, office visit benefits are usually based on a specified dollar limit per visit after a specified number of visits have been applied to the waiting period. The waiting period is often on a per illness basis. That is, a specified number of visits are not paid for under Basic Benefits for each illness. After the specified number of visits has been accumulated, Basic Benefits begin. The waiting period may be based on the illness, or it may be cumulative for all conditions based on a period of disability.

## Surgery, Assistant Surgery, and Anesthesia

For surgery, assistant surgery, and anesthesia, determination of the Basic Benefit is based on the RVS and plan designated conversion factors. The assistant surgeon's allowance is almost always 20% of the surgeon's basic allowance. Consequently, the conversion factors are the

### Practice Pitfalls

Frank Fryeburger broke his arm while skateboarding. His XYZ contract allows $7 for each visit after three visits. He sees the doctor five times during the treatment of his broken arm. Therefore, the first three visits to the doctor for treatment of the broken arm would not be covered under Basic Benefits. However, the last two visits would be covered at $7 per visit under Basic Benefits. All remaining amounts on these charges would be processed under Major Medical.

### Practice Pitfalls

Terry Tucker, covered under the XYZ contract, had a cholecystectomy (code 47610) on 3/5. The surgery used the services of an anesthesiologist, a surgeon, and an assistant surgeon. The unit value for the surgery is 25.42 for the surgeons and 15.0 for the anesthesiologist.

The basic conversion factor for surgery is $8.50. Therefore, $216.07 (25.42 × $8.5) is payable under the Basic Benefit for the surgeon. Assistant surgeons are paid at 20% of the surgeon's amount. Therefore, $43.21 ($216.07 × 20%) is payable to the assistant surgeon.

The anesthesia conversion factor is $7.50. Therefore, $112.50 (15 × $7.5) is payable as a Basic Benefit for the anesthesiologist.

same for the surgeon and the assistant surgeon. The anesthesia benefit may have the same or a different conversion factor. To get the Basic Benefit for all of these provisions, the conversion factor is multiplied by the RVS unit value. Usually, there is a maximum amount allowed per operative session and often also for a calendar year. After the maximums are reached, these services would be covered only under Major Medical unless excluded under that contract's provisions.

## Order of Basic Benefit Payments

To best use the funds available for Basic Benefits, benefits should be applied in the following order:

1. Hospital benefits.
2. Surgery, assistant surgery, and anesthesia benefits.
3. Physician's visits (in- or outpatient).
4. DXL benefits.
5. Supplemental accident benefits.

## Basic Major Medical Benefits

On a Basic only plan, expenses not paid by the Basic Benefits would not be payable at all. With a Basic-Major Medical Plan, expenses not paid by the Basic portion of the contract may be payable under the Major Medical portion. Different limitations or restrictions may apply to Basic Benefits than to Major Medical benefits. Generally, the following guidelines apply:

1. Pay all applicable Basic Benefits.
2. Refer to the policy or plan document to see whether the excess amounts not paid under the

## Practice Pitfalls

For Terry Tucker (from previous example), let's assume that this is Terry Tucker's first visit this year and no deductible has been satisfied. If the surgeon billed $1,500 for the surgery, and the allowed amount was $1,100, this is how the claim would be processed:

| | |
|---|---|
| Billed amount | $1,500.00 |
| Allowed amount | $1,100.00 |
| Excluded amount | $400.00 |
| Basic Benefit | $216.07 |
| Major Medical amount | $883.93 |
| Deductible amount | $125.00 |
| Remaining | $758.93 |
| Major Medical (payment at 80%) | $607.14 |
| Payment (MM + Basic) | $823.21 |

Basic plan would be eligible under Major Medical.

3. Apply all Major Medical limitations, deductibles, UCR maximums, and other limitations.
4. Add the Basic allowance to the Major Medical allowance to determine the total claim payment.

Usually, the Major Medical portion has a specified dollar deductible amount that must be satisfied yearly before any payments are made. In addition, expenses under Major Medical are not usually paid at 100%, at least not initially. Normally, payments are calculated at 80%, 70%, and so on (this can be any percentage).

With a Basic-Major Medical plan, all Basic Benefits will have two limitations (assuming the services are covered under both the Basic provisions and the Major Medical provisions):

1. The Basic Benefit limitation.
2. The Major Medical UCR or plan limitation.

This will become easier and clearer as you gain practice processing claims.

## Comprehensive Major Medical Benefits

The comprehensive Major Medical plan does not have Basic Benefits per se. However, there may be supplemental or built-in benefits that act the same as a Basic Benefit. In other words, some charges may be covered at 100%, the same as in a Basic plan. All of the definitions previously covered also apply to this type of plan.

All services would be subject to the Major Medical deductible (unless it is waived for certain types of services) and would then be paid at the designated coinsurance rate. Limitations are usually based on a lifetime maximum or calendar year maximum.

## Computing Stoploss

Many Major Medical contracts have a provision that provides for a greater reimbursement percentage (usually 100%) after payment of a certain dollar amount for a calendar year period. This provision limits the amount of money that the member/patient will be responsible for on allowable charges. Such a provision applies only toward "allowable" charges. Expenses not allowed under the plan, such as UCR excess amounts, noncovered expenses, and sometimes those expenses not paid at the regular plan benefit level, such as 50% benefits, would not be applied toward the stoploss. The patient would remain responsible for payment of these charges. An example of such contract wording would be "80% of the first $5,000, 100% thereafter."

To compute stoploss:

### Example 1

The plan coinsurance rate is 90%.
Stoploss is $6,000.

Major Medical paid to date for the year is $5,200.
Claim: $2,225 eligible under Major Medical.

**Step 1.** Subtract the Major Medical amount paid to date for the year from the plan's stoploss limit.

$$\begin{array}{r} \$6,000 \\ -5,200 \\ \hline \$800 \end{array}$$

$800 is 90% of the amount that must be considered by the payer to max the stoploss for the year.

**Step 2.** Calculate the amount that $800 is 90% of to determine the amount of eligible charges subject to the coinsurance stoploss limit. This is done by dividing the remaining amount by the coinsurance percentage.

$800 divided by .90 = $888.89
$888.89 will be covered at 90% to meet the stoploss limitation.

**Step 3.** Subtract the amount covered at 90%, $888.89, from the allowable charges on the claim to determine the amount that will be paid at 100% because the stoploss limit has been met.

| Description | Allowed Amount | Paid at 90% | Paid at 100% |
|---|---|---|---|
| Visit | $100 | $100.00 | 0 |
| Lab Tests | $125 | $125.00 | 0 |
| Surgery | $2,000 | $ 663.89 | $1,336.11 |
| Total | $2,225 | $ 888.89 | $1,336.11 |

**Step 4.** Calculate all remaining items normally. However, since the plan's stoploss has now been met, all subsequent allowable charges will be payable at 100% (there are some exceptions on some plans). Some types of expenses, such as nervous and mental, remain at a specific coinsurance rate regardless of whether the coinsurance limit has been met.

## Example 2

The plan's coinsurance rate is 80%. Stoploss is $6,000. Major Medical paid to date for the year is $5,700. Claim: $2,000 eligible under Major Medical.

**Step 1.** Subtract the amount applied to the Major Medical stoploss limit to date.

$$\begin{array}{r} \$6,000 \\ -5,700 \\ \hline \$300 \end{array}$$

**Step 2.** Calculate the amount that $300 is 80% of to determine the amount of eligible charges subject to the coinsurance stoploss limit. This is done by dividing the remaining amount by the coinsurance percentage.

$300 divided by .80 = $375

$375 will be covered at 80% to meet the stoploss limitation.

**Step 3.** Subtract the amount covered at 80%, $375, from the allowable charges on the claim to determine the amount that will be paid at 100% because the stoploss limit has been met.

| Description | Allowed Amount | Paid at 80% | Paid at 100% |
|---|---|---|---|
| Visit | $100 | $100 | 0 |
| Lab Tests | $75 | $75 | 0 |
| Surgery | $1,825 | $200 | $1,625 |
| Total | $2,000 | $375 | $1,625 |

**Step 4.** Calculate all remaining items normally. However, since the plan's stoploss has now been met, all subsequent allowable charges will be payable at 100% (there are some exceptions on some plans). Some types of expenses, such as nervous and mental, remain at a specific coinsurance rate regardless of whether the coinsurance limit has been met.

## Example 3

The plan's coinsurance rate is 70%.
Stoploss is $5,000.
Major Medical paid to date for the year is $4,000.
Claim: $4,500 eligible under Major Medical (Total submitted charges: $5,000).
This is a Basic/Major Medical contract.

**Step 1.** Subtract the amount applied to the Major Medical stoploss limit to date.

$$\begin{array}{r} \$5,000 \\ -4,000 \\ \hline \$1,000 \end{array}$$

**Step 2.** Calculate the amount that $1,000 is 70% of to determine the amount of eligible charges subject to the coinsurance stoploss limit. This is done by dividing the remaining amount by the coinsurance percentage.

1,000 divided by .70 – $1,428.57

$1,428.57 will be covered at 70% to meet the stoploss limitation.

**Step 3.** Subtract the amount covered at 70% ($1,428.57), from the allowable Major Medical charges on the claim to determine the amount that will be paid at 100%, since the stoploss limit has been met. Remember that Basic Benefits are paid first. Therefore, the amount of the Basic Benefits will be subtracted from the allowed amount to determine the Major Medical amount.

| Desc | Allowed Amount | Basic Benefit | Paid at 70% | Paid at 100% |
|---|---|---|---|---|
| Visit | $100 | $15.65 | $84.35 | 0 |
| Lab | $500 | $110.78 | $389.02 | 0 |
| Surgery | $3,900 | $232.16 | $955.20 | $2,712.64 |
| Total | $4,500 | $358.59 | $1,428.57 | $2,712.64 |

Even though the Basic Benefit and the stoploss benefit are paid at the same amount (100%), they are broken into separate columns on the claim form. This allows anyone reviewing the payment worksheet to see the amounts paid under each benefit.

**Step 4.** Calculate all remaining items normally. However, since the plan's stoploss has now been met, all subsequent allowable charges will be payable at 100% (there are some exceptions on some plans). Some types of expenses, such as nervous and mental, remain at a specific coinsurance rate regardless of whether the coinsurance limit has been met.

The amount(s) paid at the coinsurance percentage will be placed in the Maj Med (Major Medical) column and the amount(s) paid at 100% will be placed in the last column.

# Usual, Customary, and Reasonable (UCR)

Benefit plans define covered expenses as charges for the following services and supplies:

- Those that are medically necessary for the treatment or diagnosis of an injury or illness.
- Those that are ordered or prescribed by a licensed provider.
- Those that do not exceed the usual, customary, and reasonable (UCR) fee generally charged by like providers in the same geographic area for the same procedure.

At one time insurance companies covered a straight percentage of whatever the doctor charged. Over time, however, they found that some doctors were charging a much higher amount for the same procedure than other doctors. This was because doctors were setting their fees based on their perceived needs. For example, a doctor might decide to set his fees according to the personal expenses he had to cover, rather than the actual costs of the procedures. Because of this, fees were increasing at an alarming rate. Eventually, insurance carriers decided to establish a system called **Usual, Customary, and Reasonable (UCR)** to limit their payments. Insurance carriers limit payment to a specified amount based on the UCR system. The **allowed amount** is what the insurance company considers to be a reasonable charge for the procedure performed, and is often less than the amount that the doctor bills.

However, costs in one area of the country are often much less than those in another area of the country. Thus, insurance carriers began compiling data based on the usual amounts charged by doctors in different areas. The information on the average fees charged for a given service in a given area was developed, and fee schedules (or lists of amounts for each procedure) were developed. Eventually the RVS/Conversion Factor method was developed. This system bases amounts on the procedure performed, the geographic location (zip code area) of the provider of service's office, and the date the service was performed.

There are several sources that compile and publish UCR data. Using this data or compiling their own data, third-party administrators and insurance carriers determine the UCR allowances for their plans or clients. Amounts in excess of UCR are not considered to be an allowable expense under the plan and are therefore excluded from all benefit calculations.

UCR is usually applicable only to professional services or to hospital billings that give CPT®/RVS codes. Individually, some administrators are establishing daily UCR amounts for hospital services.

Not all procedures have a UCR fee. For instance, new procedures, experimental procedures, and very unusual and complex procedures may not have an established UCR amount. UCR can be established only when enough procedures of a particular type have been performed in a

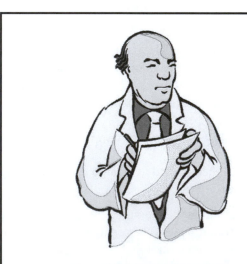

"Let's see, I need new hair implants so I think the insurance carrier should pay me $25 for an aspirin, $100 for taking a pulse..."

geographic area to allow for an "average" or "usual" amount to be determined. Usually, a minimum of 50 operations is required to provide even a rough estimate of the amount that should be considered as usual.

There are several reasons why a UCR amount will not be available, including the following:

- The CPT® code is a BR (By Report) procedure. The value of this service is based on the operative or other lab reports because the service is too unusual or variable to be assigned a unit value.

- The code entered is an RNE (Relatively Not Established) procedure. This indicates new or infrequently performed services for which sufficient data have not been collected to allow an establishment of a relative value.

- The code entered is not listed in the most recent Current Procedural Terminology (CPT®) book because it is a new procedure.

# Resource-Based Relative Value Study

At one time providers were paid based on not only the procedure performed, but also on the degree or title of the provider. For example, an M.D. and a D.C. would receive different amounts for the same procedure.

With the passage of OBRA 90-Public Law 101-608, major changes for physician payment reform took place. One change was the implementation of a fee schedule for physician payment. This fee schedule is based on relative value units that reflect the resources required to provide a service. The fee schedule is based on national uniform relative values for all physicians without respect to area of specialization. See **Table 4–1** for an example of a Relative Value Study.

The **Relative Value Units (RVUs)** represent the total RVS for components of the schedule. Components for resource-based RVS include:

- **Physician's Work Component**—reflects the resources required to furnish the professional service, including the time and the intensity of effort.

- **Overhead or Practice Expense Component**—reflects customary practice expenses (i.e., rent, salaries, staff, equipment cost, and so on).

- **Malpractice or Professional Liability Component**—reflects the risk inherent in providing various procedures. This component does not reflect any specialties but reflects that some procedures are performed routinely by physicians with specialty training in the procedure.

The RVS are to be adjusted for various locales by a geographic adjustment factor. These factors are often referred to as conversion factors.

# Calculating UCR

**UCR calculation** is the process of determining the fee usually charged by similar providers for the same procedure in the same geographic area during a specified period of time.

## Conversion Factors

The **conversion factor** is a dollar amount based on the geographic area (referred to as a **region**) in which the provider practices. For example, Los Angeles may have a surgical conversion factor of $50.64, whereas Bismarck, North Dakota's surgical conversion factor may be $28.

In determining UCR, the listed procedure unit value is multiplied by the plan's appropriate conversion factor or factors. Often there are separate conversion factors for medicine, surgery, diagnostic x-ray and laboratory (DXL), and anesthesia charges. **(see Table 4–2)**.

The appropriate conversion factor is determined by the CPT® code for the procedure, not the description of the service. The ranges of conversion factor categories are:

| | |
|---|---|
| • Medicine | 90000–99499 |
| • Anesthesia | 00100–01999 |
| • Surgery | 10000–69999 |
| • DXL | 70010–89999 |

# Relative Value Study

| CPT ®/HCPCS | Description | Total RVUs | Follow-up Days |
|---|---|---|---|
| 00215 | ANESTHESIA FOR CRANIOPLASTY | 9.0 | -- |
| 00400 | ANESTHESIA, INTEGUMENTARY SYSTEM, EXTREMITIES | 3.0 | -- |
| 00520 | ANESTHESIA FOR CLOSED CHEST PROCEDURES | 6.0 | -- |
| 00534 | ANESTHESIA FOR TRANSVENOUS INSERTION | 7.0 | -- |
| 00868 | ANESTHESIA FOR RENAL TRANSPLANT | 10.0 | -- |
| 01230 | ANESTHESIA FOR UPPER 2/3 OF FEMUR, OPEN | 6.0 | -- |
| 01480 | ANESTHESIA, ON BONES OF LOWER LEG, OPEN | 30 | -- |
| 01990 | PHYSIOLOGICAL SUPPORT, BRAIN-DEAD PATIENT | 7.0 | -- |
| 15570 | FORMATION OF DIRECT OR TUBED PEDICLE | 10.0 | 90 |
| 15952 | EXCISION TROCHANTERIC PRESSURE ULCER | 8.0 | 90 |
| 19125 | EXCISION OF BREAST LESION | 7.0 | 30 |
| 19126 | EXCISION OF BREAST LESION, EACH ADDITIONAL | 3.5 | 30 |
| 20205 | BIOPSY, MUSCLE, DEEP | 2.4 | 15 |
| 21800 | CLOSED TREATMENT OF RIB FRACTURE, EACH | 18.0 | 90 |
| 24102 | ARTHROTOMY, ELBOW WITH SYNOVECTOMY | 14.5 | 90 |
| 25622 | CLOSED TREAT OF CARPAL SCAPHOID FRACTURE | 3.5 | 60 |
| 27350 | PATELLECTOMY OR HEMIPATELLECTOMY | 12.0 | 60 |
| 27372 | REMOVAL OF FOREIGN BODY, DEEP, THIGH REGION | 5.2 | 30 |
| 27758 | OPEN TREATMENT OF TIBIAL SHAFT FRACTURE | 12.7 | 30 |
| 27784 | OPEN TREATMENT OF PROXIMAL FIBULA SHAFT FX | 12.7 | 90 |
| 28456 | PERCUTANEOUS SKELETAL FIXATION OF TARSAL BONE FX | 3.9 | 90 |
| 30125 | EXCISION DERMOID CYST NOSE, UNDER BONE | 8.5 | 30 |
| 31200 | ETHMOIDECTOMY | 7.0 | 90 |
| 31225 | MAXILLECTOMY WITHOUT ORBITAL EXENTERATION | 22.5 | 120 |
| 32800 | REPAIR LUNG HERNIA THROUGH CHEST WALL | 12.0 | 30 |
| 33217 | INSERTION OF A TRANSVENOUS ELECTRODE | 9.5 | 15 |
| 33225 | INSERTION OF PACING ELECTRODE | BR | -- |
| 33240 | INSERTION OF SINGLE OR DUAL CHAMBER PACING | 0.7 | 15 |
| 36430 | TRANSFUSION, BLOOD | 0.4 | 00 |
| 38100 | SPLENECTOMY, TOTAL | 16.0 | 45 |
| 39520 | REPAIR, DIAPHRAGMATIC HERNIA | 17.0 | 90 |
| 39545 | IMBRICATION OF DIAPHRAGM FOR EVENTRATION | 12.0 | 90 |

**Table 4–1  RVS Schedule**                                      *(continued on next page)*

| 40808 | BIOPSY, VESTIBULE OF MOUTH | 0.7 | 00 |
|---|---|---|---|
| 43840 | GASTRORRHAPHY, SUTURE PERFORATED ULCER | 14.0 | 45 |
| 47630 | BILIARY DUCT STONE EXTRACTION | 7.0 | 45 |
| 49560 | REPAIR INITIAL INCISIONAL OR VENTRAL HERNIA | 11.5 | 45 |
| 52500 | TRANSURETHRAL RESECTION OF BLADDER NECK | 10.0 | 90 |
| 58700 | SALPINGECTOMY, COMPLETE OR PARTIAL | 11.4 | 90 |
| 59400 | ROUTINE OBSTETRIC CARE | 20.0 | 45 |
| 59820 | TREATMENT OF MISSED ABORTION | 4.5 | 30 |
| 61703 | SURGERY OF INTRACRANIAL ANEURYSM | 13.0 | 90 |
| 62000 | ELEVATION OF DEPRESSED SKULL FRACTURE | 8.3 | 90 |
| 65800 | PARACENTESIS OF ANTERIOR CHAMBER OF EYE | 3.0 | 00 |
| 69400 | EUSTACHIAN TUBE INFLATION | 0.3 | 00 |
| 70250 | RADIOLOGIC EXAM, SKULL | 3.1 | -- |
| 70260 | RADIOLOGIC EXAM, SKULL, COMPLETE | 5.0 | -- |
| 70450 | CAT SCAN, SKULL | 21.7 | -- |
| 71020 | RADIOLOGIC EXAM, CHEST | 3.2 | -- |
| 73100 | RADIOLOGIC EXAM, WRIST | 2.5 | -- |
| 73130 | RADIOLOGIC EXAM, HAND, MINIMUM 3 VIEWS | 2.8 | -- |
| 73550 | RADIOLOGIC EXAM, FEMUR | 2.8 | -- |
| 73590 | RADIOLOGIC EXAM, TIBIA AND FIBULA | 2.5 | -- |
| 73718 | MRI LEG | 55.0 | -- |
| 74250 | RADIOLOGIC EXAM, SMALL INTESTINE | 6.6 | -- |
| 76090 | MAMMOGRAPHY, UNILATERAL | 4.5 | -- |
| 76092 | SCREENING MAMMOGRAPHY, BILATERAL | 4.5 | -- |
| 76870 | ECHOGRAPHY, SCROTUM AND CONTENTS | 8.0 | -- |
| 76872 | ECHOGRAPHY, TRANSRECTAL | 13.8 | -- |
| 78810 | TUMOR IMAGING | 100.0 | -- |
| 80048 | BASIC METABOLIC PANEL | 1.3 | -- |
| 80053 | COMPREHENSIVE METABOLIC PANEL | 1.6 | -- |

**Table 4–1**   (*continued*)

| 81000 | URINALYSIS | 0.7 | -- |
|-------|-----------|-----|-----|
| 82310 | CALCIUM, TOTAL | 1.0 | -- |
| 83540 | IRON | 1.6 | -- |
| 85025 | BLOOD COUNT, COMPLETE, AUTOMATED | 0.8 | -- |
| 85610 | PROTHROMBIN TIME | 0.6 | -- |
| 86901 | BLOODTYPING, RH (D) | 1.1 | -- |
| 87040 | CULTURE, BACTERIAL; BLOOD | 1.2 | -- |
| 87070 | CULTURE, BACTERIAL OTHER SOURCE | 1.3 | -- |
| 88150 | CYTOPATHOLOGY, SLIDES, CERVICAL OR VAGINAL | 0.9 | -- |
| 90782 | THERAPEUTIC, INJECTION | 2.5 | -- |
| 93000 | EKG | 7.8 | -- |
| 93545 | INJECTION DURING ANGIOGRAPHY | 22.0 | -- |
| 94060 | BRONCHOSPASM EVALUATION | 20.0 | -- |
| 97116 | GAIT TRAINING | 7.0 | -- |
| 99201 | OFFICE OR OTHER OUTPATIENT VISIT, NEW | 6.5 | -- |
| 99213 | OV ESTABLISHED PATIENT, EXPANDED | 9.0 | -- |
| 99284 | EMERGENCY VISIT, DETAILED | 25.0 | -- |
| 99285 | EMERGENCY VISIT, COMPREHENSIVE | 37.0 | -- |

**Table 4–1** *(continued)*

## Practice
# Pitfalls

Tonsillectomy, 42820, RVS, Unit Value = 16.39. Geographic conversion factor for San Francisco (zip code 940XX) is $39.54. To determine UCR for this procedure, multiply the RVS unit value of 16.39 by the conversion factor of $39.54 (for 940XX, San Francisco). The total UCR amount is $648.06. This amount would be placed in the Allowed Amount column on the Payment Worksheet (see Medical Claims Administration chapter).

On a Basic-Major Medical plan, two limits must be calculated:

- Basic allowed amount, and
- Total plan or major medical allowed amount.

The basic benefit usually has a dollar conversion factor specified in the plan document. Consequently, all providers, regardless of their geographic location or when the service is performed, receive the same basic allowance for a specific procedure. Also, the basic allowance is usually paid at 100%. Conversely, the UCR allowance under Major Medical is not normally specified in the plan document because it is usually upgraded periodically due to inflation.

# UCR Conversion Factor Report

The following list of UCR Conversion Factors is intended to be used for training and reference purposes only.

| Zip | Area | Including Zip Codes | Surgery | Medicine | X-Ray & Lab (DXL) | Anesthesia |
|-----|------|---------------------|---------|----------|-------------------|------------|
| 006 | Puerto Rico | 006-009 | 35.58 | 31.13 | 26.68 | 22.14 |
| 039 | Maine | 039-049 | 31.01 | 27.13 | 23.26 | 31.34 |
| 100 | New York City | 100-102 | 66.02 | 57.77 | 49.51 | 30.30 |
| 125 | Poughkeepsie, Monticello, NE NY | 125, 127-129, 136 | 40.71 | 35.62 | 30.53 | 32.71 |
| 153 | Southwestern PA | 153-158 | 36.76 | 32.16 | 27.57 | 25.25 |
| 210 | Baltimore Area | 210, 211, 214 | 48.00 | 42.00 | 36.00 | 35.35 |
| 255 | Huntington, Wheeling, Parkesburg, Morgantown | 255, 257, 260, 261, 265 | 32.94 | 28.82 | 24.70 | 31.14 |
| 302 | Atlanta | 302, 303 | 38.86 | 34.00 | 29.14 | 47.43 |
| 354 | Alabama-miscellaneous | 354-357, 359-360, 363-365, 368, 324 | 30.90 | 27.04 | 23.18 | 32.06 |
| 441 | Cleveland, Youngstown Area | 441, 444 | 37.10 | 32.46 | 27.83 | 38.69 |
| 480 | Detroit | 480-482, 485 | 36.63 | 32.05 | 27.47 | 31.41 |
| 550 | Minneapolis-St Paul Area | 550, 551, 553 | 26.42 | 23.12 | 19.81 | 29.46 |
| 580 | North Dakota | 580-588 | 28.00 | 24.50 | 21.00 | 23.12 |
| 606 | Chicago | 606 | 45.64 | 39.94 | 34.23 | 49.57 |
| 640 | Kansas City Area | 640-641, 661-662 | 33.48 | 29.29 | 25.11 | 40.30 |
| 770 | Houston | 770,772,775 | 40.60 | 35.52 | 30.45 | 42.66 |

**Table 4–2** Conversion Factor Report

(continued on next page)

| 777 | Austin & Beaumont | 777,779,787,788 | 33.10 | 28.96 | 24.82 | 50.31 |
|---|---|---|---|---|---|---|
| 801 | Denver, CO Springs, Alamosa, Glenwood Springs Area | 801-803,806,808, 811,816 | 32.32 | 28.28 | 24.24 | 41.69 |
| 890 | Reno & Area | 890, 895, 897 | 34.38 | 30.08 | 25.78 | 49.11 |
| 904 | Santa Monica, Long Beach, Glendale | 904, 908, 912 | 45.18 | 39.53 | 33.89 | 47.94 |
| 970 | Portland & Western OR | 970, 971, 974, 975 | 30.87 | 27.01 | 23.15 | 34.20 |

**Table 4–2** *(continued)*

# On the Job Now

**Directions:** Using the Conversion Factor Report (**see Table 4–2**), list the Surgery, Medicine, DXL, and Anesthesia conversion factors for the following zip codes.

| Zip Code | Surgery | Medicine | DXL | Anesthesia |
|---|---|---|---|---|
| 1. 12745 | _____ | _____ | _____ | _____ |
| 2. 77539 | _____ | _____ | _____ | _____ |
| 3. 97123 | _____ | _____ | _____ | _____ |
| 4. 78793 | _____ | _____ | _____ | _____ |
| 5. 04064 | _____ | _____ | _____ | _____ |
| 6. 89556 | _____ | _____ | _____ | _____ |
| 7. 21438 | _____ | _____ | _____ | _____ |
| 8. 66245 | _____ | _____ | _____ | _____ |
| 9. 81679 | _____ | _____ | _____ | _____ |
| 10. 00615 | _____ | _____ | _____ | _____ |

11. 55332  _____  _____  _____  _____

12. 77785  _____  _____  _____  _____

13. 90812  _____  _____  _____  _____

14. 26593  _____  _____  _____  _____

15. 97480  _____  _____  _____  _____

16. 36845  _____  _____  _____  _____

17. 30267  _____  _____  _____  _____

18. 58655  _____  _____  _____  _____

19. 89754  _____  _____  _____  _____

20. 15543  _____  _____  _____  _____

21. 30378  _____  _____  _____  _____

22. 91245  _____  _____  _____  _____

23. 64145  _____  _____  _____  _____

24. 03945  _____  _____  _____  _____

25. 25576  _____  _____  _____  _____

26. 55378  _____  _____  _____  _____

27. 44127  _____  _____  _____  _____

28. 80675  _____  _____  _____  _____

29. 58356  _____  _____  _____  _____

30. 97439  _____  _____  _____  _____

## Basic Allowance

Refer to the contract for XYZ Corporation. As indicated, this is a Basic-Major Medical plan. For office visits, the conversion factor is $7.50, and for DXL it is $7. To calculate the Basic payment:

1. Look up the procedure code and determine the relative unit value that applies to the procedure for the specified schedule.

2. Multiply the RVS unit value by the plan basic conversion factor. (In the case of XYZ, it would be $7 for DXL or $7.50 for office visits.)

## Practice Pitfalls

A claim is submitted with a charge for a bacterial culture, blood (87040). This has a unit value of 1.2. The basic conversion factor of $7 for DXL (XYZ contract) is multiplied by the 1.2 basic unit value for a basic allowance amount of $8.40.

The resulting figure will be the amount payable at 100% under Basic Benefits.

## Major Medical UCR

To calculate the Major Medical UCR limit:

1. Look up the procedure code and determine the relative unit value that applies to the procedure for the specified schedule.

2. Multiply the RVS unit value by the plan (or Major Medical) conversion factor based on:

   a. The specific time period during which the services were provided.

   b. The geographic location of the provider (using the first three digits of the zip code).

   c. The type of service being performed (i.e., surgery, medical). This will give you the allowed amount for the procedure.

3. Then subtract any amounts paid at the basic rate. This will give you the Major Medical amount.

## Practice Pitfalls

A claim is submitted with a charge for a bacterial culture, blood (87040). This has a unit value of 1.2. The provider lives in Atlanta, GA, zip code 30325. The DXL conversion factor for zip codes starting with 303 is $29.14. Therefore, the conversion factor of $29.14 for DXL is multiplied by 1.2 for an allowed amount of $34.97. The basic amount (figured above) is $8.40. This amount is subtracted from the $34.97, leaving $26.57 (the Major Medical amount).

The figure arrived at will be the maximum amount allowed under the plan. "Allowed" does not necessarily mean the same as "paid."

Amounts over the Major Medical UCR allowance are not considered covered by the plan. The UCR amount or the lesser amount (if the amount is lower than the UCR amount) is applied toward all of the plan limitations, including the deductible and coinsurance. The amounts not covered by the plan are the patient's sole responsibility.

Normally, if the provider's charge exceeds the UCR allowance by more than 20% or 25%, a Peer Review (consultant) may be required.

# On the Job Now

1. What does UCR mean? _____

2. What is UCR based on? _____

_____

_____

3. Explain why a procedure may not have a UCR allowance. _____

_____

_____

4. How do you calculate Major Medical UCR? _____

_____

5. How do you calculate the basic allowance? _____

_____

6. (True or False?) The maximum amount allowed under the plan will always be the amount paid. _____

7. Are amounts in excess of the UCR allowance considered covered by the plan? _____

## Special Services

The services in the procedure code range of 99000–99199 are considered special services. Regardless of the type of service provided, the UCR calculation is based on the medicine conversion factor category.

## Modifiers

When using modifiers the unit value or UCR amount should be increased or decreased based on the special circumstances which the modifier represents. For example, modifier –80 indicates that the person submitting the claim is the assistant surgeon, not the surgeon. Since the assistant surgeon is not responsible for the preoperative or postoperative care, is not responsible for the life of the patient, and only assists the surgeon during the surgery, the assistant surgeon is paid at 20% of the amount allowed for the surgeon. Thus, the UCR for an assistant surgeon would be calculated as RVS unit value multiplied by conversion factor × 20%.

There may also be adjustments based on whether or not there were multiple or asterisk procedures.

For standard adjustments on modifiers, consult the CPT® book. For those modifications not listed, the adjustment will vary according to the insurance carrier's policy and the contract provisions. We have listed the most common modifiers in the appropriate chapter (i.e., the surgical modifiers are included in the Surgery and Anesthesia Claims chapter).

# On the Job Now

**Directions:** Using the ABC Corporation contract, calculate the plan UCR amounts. Use the conversion factor for zip code 90820.

| Procedure Code | Description | Conversion Factor | Units | Amount |
|---|---|---|---|---|
| 1. 15952 | Excision Trochanteric Pressure Ulcer | _____ | _____ | _____ |
| 2. 93000 | EKG | _____ | _____ | _____ |
| 3. 27372 | Removal of Foreign Body, Deep, Thigh | _____ | _____ | _____ |
| 4. 78810 | Tumor Imaging | _____ | _____ | _____ |
| 5. 70250 | Radiologic Exam, Skull | _____ | _____ | _____ |
| 6. 19125 | Excision of Breast Lesion | _____ | _____ | _____ |
| 7. 36430 | Transfusion, Blood | _____ | _____ | _____ |
| 8. 87040 | Culture, Bacterial; Blood | _____ | _____ | _____ |
| 9. 40808 | Biopsy, Vestibule of Mouth | _____ | _____ | _____ |
| 10. 20205 | Biopsy, Muscle, Deep | _____ | _____ | _____ |
| 11. 47630 | Bilary Duct Stone Extraction | _____ | _____ | _____ |
| 12. 59820 | Treatment of Missed Abortion | _____ | _____ | _____ |
| 13. 86901 | Blood Typing, RH (D) | _____ | _____ | _____ |
| 14. 69400 | Eustachain Tube Inflation | _____ | _____ | _____ |
| 15. 32800 | Repair Hernia Through Chest Wall | _____ | _____ | _____ |

# On the Job Now

**Directions:** Using the Ninja Enterprises contract, calculate the plan UCR amounts. Use the conversion factor for zip code 36810.

| Proc. Code | Description | Conversion Factor | Units | Amount |
|---|---|---|---|---|
| 1. 15952 | Excision Trochanteric Pressure Ulcer | _____ | _____ | _____ |
| 2. 93000 | EKG | _____ | _____ | _____ |
| 3. 27372 | Removal of Foreign Body, Deep, Thigh | _____ | _____ | _____ |
| 4. 78810 | Tumor Imaging | _____ | _____ | _____ |
| 5. 70250 | Radiologic Exam, Skull | _____ | _____ | _____ |
| 6. 19125 | Excision of Breast Lesion | _____ | _____ | _____ |
| 7. 36430 | Transfusion, Blood | _____ | _____ | _____ |
| 8. 87040 | Culture, Bacterial; Blood | _____ | _____ | _____ |
| 9. 40808 | Biopsy, Vestibule of Mouth | _____ | _____ | _____ |
| 10. 20205 | Biopsy, Muscle, Deep | _____ | _____ | _____ |
| 11. 47630 | Bilary Duct Stone Extraction | _____ | _____ | _____ |
| 12. 59820 | Treatment of Missed Abortion | _____ | _____ | _____ |
| 13. 86901 | Blood Typing, RH (D) | _____ | _____ | _____ |
| 14. 69400 | Eustachain Tube Inflation | _____ | _____ | _____ |
| 15. 32800 | Repair Hernia Through Chest Wall | _____ | _____ | _____ |

# On the Job Now

**Directions:** Using the XYZ Corporation contract, calculate both basic and plan UCR amounts. Use the conversion factor for zip code 04143.

| Proc. Code | Description | Conversion Factor | Units | Basic Allowance | Major Medical Allowance |
|---|---|---|---|---|---|
| 1. 15952 | Excision Trochanteric Pressure Ulcer | _____ | _____ | _____ | _____ |
| 2. 93000 | EKG | _____ | _____ | _____ | _____ |
| 3. 27372 | Removal of Foreign Body, Deep, Thigh | _____ | _____ | _____ | _____ |
| 4. 78810 | Tumor Imaging | _____ | _____ | _____ | _____ |
| 5. 70250 | Radiologic Exam, Skull | _____ | _____ | _____ | _____ |

| Proc. Code | Description | Conversion Factor | Units | Basic Allowance | Major Medical Allowance |
|---|---|---|---|---|---|
| 6. 19125 | Excision of Breast Lesion | _____ | _____ | _____ | _____ |
| 7. 36430 | Transfusion, Blood | _____ | _____ | _____ | _____ |
| 8. 87040 | Culture, Bacterial; Blood | _____ | _____ | _____ | _____ |
| 9. 40808 | Biopsy, Vestibule of Mouth | _____ | _____ | _____ | _____ |
| 10. 20205 | Biopsy, Muscle, Deep | _____ | _____ | _____ | _____ |
| 11. 47630 | Bilary Duct Stone Extraction | _____ | _____ | _____ | _____ |
| 12. 59820 | Treatment of Missed Abortion | _____ | _____ | _____ | _____ |
| 13. 86901 | Blood Typing, RH (D) | _____ | _____ | _____ | _____ |
| 14. 69400 | Eustachain Tube Inflation | _____ | _____ | _____ | _____ |
| 15. 32800 | Repair Hernia Through Chest Wall | _____ | _____ | _____ | _____ |

## Fee Schedules

Some plans have established their own calculations of the amount payable for particular services. These amounts are listed on what is commonly called a **fee schedule (see Table 4–3)**. Fees are assigned according to the particular CPT® code, and this is considered the allowable amount for that particular procedure.

If a fee schedule is used, the claims examiner looks up the appropriate code to obtain the allowed amount. This eliminates the need for numerous calculations and can speed up the process of claims examining. However, the compensation with the schedules is the same in a large city as it is in outlying areas.

## Fee Schedule

| CPT® Code | Description | Allowed Amount | Follow-up Days |
|---|---|---|---|
| 00400 | ANESTHESIA, INTEGUMENTARY SYSTEM, EXTREMITIES | 98.13 | -- |
| 19126 | EXCISION OF BREAST LESION, EACH | 142.49 | 30 |
| 24102 | ARTHROTOMY, ELBOW WITH SYNOVECTOMY | 590.30 | 90 |
| 28456 | PERCUTANEOUS SKELETAL FIXATION OF TARSAL BONE FX | 158.77 | 90 |
| 36430 | TRANSFUSION, BLOOD | 16.28 | 00 |
| 49560 | REPAIR INITIAL INCISIONAL OR VENTRAL HERNIA | 468.17 | 45 |
| 59820 | TREATMENT OF MISSED ABORTION | 183.20 | 30 |
| 65800 | PARACENTESIS OF ANTERIOR CHAMBER OF EYE | 122.13 | 00 |
| 70250 | RADIOLOGIC EXAM, SKULL | 94.64 | -- |
| 76090 | MAMMOGRAPHY, UNILATERAL | 137.39 | -- |
| 80053 | COMPREHENSIVE METABOLIC PANEL | 48.85 | -- |
| 99201 | OFFICE OR OTHER OUTPATIENT VISIT, NEW | 264.61 | -- |

**Table 4–3  Fee Schedule (sample of various codes)**

# Cost Containment Programs

Until the tremendous growth in healthcare costs triggered the need for new approaches, plan sponsors had been primarily concerned with improving employees' access to quality medical care. As a result of the increased healthcare costs of the last 40 years, many employers have been struggling to provide adequate care for their employees at an affordable cost. Because of this, a variety of programs have been developed to slow down the rate of increase in both the premiums and the cost of healthcare.

Some of the more popular methods used in trying to slow down spiraling healthcare costs include the following:

- Preadmission Testing (PAT).
- Precertification of Inpatient Admissions.
- Utilization Review (UR).
- Second Surgical Opinion (SSO) Consultation.
- Preferred Provider Organizations (PPO).
- Health Maintenance Organizations (HMO).

Other cost containment programs include:

**Preauthorization**—A number of insurance carriers will require that certain benefits be preauthorized before the services are received. Preauthorization means to gain approval of the services that are to be performed, as well as to obtain an understanding of whether or not the insurance carrier will provide coverage for these services.

**Predetermination**—An estimate of maximum benefits that may be paid under the plan for the services. It is not, however, a guarantee that benefits will be paid.

## Preadmission Testing

Preadmission testing (PAT) was designed to reduce the duration of elective hospital confinements. This benefit is appropriate for scheduled, nonemergency hospital admissions that require the standard prerequisite testing before surgery. As a rule, this type of testing is restricted to a period of three to seven days before admission. Additionally, some plans limit the place of testing to either the hospital where the surgery is performed or the patient's regular provider of services.

No payments under PAT are made for preadmission tests that are performed during the hospitalization, or those results that are rejected by the physician as unreliable. Since preadmission testing generally serves to reduce costs, most plans offer an incentive to the member to use PAT by paying these charges at a higher coinsurance level than regular testing or hospital-related services.

**Example:** Outpatient diagnostic tests performed prior to inpatient admission paid at 100% whether through a network provider or not.

## Precertification of Inpatient Admissions

**Precertification** means preapproval for admission on an elective, nonemergency hospitalization. Contact is made either with the plan administrator or to some other entity sanctioned to determine the necessity of the admission. Most often, these entities are comprised of a specialized group of nurses working under the direction of a physician. The nurses deal directly with the physician's office and the facility to determine whether the admission is necessary and whether the number of days of care is medically necessary. If the patient stays longer than the approved number of days, the additional days of care may not be covered or the usual payment may be reduced by a percentage specified in the plan document. The objective of this program is to prevent unnecessary admissions and to get the patient out of the hospital as soon as is medically appropriate.

Some programs provide for precertification only prior to or on the day of hospitalization. Other programs provide for a complete approach to managing the care, which entails a utilization review program.

As part of HIPAA, the Federal Government has mandated that no precertification can be required on maternity confinements. The law stipulates a confinement for a normal delivery cannot be limited to less than 48 hours (two days) or in the case of a cesarean section 96 hours (four days). The law, however, does not state that a concurrent review cannot be required. Therefore, if the patient stays hospital-confined beyond the two days for a normal delivery or four days for a cesarean section and the plan has concurrent review and extended stay provisions, applicable penalties can be imposed on those extra days.

## Utilization Review

As previously indicated, precertification or a prospective review determines the need and appropriateness of the recommended care. **Utilization review (UR)** is a process whereby insurance carriers review the total treatment of a patient and determine whether or not the costs will be covered. A complete Utilization Review program contains the following three components:

1. Precertification (prior to) or prospective review.
2. Concurrent review (during the confinement).
3. Retrospective review (after termination of confinement).

**Concurrent review** determines whether the estimated length of time and scope of the inpatient stay is justified by the diagnosis and symptoms. This review is conducted periodically during the projected length of stay. If the length of stay exceeds the criteria or if there is a change in treatment, the matter is referred to the medical consultant for review. This consultant at no time dictates the method of treatment or the length of stay. These decisions are left entirely to the patient and the attending physician. However, the consultant is entitled to inform the patient, physician, and facility that the continued stay exceeds the approved number of days and may not be covered by the plan as medically necessary. It is then the patient's responsibility to decide what action to take.

**Retrospective review** is used to determine after discharge whether the hospitalization and treatment were medically necessary and covered by the terms of the benefit program. This type of review may be used as a substitute for admission and concurrent reviews when the failure to notify the UR program of an admission prevents the regular review procedures. However, the main drawback to the retrospective review is that the patient and providers are not notified about the services that will not be covered until after they have been provided. The best programs always work most effectively when the patient is notified beforehand that he or she will be primarily responsible for payment of services. This approach deters the member from incurring unanticipated expenses.

## Second Surgical Opinion Consultations

Surgical claims represent the second highest categorical cost to benefit plans (hospitalization ranks first). The United States has the world's highest rate of surgical treatment because neither the physician nor the patient has any financial incentive to consider less expensive alternatives.

About 80% of all surgeries can be considered "elective." That is, they are not required because of a life-threatening situation. The objective of a Second Surgical Opinion Consultation (SSO) is to eliminate elective surgical procedures that are classified as unnecessary.

**Unnecessary surgery** is that which is recommended as an elective procedure when an alternative method of treatment may be preferable for a number of reasons, including:

- The surgery itself may be premature, taking into consideration all pathologic indications.
- The risk to the patient may not justify the benefits of surgery.
- An alternative medical treatment may be superior for both medical and cost-effective reasons.
- A less severe surgical procedure may be preferable under the circumstances. Or, no medical or surgical procedure may be necessary at all.

In this program, the plan participant consults an independent specialist to determine whether the recommended elective surgical procedure is advisable. This process is not intended to interfere with the patient-physician relationship or to prevent the participant from receiving necessary elective operations. This program may be administered in one of two ways:

1. A **mandatory program** requires the patient to obtain an SSO for specific procedures, or there is an automatic reduction or denial of benefits. For an example of this type of program, see the Ninja Enterprises contract.
2. A **voluntary program** encourages participants to have an SSO, but there is no automatic reduction of benefits if the patient does not comply.

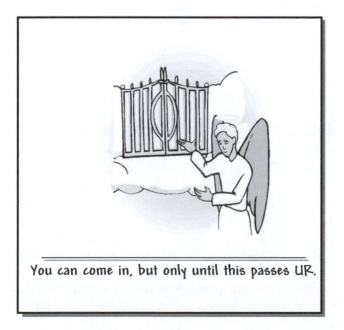

You can come in, but only until this passes UR.

In both approaches, the SSO and related tests are usually paid at 100% so that the patient will not have any out-of-pocket expenses for conforming to the program.

The SSO program has met with much criticism because it has not effectively reduced the number of elective surgeries. One of the main reasons for this ineffectiveness is that physicians may be reluctant to tell a patient that a surgery is not necessary. This attitude stems from the growing number of malpractice lawsuits. For example, if a physician indicates that a patient does not need surgery and a sudden emergency situation arises that is related to the original need for surgery, the physician may be held liable under a malpractice suit. Consequently, many plans are abandoning the SSO plan provision.

# Managed Care

**Managed care** is a strategy for reducing or controlling healthcare costs by closely monitoring and restricting the use and cost of services. With this type of system, the insurer manages the delivery of healthcare and controls costs by emphasizing primary and preventive care services. Managed care plans use quality assurance and utilization review to ensure the appropriate delivery of care. Preferred provider organizations, HMO's, and point-of-service plans are examples of managed care plans. An **in-network** provider is a physician or other service provider who is contracted with a managed care plan. An **out-of-network** provider is a healthcare provider with whom a managed care organization does not have a contract to provide healthcare services.

## Preferred Provider Organizations

A **Preferred Provider Organization (PPO)** is a group of healthcare providers who agree to provide services to a specific pool of patients for an agreed fee (contractual). PPOs include doctors, dentists, hospitals, and any provider group that contracts with another entity to provide services at competitive fees.

PPO packages may involve contractual agreements for a limited number of healthcare services or for a full range of inpatient and outpatient medical services. Because the PPO group has agreed to specific benefits, they usually have their own utilization review committees or guidelines to reduce the amount of testing performed, hospitalizations, and other services.

In some cases, a health plan may continue to offer standard indemnity coverage but may also offer special PPO arrangements in which the PPO provider is paid more quickly and at a higher rate than non-PPO providers. In such a case, the plan participant saves money because out-of-pocket expenses are also reduced. The Ninja contract is an example of a PPO contract.

Many PPO providers are available. The benefits of a PPO provider compared with a non-PPO provider vary greatly from plan to plan. However, generally both the patient and the plan reduce costs by being members of a good PPO.

Some of the advantages for the patient associated with being in a PPO are:

- Reduced healthcare costs with no restriction (or with only minimal restrictions) of freedom of choice of providers. Reduced healthcare costs mean reduced out-of-pocket expenses.
- Less paperwork in filing claims because the PPO submits the claim directly to the payer and payment is made directly to the PPO.
- Treatment only for services that are medically necessary because there is usually a formal utilization review program.

Some of the advantages to the provider associated with being in a PPO are:

- Increased patient volume.
- Prompt claim payment.
- Reduced financial risk due to automatic assignment of benefits.
- Active participation in local cost-containment efforts.

Some of the advantages to the benefit plan associated with being in a PPO are:

- Reduced healthcare cost.
- Better utilization control.

## Health Maintenance Organizations

A **Health Maintenance Organization (HMO)** is a type of prepayment policy in which the organization bears the responsibility and financial risk of providing agreed-on healthcare services to the members enrolled in its plan, in exchange for a fixed monthly membership fee. This fee can be paid by the member himself, or it can be paid on his behalf by his employer or government-sponsored plan.

If services are available through the HMO but the insured does not go through the HMO provider, either the benefit will be reduced or the member will be entirely responsible for the payment of care received. Any services provided outside the HMO network must be preapproved by the HMO to be covered. If services are not approved, the HMO usually will not pay the charges.

The main difference between a PPO and an HMO is that an HMO provider receives a monthly fee based on capitation (number of covered plan members), whereas a PPO provider is paid only when a member is treated. A disadvantage of the HMO arrangement is the limitation of the patient's freedom of choice of physicians. In addition, the location of the HMO facilities may be limited or inconvenient for many plan members.

## Exclusive Provider Organizations

In the **Exclusive Provider Organization (EPO)**, the patient must select a primary care provider and can only use physicians who are part of the network or who are referred by the primary care physician. EPO physicians are paid as services are rendered, after which they get a capitation or utilization bonus from the carrier.

## Gatekeeper PPO

In the **Gatekeeper PPO**, the member chooses a family provider or physician and must see him or her before being referred to a specialist. The specialist may or may not be within the network. In essence, the family physician is the "gatekeeper" to alternative services and can choose to refer the patient or not.

## Physician Hospital Organizations

A **Physician Hospital Organization (PHO)** is an organization of physicians and hospitals that bands together for the purpose of obtaining contracts from payer organizations. The PHO bargains as an entity for preferred provider status with various payers. The organization also refers clients to each other.

## Management Service Organizations

A **Management Service Organization (MSO)** is a separate corporation set up to provide management services to a medical group for a fee. Individual physicians and providers contract with the MSO for services. An MSO may be owned by a single hospital, several hospitals, or investors.

## Medical Case Management

**Medical Case Management (MCM)** is the process of evaluating the effectiveness and frequency of medical treatments by reviewing services to determine whether the care that is being rendered or that is going to be rendered is appropriate. When a situation arises in which the potential for high claims payment exists based on the diagnosis or the type of services needed by the claimant, the case is generally referred to the Medical Case Management Department. The MCM (in some instances, an outside company performs this function) reviews these cases and tries to minimize the company's loss by finding alternative solutions for patient care. This may necessitate providing the patient with equipment or care that is normally not covered under the plan if it is more cost-effective for the plan and also beneficial to the patient to make these provisions. MCM usually focuses on high dollar claims involving inpatient hospital confinements. Less costly alternatives, such as hospice, nursing home, and home healthcare with discounted nursing or equipment, are explored.

An important goal of MCM is to save costs for the insured, the patient, the plan, the healthcare providers, and the administrator. Furthermore, this process can result in higher quality care.

Under most plans, MCM is a voluntary process. To be successful, the cooperation of the patient and family is important.

Situations that may indicate possible claims for MCM are included in Appendix C. The health claims examiner should watch carefully for certain factors that may indicate that a claim file is a good candidate for MCM. These factors include:

1. Pattern of repeated hospital admissions (or two within six months).

2. Outpatient therapies of more than six weeks (including nursing services).

3. Home care by an RN of more than four hours per day.

4. Skilled nursing care in an extended care facility of more than six weeks.

5. Any hospital interim bill (excessive length of stay).

6. Any terminal or progressive disease requiring long-term skilled care.

Use experience and common sense to identify claims that are unusual and may become "catastrophic" by virtue of chronicity or immediately high cost.

# CHAPTER REVIEW

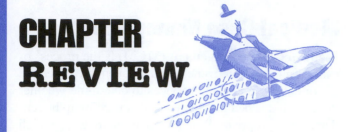

## Summary

- The three major types of indemnity coverage currently available are:
  1. Basic only.
  2. Basic-Major Medical.
  3. Comprehensive Major Medical.
- It is important to understand the terminology associated with contracts and how benefit payments are calculated under each type of coverage.
- Quick and accurate benefit payments are what make a health claims examiner a valuable employee.
- The concept of usual, customary, and reasonable charges allows a payer to determine allowable charges based on what is considered to be a usual and reasonable charge for a given service performed in a given area.
- This prevents the paying of excessive benefits to doctors who may charge high fees on their bills.
- UCR allows for the payment of higher rates in areas in which there is a higher cost of doing business (i.e., building costs, personnel) and lower rates in areas in which there is a lower cost of doing business.
- The cost of healthcare coverage in general is increasing faster than any other segment of service or commodity in our society.

- In general, although overall inflation has been very low in the last few years, the medical inflation rate, particularly as it relates to health insurance, has increased by double digits. Because of these factors, it is essential to the survival of the health insurance industry that cost containment provisions be implemented to help reverse this trend.

## Assignments

Complete the Questions for Review.
Complete Exercises 4–1 through 4–3.

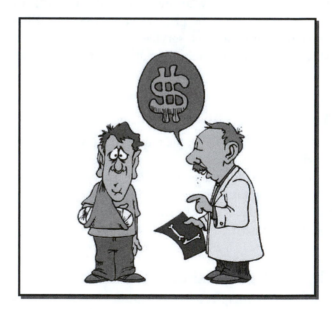

## Questions for Review

**Directions:** Answer the following questions without looking back at the material just covered. Write your answers in the space provided.

1. Name the three major types of coverage which are currently available.

   1. _____

   2. _____

   3. _____

2. _____ is the arrangement by which both the member and the plan share in a

specified ratio of the covered losses under a policy.

3. _____ are those expenses that are allowable under the plan.

4. What is an individual deductible? _____

_____

5. A _____ provides a specified allowance for a certain type of service.

6. (True or False?) Expenses not paid by the Basic portion of the contract may be payable under the Major
Medical portion. _____

7. Define accumulation period. _____

_____

8. Define automatic annual reinstatement. _____

_____

9. Explain the three-month carryover provision. _____

_____

10. What is the procedure code range for special services? _____

11. What do BR and RNE stand for and what is the difference between them? _____

_____

12. _____ is routine laboratory and x-ray tests performed on an outpatient basis

before a scheduled inpatient admission.

13. To _____ means to get preapproval for an admission on an elective,

nonemergency hospitalization.

14. List the two ways that second surgical opinion programs may be administered.

1. _____

2. _____

15. A _____ is a type of prepayment policy in which providers agree to charge

members for their services in accordance with a fixed schedule of rates.

If you were unable to answer any of these questions, refer back to that section and then fill in the answers.

# Exercise 4-1

**Directions:** Find and circle the words listed below. Words can appear horizontally, vertically, diagonally, forward, or backward.

```
W C U M U L A T I V E B E N E F I T Q A
W E W A O H N E C S D N S K W O C S G U
E X I H C O I N S U R A N C E V Z G M T
I T M V N O I G E R B R E O E T R T A I
V E A P E S U Z Z M U F P Y Y E I S R L
E N N Y Q R B E A K B N X P G F G E G I
R D A H E I E P D I D C E A E O C D O Z
T E G N M M R V G C O O T N I B R O R A
N D E M O M I Y I P F E E Y D Z M C P T
E B D J E M J V A T D B K V M V I R Y I
R E C X V I I Y R E C M C P V X X E R O
R N A C F A M E D I W E O M J Z B I A N
U E R D B E A U S F R S P J I L H F T R
C F E G N T C A I X Q G F S F S A I N E
N I V T M T B Q M Z K X O R O L E D U V
O T L E I U F U B V P L T X A R F O L I
C S N B I I T F B H T Q U N U R T M O E
B T L D Q O M W M Z M D O C G P X E V W
S E Y R U J N I L A T N E D I C C A R Z
G N I T S E T N O I S S I M D A E R P G
```

1. Accidental Injury
2. Concurrent Review
3. Cumulative Benefit
4. Extended Benefits
5. Managed Care

6. Out-of-Pocket Expense
7. Region
8. Retrospective Review
9. Utilization Review
10. Voluntary Program

# Exercise 4-2

**Directions:** Complete the crossword puzzle by filling in a word from the keywords that fits each clue.

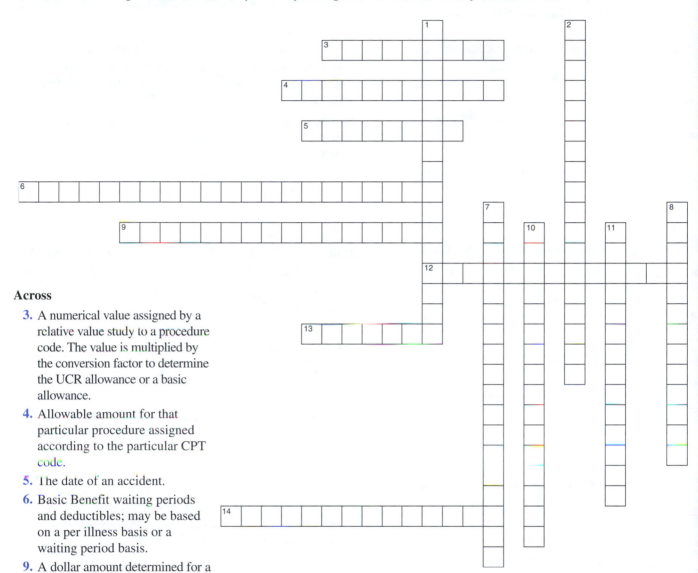

**Across**

3. A numerical value assigned by a relative value study to a procedure code. The value is multiplied by the conversion factor to determine the UCR allowance or a basic allowance.

4. Allowable amount for that particular procedure assigned according to the particular CPT code.

5. The date of an accident.

6. Basic Benefit waiting periods and deductibles; may be based on a per illness basis or a waiting period basis.

9. A dollar amount determined for a specific service type or a particular region. Each region may have a unique set of these dollar amounts, and each service type may be assigned a specific dollar amount.

12. In this PPO, the member chooses a family provider or physician and must see him or her before being referred to a specialist. The specialist may or may not be within the network.

13. The greatest amount payable by the plan.

14. Any expense which is allowable under the plan.

**Down**

1. Requires the patient to obtain an SSO for special procedures, or there is an automatic reduction or denial of benefits.

2. The period of time in which to satisfy the deductible, accumulate COB credit reserves, reach maximums, and so on.

7. Surgery recommended as an elective procedure when an alternative method of treatment may be preferable for a number of reasons.

8. An amount usually charged by most providers within a geographic region for a specified service.

10. To get preapproval for admission on elective, nonemergency hospitalization.

11. The process of determining the fee usually charged by similar providers for the same procedure in the same geographic area during a specified period of time.

# Exercise 4-3

**Directions:**  Match the following terms with the proper definition by writing the letter of the correct definition in the space next to the term.

1. _____ Automatic Annual Reinstatement

2. _____ Common Accident Provision

3. _____ Exclusive Provider Organization

4. _____ Health Maintenance Organization

5. _____ Management Service Organization

6. _____ Medical Case Management

7. _____ Nondisabling or Per Visit Benefit

8. _____ Out-of-Network

9. _____ Physician Hospital Organization

10. _____ Preferred Provider Organization

11. _____ Relative Value Units

12. _____ Three-Month Carryover Provision

13. _____ Usual, Customary, and Reasonable

a. Eligible charges incurred in the last quarter of the calendar year and applied toward the member's deductible will also count toward the following year's deductible.

b. A healthcare provider with whom a managed care organization does not have a contract to provide healthcare services.

c. An amount usually charged by most providers within a geographic region for a specified service.

d. In this type of benefit, there is a waiting period, a daily maximum, and a calendar year maximum.

e. Represent the total RVS for components of the schedule.

f. A group of healthcare providers who agree to provide services to a specific pool of patients for an agreed fee.

g. An organization of physicians and hospitals that bands together for the purpose of obtaining contracts from payer organizations.

h. A corporation set up to provide management services to a medical group for a fee.

i. A type of prepayment policy in which the organization bears the responsibility and financial risk of providing agreed-on healthcare services to the members enrolled in its plan, in exchange for a fixed monthly membership fee.

j. The process of evaluating the effectiveness and frequency of medical treatments by reviewing to determine whether the care that is being rendered or that is going to be rendered is appropriate.

k. A contractually specified amount of money that may be added to the balance of available lifetime benefits.

l. The patient selects a primary care giver and can use only physicians who are part of the network or who are referred by the primary care physician.

m. A provision whereby only one deductible is taken for all members of a family involved in the same accident.

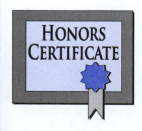

## Honors Certification™

The Honors Certification™ challenge for this chapter constitutes a written test. You will be presented with general information and asked to make the calculations discussed in this chapter. Each incorrect response will result in a deduction of up to 5% from your grade. You must score 80% or higher to pass this test. If you fail the test on your first attempt, you may retake the test one additional time. The items included in the second test may be different from those in the first test.

# SECTION 3

## MEDICAL CLAIMS EXAMINING GUIDELINES AND PROCEDURES

# 5
# Medical Claims
## Administration

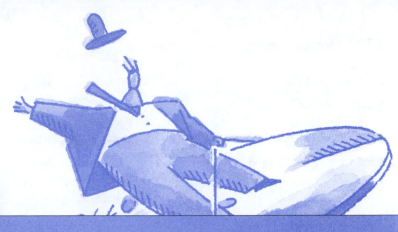

## After completion of this chapter
### you will be able to:

- Describe the way claim files are usually kept.
- List the rules for proper documentation of claim files.
- Identify claims that should be referred to consultants or technical personnel.
- Properly pend a claim using a given scenario.
- Identify the five guidelines to be used when processing claims.
- Properly process a claim using the payment worksheet.
- Properly process a drug/prescription claim using the payment worksheet.
- Define and explain the purpose of coordination of benefits.
- Recognize and define terms related to COB.

- Properly determine primary, secondary, and tertiary payers based on the OBD rules.
- Recognize and investigate potential COB situations.
- Compute the correct secondary benefit and credit reserve.
- Describe the differences between primary and secondary payers.
- Determine COB benefits as they apply to PPO and HMO plans.
- Properly define and explain the four different types of adjustments.
- State the ways that reimbursement may be obtained on an overpayment.
- List the situations in which the collection of an overpayment should not be attempted.

## Keywords and concepts
### you will learn in this chapter:

- Adjustment
- Allowable Expense
- Assignment of Benefits
- Batch Files
- Claim Determination Period
- Claim Files

- Claim Investigation
- Claim Processing
- Coordination of Benefits (COB)
- Credit Reserve (CR)
- Documentation

- Electronic Claims
- Electronic Claims Submission
- Explanation of Benefits (EOB)
- Family Files
- Full Credit Adjustment

- Gender Rule
- Global COB
- Insular COB
- Member Files
- Normal Liability (NL)
- Order of Benefit Determination Rules (OBD)

- Overinsurance
- Partial Credit Adjustment
- Pended Claims
- Primary Plan
- Provider of Service (Provider)
- Rebundling

- Referral
- Secondary Plan
- Statistical Adjustment
- Supplemental Adjustment
- TRICARE (formerly CHAMPUS)
- Unbundling

The claims examiner's job entails a wide variety of administrative duties to ensure proper claims handling. In this chapter, we will address the importance of the following: verification of coverage and eligibility, accurate claim file documentation, investigation, referrals, and pending claims. Company guidelines vary from payer to payer, so please review your company guidelines when making claim determinations.

# Maintenance of Claim Files

When a claim is received by a payer, the department (the name of the department varies from company to company) documents the receipt of the claim usually via a microfilm medium that copies the claim and assigns it a claim number, which includes the date. The date is used to keep all the claims received in chronological order so that the oldest mail can be processed first. After the claim has been documented and received, it is routed to the claims processor for handling.

**Claim Files** are files for holding claims and other processing information. Some claims payers prefer to have a manual filing system in which the physical claims are kept for ready access by examining personnel. Although manual filing systems may vary, they usually entail the maintenance of family files, member files, or batch files.

## Family Files

**Family files** are folders of claims that are kept for each family of claimants. The claimants are usually identified by the same subscriber identification number. This identification number is used to group the members of a family together into a single file or folder. Most companies use the member's social security number as the identification number.

Within the family folder, each member's information and claims are grouped separately. This grouping is based on the calendar year in which the charges were incurred, the date the expenses were processed, and whether the claim is completed or pended for additional information.

Therefore, each member will have a separate interfamily subfile for each calendar year. Within this subfile, completed claims are usually arranged with the claims processed earliest in a calendar year placed at the bottom of the file and the claims processed later in the year placed on top. In addition, there may be a separate correspondence subfile and a separate pended claim file by year, or there may be only one of each of these subfiles for each member with all years combined together. However, as with the completed claims, the correspondence or pending claims are usually arranged chronologically so that those received the earliest are placed at the bottom and those received later are placed at the top of the stack.

## Member Files

An alternative to having family files is to have member files. **Member files** are files that contain only one member's claim documents per file, and include documents for all years. Therefore, unlike the family files, in which the entire family is accessed when a claim or phone call is received for a family member, only a single member's file is accessed. Correspondence and pended claims are kept separate from completed claims, and all information is arranged chronologically according to the date of handling.

Unfortunately with the individual member file, it is difficult for the examiner to track trends, fraud, overutilization, and other abuses being practiced by a family or provider, since the information is located in multiple files. However, member files tend to be neater and easier to handle than family files.

## Batch Files

**Batch files** are batches of claims grouped together according to the date they were processed and the person who processed them. Every claim processed by an individual each day is placed in the same folder or secured together and filed. The claims are usually placed in order by claim number. Pended claims and correspondence are usually kept in separate files. When a pended claim is completed, it is placed in the batch file according to the date of completion.

With the batch system, when claims for one person need to be accessed, multiple batch files may need to be accessed as well. This process tends to be labor-intensive. In addition, as with member files, trends and abuses cannot be easily recognized by examining personnel.

# On the Job Now

1. Name the three types of manual claim files that may be used in a claim processing system.

　1. _____

　2. _____

　3. _____

## Claim File Documentation

**Documentation** is the orderly organization and communication of important facts that can be used to furnish decisive evidence of claim handling or processing. Documenting the claim file with pertinent information is an important job of the claims examiner. If the claim cannot be processed upon receipt, the claim file must be documented as to the disposition of the claim. The most common reason a claim cannot be processed is that additional information is needed from the provider or the member. The claims examiner's responsibility is to indicate in the claim file the information requested and the date of the request. The date that the follow-up letter should be sent (in the event that the information is not received within a certain amount of time) should also be included in the claim file.

This documentation enables the examiner to refresh his or her memory at a future date. Since you may not be the person who follows up on the claim or receives the information requested, be sure that the documentation is understandable and that it provides concise, informative, and pertinent information. Refrain from marking claim documents unnecessarily, since this may be very confusing to others reviewing

the claim at a later date. Proper documentation should have the following attributes:

1. **Clean claim files.** Never include any derogatory references to the member. Never write down personal remarks. Likewise, there should never be any reference to ethnic origin unless the information is relevant to the case. Always keep your information objective. Do not highlight or mark in any way sections, passages, or words of a narrative report or claim form. As innocent as it may seem, a judge, jury, or plaintiff's attorney may see it as singling out, bad faith, or discriminatory and arbitrary.

2. **Document the files properly and show the basis for your decision.** Careless or poorly worded claim files can give an appearance of bad faith or a conscious disregard of the claimant's rights. The representations made must not only be fair and reasonable but must also create a claim file that shows fairness, reasonableness, and factual accuracy when read by a jury. Always correctly record the basis for all claims decisions. Such a practice should also force you to carefully consider your every action before taking it, and to

discover and correct errors before any serious damage has occurred.

3. **Be careful when using words of the trade.** Sometimes such words or phrases may be taken out of context and used to give a bad connotation. Be particularly aware of words that may have a double meaning, especially if taken out of context.

4. **Give initial, factual information to an attorney involved on behalf of the claimant, if there is one involved.** If the attorney requests further information, questions concerning the extent and nature of that information should be discussed with a member of your company's legal department or a supervisor before responding to the attorney. All information or copies of documents should be clearly documented in the file.

Some companies retain specialists to handle attorney claims. In such instances, the case should be referred immediately to the specialist. Nothing should be said or sent to the attorney regarding the case unless you are directed to do so by the specialist. Since the handling of these claims differs significantly from company to company, always request clarification on the handling of such claims before taking any action.

1. **All information regarding the claim should be put in writing.** This means that phone conversations should always be documented and summarized in writing. A Telephone Information Sheet is sometimes used to record this information. A sample copy of a Telephone Information Sheet is shown as **Figure 5–1**. Also, base what you have to say about a case or an individual on factual information and express no opinion either in oral or written communications.

2. **Be careful when asked to furnish information.** Information furnished by a doctor or provider with regard to a claim may be privileged information. If medical information is requested by the claimant, normally the claimant should be advised to contact the provider directly. The fact that the claimant is a patient of the provider does not necessarily entitle him or her to the information that has been furnished.

# Claim Investigation

**Claim investigation** is making a detailed inquiry to verify facts pertaining to a submitted claim. When a claim is received, the minimal information that should be ob-

tained is a diagnosis, services rendered, the age, marital status, and student status (if applicable) of the claimant. Reasons for investigation may include possible preexisting conditions, fraud, work-related injuries, and coordination of benefits. When making your request for information, be as specific as possible regarding the type of information needed. Request information in such a way that you get narrative answers rather than yes or no answers. Avoid sending several requests for different information to the same provider or member. Request all information at once so that claims are not unnecessarily delayed. Always attach an Authorization to Release Information with your request.

# Referrals

Upon receipt of the information requested, you may find that the claim decision is beyond your level of expertise or authorization. When this occurs, the claim must be referred and reviewed by a technical claims person. This person may be a lead examiner, supervisor, medical review person, or consultant.

This **referral** process ensures that there is a consistent approach to unusual situations, and maintains an avenue of communication to higher levels in the case of sensitive issues. Following is a list of claims that are usually referred to technical personnel:

1. **Lawsuits, legal actions, or legislative issues.** An attorney letter may be received demanding payment or making reference to insurance law, a summons, a Notice of Complaint, or other lawsuit notification correspondence.

2. **Providers who have been flagged.** Flagged providers are those who have been identified as being questionable; therefore, special handling is required. Providers may be flagged for questionable billing practices, overuse of certain benefits (i.e., chiropractic services, biofeedback), new providers pending state approval to perform qualified services (i.e., surgi-center), or other issues.

3. **Fraud.** Providers have submitted claims in which indications of fraud have been identified and the claims are pending for verification.

When claims are received for the above situations, a referral form should be completed and routed to the appropriate department. It is important that copies of all documents, letters, and forms be sent along with the referral claim.

**Figure 5–2** is an example of a claim referral form.

**ANY INSURANCE CARRIER, INC.**
123 Any Drive
Anywhere, USA 12345
(800) 555-1234

## TELEPHONE INFORMATION SHEET

Date: _____

Claim Identification: _____

_____

_____

Person making inquiry: _____

Person supplying information: _____

Telephone Number: _____

Briefly state information received or desired: _____

_____

_____

Indicate additional handling, if any: _____

_____

_____

This form, when completed should be placed in the claim file.

■ **Figure 5–1** Telephone Information Sheet

## Claim Office Referral Sheet

To _____

From _____    Date _____

Policy #    Soc. Sec. #    Employee's Name    Dependent's Name

Eff. Date    Term. Date    Patient's Age    Provider of Service

**Reason for Referral:**

_____

_____

_____

**Attachments:**

( ) □ Denial/□ Attorney Letters    ( ) Preop Photos    ( ) □ Policy/□ Booklet Page
( ) Special Correspondence    ( ) Op/Anesthesia/Path Report    ( ) Billings
( ) □ Hospital/ □ Dr. Records    ( ) X-rays    ( ) Other:

Please make sure that all materials referenced in any appeal letter (insured/provider/attorney) are enclosed with this file.

**Reply:**

_____

_____

_____

_____

Signature _____    Date _____

**ANY INSURANCE CARRIER, INC.**

■ **Figure 5–2** Claim Referral Form

## Pended Claims

**Pended claims** are claims that have not been completely adjudicated or closed. These claims may require follow-up investigation so that correct and prompt liability decisions can be made, which comply with legislative or regulatory requirements for fair claim handling.

When requesting information, make sure that you request all the information needed to complete processing of the claim to ensure that an additional delay does not occur. Send a letter notifying the claimant and the provider that additional information is needed before the claim will be processed. Many companies use a standard form letter requesting further information. **Figures 5–3** and **5–4** are examples of standard request forms.

The first follow-up date should be scheduled three to four weeks after the original request. If the requested information is not received within the scheduled follow-up period, send a second notice letter with follow-up scheduled for three to four weeks. If the requested information is not received within 60 days, it may be necessary to close the claim. Send a final letter advising the insured and the provider that because information requested has not been received, the claim is being closed. Also indicate that if the requested information is received within a reasonable length of time, you will be happy to reopen the claim. If the company has a statute of limitations on filing a claim, this information should be indicated in the letter.

## Claim Processing

Some claims are submitted manually to insurance carriers; however, many claims are routinely submitted electronically for processing. These types of claims are called **electronic claims**. **Electronic claims submission** is a process whereby insurance claims are submitted via computerized data (either by data diskette or modem) directly from the provider to the insurance company. When claims are submitted electronically, the claim data is entered directly through the phone lines into the insurance carriers' computer system. The Administrative Simplification and Compliance Act

**ANY INSURANCE CARRIER, INC.**
**123 Any Drive**
**Anywhere, USA 12345**
**(800) 555-1234**

Control No. ____________

Name ____________

**Please refer to the paragraph checked below.**

□ Careful attention is being given to this claim. We will write you further about it in a short time.

□ As you requested, we are returning the ____________

□ Please let us know whether this claimant has returned to work and if so, when ________ If not, does total disability still exist? ________ Will proofs of claim be submitted? ________ Information as to the claimant's present condition will be appreciated.

□ Please have the ________ statement completed and return the attached form to us.

□ Consideration of further benefits can be given only after we receive the ____________

□ The attached furnished our first knowledge of this claim. Will you please arrange for submission of the required proofs of claim if this is properly covered under our insurance.

**Figure 5–3** Request for Additional Information Letter

ANY INSURANCE CARRIER, INC.
123 Any Drive
Anywhere, USA 12345
(800) 555-1234

Request Form
☐ Medical ☐ Dental

Please return requested information to: _____

☐ **First Request** ☐ **Second Request**     ☐ **Third and Final Request**

Insured: _____     Date: _____

Patient: _____

**BEFORE WE CAN PROCESS YOUR CLAIM, WE WILL NEED THE ADDITIONAL INFORMATION CHECKED BELOW:**

☐ Please complete in full the member portion of the claim form. Dental (employee section).

☐ Itemized Statements from: _____

☐ Copies of other Insurance Payments from: _____

☐ Full-time Student Eligibility Form Request: Please have the Registrar of the College or University that _____ attends complete the attached Student Eligibility Form for the _____ Semester/Quarter.

☐ Other: _____

☐ THE FOLLOWING EXPENSES WILL BE HELD UNTIL THE ABOVE REQUESTED ITEMS ARE RECEIVED IN THIS OFFICE _____

☐ We have attempted on _____ to obtain the above necessary information to properly process your claim. As of this date it has not been received. The file will **now** be considered **closed** until such time the information is received and proper evaluation can be given your claim.

Thank you,

**■ Figure 5–4** Request for Additional Information Letter

(ASCA) requires claims to be submitted to Medicare electronically, with some exceptions.

Claims submitted electronically usually contain fewer errors; because they eliminate the need for data entry personnel to reenter the information, payment is also generated more quickly. In addition, insurance carriers reduce their management and overhead costs by allowing electronic claims submission. Most payers also process electronic claims faster than paper claim submissions.

Generally, electronic claims submission is performed on a weekly basis by the provider. Once a week, the medical biller contacts the insurance carrier using the computer and downloads the information. Because electronic claims submission does not allow the opportunity for the physician to sign the claims, a physician's signature on the agreement will be accepted in lieu of a signature on the claim form. It is also imperative to have a

patient signature on file for Authorization to Release Information and Assignment of Benefits.

**Claim Processing** means to determine benefit amounts and pay, pend, or deny a claim. In the following paragraphs, we will discuss coverage and guidelines for processing claims. These guidelines are generalized, and company guidelines will always supersede any of the guidelines discussed in this chapter. Use the guidelines when processing the claims in this book.

## Claim Analysis

A good claims examiner must have a thorough and systematic process for analyzing claims. The same process is used on each claim no matter how simple or complex. This is how consistency and accuracy are developed. The following model may be used in the development of a systematic approach. Identify the issues involved in the claim. There may be many issues, including the following eight:

1. Eligibility:

   a. Has the policy lapsed for nonpayment of premiums?

   b. At the time of service, was the claimant currently enrolled under the plan?

   c. If a dependent, is the claimant within the proper age limit? If not, is the dependent a full-time student or otherwise within the extended age limit?

   d. Have all eligibility requirements set forth in the policy been met?

   e. Was any material misrepresentation made in the original application for coverage?

2. Possible other coverage:

   a. Is an injury involved? If so, do you have the date, place, and circumstances of the injury on file?

   b. Is there evidence of other insurance? Could TPL be involved?

   c. Is the injury work-related? If so, has a Workers' Compensation claim been filed?

   d. Does the claimant have other insurance that might cover these services?

3. Determine what the policy/plan language provides:

   a. What is the definition of total disability?

   b. What is the contract definition of accident and sickness?

   c. What plan provisions could apply to this claim? What plan limitations and maximums could apply to the claim?

   d. Is there a preexisting limitation on the plan and, if so, how is it applied?

4. Is there any information missing from the claim which is necessary for determination of payment (diagnosis, patient, provider licensing, etc.)?

5. Obtain all relevant facts. Request all missing information or documentation at one time. Thoroughly investigate all available data. Do not pend a claim again and again, to request information that should have been initially requested.

6. Make an honest evaluation of the facts and the plan benefits. Seek assistance from supervisors or lead examiners when necessary, before, not after, pending or denying a claim.

7. Keep the member informed. Each time a claim is pended or denied, a letter must be sent. In addition, usually every 30 days a follow-up letter should be sent on a claim remaining pended.

8. No decision is final. If the benefits are denied, there should always be an opportunity for reevaluation of the claim if new or different information is received.

## Good Claim Practices

Consider the following five guidelines when processing claims:

1. **Fully analyze the claim initially.** Consider all possible reasons for acceptance or denial. Look for a way to pay a claim, not deny it. Often an initial review of a claim will reveal clear and obvious grounds for denial. Sometimes the obvious grounds disappear later when the denial is questioned. Always clearly document the grounds for denial. Resist the natural temptation to deny a claim without a complete investigation and without considering all other possible grounds for acceptance.

2. **Thoroughly investigate and document the facts within the claim file.** This may be one of the most important steps that each examiner needs to take before paying or denying a claim. The lack of a proper investigation or documentation has probably resulted in more bad faith lawsuits than any other individual factor.

   a. Investigate and thoroughly document all aspects under investigation before taking a position on the status of a claim.

   b. After investigation, evaluate the facts in an impartial and objective manner. If the facts are technical, seek assistance from a lead examiner or supervisor.

   c. Verify the authenticity of the date. Is the person providing the information a qualified provider or other qualified person?

   d. Never rely on incomplete or ambiguous claim forms or inspection reports.

   e. Consider all policy provisions.

3. **Handle claims promptly and keep claimants informed.**

   a. Give priority to delayed/pended claims.

**b.** Resolve conflicting evidence or information promptly.

**c.** Do not withhold or delay payments in hope of a compromise.

**d.** Be sure to indicate the date and other documentation for the following: when claims are received or processed, when correspondence is received or sent, and when telephone calls are received or made.

**4. Make proper use of medical evidence.**

**a.** Always contact the doctor to clear up any medical questions concerning the claimant.

**b.** When a second medical opinion is required, the proper selection of an independent medical examiner is very important. A specialist should be chosen for the specific disease or injury. The medical examiner must always be provided with all the claimant's relevant medical information and records, whether they are favorable or unfavorable. Also, the examiner cannot provide a correct conclusion unless the correct questions are asked. Sometimes asking the correct questions is the most difficult part of preparing a case for review.

**5. Be observant in looking for excessive charges.**
There are a few doctors who will indicate a long list of diagnoses to match up the wide variety of tests given, so that the claim will be covered by the insurance carrier. Some situations to watch for are:

**a.** High charges, a long list of diagnoses, and no subsequent visits.

**b.** Multiple diagnoses involving multiple bodily functions.

**c.** Services described in very technical and nonstandard medical terminology, especially in connection with exotic extensive medical testing.

**d.** Vague or ambiguous diagnoses.

**e.** Diagnoses involving extensive testing, beginning with hyper- or hypo- (i.e., hypoglycemia, hypercholesterolemia, hypomineralism).

**f.** Claims or bills that appear to be preprinted or that include wordy descriptions of services either on the claim or enclosed with the bill.

These are only a few of the instances that should alert the attention of a good claims examiner. If necessary, medical records should be requested to investi-

gate the patient's history and chief complaints, the tests performed, and their results.

In questionable cases, use common sense and seek advice early. Often a second opinion or different point of view can clarify the situation. Do not hesitate to seek the opinions of your supervisor or lead examiner. Two areas in which help is often needed are in questioning preexisting conditions and usual and customary charges. Your responsibility is to make decisions, but prudent decisions come with time and experience. Until you have experience, consider asking questions as a part of your learning and training.

# Unbundling of Services

**Unbundling** (also called fragmentation or code splitting) is the billing of multiple procedure codes for a group of procedures that are covered by a single comprehensive code. It encompasses surgery, pathology and lab charges, radiology, and medical services. Coding manipulations are often used to inappropriately increase claim reimbursements. The allowable charge determination will be based upon the single comprehensive code which includes the entire procedure.

The component parts of the procedure are to be denied as already included within the allowable charge for the single procedure. This process is referred to as "**rebundling**."

Examples of unbundling include the following:

- Fragmenting one service into component parts and coding each component part as if it were a separate service. For example, the correct CPT® comprehensive code to use for upper gastrointestinal endoscopy with biopsy of stomach is 43239. Separating the service into two component parts, using CPT® code 43235 for upper gastrointestinal endoscopy and CPT® code 43600 for biopsy of the stomach, is inappropriate.

- Reporting separate codes for related services when one comprehensive code includes all related services. An example of this type of unbundling is coding a total abdominal hysterectomy with or without removal of tubes, with or without removal of ovaries (CPT® code 58150) plus salpingectomy (CPT® code 58700) plus oophorectomy (CPT® code 58940) rather than using the comprehensive CPT® code 58150 for all three related services.

- Breaking out bilateral procedures when one code is appropriate. For example, bilateral mammography is coded correctly using CPT® code 76091 rather than incorrectly submitting CPT® code 76090-RT for the right mammography and CPT® code 76090-LT for left mammography.
- Downcoding a service in order to use an additional code when one higher level, more comprehensive code is appropriate. A laboratory should bill CPT® code 80048 (basic metabolic panel), when coding for a calcium, carbon dioxide, chloride, creatinine, glucose, potassium, sodium, and urea nitrogen performed as automated multichannel tests. It would be inappropriate to report CPT® codes 82310, 82374, 82435, 82565, 82947, 84132, 84295 and/or 84520 in addition to the CPT® code 80048 unless one of these laboratory tests was performed at a different time of day to obtain follow-up results, in which case a modifier -91 would be utilized.
- Separating a surgical approach from a major surgical service. For example, a provider should not bill CPT® code 49000 for exploratory laparotomy and CPT® code 44150 for total abdominal colectomy for the same operation because the exploration of the surgical field is included in the CPT® code 44150.

## Mutually Exclusive Code Pairs

These codes represent services or procedures that, based on either the CPT® definition or standard medical practice, would not or could not reasonably be performed at the same session by the same provider on the same patient. Codes representing these services or procedures cannot be submitted together.

Examples of mutually exclusive code pairs include the following:

- When the repair of the organ can be performed by two different methods. One method must be chosen to repair the organ and that is the code that must be used.
- The billing of an "initial" service and a "subsequent" service. A service cannot be initial and subsequent at the same time. If a physician reports "mutually exclusive" coding combinations, the carrier will pay for the procedure with the lowest work relative value unit and deny the other code(s).

- A vaginal hysterectomy (procedure code 58260) and a total abdominal hysterectomy (procedure code 58150) are mutually exclusive — either one or the other, but not both procedures, is performed.
- CPT® codes 13100 and 13101 for the complex repair of the trunk. If multiple wounds of the trunk are repaired in the same operative session, coding is based on the total length of all the repairs.
- Complex Treatment Device CPT® Code 77334 billed on the same date of service (DOS) as the Simple Treatment Device Code 77332. Only one treatment device code should be paid because they are mutually exclusive on the same date of service. If these codes are billed on the same DOS, many payers will deny the major code as a duplicate and pay only the lesser code.

## Separate Procedures

Although certain CPT® codes are identified as "separate procedures," it has been determined that these codes may occasionally be provided as part of a more comprehensive procedure. Under such circumstances, the more comprehensive procedure code should be billed.

By definition, the "separate procedure" is commonly performed as part of a larger service and usually represents a procedure that the physician performs through the same incision or orifice, at the same site, or using the same approach. For example, an excision of a flexor tendon of the finger (CPT® code 26180) is performed with another surgery code from the 20000 section. The excision of the tendon (separate procedure) should not be billed.

**Note:** Separate procedure codes can only be billed when the separate procedure is the only procedure performed.

## Payment Worksheet

Whenever claims are processed manually, a payment worksheet must be completed by the examiner. This worksheet explains to the member how the benefits on the claim were calculated. Although worksheets vary from company to company, the general format and requirements remain the same. Following are explanations of the various fields on the payment worksheet **(see Figure 5–5 and Figure 5–6)**.

# Payment Worksheet

| Eligible Employee: | Nancy Normal | Accident Benefit: | $ | 0.00 | (CCYY) |
|---|---|---|---|---|---|
| Company: | XYZ Corporation | Lifetime Max: | $ | 109.46 | |
| Insured's ID Number: | 777 77 XYZ | Deductible: | $ | 125.00 | (CCYY) |
| Patient: | Normal Nancy | Carryover Ded: | $ | 0.00 | (CCNY) |
| Relationship: | Self | Coinsurance: | $ | 11.74 | (CCYY) |
| Provider's Zip Code: | 89578 | Date of Injury: | | | |

| Procedure Type of Service | Dates of Service | Billed Amount | Excluded Amounts* | Allowed | Basic/ Accident 100% | Maj. Med. ____% | ____% | UCR Calcula-tions |
|---|---|---|---|---|---|---|---|---|
| 1.    99201 | 2/5/CCYY | $ 220.00 | $ 24.48 | $ 195.52 | $ 48.75 | $ 146.77 | | 6.5 x 30.08 |
| 2.    85025 | 2/5/CCYY | $ 40.00 | $ 19.38 | $ 20.62 | $ 5.60 | $ 15.02 | | 0.8 x 25.78 |
| 3.    87040 | 2/5/CCYY | $ 30.00 | $ 0.00 | $ 30.00 | $ 8.40 | $ 21.60 | | 1.2 x 25.78 |
| 4. | | | | | | | | |
| 5. | | | | | | | | |
| 6. | | | | | | | | |
| ⇩Remarks: | Totals: | $ 290.00 | $ 43.86 | $ 246.14 | $ 62.75 | $ 183.39 | | |
| Deductible has been satisfied. | Deductible: | | | | $ 0.00 | $ 125.00 | | |
| | Amount Subject to Coinsurance: | | | | $ 62.75 | $ 58.39 | | |
| | Coinsurance: | | | | $ 0.00 | $ 11.68 | | |
| | Amount Subject to Adjustment: | | | | $ 62.75 | $ 46.71 | | |
| | Adjustment (See Remarks): | | | | $ 0.00 | $ 0.00 | | |
| | Payment Amount: | | $ 109.46 | | $ 62.75 | $ 46.71 | | |

| *Denial Reasons | |
|---|---|
| 1. | $ 24.48 not covered — Exceeds amount allowed by your plan. |
| 2. | $ 19.38 not covered — Exceeds amount allowed by your plan. |
| 3. | |
| 4. | |
| 5. | |
| 6. | |

| Payees | |
|---|---|
| 1. | $ 90.00 — Dee N. Aee, M.D. |
| 2. | $ 19.46 — Nancy Normal |
| 3. | |
| 4. | |
| 5. | |
| 6. | |

If you disagree with our decision on your claim, you have the right by law to request that your claim be reviewed by your plan administrator. This request must be made in writing within 60 days of receipt of this notice. If you wish, you may submit your written comments and views. Please consult your plan's claim review procedures. See your employer regarding any other ERISA questions.

■ **Figure 5–5** Payment Worksheet (References Figure 2–1)

# Payment Worksheet

| Eligible Employee: | Betty Bossy | Accident Benefit: | $ | 0.00 | (CCYY) |
|---|---|---|---|---|---|
| Company: | Ninja Enterprises | Lifetime Max: | $ | 8,996.00 | |
| Insured's ID Number: | 999-99 NIN | Deductible: | $ | 0.00 | (CCYY) |
| Patient: | Self | Carryover Ded: | $ | 0.00 | (CCNY) |
| Relationship: | Self | Coinsurance: | $ | 1,250.00 | (CCYY) |
| Provider's Zip Code: | 12890 | Date of Injury: | | | |

| Procedure Type of Service | Dates of Service | Billed Amount | Excluded Amounts* | Allowed | Basic/ Accident 100% | Major Medical 80 % | ___ % | UCR Calcula- tions |
|---|---|---|---|---|---|---|---|---|
| 1.   R&B | 02/06/YY- 02/14/YY | $3160.00 | | $ 3160.00 | | 3160.00 | | |
| 2.   MISC | 02/06/YY- 02/14/YY | $7086.00 | | $ 7086.00 | | 7086.00 | | |
| 3. | | | | | | | | |
| 4. | | | | | | | | |
| 5. | | | | | | | | |
| 6. | | | | | | | | |

| ⇩Remarks: | Totals: | $10246.00 | $ | $10246.00 | $ | $10246.00 | |
|---|---|---|---|---|---|---|---|
| Network Provider paid at 80% | Deductible: | | | | $ | $   150.00 | |
| | Amount Subject to Coinsurance: | | | | $ | $10096.00 | |
| Precertification performed. | Coinsurance: | | | | $ | $ 1250.00 | |
| | Amount Subject to Adjustment: | | | | $ | $ 8846.00 | |
| | Adjustment (See Remarks): | | | | $ | $ | |
| | Payment Amount: | | $ 8846.00 | | $ | $ 8846.00 | |

| *Denial Reasons |
|---|
| 1. |
| 2. |
| 3. |
| 4. |
| 5. |
| 6. |

| Payees |
|---|
| 1.   $8846.00—Abe Domin, M.D. |
| 2. |
| 3. |
| 4. |
| 5. |
| 6. |

If you disagree with our decision on your claim, you have the right by law to request that your claim be reviewed by your plan administrator. This request must be made in writing within 60 days of receipt of this notice. If you wish, you may submit your written comments and views. Please consult your plan's claim review procedures. See your employer regarding any other ERISA questions.

■ **Figure 5–6** Payment Worksheet (References Figure 2–5)

## Header Information

The header area is where the member and plan identification information are indicated. It is composed of the following fields:

**Eligible Employee.** The insured or employee's full name.

**Company.** The name of the employer or company.

**Insured's Identification Number.** The insured or employee's social security number.

**Patient.** The patient/claimant's name.

**Relationship.** The relationship of the patient to the insured.

The following information should be filled in after completing the claim payment worksheet:

**Accident Benefit.** Amount of accident benefit year to date.

**Lifetime Max.** Amount of lifetime maximum to date.

**Deductible.** Amount of deductible, year to date.

**Carryover Deductible.** Amount of deductible carried over from the previous year.

**Coinsurance.** Amount of coinsurance paid, year to date.

## Claim Data Information

The body of the worksheet is where the billed services are itemized, indicating the amount allowed for each service, the amount excluded, and the percentage at which the amount allowed is payable. This section includes the following fields:

**Procedure/Type of Service.** The applicable CPT® code or English language description of service.

**Dates of Service.** Date of service for this particular single line of coding.

**Billed Amount.** The total amount of charges for the services indicated on this single line of coding.

**Excluded Amounts.** The amount of charges for this single line of coding that is not allowable under the plan. An explanation should be placed under Denial Reasons.

**Allowed.** The amount remaining after the excluded expenses are subtracted from the billed amount.

**Basic 100%.** The amount of the allowed expense that is payable at 100%. If there are multiple applicable plan percentages for a single charge, the allowed expense should be broken up based on the amount payable at each specific percentage.

**Maj. Med %.** The Major Medical amount allowed after any higher benefits such as Basic have been subtracted from the allowed expense.

**%.** Any additional applicable percentage rate that may apply to an allowed amount. This can be due to OOP maximums, SSO not performed, and so on.

**Totals.** The totals of all amounts within that column.

**Deductible.** The amount of the charges applied to the plan deductible.

**Amount Subject to Coinsurance.** Amount payable at the plan coinsurance rate after any deductible is taken.

**Coinsurance.** The coinsurance rate that is the patient's liability.

**Amount Subject to Adjustment.** The amount that would need to be adjusted because of COB, overpayment, or any other type of adjustment.

**Adjustment (see Remarks).** The actual adjustment being made.

**Payment Amount.** The payment amount that would be made for this claim.

**Remarks.** This space is used to explain the type and reason for any adjustments being made. This space is also used to detail any other patient information related to the handling of this claim.

**Denial Reasons.** A reason for the denial, which must be explained to the member whenever a charge or portion of a charge is not covered under a plan. The reason should be entered in this area and referenced by line item.

**Payees.** This indicates the amount of the claim payment and who is to be paid.

## Processing the Claim

After determining that the claim is properly completed, the claimant is covered, the provider is appropriate, there is no other insurance, and that the services are covered, it is time to begin processing the claim.

The claim information is taken from the sample CMS-1500 found in the Billing Forms and Resource Manuals chapter (**Figure 2–1**). This information is shown on the claim form, and on the description in parentheses. The information shown in brackets is either the calculation used to arrive at an amount, or the block on the CMS-1500 that contains the information. We will be using the XYZ Corporation contract from Appendix A, and the RVS Schedule and Conversion Factor Report from Appendix B.

## Completing the Payment Worksheet

The claim payment worksheet is equivalent to an explanation of benefits. A copy of this worksheet will be sent to the member to explain the benefit payment for the claim. Therefore, each section should be filled out accurately and completely.

The claim payment worksheet used for this course is intended to be an example only. It contains the information in much the same format as most insurance carriers' EOBs. This worksheet and the guidelines for completing it are to be used for training and reference purposes, since the particular company or plan worksheets and guidelines may differ.

The following information will explain how to complete the sections of the payment worksheet.

**Step 1.** Complete the information regarding the patient and insured first. This information is contained in the box in the upper-left-hand corner of the payment worksheet.

| Payment Worksheet Field | CMS-1500 | CMS-1500 Block Number | UB-92 | UB-92 Form Locator | Practice Pitfalls |
|---|---|---|---|---|---|
| Eligible Employee | Nancy Normal | Block 4 | Betty B. Bossy | FL 58 | |
| Company | XYZ Corporation | Block 11b | Ninja Enterprises | FL 65 | |
| Insured's Identification Number | 777-77-XYZ | Block 1a | 999-99 NIN | FL 60 | |
| Patient | Nancy Normal | Block 2 | Bossy Betty B | FL 12 | |
| Relationship | Self | Block 6 | 18 (self) | FL 59 | |
| Provider's Zip Code | 89578 | Block 33 | 12890 | FL 1 | |

**Step 2.** Next, each CPT® code should be listed in the "Procedure Type of Service" column. Only codes that are the same should be combined together, otherwise list one code per line, regardless of whether this means using more than one payment worksheet.

| Procedure Type of Service | 1. 99201<br>2. 85025<br>3. 87040 | Field 24D | 111<br>(inpatient<br>hospital claim) | FL 4 | |
|---|---|---|---|---|---|

**Step 3.** List the date(s) of service in the "Dates of Service" column.

| Dates of Service | 1. 02/05/CCYY<br>2. 02/05/CCYY<br>3. 02/05/CCYY | Field 24A | 02/06/CCYY<br>through<br>02/14/CCYY | FL 6 | |
|---|---|---|---|---|---|

**Step 4.** Enter the amount the provider billed in "Billed Amount" column.

| Billed Amount | 1. $220.00<br>2. $40.00<br>3. $30.00 | Field 24F | $10,246.00 | FL 55 | |
|---|---|---|---|---|---|

**Step 5.** Determine the allowed amount for the service or procedure. Using the Relative Value Study shown in Appendix B, locate the unit value for the CPT® code assigned to each service provided. The unit value for the procedure is located in the right-hand column titled "Total RVU's." Next, determine the conversion factor for the procedure from the UCR Conversion Factor Report (see Appendix B).

Using the first three numbers of the provider's zip code, locate the type of service. Four categories are listed next to the zip code location. The categories are:

1. Surgery
2. Medicine
3. X-ray/Lab
4. Anesthesia

Multiply the appropriate conversion factor by the unit value for the procedure. The appropriate category is determined by the CPT® code, not the description of service. This total is the allowed amount. If the billed amount is less than the allowed amount, the billed amount is considered to be the allowed amount.

Thus, you will have: (195.52, 20.62, and 30.94) (6.5 [RVS] x 30.08 [Medicine Conversion factor for zip codes starting 895] = 195.52), (0.8 [RVS] x 25.78 [x-ray/lab conversion factor] = 20.62), (1.2 [RVS] x 25.78 (x-ray/lab conversion factor) = 30.94). However, since the billed amount for line three is less than the UCR amount, the allowed amount will be the billed amount.

Skip to the Allowed column and enter the allowed amounts as figured above.

| Payment Worksheet Field | Calculation | | UB-92 Input | UB-92 Form Locator Field | Practice Pitfalls |
|---|---|---|---|---|---|
| Allowed | 1. $195.52<br>2.  $20.62<br>3.  $30.00 | | 1. $3160.00<br>2. $7086.00 | | |

**Step 6.** Next, subtract the allowed amount from the billed amount. The resulting figure is the excluded amount that should be placed in the Excluded Amounts column. Remember, if the allowed amount is greater than the billed amount, the billed amount will be the allowed amount. Therefore, the excluded amount will be: ($24.48, $19.38, 0.00) ($220.00 [billed amount] − $195.52 [allowed amount] = 24.48, $40.00 − $20.62 = 19.38, $30.00 − $30.00 = 0.00)

| Excluded Amounts | 1. $24.48<br>2. $19.38<br>3.   $0.00 | | | | |
|---|---|---|---|---|---|

**Step 7.** Each explanation of benefits must list any amounts that are denied and the reason for the denial. Skip to the Denial Reasons section and enter a denial reason on the corresponding line in the denial reasons section. Usually, a brief explanation such as "$24.48 not covered — charge exceeds amount covered by your plan" is sufficient. If the service is not covered, the corresponding code (or description) and an explanation should be listed in the same manner (i.e., $300.00 not covered—cosmetic services are not covered by your plan). See Appendix B for a list of denial reasons to use.

| Denial Reasons | 1. $24.48 not covered<br>—Exceeds amount<br>allowed by your plan<br>2. $19.38 not covered<br>—Exceeds amount<br>allowed by your plan. | | | | |
|---|---|---|---|---|---|

**Step 8.** If the plan has a basic allowance, the unit value should be multiplied by the basic allowance listed in the contract. For example, if the contract stipulates that the basic allowance for an office visit is $7.00 and the CPT® has a unit value of 1.0, then the basic allowance would be $7.00. The basic allowance amount would be placed in the Basic/Accident 100% column. ($48.75, $5.60, $8.40) ($7.50 [Outpatient Physicians Visits basic conversion factor from contract] x 6.5 [RVS units] = $48.75, $7.00 [x-ray and laboratory basic conversion factor from contract] x 0.8 [RVS units] = $5.60, $7.00 [x-ray and laboratory basic conversion factor from contract] x 1.2 [RVS units] = 8.40).

| Basic/Accident 100% | 1. $48.75 | | | | |
|---|---|---|---|---|---|
| | 2. $5.60 | | | | |
| | 3. $8.40 | | | | |

**Step 9.** The basic allowance is subtracted from the allowed amount and the remainder is placed in the Major Medical column. ($146.77, $15.02, $21.60) ($195.52 [major medical allowed amount] − $48.75 [basic amount] = $146.77, $20.62 [allowed amount] − $5.60 [basic amount] = $15.02, $30.00 [allowed amount] − $8.40 [basic amount] = $21.60).

| Major Medical | 1. $146.77 | | 1. $3160.00 | | |
|---|---|---|---|---|---|
| | 2. $15.02 | | 2. $7086.00 | | |
| | 3. $21.60 | | | | |

**Step 10.** After all the charges have been figured individually, the total for each column is added up and placed at the bottom of the column in the "Totals" row. ($43.86, $246.14, $62.75, $183.39)

Check your totals for accuracy by adding the Major Medical amount to the Basic amount. These two figures should total the Allowed Amount. Then add the Allowed Amount to the Excluded Amount. The total of these two figures should match the Billed Amount column and the total amount of the claim.

If the contract allows different percentages based on the type of service (i.e., Basic Benefits at 100%, Major Medical at 80%, Accidents at 100%, etc.), then each different type of benefit (i.e., Basic, Major Medical, Accident) should be placed in a different column. If there are not enough columns on the payment worksheet, all services paid at the same percent may be placed together in a single column. There is also an additional untitled column to allow for varying percentages.

| Totals | 1. $43.86 | | 1. $3160.00 | | |
|---|---|---|---|---|---|
| | 2. $246.14 | | 2. $7086.00 | | |
| | 3. $62.75 | | | | |
| | 4. $183.39 | | | | |

**Step 11.** Now it is time to calculate the actual benefit payment. At the top of each payment column (Basic/Accident, Major Medical and Untitled), place the coinsurance percentage amount that applies to the figures in that column if it is not indicated (i.e., 100%, 80%).

**Step 12.** Check the contract for the deductible amount and the Beginning Financials if applicable, for any previously paid deductible amounts. The following questions should also be answered.

- Is there a deductible amount for basic benefits?
- Has the deductible for this individual been satisfied?
- Does the deductible combine the medical plan with a dental plan (the plans are integrated)?

- If so, has the deductible been satisfied under the medical or dental portion of the contract?
- Has the family deductible been satisfied?
- Is there any carryover deductible from the previous year that should be applied?

Using the above questions and information, calculate both the basic and the major medical deductible amounts. The deductible amount on the basic portion of a plan will only usually be for hospital services.

| Deductible | 1.　$0.00 | | | | |
|---|---|---|---|---|---|
| | 2.　$125.00 | | $150.00 | | |

**Step 13.** To calculate the Basic Benefits, first, enter the amount of the deductible in "Deductible" row in the basic benefits column. In this case there is no basic deductible on the services for Nancy Normal. The only basic deductible stated in the contract is a $50 inpatient hospital deductible, however, this claim is not for inpatient hospital services.

| Deductible | $0.00 | | | | |
|---|---|---|---|---|---|

**Step 14.** Next, subtract the deductible amount from the total of the column and place the resulting amount in the "Amount Subject to Coinsurance" row. Since the deductible amount is $0.00, the amount to be placed here is $62.75 ($62.75) [$62.75 − $0.00 = $62.75]

| Amount Subject to Coinsurance | $62.75 | | | | |
|---|---|---|---|---|---|

**Step 15.** Next, multiply the amount subject to coinsurance by the insured's portion of the coinsurance amount (the remaining amount needed to reach 100%). For example, if the plan's coinsurance amount is 80%, then the insured's responsibility is 20%. For this column, the payment amount is 100%, so there is no coinsurance amount for the patient. ($62.75) [$62.75 x 0% = $0.00]

| Coinsurance | $0.00 | | | | |
|---|---|---|---|---|---|

**Step 16.** Finally, subtract the coinsurance amount from the amount subject to coinsurance. The remaining balance is the amount subject to adjustment and goes in the next column. ($62.75) [$62.75 − $0.00 = $62.75]

　　We will cover the rows "Adjustment (See Remarks)," and "Payment Amount" in Steps 22 and 23.

| Amount Subject to Adjustment | $62.75 | | | | |
|---|---|---|---|---|---|

**Step 17.** To calculate the Major Medical benefits, first, calculate the Major Medical deductible that should be applied on this claim. Since this treatment is for a new patient visit at the beginning of the year, we will conclude that Nancy Normal has not yet paid any of her deductible. Therefore, we will place $125.00 in the "Deductible" row of the Major Medical column. ($125.00)

**Note:** If any individual or family deductible or coinsurance amounts are met on this claim, an asterisk should be placed beside the deductible or coinsurance amount and a notation made in the remarks box (i.e., CCYY individual deductible has now been met).

| Deductible | $125.00 | | | | |
|---|---|---|---|---|---|

**Step 18.**  Next, subtract the deductible amount from the total of the column and place the resulting amount in the "Amount Subject to Coinsurance" row. (58.39) [$183.39 − $125.00 = $58.39]

If the amount in the "Deductible" field equal the amount in the "Totals" field, then the "Amount Subject to Coinsurance would be $0, and no major medical payment will be made on the claim.

| Amount Subject to Coinsurance | $58.39 | | $10096.00 | | |
|---|---|---|---|---|---|

**Step 19.**  Next, multiply the amount subject to coinsurance by the insured's portion of the coinsurance amount (the remaining amount needed to reach 100%). For example, if the plan's coinsurance amount is 80%, then the insured's responsibility is 20%. ($11.68) [$58.39 x .2 = $11.68]

| Coinsurance | ($11.68) | | ($1250.00) | | |
|---|---|---|---|---|---|

**Step 20.**  Next, ask the following questions:

- What is the maximum coinsurance amount listed in the contract?
- Has this coinsurance limit been met?
- If the individual coinsurance limit has not been met, has the family coinsurance limit been met?

If any coinsurance limits have been met, the coinsurance amount should be adjusted accordingly. For example, if the individual coinsurance limit is $1,500 and $1,495 has been paid by the individual, the coinsurance amount would be $5.

**Step 21.**  Finally, subtract the coinsurance amount from the amount subject to coinsurance. The remaining balance is the amount subject to adjustment and goes in that row. ($46.71) [$58.39 − $11.68 = $46.71]

| Amount Subject to Adjustment | $46.71 | | $8846.00 | | |
|---|---|---|---|---|---|

**Step 22.**  Ask the following questions:

- If there is other insurance, what is the amount paid by the other insurance company?
- Are there any other reasons why there would be an adjustment to this claim?
- If so, what is the proper adjustment amount?

If there is an adjustment, the amount of the adjustment should be placed in the row "Adjustment (See Remarks)," and an explanation should be placed in the "Remarks" box to the left. See Appendix B for a list of remarks to use. Many claims will not have an adjustment amount. If there is an adjustment amount, the amount of the adjustment cannot be more than the amount shown in the "Amount Subject to Adjustment." For example, if there was an adjustment of $100 on Nancy's claim, $62.75 would be placed in the first column and $37.25 would be placed in the second column. Since there is no adjustment on this claim, we will place 0.00 in these boxes for both the Basic and Major Medical columns.

| Adjustment (See Remarks) Remarks | 1.  $0.00  2.  $0.00 | | $   0.00 | | |

**Step 23.**  The adjustment amount if any, should then be subtracted from the amount subject to adjustment, and the resulting amount would be placed in the "Payment Amount" row. For the Basic Benefits column this amount is $62.75 and for the Major Medical column this amount is $46.71.

| Payment Amount | 1.   $62.75  2.   $46.71 | | $8846.00 | | |

**Step 24.**  Add up the payment amount from all columns. The resulting payment amount should be placed in the box immediately to the right of the words "Payment Amount." This is the amount of the benefits being paid by the insurance carrier for this claim. ($109.46) ($62.75 + 46.71 = $109.46)

| Payment Amount | $109.46 | | $8846.00 | | |

**Step 25.**  In this case, Nancy has paid $200 on the claim, leaving a balance of $90 owed to the provider. Since the provider should not be paid more than he has charged, the payment must be split. $90 will be paid to the provider and the remaining $19.46 will be reimbursed to Nancy. This information is placed in the "Payees" section.

| Payees | 1. $90.00—Dee N. Aee, M.D.  2. $19.46— Nancy Normal | | 1. $8846.00— Abe Domin, M.D. | | |

**Step 26.**  In this case, this is the first claim for Nancy. Thus, the following amounts are listed in her updated history:

**Accident Benefit:**  $0.00 (CCYY) [This was not an accident claim, so no accident benefits were paid.]

**Lifetime Max:**  $109.46 [This is the total amount of all claims paid on Nancy during her lifetime. Since this is her first claim, it is just the amount from this claim.]

**Deductible:**  $125.00 (CCYY) Nancy paid $125 in deductible on this claim. She has now met the CCYY year deductible.]

**Carryover Ded:**  $0.00 (CCNY) [This claim was not paid in the last three months of the year so there is no carryover deductible.]

**Coinsurance:**  $ 11.74 (CCYY) [This is the amount of Nancy's copayment on this claim.]

**Date of Injury:**  [This would not apply since this claim is not an accident.]

You have now finished processing this claim!

| Accident Benefit | $0.00 | | $0.00 | | |
| Lifetime Max | $109.46 | | $8,846.00 | | |
| Deductible | $125.00 | | $150.00 | | |
| Carryover Ded | $0.00 | | $0.00 | | |
| Coinsurance | $11.74 | | $1,250.00 | | |
| Date of Injury | NA | | N/A | | |

## ERISA

Federal ERISA requirements affect all claim denials. The ERISA Right of Review statement must be included with every claim denial and on every EOB where all or part of a claim is denied. The following is wording that may be used on the EOB or statement:

"If you disagree with our decision on your claim, you have the right by law to request that your claim be reviewed by your plan administrator. This request must be made in writing within 60 days of receipt of this notice. If you wish, you may submit your written comments and views. Please consult your plan's claim review procedures. See your employer regarding any other ERISA questions."

## Payees

Now all that is left to do is to determine whom to pay, and to update the financial history. Look back on the claim form. Benefits may be assigned to the provider of services by the member. The assignment must bear the member's written signature on a form that authorizes benefits payable directly to the provider of service. An **assignment of benefits** is a statement, usually included on the claim form, which permits the member to authorize the administrator to pay benefits directly to the person or institution that provided the service. A **provider of service** (often just **provider**) is the physician, chiropractor, dentist or other healthcare professional or establishment (hospital, nursing home, etc.) that provides healthcare services. The examiner is required to honor all valid assignments made by the member.

When reviewing a claim, note whether an assignment has been made. If payment is made because of failure to honor an assignment and benefits are released to the member, the provider of service can also request payment, and payment must be made to the provider as well. The incorrect payment made to the member will have to be recouped (this will be covered later in the section on Adjustments). Ensuring that all valid assignments are honored is a basic part of good claim handling.

When processing a claim, ask yourself, did the insured authorize payment directly to the provider of services or is there a mandatory assignment of benefits?

- If not, the payee would be the insured.

- If so, check the billed amount from the claim and the amount (if any) that the patient/insured has already paid. If the difference between the billed

amount and the amount that the patient or insured paid (balance due) is less than the benefit payment amount, the payee would be the provider of services up to the balance due. Any remaining funds would then be paid to the insured.

## Updating History

Updating the payment history is vitally important to ensure that proper benefit payments are calculated. Each preceding question that related to previous payments of deductibles, coinsurance amounts, satisfaction of individual or family limits, accident benefits, and other accumulated amounts will change with the processing of each claim. On our payment worksheet, the updated history appears in the upper-left-hand corner of the sheet. If claims are processed by computer, the computer should handle the updating of the history for you.

If accident benefits were paid on this claim, add the payment amount of the accident benefits to any previous accident benefit amounts paid on this individual for this accident. This amount goes on the first line. The amount paid on all accidents in this calendar year should be placed to the right of this amount, along with the current year (in parentheses).

The amount of the benefits paid under Major Medical should be added to all previous major medical benefits paid. If the plan has a calendar year maximum rather than a lifetime maximum, the amount of the benefits paid should be added to all previous benefits paid during that calendar year. The result should be placed in the lifetime maximum space on the next line. Usually, Basic benefits on Basic and Major Medical plans do not apply to lifetime paid amounts. Check the contract to see whether there are separate maximums for Basic and Major Medical payment amounts. If the plan calls for a calendar year maximum, the word "lifetime" should be replaced by the words "calendar year" and the current year should be included.

The amount of any deductibles calculated on this claim should be added to any previously paid deductible amounts and the result placed in the deductible space with the current year.

If any of the dates of service on this claim fall within the last three months of the calendar year and the contract includes a carryover provision, the amount of deductible paid on these services should be placed on the line labeled "carryover deductible," along with the year. If there is more than one date of service and if some are in the last three months and others are not, the deductible amount should be taken from the amount or amounts of the services in the order in which they are received.

**Example:** An exam was performed on 9/18/CCYY. Two moles were found and removed on 10/10/CCYY. The allowed amount was $40 for the exam and $120 for the mole removal. The patient had previously satisfied $25 of the $100 deductible. The total paid deductible amount would be $75 on this claim. Forty dollars of the deductible would be for the first service and $35 would be for the mole removal. Therefore, $35 would be considered the carryover deductible amount.

Finally, add the amount listed on the coinsurance line with any previous coinsurance amounts for the calendar year. The total, along with the year, should be placed on the coinsurance line of the financial history box. You have now completed payment on this claim.

# Quick Reference Formulas

The following quick reference formulas will help you remember the calculation included on a payment worksheet.

## Plan UCR

Unit value × plan conversion factor = plan UCR.

Anesthesia: Time units + procedure unit value × plan conversion factor.

$$(TU + UV) \times CF = ANES. ALLOW.$$

Multiple Surgery: 100% of the basic or UCR allowance for the major procedure.

## Noncovered Charges

Total charges minus allowable amounts (UCR).

$$TC - UCR = NC$$

## Basic Allowance

Procedure unit value × basic conversion factor.

$$UV \times BCF = BASIC$$

## Major Medical Allowance

Plan UCR allowance minus basic allowance.

$$UCR - BASIC = MM\ ALLOWABLE$$

## Major Medical Payment

Plan UCR minus basic allowance minus applicable deductibles multiplied by plan coinsurance rate.

$$(UCR - BASIC) - DEDS \times \% = MM\ PAYMT$$

## Total Payment

Major Medical payment plus basic payment.

$$MM + Basic = TP$$

# Claim Office Administration

Several forms are helpful to the claims examiner in tracking their calculations and recording important information for easier use. The Inventory/Production Sheet (**Figure 5–7**) is a form on which the claims examiner records all the claims processed or pended and the finished correspondence and phone calls, as well as all the received claims that are not yet processed and unfinished correspondence, for that work week. The Family Benefits Tracking Sheet (**Figure 5–8**) is a form designed to keep track of the benefits that have been paid to date on each member of a family, so that a claims examiner is able to quickly calculate any remaining aggregate and nonaggregate deductible amounts and coinsurance limits on a given family contract.

# Inventory/Production Sheet

Name: _____
Department: _____
Week of: _____

| | Medical Claims Processed | Hospital Claims Processed | Dental Claims Processed | Pended Claims | Correspondence Handled or Written | Phone Calls Made | Downtime |
|---|---|---|---|---|---|---|---|
| **Day 1** | | | | | | | |
| **Day 2** | | | | | | | |
| **Day 3** | | | | | | | |
| **Day 4** | | | | | | | |
| **Day 5** | | | | | | | |
| **TOTALS** | | | | | | | |

| | Unprocessed Medical Claims | Unprocessed Hospital Claims | Unprocessed Dental Claims | Pended Claims | Unfinished Correspondence |
|---|---|---|---|---|---|
| **Day 1** | | | | | |
| **Day 2** | | | | | |
| **Day 3** | | | | | |
| **Day 4** | | | | | |
| **Day 5** | | | | | |
| **TOTALS** | | | | | |

■ **Figure 5–7** Inventory/Production Sheet

# FAMILY BENEFITS TRACKING SHEET

**FAMILY DEDUCTIBLE**

| Patient Name | Document # | Amount | Total |
|---|---|---|---|
|  |  |  |  |
|  |  |  |  |
|  |  |  |  |
|  |  |  |  |
|  |  |  |  |
|  |  |  |  |
|  |  |  |  |
|  |  |  |  |
|  |  |  |  |

Contract: _____

Ind. Ded.: _____

Family Ded.: _____

  Aggregate  Nonaggregate

Coins. Limit: _____

Family Coins. Limit: _____

  Aggregate  Nonaggregate

| Document # | Individual Deductible | | Coinsurance | | Lifetime Maximum | |
|---|---|---|---|---|---|---|
|  | Amount | Total | Amount | Total | Amount | Total |

**Patient Name:**

| Prior C/O | ------ | | ------- | | ------- | |
|---|---|---|---|---|---|---|
|  |  |  |  |  |  |  |
|  |  |  |  |  |  |  |
|  |  |  |  |  |  |  |
|  |  |  |  |  |  |  |
|  |  |  |  |  |  |  |

**Patient Name:**

| Prior C/O | ------ | | ------- | | ------- | |
|---|---|---|---|---|---|---|
|  |  |  |  |  |  |  |
|  |  |  |  |  |  |  |
|  |  |  |  |  |  |  |
|  |  |  |  |  |  |  |
|  |  |  |  |  |  |  |

**Patient Name:**

| Prior C/O | ------ | | ------- | | ------- | |
|---|---|---|---|---|---|---|
|  |  |  |  |  |  |  |
|  |  |  |  |  |  |  |
|  |  |  |  |  |  |  |
|  |  |  |  |  |  |  |
|  |  |  |  |  |  |  |

**Patient Name:**

| Prior C/O | ------ | | ------- | | ------- | |
|---|---|---|---|---|---|---|
|  |  |  |  |  |  |  |
|  |  |  |  |  |  |  |
|  |  |  |  |  |  |  |
|  |  |  |  |  |  |  |
|  |  |  |  |  |  |  |

■ **Figure 5–8** Family Benefits Tracking Sheet

# Prescription Drug Claims

Many health plans cover expenses for prescription drugs. However, these drugs must often meet the following three criteria:

1. They must be prescribed by the member's physician. This physician must be duly licensed and able to prescribe medications in the state in which the prescription was issued.

2. They must be prescription medications (i.e., they must, by law, require a prescription from a licensed physician for their dispensation).

3. They must be prescribed to treat a disease, bodily injury, or a mental or nervous disorder.

Some plans may cover prescriptions that do not meet the above criteria. These can include antacids, eye and ear medications, compounded dermatalogic preparations, or other medications. If these drugs are listed, they will be specifically indicated in the policy.

Nonprescription drugs are generally not covered under the provisions of a contract. In addition, some prescription drugs may not be covered. These can include:

- Contraceptives prescribed for contraception.
- Dietary supplements, health foods, or vitamins (including prenatal vitamins).
- Appetite suppressants.

The *Physicians' Desk Reference* should be consulted to determine whether a drug is a prescription or a nonprescription drug.

## "Red Book" and "Blue Book"

Some plans have separate drug subcoverage. Drugs on these plans are often paid according to a set price schedule, regardless of the amount charged by the pharmacy or dispensing physician. These schedules are often based on the *Blue Book* or the *Red Book*. These two books list wholesale prices of drugs.

Often the plan provisions will specify payment at 150% or 175% of the *Blue Book* or *Red Book* price.

To find the correct payment amount, first determine the manufacturer of the drug. If the drug manufacturer is not listed, the information should be looked up using the *Physicians' Desk Reference*. The least expensive generic drug should be used to calculate benefits.

Determine the charge for the smallest quantity listed, and then determine the price per unit. The unit may be indicated in quantification by tables, by ounces, or by some other measurement. If the drugs are listed in metric units and the prescription is issued in nonmetric units, the metric units must be converted to nonmetric units (or vice versa). Metric conversion tables can be found in most medical dictionaries.

Multiply the price per unit by the number of units dispensed. This is the wholesale price for the drug. This wholesale price should be multiplied by the ×% (150% or 175%) indicated by the plan. Then, add any amount indicated as $A ($1.35, $1.50, or $1.65). If this amount is more than the amount charged, the amount charged should be used. If not, this amount is considered the allowable amount. This allowed amount is then paid at the (50%, 75%, or 100%) amount at which benefits are payable.

## Guidelines for Handling Prescription Drug Claims

Prescription drugs can be issued on an outpatient or inpatient basis. For the guidelines regarding payment for inpatient drugs (including those issued for take home), see the Physician's, Clinical, and Hospital Services Claims chapter.

For outpatient drug claims, certain guidelines should be followed. These include the following:

1. A valid claim form must be on file showing the eligible diagnosis for which the drugs are being prescribed. This form shows that the patient was under the care of a physician for the covered diagnosis when the prescription was issued. After a valid claim form has been accepted, it is not necessary for a new claim form to accompany each drug claim as long as the patient is still under the doctor's care and the diagnosis is still valid. For example, if the diagnosis is of a chronic nature, drugs will often be refills of earlier prescriptions.

2. The pharmacy bill, receipt, or pharmacy statement for each prescription must accompany the request for payment.

3. All drug receipts or pharmacy bills must show the prescription number, the name of the physician, the name of the patient, the date of issuance, and the amount charged. If any of these items are omitted, the validity of the prescription should be checked prior to payment of the claim. Some receipts may also list the type of drug. This is helpful for determining whether the drug is a prescription drug or an over-the-counter drug.

4. The drugs must be appropriate for the condition being treated, the amount of time since the first diagnosis of the condition, and the amount of drug prescribed. For example, persons suffering from a serious heart disease or diabetes may require large amounts of drugs over an extended period of time, whereas a patient suffering from an ear infection would require a small amount of drugs over a much shorter period of time.

5. If prescriptions are questionable, further information should be obtained from the prescribing physician, not from the patient. Causes for review include:

   a. The amount of the prescription expense is not appropriate to the condition being treated.

   b. The drugs are generally used to treat conditions that are not covered under the policy (i.e., exogenous obesity, contraception).

   c. The claim is for contraceptive medications. If the woman is over the age of 45, many doctors prescribe contraceptive medications for hormone imbalance. Some plans may cover contraceptives issued for these reasons but not for contraceptive reasons.

   d. A large number of prescription claims is submitted at one time. This may indicate claims being submitted for prescriptions that were issued to more than one person.

   e. The prescription or information on any claim appears to have been altered.

6. If a receipt or statement is received for more than one drug, care should be taken to determine which drugs are covered and which are not. Often several types appear on the same claim.

7. Plan provisions should be checked to determine which drugs are covered and which are not. Also, drugs issued for a noncovered diagnosis should be denied as not covered.

   **Example:** Morphine would be covered for heart surgery but not for cosmetic surgery.

8. Check the licensure of the prescribing doctor. In many states, physicians, dentists, podiatrists, and psychiatrists are allowed to prescribe medications. However, chiropractors, naturopaths, optometrists, and psychologists are not. These doctors may suggest or dispense nonprescription medications, food supplements, or vitamins. However, since these items are not generally covered under the plan, no benefits would be payable. If the drug appears to be a prescription drug, but the physician indicated is not a physician, dentist, podiatrist, or psychiatrist, further investigation is warranted.

9. Finally, check the appropriate coverages for drug claims. Most prescription drugs are covered under Major Medical benefits and would be processed according to the general guidelines provided in the Major Medical plan. However, there may be specific plan provisions on medications. Care should also be taken to check the exclusions listed in the policy because this is usually where the exclusions to types of drugs and diagnoses will be listed.

## Coordination of Benefits

**Coordination of benefits (COB)** is a process that occurs when two or more plans provide coverage on the same person. Coordination between the two plans is necessary to allow for payment of 100% of the allowable expense but no more. This process was developed in response to a growing problem of overinsurance.

**Overinsurance** occurs when a person is covered under two or more policies and is eligible to collect an accumulation of benefits that actually exceeds the amount charged by the provider. The purpose of COB is to allow coverage and usually payment of 100% of allowable expenses without the covered member or members "making" money over and above the total costs for care.

In response to the diversity of handling procedures used by various carriers and administrators in coordinating coverages, the National Association of Insurance Commissioners (NAIC) developed a standardized model for COB administration. Most benefit plans follow this model, but it is not mandatory. Therefore, the plan provisions must be checked before processing COB claims, since the handling procedures may vary according to whether or not the NAIC guides are used.

## Definitions

To process COB claims correctly, the following definitions must be understood:

**Group Plan**—A form of coverage with which coordination of benefits is allowed. A plan may include:

1. Group, blanket, or franchise insurance policy or plan if not individually underwritten.

2. Health maintenance organization, hospital, or medical service prepayment policy available through an employer, union, or association.

3. Trustee policy or plan, union welfare policy or plan, multiple employer policy or plan, or employee benefit policy or plan.

4. Governmental programs (Medicare) or policies or plans required by a statute, except Medicaid or Medi-Cal.

5. "No-fault" auto policy or plan. (Applies to some plans only. The plan must specify whether or not this is applicable.)

**Primary Plan**—The benefit plan that determines and pays its benefits first without regard to the existence of any other coverage.

**Secondary Plan**—The plan that pays after the primary plan has paid its benefits. The benefits of the secondary plan take into consideration the benefits of the primary plan and may reduce its payment so that only 100% of allowable expenses are paid.

**Allowable Expense**—Any necessary, reasonable, and customary item of a medical or dental expense, at least partly covered under at least one of the plans covering the person for whom a claim is made. Items that are excluded by the secondary plan, such as dental services and vision care services, would not be considered allowable. Conversely, amounts that are limited under the secondary plan would be considered allowable (the entire charge). For example:

1. Each plan provides a limit of $35 per visit for outpatient psychiatric care. The psychiatrist charges $50 per visit. Since both plans limit payment to $35 per visit, only $35 would be considered an allowable expense under COB.

2. Based on the primary plan's UCR guidelines, the amount allowable for surgery is $1,200. The secondary plan's UCR for the same surgery is $1,000. When coordinating benefits, the secondary plan would allow the greatest amount allowed by at least one of the plans.

Therefore, the allowable amount when coordinating benefits would be $1200. Bear in mind that this amount has nothing to do with how the secondary plan calculates its usual payment. You will see how the two amounts interact later.

**Claim Determination Period**—Usually a calendar year. It does not include any part of a year before the effective date of duplicate coverage under the secondary plan. It does not include any remaining amount during a calendar year occurring after the termination date of the primary plan. As long as the secondary plan is not terminated, COB continues to be performed even though there are no longer multiple coverages.

**Normal Liability (NL)**—The amount payable under the secondary plan's provisions without regard to any other coverage (what would regularly have been paid if there were no other insurance). This is not necessarily the amount that will actually be paid.

**Example:** The secondary plan pays 80% of UCR after a $100 deductible. The first claim is paid as follows: (OIS= Other Insurance Payment):

| | |
|---|---|
| Charge | $200 |
| Deductible | $100 |
| OIS payment | $160 |
| Secondary plan's NL | $80 |
| Secondary plan's actual payment | $40 |

**Credit Reserve (CR) (benefit credit, credit savings, etc.)**—A cumulative amount within a claim determination period that is derived from the amount of funds that a plan has saved by being the secondary carrier. The credit reserve does not carry over from one calendar year to another. Each year, the balance begins at $0. A running total is kept for each separate determination period (calendar year).

**Example:** Same benefits as above.

| | |
|---|---|
| Charge | $200 |
| Deductible | $100 |
| OIS payment | $100 |
| Secondary plan's NL | $80 |
| Secondary plan's Actual payment | $40 |

CR = NL – AP, or $80 – $40 = $40 in savings.

**Insular COB**—COB applied separately to medical and dental charges. All savings are kept separately.

**Global COB**—COB applied to both medical and dental charges combined. All savings are kept intermingled.

**Explanation of Benefits (EOB)**—An explanation of benefits letter from a payer indicating how a member's benefits have been applied in response to the submission of a claim for services. The EOB indicates deductibles, coinsurance amounts, nonallowable amounts, UCR limitations, and other pertinent information. An EOB is required by law to be generated on each claim submission showing the disposition of the claim (i.e., how it was paid, denied, pending for additional information, etc).

## Order of Benefit Determination Rules

**Order of Benefit Determination Rules** were established to provide standardized rules for coordination among health plans. Since each plan would prefer to pay as the secondary payer, it became necessary to develop rules to determine when a plan should pay as primary, secondary, or tertiary.

The 14 rules determining the order of payment are referred to as the **Order of Benefit Determinations (OBD)** (see Table 5–1)

## Order of Benefit Determination Rules

| Rule # | Description |
|---|---|
| 1 | The plan without a COB provision will be primary to a plan with a COB provision. |
| 2 | When a plan does not have OBD rules, and as a result the plans do not agree on the OBD, the plan without these OBD rules will determine the order of payment. |
| 3 | The plan that covers an individual as an employee will be primary to a plan that covers that individual as a dependent. |
| 4 | If an individual is an employee under two plans, the primary is the one under which the employee has been covered the longest. |
| 5 | If an employee is an active employee under one plan and a retiree (or laid off) under another, the active plan will pay as primary. |
| **The parent birthday rule, explained in #6 and #7, affects the OBD for dependent children of parents who are living together and married (not divorced or legally separated).** | |
| 6 | The plan of the parent whose birthday (based on month and day only) occurs first during the calendar year, is the primary plan. |
| 7 | When both parents' birthdays are the same (based on month and day), the plan that covered one parent the longest is the primary plan. |
| **For dependents of legally separated or divorced parents and those whose parents have remarried, the order of benefits determination is based on the following rule:** | |
| 8 | The plan of the parent specified as having legal responsibility for the healthcare expense of the child is the primary plan. |
| **For dependents of separated parents with no court decree:** | |
| 9 | The plan of the parent with custody is prime. |
| 10 | The plan of the step-parent (if any) with whom the child resides is secondary. |
| 11 | The plan of the natural parent without custody is tertiary. |
| 12 | The step-parent (if any) who does not reside with the child has no legal right to declare dependency. Therefore, no coordination should be performed because the child is probably not an eligible dependent under the plan. |
| 13 | For joint custody, with no additional responsibility designation, the plan of the parent whose coverage has been in effect the longest would be the primary payer. However, this rule may vary by administrator. Some parents pay costs on a 50/50 basis, thereby sharing equally in the healthcare risk. |
| 14 | A few rare plans do not use the birthday rule as previously described. These plans generally use the **gender rule**; which states that the plan covering the male employee is primary, and the plan covering the female employee is secondary. |

**Table 5–1** Order of Benefit Determination

# On the Job Now

1. Define COB. _____

   _____

2. What is the purpose of COB? _____

   _____

3. The _____ is the benefit plan that determines and pays its benefits first without regard to the existence of any other coverage.

4. The _____ is the plan that pays after the primary plan has paid its benefits.

## Right to Receive and Release Information

Certain facts are needed to determine and apply the appropriate COB rules. Therefore, plan representatives have the right to decide which facts are required and to obtain the needed facts from, or give the facts to, any other organization. The plan should get the insured's consent to do this. In addition, each person claiming benefits under a plan must give the facts required to properly process a claim. It is also important to realize that most providers of care do not release any information to a payer without a signed release from the member. Information should be requested or released to others only when absolutely necessary to determine benefits under the plan. The unnecessary request or release of information could be a violation of the right to privacy, which is punishable by law. Therefore, request only what is necessary, and routinely request a written authorization from the member to release information.

## Right of Recovery

If the amount of the payments made by the plan is more than it should have paid under the COB provision, the plan may recover the excess from one or more of the following:

1. The person or persons it has paid or on behalf of whom it has paid.
2. Other insurers/plans.
3. Other organizations.

The "amount of the payments made" includes the reasonable cash value of any benefits provided in the form of services.

## Practice Pitfalls

Following are some miscellaneous guidelines:

- The difference between the cost of a private and a semiprivate hospital room is not considered an allowable expense unless the patient's stay in a private room was medically necessary either as generally accepted medical practice or as specifically defined in the plan.

- Items of expense under coverages such as dental care, vision care, prescription drug, or hearing aid programs may be excluded from the definition of allowable expense. A plan that provides only benefits for such items may limit its definition of allowable expense to like items.

- A medical plan may have COB with medical expenses only, and a dental-only plan may limit COB to other dental plans only.

- An item of expense covered under the primary plan may be considered an allowable expense under the secondary plan even though that plan does not provide such a benefit. For example, if the primary plan covers routine examinations and the secondary plan excludes routine examinations, routine exams may be considered an allowable expense by the secondary carrier in this instance.

- This COB rule varies widely from payer to payer. As previously indicated, some payers do not consider excluded expenses as allowable; others do. Therefore, the COB provisions and administrative handling rules must be verified. (Remember that we are talking about the amount considered as an allowable expense under COB, not the amount used to determine the secondary plan's normal liability.)

# Health Maintenance Organizations

A **health maintenance organization (HMO)** is a type of prepayment plan in which providers agree to charge members for their services in accordance with a fixed schedule of rates. The HMO member (insured) usually pays a specified copayment at the time the service is rendered. The patient and the doctor are usually not involved in having to complete the claim forms for submission to a payer. Instead, the HMO is billed directly, or the HMO pays a monthly retainer fee (capitation) to the physician for membership plus other specified fees.

If the required medical services are available through the HMO but the insured does not go to an HMO provider for the treatment, he or she may be held entirely responsible for all the expenses.

Prepayment plans are included in the definition of the type of policies to which COB provisions apply. However, many HMO's do not have COB provisions, although more are starting to incorporate the COB concept because of the spiraling costs of medical care.

An example of an HMO is Kaiser Permanente. Kaiser provides a prepayment policy for hospital and professional medical services at no cost or at a small fee, as long as the member goes to a Kaiser facility. Subsequently, the HMO provides the member with a "reasonable cost statement," which represents what would have been charged to a nonmember. If the HMO does not have the COB provision, the HMO would be considered the primary payer. To coordinate benefits, a request must be made for receipts or statements showing the actual "out-of-pocket" expense. The secondary plan would pay no more than the amount that would be considered the allowable expense. If the HMO does have a COB provision, the regular OBD determination rules should be applied.

# Preferred Provider Organizations

As previously covered, **preferred provider organizations (PPOs)** are special arrangements in which members are responsible for expenses based on specific contractual UCR arrangements. Some services may be covered at a higher rate than others, and some may not be covered at all. Usually, COB will apply to PPO claims. The main difference between going to a regular provider is reflected in the patient's liability. That is, if the member goes to a PPO provider, the member is not responsible for any amounts in excess of the PPO contractual UCR amount.

In addition, depending on the payer, the plan, and the PPO, the secondary payer may not be held responsible for any amounts in excess of the contractual PPO amount, even though the secondary payer is not a party to the contract. This handling is based on the premise that if the member is not responsible for anything over the PPO rate, then neither is the secondary plan. Once again, this handling varies.

A PPO's EOB usually specifically states the member's responsibility. By referring to the appropriate field on the EOB, the secondary carrier can tell what amount to use to determine the allowable expense. Anything in excess of the patient's liability amount is not considered allowable.

If the member does not go to a PPO provider, the member is responsible for all the charges, including the amounts in excess of the primary plan's UCR. In addition, most plans penalize their members for not going to PPO providers by reducing the plan's payment (i.e., the coinsurance percentage paid by the plan is reduced from 80% to 70%, or even lower).

# TRICARE

**TRICARE** (formerly CHAMPUS) provides a comprehensive program of healthcare benefits for active duty and retired services personnel, their dependents, and the dependents of deceased military personnel. TRICARE is secondary to all other insurance or health policies except Medicaid and TRICARE supplemental insurance. However, because many services are provided free of charge or with only a minimal fee, many examiners never see a TRICARE EOB.

# On the Job Now

**1.** What is a PPO? _____

**2.** What does HMO stand for? Describe what an HMO is. _____

_____

_____

**3.** What is TRICARE? _____

_____

_____

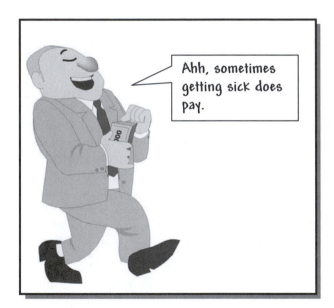

Ahh, sometimes getting sick does pay.

## Recognizing the Presence of Dual Coverage

The possibility that a claimant may have dual coverage is indicated in the following two examples:

1. The greatest likelihood of dual coverage occurs when the spouse is employed. Claim forms usually request the name of the employee's spouse, and the name and address of the spouse's employer. The claim form defines what is meant by other group insurance and asks the claimant to designate which type of other insurance exists.

2. Even when the claimant states that there is no other coverage, additional inquiries should be made in the following instances:

- In claims that involve married employees or their dependents, often the spouse also has group coverage on the family.

- The claim form indicates that the spouse is not employed. Under the policy held by the spouse's previous employer, extended benefits or a provision for COBRA may be available.

- The claim is for a dependent child, but the area on the form requesting other insurance information has been left blank.

- Notations on the hospital bills or claim papers show that some other insurer/plan has paid benefits or that there is other employment within the family.

- The claimant does not assign hospital benefits. This may indicate that the claimant has used other benefits to pay the provider and thus does not want a duplicate payment to be made (to the provider).

- It is known from a group's local sources that a patient is covered under another plan.

- Photocopies of bills are submitted. Usually, the original is submitted, and a copy is kept by the member. The originals may have been submitted to another payer.

- The provider charges for the completion of a claim form, but the submitted form was not received from the provider. The charge may have been for completing a form for another payer.

- Requests for information are received from other policyholders/plans or insurers.

- The occupation of the claimant, spouse, or dependent suggests coverage through a union or other professional affiliation.
- A hospital or surgeon's bill makes reference to other coverage.
- A bill showing a substantial credit or adjustment to the account.
- The claim submitted is the first maternity bill for the subscriber's spouse. In such a case, the wife may have been regularly employed until her pregnancy, and benefits may be available through the extension of benefits provision of her previous policy.
- The claim is submitted on another carrier's claim form, or an EOB is attached.
- A duplicate coverage inquiry (DCI) is received. This is an industry-approved form designed to establish the existence of other coverage.
- An HMO requests reimbursement for the value of service provided to one of their patients.

- Claim history shows COB payments or secondary carrier payments in the past, but claims are now being paid as primary with no explanation.

Pursuit of details pertaining to other coverage can be through a variety of sources. If the claim form indicates that the insured's spouse is employed and includes the name and address of the spouse's employer, contact that employer to determine whether there is other group coverage. If the claim form does not indicate the name and address of the spouse's employer, request the missing information from the subscriber.

Additional sources of information regarding the existence of dual coverage include:

- Files from hospital admissions.
- City directories listing members of a family, their occupations, and places of employment.
- Information cards compiled by the Benefits Office for local employer plans.

# On the Job Now

1. (True or False?) The plan without a COB provision is secondary to a plan with a COB provision. _____

2. Define Global COB. _____

_____

3. _____ applies separately to medical and dental charges. All savings are kept separate.

## COB Worksheet

The COB worksheet is used to help calculate the proper benefits when there is COB between more than one health plan. **Figure 5–9** is a sample COB

worksheet. To begin, calculate the allowable amount that would be paid on this claim if there was no other insurance. Then, follow the instructions on the bottom of the COB Calculation Worksheet.

## Coordination of Benefits Calculation Worksheet

Patient's Name: _____ Year: _____

**Payment Calculation:**

1. Total allowable amount for this claim is the higher of either the primary plan's
   allowable amount or the secondary plan's allowable amount. _____

2. Total primary insurance carrier payment for this claim. _____

3. Difference between Line 1 and Line 2. _____

4. Secondary insurance carrier's normal liability for this claim. _____

5. The lesser of Line 3 or Line 4.
   This is the amount of the secondary insurance carrier actual payment on this claim. _____

**Credit Reserve:**

6. Normal liability for this claim (Line 4 above). _____

7. Actual payment for this claim (line 5 above). _____

8. Subtract Line 7 from Line 6. _____

9. Credit reserve on all previous claims for this patient. _____

10. Total credit reserve (add Line 8 and Line 9). _____

**Instructions:**

Place the patient's name and the year that services were rendered in the box on the top of the COB calculation sheet.

1. Enter the total allowable amount on this claim. The total allowable amount is the greater of either the primary plan's allowable amount or the secondary plan's allowable amount.
2. Enter the total amount that other insurance companies have paid on this claim.
3. Subtract Line 2 from Line 1.
4. Enter the normal liability amount for this insurance company for this claim.
5. Enter the lesser of either Line 3 or Line 4. This is the actual amount of the secondary insurance payor on this claim.

**To Calculate Credit Reserve:**

6. Enter the normal liability amount for the secondary insurance carrier for this claim.
7. Enter the actual payment for the secondary insurance carrier for this claim.
8. Subtract Line 7 from Line 6. This is the amount of money the secondary carrier has saved by paying secondary on this claim. This amount becomes part of the credit reserve.
9. Enter the credit reserve amount for all previous claims for this patient.
10. Add Line 8 and Line 9. This is the total credit reserve for this patient.

■ **Figure 5–9** Coordination of Benefits Calculation Worksheet

# Adjustments

An **adjustment** is the reprocessing of a claim to correct prior errors. Although the terminology may vary from company to company, the concepts behind each type are basically the same. The four basic types of adjustments are:

1. **Statistical Adjustment**—An adjustment that changes the claim data (i.e., procedure coding, type of benefit paid, diagnosis) but does not increase or decrease the original claim payment.

2. **Supplemental Adjustment**—An adjustment that increases the original claim payment. A statistical adjustment may also be involved (often but not always) since the original claim coding may have caused the incorrect payment.

3. **Full Credit Adjustment**—An adjustment that completely reverses a claim payment because the original submission should not have been paid at all.

4. **Partial Credit Adjustment**—An adjustment that partially reverses a claim payment. The original claim was overpaid.

## Statistical Adjustment

A **statistical adjustment** changes claim data but does not increase or decrease the claim payment. As the name implies, this type of adjustment is required to correct historical data only. The original payment is not affected by the corrected data.

The following are some of the more common reasons for requiring a statistical adjustment:

1. The claim was processed under an incorrect member identification (ID) number.

2. The claim was processed on an incorrect claimant but under the correct ID number.

3. The claim payment was issued to an incorrect provider of service. The provider's tax identification number or social security number was input incorrectly, or a totally wrong provider was paid. If the provider paid was in the same medical group, a statistical adjustment may be sufficient. However, if a completely separate and unaffiliated provider was paid, a full-credit adjustment is probably required with a new payment issued to the correct provider.

4. The claim was processed under an incorrect group number, but the payment remains the same.

5. The claim was erroneously denied; charges should have been applied to the deductible. (No payment will be made even when processed correctly.)

6. Charges were applied to the deductible but should have been denied.

## Supplemental Adjustment

A **supplemental adjustment** is performed to increase an original claim payment. Often, a supplemental adjustment is required because the original claim was coded incorrectly. Therefore, a statistical adjustment is usually involved, but the changes are such that a payment or an additional payment will result. The following are some of the more common reasons why a supplemental adjustment may be required:

1. The original claim was erroneously denied when benefits should have been paid.

2. Charges were applied to the deductible in error; benefits should have been paid. This usually occurs when the deductible applies to specific types of expenses, but not to all types.

3. Some benefits were paid, but additional benefits should have been paid.

4. Late charges are received.

5. Corrected billing or other information is received.

6. The claims examiner or adjuster applied incorrect benefits.

7. The examiner coded the diagnosis or procedure incorrectly, thus causing an incorrect UCR allowance or other limitation.

Whenever an underpayment is found, an adjustment should be preformed for the corrected amount. Either a letter or full explanation on the new EOB should be sent to the proper parties.

## Full-Credit Adjustment

A **full-credit adjustment** completely reverses the original claim payment. Usually, this type of adjustment is not performed until the original monies paid out have been returned in full to the payer. When an incorrect provider is paid and the money is returned, many companies consider this to be a full-credit adjustment with a subsequent payment remitted to the correct provider. Regardless of whether or not a subsequent corrected payment is issued, the original payment is received back in the claims office and is reversed in the system. Following are some reasons why full-credit adjustments may be required:

1. A duplicate claim is received and paid in error.
2. The member is not eligible for benefits under the plan.
3. Claim benefits are paid incorrectly, or plan limitations are not adhered to.
4. An incorrect provider is paid who is unaffiliated with the correct provider of service.

## Partial Credit Adjustment

A **partial credit adjustment** partially reverses a claim payment. In this case, part of the original payment is correct and part is incorrect. The common reasons why partial credit adjustments are performed include:

1. When a greater payment was made on a claim than what should have been made according to the plan provisions and limitations.
2. Because the claims examiner applied benefits incorrectly either through incorrect coding, duplication of payment, inappropriate application of benefits, or some other error.

## Collecting Overpayments

Even the best claims examiners may make errors. When this happens, an overpayment of benefits may occur. Under most circumstances, every attempt should be made to recover overpayments when they are discovered. Most insurance companies have a standard adjustment form letter to send the member in order to inform them of an adjustment to their claim; see **Figure 5–10** for an example. However, there are

times when the recovery of overpayments is not feasible or cost-effective. The following are guidelines only and apply to situations in which overpayment recovery should not be attempted:

- The overpayment is under $25.
- The overpayment occurred more than 12 months ago and is under $200.
- The claimant is deceased and the overpayment is under $200.

There are normally three ways to obtain reimbursement of an overpayment.

1. Deduct the overpayment from future benefits of the family member for whom the overpayment occurred. You cannot deduct an overpayment on one family member's claim from benefits due on another family member's claim unless specifically requested by the insured and confirmed in writing. It is not necessary to obtain permission to deduct benefits for the member for whom the overpayment occurred, but advise the claimant of the circumstances of the overpayment and the method that will be used for recoupment.
2. Arrange with the insured for a lump sum payment or establish a payment plan to recoup the overpayment.
3. Obtain reimbursement from a third party, usually another carrier where COB is involved.

Remember that benefits cannot be taken from charges that have been assigned to the provider of services. When a refund is received or offered, accept or pursue all such refunds, regardless of the amount of overpayment or the time that has elapsed since the overpayment occurred.

**Any Insurance Carrier, Inc.**
**123 Any Drive**
**Anywhere, USA 12345**
**(800) 555-1234**

Dear Member:

An error was inadvertently made during the processing of your claim. The attached explanation of benefits shows the corrected payment amount.

The reason for the adjustment is:

☐ Incorrect deductible taken.
☐ Allowed amount figured improperly.
☐ Benefits are not allowed for this procedure.
☐ Incorrect coinsurance amount was applied.
☐ The patient was listed incorrectly.
☐ Other: _____

_____

_____

The following action will be taken to correct this error:

An underpayment was previously made on your claim.
☐ A check is enclosed for $_____ .
☐ Benefits were assigned on this claim. A check in the amount of $_____ has been forwarded to the provider of services.

An overpayment was previously made on your claim and a check was issued to you.
☐ Please remit payment of $_____to our office immediately.
☐ Payment will be subtracted from our next payment to you.

An overpayment was previously made on your claim. Benefits were assigned on this claim and therefore payment was made to the provider of services. Your provider may bill you for amounts refunded to us.
☐ A request for repayment had been sent to your provider.
☐ Payment will be subtracted from your next payment to this provider.
☐ Other: _____

_____

We are sorry for any inconvenience this may have caused.

Sincerely,

■ **Figure 5–10** Adjustment Form Letter

# On the Job Now

1. List the four basic types of adjustments.

   1. _____

   2. _____

   3. _____

   4. _____

2. A _____ adjustment changes claim data but does not increase or decrease a claim payment.

3. A _____ adjustment is performed to increase an original claim payment.

4. A _____ adjustment reverses the original claim payment.

5. A _____ adjustment partially reverses a claim payment.

# On the Job Now

**Directions:** Using the following information, complete a COB calculation worksheet.

1. Patient's Name: Betty Bossy. Year: CCYY. Total submitted expenses = $1,600. Primary plan, A, considers the allowable amount to be $1,450 and has made a payment of $1,160 on this claim. Secondary plan, B, considers the allowable amount to be $1,495. Both calculate benefits at 80%. Neither plan has made any previous payments or had any previous allowable amounts. Prior credit reserve amount is $487.

2. Patient's Name: Danny Dingbat. Year: CCYY. Total submitted expenses = $1,200. Primary plan, A, considers the allowable amount to be $1,000 and has made a payment of $800 on this claim. Secondary plan, B, considers the allowable amount to be $1,200. Both calculate benefits at 80%. Prior credit reserve amount is $595.

3. Patient's Name: Patty P. Patient. Year: CCYY. Total submitted expenses = $1,400. Primary plan, A, considers the allowable amount to be $1,400 and has made a payment of $1,120 on this claim. Secondary plan, B, considers the allowable amount to be $1,200. Plan A calculates benefits at 80%. Plan B limits payment to 50% of the allowable amount to a calendar year maximum of $500; $450 has already been paid. Prior credit reserve amount is $740.

# CHAPTER REVIEW

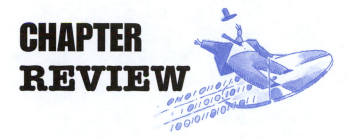

## Summary

- There are many important responsibilities of the claims examiner.
- By applying basic guidelines, the examiner will establish a practice that will enable him or her to routinely make clear and concise claim decisions.
- Coordination of benefits is necessary to ensure that when charges are covered by more than one carrier, the total payment does not exceed more than 100% of the bill.
- These guidelines should be considered whenever there is the possibility of dual coverage or a third party payer.
- Learn to identify the possible existence of another payer by applying the guidelines and rules that were covered in this chapter.
- Remember that most adjustments affect the monies that the subscribers, members, or providers receive. This is always a sensitive situation. Therefore, always be sure that an adjustment is necessary and is performed correctly so that a second or third adjustment is not required.
- Follow the procedures established by the payer for handling adjustments, and give the affected parties adequate notification.
- Failure to follow such procedures significantly increases the likelihood of subsequent ill will or legal action. If in doubt, request assistance before making an adjustment.

## Assignments

Complete the Questions for Review.
Complete Exercises 5–1 through 5–3.

## Questions for Review

**Directions:**  Answer the following questions without looking back at the material just covered. Write your answers in the space provided.

1. If the claim cannot be processed upon receipt, the claim file must be _____

_____

2. Referrals should be made for which three types of claims?

   1. _____

   2. _____

   3. _____

3. What is electronic claims submission? _____

_____

4. Briefly explain the pended claim follow-up procedure. _____

_____

_____

_____

5. Why is it important to update payment history? _____

_____

If you were unable to answer any of these questions, refer back to that section and then fill in the answers.

# Exercise 5-1

**Directions:** Find and circle the words listed below. Words can appear horizontally, vertically, diagonally, forward, or backward.

```
C R F A E V X M O K L K D L W C R C R T R M
H R Z M L W P L T G W O M L H R W L P U U O
C D M O X L O Z D I C D U F T E X T X K B A
C S O M B L O C Z U M N Z J O D V O I T K W
T X U G F Y R W M R S J W X S I I I E M R N
W L Q H W C J E A M N X X E N T R M F P Z U
Q R C V R C N R Y B W E L T N R H I V F O N
J V P G Z T O R G E L K Y F P E V D K S N G
Y Y Q U A V S D Y Q N E Z O H S D Y Q M K W
U O C T M E W W H P F A E G I E G A O D X E
E G I X F N K Z O F N M L X S R W L L D F L
S O S G A A U F Z C E E Q P P V D N N Y M U
N E C N A R U S N I R E V O Y E E V N S S R
T O L F M W I J P A Y X J L D R N R A X R R
M Q L E W Z A V C D U V D M D V A S D R G E
S T A T I S T I C A L A D J U S T M E N T D
U P E H K S R H U O U X W A L Y C M I V Q N
K M J S G T X L W D P M N G J I Y K X R V E
J K I R R F V K A Z N T X S O I K Q O H P G
V P F P F W I C R W Q K I P O L B A P S F R
I P Q T N U T H O J K L Y R I M K Q K N X R
V A T C D P O D P R A W N R Z G Q R I Q P B
```

1. Allowable Expense
2. Credit Reserve
3. Documentation
4. Gender Rule

5. Overinsurance
6. Primary Plan
7. Statistical Adjustment
8. TRICARE

# Exercise 5-2

**Directions:** Complete the crossword puzzle by filling in a word from the keywords that fits each clue.

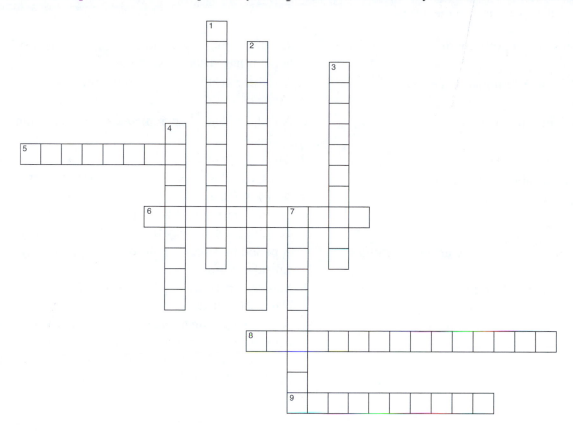

## Across

**5.** To send a claim to be reviewed by a technical claims person.

**6.** Folders of claims that are kept for each family of claimants.

**8.** The amount payable under the secondary plan's provisions without regard to any other coverage.

**9.** Files which are kept in batches or groups based on the date they were processed and the person who processed them.

## Down

**1.** Claims that have not been completely adjudicated or closed.

**2.** The plan that pays after the primary plan has paid its benefits.

**3.** The reprocessing of a claim to correct prior errors.

**4.** COB applied to both medical and dental charges combined. All savings are kept intermingled.

**7.** COB applied separately to medical and dental charges. All savings are kept separately.

# Exercise **5-3**

**Directions:** Match the following terms with the proper definition by writing the letter of the correct definition in the space next to the term.

1. _____ Assignment of Benefits

2. _____ Claim Determination Period

3. _____ Claim Investigation

4. _____ Coordination of Benefits

5. _____ Explanation of Benefits

6. _____ Full Credit Adjustment

7. _____ Order of Benefit Determination Rules

8. _____ Partial Credit Adjustment

9. _____ Supplemental Adjustment

a. A letter from a payer, indicating how a member's benefits have been applied.

b. An adjustment that increases the original claim payment.

c. An adjustment that completely reverses a claim payment.

d. An adjustment that partially reverses a claim payment.

e. Fourteen rules determining the order of payment.

f. A process that occurs when two or more group plans provide coverage on the same person so that the insured does not make money from an illness or injury.

g. A period in which COB is determined, usually a calendar year.

h. Making a detailed inquiry to verify facts pertaining to a claim submitted.

i. A statement, usually included on the claim form, which permits the member to authorize the administrator to pay benefits directly to the person or institution that provided the service.

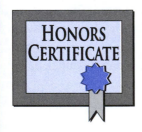

## Honors Certification™

The Honors Certification™ challenge for this chapter constitutes a written test of the information contained within this chapter, including the formulas on how to calculate benefits. There will also be three COB claims to process. Each incorrect answer will result in a deduction of up to 5% from your grade. You must achieve a score of 85% or higher to pass this test. If you fail the test on your first attempt, you may retake the test one additional time. The items included in the second test may be different from those in the first test.

# 6

# Physician's, Clinical,
## and Hospital Services Claims

## After completion of this chapter
**you will be able to:**

- Identify services that are within the medical/physician's services 90000 code range of the *CPT*®.
- Explain how the physician's services section is broken down, when codes should be used, and which providers may bill using these codes.
- Properly code and process physician's services claims.
- Identify codes that fall within the DXL range of the *CPT*®.
- Explain component charges and how they are calculated.
- Explain what panel tests are.
- Discuss unbundling and show how to combine an unbundled charge.
- Identify institutions that are considered to be "hospitals" in claims processing.
- Identify common types of hospital services.

- Separate hospital room and board charges from ancillary charges.
- Identify and explain other facilities that may bill using a UB-92, and may be considered for hospital benefits.
- List the guidelines which determine when a medical emergency exists.
- Identify ambulance services charges.
- State and describe the general guidelines for ambulance coverage.
- Determine proper ambulance benefits.
- Process ambulance claims.
- Define and explain what qualifies as durable medical equipment.
- List guidelines for DME benefit payments.
- Determine proper benefit payment for DME benefits.
- Identify common criteria for equipment covered under the DME provisions.

# Keywords and concepts
## you will learn in this chapter:

- Acupuncture
- Air Ambulance
- Alternative Birthing Centers (ABC)
- Ambulance Expenses
- Ambulatory Surgical Centers (also called Surgi-centers)
- Ancillary Expenses
- Biofeedback
- Consultation
- Convalescent Facilities
- CT (Computed Tomography) Scans
- Custodial Care
- Day Care Centers
- Diagnostic Charges
- Diagnostic X-rays
- Dialysis
- Durable Medical Equipment (DME)
- Emergency Medical Technician (EMT)

- Facility Services
- Hospice Care
- Hospital Services
- Inpatient Care
- Laboratory Examinations
- Maintenance Therapy
- Medical Management
- Medically Oriented Equipment
- Miscellaneous Services
- Mobile Intensive Care Unit
- Necessity
- Night Care Centers
- Nuclear Medicine
- Nursing Homes
- Office or Other Outpatient Visits
- Ophthalmology Care
- Orthoptics
- Osteopathic Treatment
- Outpatient
- Panel Tests

- Papanicolaou or "Pap Smear"
- Paramedics
- Personal Items
- Physical Medicine
- Professional Component
- Professional Services
- Prosthetic Devices
- Radiation Oncology
- Reasonableness
- Rehabilitation Facilities
- Second Opinion or Confirmatory Consultation
- Speech Therapy
- Stat Fees
- Take-Home Prescriptions
- Technical Component
- Telemetry Charges
- Ultrasonography
- Urgent Care Center
- Van Transportation Units
- X-rays

---

The most common services billed by a physician are office and hospital visits. We will review and discuss some specific physician's services and basic guidelines and coverage for these services. When referring to medical services, there are three basic categories:

1. Professional services.
   a. Surgical
   b. Nonsurgical
2. Facility services.
3. Miscellaneous services.

**Professional services** are those performed by a licensed individual such as a medical doctor, physician's assistant, nurse, or chiropractor. **Facility services** are those services provided at a "place," for example, a hospital or clinic. Equipment usage and room fees (i.e., x-ray equipment, operating room) are considered facility expenses. **Miscellaneous services** are all other types of services not included in the previous categories. For example, prescriptions, medical equipment (i.e., wheelchairs, crutches), and ambulance charges are all considered miscellaneous types of expenses.

# CPT® Coding Evaluation & Management

In the remainder of this chapter we will discuss each of the sections of the *CPT®* and any guidelines for that section. Refer to the *CPT®* for additional information.

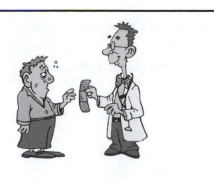

"Hmmm, I wonder if the insurance company will consider this a comprehensive, high complexity exam?"

## Office or Other Outpatient Services (99201–99215)

This section is used to report **office visits** or other encounters between a physician and patient that occur outside a hospital setting.

There are different codes for new and established patients. In general, codes for new patients (99201–99205) carry a higher unit value since the physician is expected to spend additional time completing initial paperwork on the patient and performing a more in-depth history and physical. Because of this, claims examiners should determine whether a patient has previously seen the physician before processing a claim for a new patient. A new patient is considered to be one who has not received any services from this provider, or from another provider of the same specialty who belongs to the same group practice for the last three years. If a provider is on call or is covering for another provider, the patient is classified as they would be for the provider who is not available (i.e., the one being covered for).

## Hospital Observation Services (99217–99220)

These codes are used to denote that the patient was kept in the hospital "for observation." This generally happens when there is a chance that the patient's

The first section of the *CPT*® includes the 99201–99499 series of codes for evaluation and management of a patient (**see Table 6–1**). The Medicine section of the *CPT*® is usually found toward the back of the book and includes codes 90281–99602.

| EVALUATION AND MANAGEMENT CODES | |
| --- | --- |
| Office or Other Outpatient Services | 99201 – 99215 |
| Hospital Observation Services | 99217 – 99220 |
| Hospital Inpatient Services | 99221 – 99239 |
| Consultations | 99241 – 99255 |
| Emergency Department Services | 99281 – 99288 |
| Pediatric Critical Care Patient Transport | 99289 – 99290 |
| Critical Care Services | 99291 – 99292 |
| Inpatient Pediatric Critical Care Services | 99293 – 99294 |
| Inpatient Neonatal Critical Care Services | 99295 – 99296 |
| Continuing Intensive Care Services | 99298 – 99300 |
| Nursing Facility Services | 99304 – 99318 |
| Domiciliary, Rest Home, or Custodial Care Services | 99324 – 99340 |
| Home Services | 99341 – 99350 |
| Prolonged Services | 99354 – 99360 |
| Case Management Services | 99361 – 99373 |
| Care Plan Oversight Services | 99374 – 99380 |
| Preventive Medicine Services | 99381 – 99429 |
| Newborn Care Services | 99431 – 99440 |
| Special Evaluation and Management Services | 99450 – 99499 |
| Other Evaluation and Management Services | 99499 |

**Table 6–1  Evaluation and Management Codes**

condition may worsen and the doctor wants to be sure that immediate medical help is available if that should happen.

## Hospital Inpatient Services (99221–99239)

Hospital inpatient services are visits during the course of a hospital stay. These visits are billed separately from other hospital charges.

An initial hospital visit is the first encounter with the patient by the admitting physician. Everything after this first visit is classified as a subsequent visit, regardless of whether or not the additional visit is performed by the admitting physician or by a different physician.

If a physician performs admit services at a location other than the hospital (i.e., his office), this information should be reported with the claim.

## Consultations (99241–99255)

Usually, a **consultation** is provided by a specialist who has been requested to provide an opinion only. The specialist examines the patient at the request of another physician. He or she may request diagnostic services and may make therapeutic recommendations to the referring physician. However, the specialist does not usually take over the day-to-day treatment or management of the patient. In fact, to qualify as a consultation, the consulting physician cannot be responsible for the regular management of the patient.

If the physician subsequently assumes responsibility for the routine care of the patient, the services should be coded as visits and not consultations even if billed as consultations. (The initial consultation would be allowed as such.) If the consultant is seeing the patient in addition to the regular attending physician, 99231–99233 should be used.

Modifier -32 is used to indicate that the consultation is rendered at the request of a third party (i.e., the insurer).

## Confirmatory Consultations

A **second opinion** or **confirmatory consultation** is designed as a benefit to the patient by confirming the need for surgeries that have a reputation for being done needlessly. Many plans provide a special benefit called an SSO Benefit, which provides 100% payment on services provided by a second, independent specialist whom the patient consults before the scheduling of an elective, nonemergency surgery. Normally, for an SSO benefit to be payable, the following requirements must be satisfied:

1. The second or third opinion physician must be totally uninvolved with the original recommending physician. Therefore, he or she cannot be part of the same medical group and will often be picked by the administrator, medical management firm, or payer.
2. The consultation must be completed before the scheduling of surgery.
3. The second opinion physician cannot perform the recommended surgery.

Depending on the plan, failure to obtain an SSO may result in:

1. Denial of all charges for the surgery and related services.
2. Application of a special, reduced coinsurance. For instance, instead of paying 80% of the allowed amount, 50% would be paid.
3. No change of benefits. In this case, the SSO is considered to be a benefit for the member and is not used to penalize for noncompliance.

## Emergency Department Services (99281–99288)

When a patient goes to the outpatient or emergency department of a hospital, a physician is usually in attendance that has a contract to provide professional care at the facility. The contracting physician's charges may appear on the hospital bill or may be billed separately. Many hospitals have two types of outpatient departments: the emergency room (ER), and outpatient medical clinics.

When a claim is received from a hospital for clinic charges, there is often a room charge for the use of the facility and a separate physician charge. The coding of these types of claims vary greatly from payer to payer; however, there are two main handling procedures:

1. *CPT®* services are coded separately and subject to usual, customary, and reasonable (UCR).
2. Generic or UB-92 codes are used and are not subject to UCR.

The following rules provide some common handling suggestions:

1. If a hospital is billing for professional component charges separately from the actual lab or x-ray charges, combine the two together because they represent one total service.

2. Physician treatment charges (professional fees) may be coded separately from other fees. This will depend on whether or not the payer is cost-conscious. If coded separately, the charge is usually subject to UCR, whereas if not coded separately, it will not be subject to UCR.

3. **Stat fees,** (a charge for DXL services performed on an expedited priority basis) should also be combined with the actual laboratory or x-ray charges.

These guidelines vary from payer to payer, so verification must be requested.

If the patient wants to have his regular physician in attendance and the physician is called in from outside the hospital to provide services, code 99056 should be used. If the patient visits the outpatient clinic of a facility, regular office visit coding should be used, since a clinic is conceptually the same as an office. That is, the same doctors see the same patients, visits are scheduled the same as in the office and the treatment provided is the same as what would be provided in an office. In essence, the physician is using the facility as her office.

For ER services, the facility must accept emergency patients 24 hours a day, seven days a week. No distinction is made between the first visit and subsequent visits. If the care provided is critical, then the critical care CPT® codes should be used, not the ER codes.

## Pediatric Critical Care Patient Transport (99289-99290)

These codes are used to bill for direct, face-to-face care provided by a physician during interfacility transport of a critically ill or injured pediatric patient. These codes are time-based. The first code is for the first 30–74 minutes of hands-on care. The second code is for each additional 30 minutes. The second code cannot be used without the first code.

## Critical Care Services (99291-99300)

Critical care involves the care of critically ill patients during a medical emergency that requires the constant attention of the provider. Most of the coding in this section is time-dependent (either in minutes or in days). Critical care services include the monitoring of the patient. Additional services such as suturing lacerations, setting fractures, or most other procedure are reported and allowed separately from the critical care services.

## Skilled Nursing Facility (99304-99318)

A skilled nursing facility is a specially qualified facility that has the staff and equipment to provide skilled nursing care or rehabilitation services and other related health services.

A patient may be transferred from an inpatient hospital to a nursing facility for supervised care when the patient no longer requires the skill levels of the inpatient hospital. Patients may also come directly from their home or any other environment.

If a patient is admitted to the nursing facility after receiving services in the physician's office or hospital emergency room, all evaluation and management services are considered inclusive in that visit. No separate allowance is made for an additional evaluation and management at the skilled nursing facility.

Except for hospital discharge services, any evaluation and management provided on the same day as admission to the nursing facility (whether at the facility or at a different location) are considered to be the initial admission evaluation.

## Domiciliary, Rest Home, or Custodial Care Services (99324-99340)

**Custodial care** is primarily for the purpose of meeting the personal daily needs of the patient and can be provided by personnel without medical care skills or training. For example, custodial care includes assistance with walking, bathing, dressing, eating, and other activities. Skilled nursing personnel are not required for this nonmedical type of care, which is commonly referred to as "meeting the daily living needs" of the patient. Most plans do not provide coverage for these types of services and for those that do, payment is very limited. If there is a question as to whether care is custodial, copies of the provider's nursing notes or the admit and discharge reports should be requested.

These claims may have modifier -MP or -SP to indicate whether multiple patients or a single patient were seen during the visit. This information is used most often by Medicare, but some health plans will reduce the benefit for multiple patients if they normally include transportation time in their calculations.

## Home Services (99341-99350 and 99500-99602)

These codes are used to bill for services provided to a patient in their home. Home services are often provided in lieu of hospitalization. For example, a patient who has suffered a heart attack may need extensive bed rest, with medications provided once or twice a day. If a nurse visits the home to provide the medications, there may be no need to hospitalize the patient.

Codes 99341–99350 are used by physicians to report evaluation and management procedures. Codes 99500–99602 are used by nonphysician healthcare professionals to report medical services.

Plans will often cover this type of care, especially if it represents an overall cost savings.

## Prolonged Services (99354–99360)

These codes are used to bill for prolonged or standby service that is beyond the usual service for inpatient or outpatient services. The service must be of at least 30 minutes in duration for it to be considered a prolonged service. These codes are reported in addition to the original service. Services which involve face-to-face contact are coded according to the amount of time spent with the patient, regardless of whether that time is continuous or not (i.e., a physician who checks in on their patient several times during a day).

## Case Management Services (99361–99373)

These codes are used to bill for team conferences or phone calls made by a provider in the treatment of a patient. These can include consulting with other providers, coordinating the patient's care with other professionals assigned to the patient (i.e., nurses, therapists, etc.), and any contact with other medical professionals regarding the care of the patient.

## Care Plan Oversight Services (99374–99380)

Care plan oversight is the reviewing of a patient's medical care and records usually for a patient under the care of a home health agency, hospice, or nursing home. This time is not considered to be face-to-face time with the patient.

Care plan oversight is reported according to the amount of time per month (or per 30-day period) that the physician spends reviewing the patient's treatment plan and records. Only one provider is allowed to bill for this service each month.

## Preventive Medicine Services (99381–99429)

These codes are used to bill for the evaluation and management of patients who do not have an illness or injury (i.e., annual checkup). The patient's age is often a factor in the codes in this section (i.e., checkup for an infant). This section also includes codes for risk factor assessment (i.e., suicidal tendencies, weight problems, substance abuse).

## Newborn Care Services (99431–99440)

These codes are used to bill for services provided by a physician to a newborn infant, including the immediate postpartum exam, preparation of birth and other medical records, and stabilization of a newborn infant.

## Special E/M Services (99450–99499)

These codes are used to bill for basic life or disability evaluations (i.e., follow-up evaluation for a work-related disability patient). These codes are used when the main purpose of the visit is to evaluate the patient, not to provide treatment.

Code 99499 is used to bill for evaluation and management services that are not listed elsewhere.

Coverage for these services can vary widely by payer. Check with your supervisor before processing these claims.

# CPT® Coding Medicine

The Medicine Section of the *CPT*® contains evaluation, therapeutic, and diagnostic procedures and services that are generally not invasive. The Medicine section has multiple subsections and it is important to read the subsection information and instructions that pertain to the group codes that will follow. The codes in this section range from 90281–99602, and may be used in conjunction with all other *CPT*® sections (**see Table 6–2**). Codes in this section do not include supplies used in the testing, therapy, or diagnostic treatments, unless specifically stated in the code description.

## Immune Globulins (90281–90399), Immunization Administration for Vaccines/Toxoids (90465–90474), and Vaccines, Toxoids (90476–90749)

Immunizations are the administration of a vaccine or toxoid (a weakened form of the toxin) to stimulate the immune system to provide protection against a certain disease or condition. The actual immunization administration (codes 90465–90474) is coded in addition to the immune globulins (90281–90399), and/or vaccine or toxin (90476–90749) which has been injected.

Immunizations are considered to be preventive treatment. Therefore, usually an active illness or disease is not present. Consequently, many plans do not cover such routine services except under five special circumstances:

1. Influenza virus (90655–90658)—may be covered for senior citizens who have a history of respiratory illness, or at-risk infants.

2. Rabies (90675–90676)—may be covered as active treatment of an animal bite.

3. Pneumococcal (90732)—may be covered for young or older patients with a history of respiratory illness.

4. Tetanus toxoid (90703)—may be covered when provided due to an injury such as stepping on a

nail. Some firms code this injection as 90782 rather than 90703.

5. The state in which the plan operates may have mandated laws that specify that all plans must provide specific levels of routine care for children. In such a case, the plan may be obligated to provide such benefits.

When a covered immunization is the only service provided, the evaluation and management code for a minimal service exam is also allowed.

## Therapeutic or Diagnostic Infusions (90780–90781)

These codes are used to bill for infusion services provided by a physician who was in constant attendance during the infusion. Code 90780 indicates the first hour of infusion. Code 90781 indicates each additional

| MEDICINE CODES | |
|---|---|
| Immune Globulins | 90281 – 90399 |
| Immunization Administration for Vaccines/Toxoids | 90465 – 90474 |
| Vaccines/Toxoids | 90476 – 90749 |
| Hydration, Therapeutic, Prophylactic and Diagnostic injections or infusions | 90760 – 90779 |
| Psychiatry | 90801 – 90899 |
| Biofeedback | 90901 – 90911 |
| Dialysis | 90918 – 90999 |
| Gastroenterology | 91000 – 91299 |
| General Ophthalmology Services | 92002 – 92400 |
| Otorhinolaryngologic Services | 92502 – 92700 |
| Cardiovascular | 92950 – 93990 |
| Pulmonary | 94010 – 94799 |
| Allergy and Clinical Immunology | 95004 – 95199 |
| Endocrinology | 95250 – 95251 |
| Neurology and Neuromuscular Procedures | 95805 – 96004 |
| Central Nervous System Assessments/Tests | 96101 – 96120 |
| Health and Behavior Assessment /Intervention | 96150 – 96155 |
| Chemotherapy Administration | 96401 – 96549 |
| Photodynamic Therapy | 96567 – 96571 |
| Special Dermatological Procedures | 96900 – 96999 |
| Physical Medicine and Rehabilitation | 97001 – 97799 |
| Medical Nutrition Therapy | 97802 – 97804 |
| Acupuncture | 97810 – 97814 |
| Osteopathic Manipulative Treatment | 98925 – 98929 |
| Chiropractic Manipulative Treatment | 98940 – 98943 |
| Education and Training for Patient Self-Management | 98960 – 98962 |
| Special Services, Procedures and Reports | 99000 – 99091 |
| Qualifying Circumstances for Anesthesia | 99100 – 99140 |
| Moderate (Conscious) Sedation | 99143 – 99150 |
| Other Services and Procedures | 99170 – 99199 |
| Home Health Procedures/Services | 99500 – 99600 |
| Home Infusion Procedures/Services | 99601 – 99602 |

**Table 6–2** Medicine Codes

hour up to eight hours. No coding is available for infusions that take longer than eight hours.

Even though these services take a prolonged period of time, these codes are not to be used with the codes for prolonged services. The prolonged amount of time has been included in the RVS amount for these codes.

## Therapeutic, Prophylactic, or Diagnostic Injections (90760–90761)

These codes are used to bill for the injection of a substance into the body. When these codes are used, the injected material should be specified on the claim.

These codes are used for reporting injections to health plans. Claims submitted to Medicare should use HCPCS codes to report injections.

## Psychiatry (90801–90899)

Psychiatric or mental/nervous care and treatment includes:

- Psychotic and neurotic disorders.
- Organic brain dysfunction.
- Alcoholism.
- Chemical dependency.

The language description on the claim form generally indicates "psychotherapy," "individual therapy," or "group therapy." The ICD-9-CM coding is usually in the range of 290.00–319.00. The providers of service are usually medical doctors (typically psychiatrists) or clinical psychologists.

If one of the following providers is indicated, most benefit plans require a referral by an M.D.:

1. Marriage, Family, and Child Counselor (MFCC).
2. Licensed Clinical Social Worker (LCSW).
3. Master of Social Work (MSW).

These CPT® codes are used only when psychiatric counseling or therapy is provided. If such therapy is not provided, even if the service is performed by one of the above licensed providers, a different code range should be used.

Most plans pay a reduced benefit for mental/nervous and psychiatric treatment. There may be a limit on the number of visits per year, along with a dollar limit per visit, or per calendar year. Also, many plans only cover certain provider licensing. Therefore, read the plan document carefully before processing these types of claims.

## Biofeedback (90901–90911)

**Biofeedback** is training an individual to consciously control automatic, internal bodily functions. For example, through conscious control, some body rhythms that control the constriction of blood vessels or the beating of the heart can be increased or decreased. This type of treatment can be used for a variety of illnesses or symptoms. A common use is for the control of intractable pain.

Biofeedback is controversial in that its effectiveness is very hard to prove or disprove. In addition, it does not cure anything. Instead, it is used as a tool in dealing with the symptoms of a condition, not in its treatment. Most plans do not cover biofeedback treatment, or if it is covered, it is very limited and only for certain diagnoses.

## Dialysis (90918–90999)

**Dialysis** is a treatment given to patients who have suffered acute kidney failure and must have their kidney functions taken over artificially. Notice that this is not really a treatment because it is only handling the functions normally performed by the body (however, it is still referred to generically as "treatment"). For a patient with this disease to survive, the blood cleansing function must be performed artificially by one of three processes currently available:

- Hemodialysis.
- Continuous Ambulatory Peritoneal Dialysis (CAPD).
- Transplantation of a new kidney.

Most hemodialysis is performed at private dialysis centers. A small percentage of the patients have a machine in their homes. The fees for dialysis are usually billed on a monthly basis. Either the actual dates of service should be indicated or a monthly from/through date is used. Normally, the only time you see these bills is for the first 30 months of treatment. After 30 months Medicare becomes the primary payer (refer to the Medicare and Medicaid chapter for additional information). If the dialysis is performed in an acute facility, you may be billed separately for the facility fees and the physician fees. Remember, the CPT® codes are to be used only on physician's services.

CAPD is performed by the patient at home. The peritoneum of the stomach is used to cleanse the blood. Surgery is required for the implantation of catheters and the construction of the internal bag (made of the peritoneum) to hold the dialysate fluids. Monthly supplies must be purchased, and there will be monthly examination charges by the attending physician.

A kidney transplant is the only cure for End-Stage Renal Disease (ESRD). Transplants are coded in accordance with the surgery section of the *CPT®*.

All evaluation and management services on the day of dialysis are considered to be part of the dialysis treatment. No separate allowance is made for an E/M visit, unless the E/M visit is for treatment unrelated to dialysis.

## Gastroenterology (91000–91299)

Gastroenterology services deal primarily with the esophagus, stomach, and intestines. These codes are used to bill for diagnostic services of the digestive system. The RVS allowance for these codes is for the diagnostic procedure only. The claim should also list an E/M code for the visit.

## General Ophthalmology Services (92002–92499)

**Ophthalmology care** is eye care provided either by an optometrist or an ophthalmologist (M.D.). Most health plans do not cover routine vision care services related to the refraction and subsequent prescription of glasses or contact lenses. If they are covered, the benefits are usually very limited in both the dollar allowance and frequency of services, and are often provided under a separate vision care plan or benefit. Therefore, always be sure to verify plan benefits before processing a vision claim. Also be aware that not all vision care is routine. Some vision care is essential for the proper care and treatment of eye disease. Most payers have a listing of payable diagnoses. However, prescription services for glasses or contact lenses may still be considered routine (except possibly if the lens of the eye has been removed, as in cataract surgery).

**Orthoptics** is the retraining of the muscles that control vision. Some plans allow for this therapy for certain conditions such as strabismus and binocular vision. If the plan does allow therapy, it is usually very limited and may require a second opinion from an ophthalmologist.

## Otorhinolaryngologic Services (92502–92700)

Otorhinolarygological services are those services associated with the head, or more specifically, the ear, nose, and throat. This section is for the billing of special services that are not part of a routine examination.

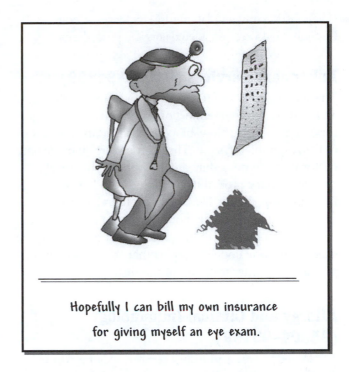

Hopefully I can bill my own insurance for giving myself an eye exam.

**Speech therapy** (codes 92507–92508) is usually for the correcting of speech that has been impaired because of sickness or injury and occurred while the individual was insured under the plan. The services must also be performed by a qualified practitioner. Conditions such as restoration of speech ability after a stroke or throat surgery would be covered. However, speech therapy for conditions such as stuttering or congenital deafness is usually not covered.

If you are unsure of the underlying need for the speech therapy services, the claim should be referred to a specialist for further review.

## Cardiovascular (92950–93990)

Cardiovascular services are services which treat the heart, arteries, and veins. Vascular studies (93875–93981) are diagnostic procedures to determine the condition of, or blood flow through an artery or vein. All cardiovascular codes should be listed in addition to the E/M services code describing the visit.

This is a very large section, and it is heavily used by the examiner. The following codes are some of the more commonly billed services:

| | |
|---|---|
| 93000 | EKG |
| 93010 | EKG Interpretation Only |
| 93015 | Cardiovascular Stress Test |
| 93224 | 24-hr EKG Monitoring |

As a rule, the codes from 93000 through 93350 and 93600 through 93981 are considered to be DXL

(Diagnostic x-ray and laboratory) expenses. Codes 93501 through 93545 are considered surgical procedures.

## Pulmonary Services (94010–94799)

These codes are used for billing procedures of the lungs and airways. These are most often diagnostic procedures for determining air flow, blood gases, and the conditions of the respiratory system. These procedures include both performing the procedure and interpreting the results.

Pulmonary procedures should be coded separately from the appropriate E/M code for the visit.

These codes include both the taking of the test and the interpretation of the results. Modifier -26 may be used with these codes to report that the physician only provided the interpretation of the results.

## Allergy and Clinical Immunology (95004–95199)

These codes are used to bill for services performed to determine a patient's allergy or sensitivity to certain substances, and the treatment of those allergies.

These codes should be reported in addition to the appropriate E/M code for the visit. Codes 99241–99245 should be used to report consultations with the patient or the patient's family regarding the management of their condition.

## Endocrinology (95250–95251)

These codes are used for the glucose monitoring of a patient. These codes should not be used with the code for collection and interpretation of physiologic data (99091).

## Neurology and Neuromuscular Procedures (95805–96004)

These codes are used to bill for procedures of the nervous system and are often reported in conjunction with consultations. A separate allowance should be made for the test and the consultation.

EEG services include both the taking of the test and the interpretation of the results. Modifier -26 may be used with EKG codes to report that the physician only provided the interpretation of the results.

## Central Nervous System Assessments/Tests (96101–96120)

These codes are used to bill for services to test the response of the central nervous system, including psychological testing, aphasia (lack of speech) testing, and developmental testing.

## Health and Behavior Assessment/Intervention (96150–96155)

These codes are used to bill for health and behavior assessment or intervention performed by a physician. Time is the major component for determining the correct code for these procedures.

## Chemotherapy Administration (96401–96549)

Chemotherapy is the treatment of cancer by use of chemicals introduced to the body. These codes are for the administration of chemotherapy agents by a physician, or by a qualified person under the direction of a physician.

These codes should be reported in addition to the appropriate E/M code for the visit. If an intra-arterial catheter is placed to facilitate the administration of the chemotherapy drugs, the appropriate code from the cardiovascular surgery section should be added.

If chemotherapy is administered by more than one technique, each technique should be reported separately.

## Photodynamic Therapy (96567–96571)

Photodynamic therapy (also called PDT) is a treatment method for some types of cancer. It uses light with a light-sensitive agent.

## Special Dermatological Procedures (96900–96999)

These codes are used to bill for treatment to the skin, including acne and other dermatologic disorders. The underlying cause for treatment must be determined to identify whether or not these services are covered, as many dermatological procedures are considered cosmetic.

## Physical Medicine and Rehabilitation Services (97001–97799)

**Physical medicine** is the manipulation and physical therapy associated with the nonsurgical care and treatment of the patient. The most common form of physical medicine is chiropractic manipulation of the spine (theoretically, any joint can be involved). The chiropractor's scope of practice is limited in most states. For instance, in some states, chiropractors are not allowed to draw blood and can only prescribe over-the-counter medications. The limitations vary by state.

Chiropractic care and billing used to be limited to manipulation of the spine and x-rays. Now, chiropractors use many different physical therapy modalities. Consequently, there has evolved an intense monitoring and restricting of payment for chiropractic services. Such restrictions may limit the number of visits per year, per month, or per condition, along with specifying daily reimbursement maximums or limiting the number of modalities that may be performed in a single visit. A wide variety of techniques have emerged to handle the overutilization of chiropractic care. As a result, it is important to check the coverage since the payment policies vary from payer to payer.

Many chiropractors use accident diagnosis, 84x.xx series, for billing purposes. Unless an accident or injury has actually occurred with a date, place, and circumstances indicated, the coding should be changed to reflect a noninjury skeletal condition, (72x.xx). (This varies by payer.) Situations that should warrant further review include:

- Possible overutilization.
- Over three physical medicine visits in a week.
- Over 12 visits in a month.
- Over three months and at least 34 visits of physical medicine visits.
- Second provider of physical medicine on the same day.
- Over four physical medicine codes per day.
- More than one initial office visit by the same physician.
- Claims when the only physical medicine charges are for modalities or massage (97010–97039 procedure codes); Modalities are a method of therapy, usually physical (i.e., a massage).
- Claims for use of an orthion table or for orthion therapy.

If a particular claim appears to be excessive, the attending physician should be contacted and the following information obtained:

- An outline of the therapy program recommended.
- A list of goals to be achieved through the program.
- A narrative description of how each procedure being performed is required to achieve one or more of the goals listed.

If the physician's reply justifies the use of therapy, frequency, and duration, process the claim accordingly. It takes time and skill to be able to interpret or determine necessity of services rendered. Therefore, if you are not sure what action should be taken after compiling the information necessary to make a claim determination, refer the information to a claims specialist. Any of these limitations would depend on the health plan and the payer's policy.

## Medical Nutrition Therapy (97802–97804)

These codes are used to bill for services to assess, counsel, and treat patients regarding their nutritional needs. The services can include body measurements and histories, nutritional counseling, and administration of medical foods or tube feedings. The diagnoses for these codes can involve weight issues, nutritional deficiency issues (whether caused by diet or by a medical condition), and diseases or conditions that require a modification in the patient's normal nutritional routine (i.e., diabetes).

Since many plans do not cover obesity or other weight issues, the patient's diagnosis and the plan guidelines should be checked before processing the claim.

## Acupuncture (97810–97814)

**Acupuncture** is the ancient Chinese practice of inserting fine needles into various points in the body to relieve pain, induce anesthesia, and to regulate and improve body functions. These codes are used to report Acupuncture services. Acupuncture codes report 15-minute increments. Time is calculated based upon the time the provider spends face-to-face with the patient, not the amount of time the needles are in place. There are different codes for needles used with electrical stimulation and those without.

## Osteopathic Manipulative Treatment (98925–98929)

**Osteopathic treatment** involves therapy based on the idea that the body can cure itself if it is in a normal state and provided with the proper environmental conditions. The appropriate code is determined by the number of body regions involved in the treatment. This therapy is often considered controversial and is not covered by many plans.

## Chiropractic Manipulative Treatment (98940-98943)

These codes are used to bill for treatment to the bones and muscles of the body, especially of the back. The codes in this section are often used in the treatment of patients involved in auto accidents or work-related injuries.

Any manipulation treatment includes a patient assessment.

Due to the high amount of abuse in this area, the diagnosis should be considered before processing chiropractic codes. Often documentation of a proposed treatment plan will be required, and a specific number of treatments will be preauthorized. If preauthorization is not obtained prior to treatment, many plans limit or deny payment for these types of claims.

## Special Services, Procedures, and Reports (99000-99091)

These codes are used to bill for special circumstances regarding services performed, such as the handling of a laboratory specimen. These codes are used in addition to the normal code that describes the procedure performed.

Proper use of this code can increase the reimbursement allowance. However, since the normal allowance for a laboratory test includes both performing the test and interpreting the results, it is important to verify the procedures performed by each provider prior to processing the claim, in order to verify that the extra allowance is appropriate.

## Qualifying Circumstances for Anesthesia (99100-99140)

For further information on this section, see the Surgery and Anesthesia Claims chapter.

## Moderate (Conscious) Sedation (99143-99150)

This section is for the billing of conscious sedation (with or without analgesia) when the actual procedure is provided by the same physician. If the physician who is performing the conscious sedation is not the physician performing the procedure, the appropriate anesthesia code should be used.

Many plans will limit additional payments for sedation provided by the provider of the actual procedure. For further information, see the Surgery and Anesthesia Claims chapter.

## Other Services and Procedures (99170-99199)

This section is used for reporting services that do not fit under any of the above categories. This can include physician attendance at hyperbaric oxygen therapy, assessment of a child for possible sexual abuse, hypothermia treatment, and many other conditions.

Since the circumstances for these procedures are widely varied, the diagnosis should be checked for determination of whether the therapy is covered by the plan.

## Home Health Procedures/Services (99500-99600)

These codes are used to bill for services provided in the patient's home by nonphysician healthcare professionals.

## Home Infusion Procedures/Services (99601-99602)

These codes are used to report per diem home visits for the purpose of administering infusions.

## Category II and III Codes

Category II codes are used to provide classification codes which will allow the collection of data for performance measurement. These codes are identified by four digits followed by the letter "F." Category III codes are for "emerging technologies." These are new procedures whose value may not yet be fully realized. Many insurance carriers consider these to be experimental procedures and exclude them. These codes are identified by four digits followed by the letter "T."

# Maintenance Therapy

**Maintenance therapy** refers to the various kinds of treatment (usually medical) given to patients to enable them to maintain their health in a disease-free or limited disease state. Maintenance services must be

# On the Job Now

**Directions:** Write the codes for each section in the space provided.

| Section | Codes |
|---|---|
| Consultations | _____ |
| Emergency Department Services | _____ |
| Domiciliary, Rest Home, or Custodial Care Services | _____ |
| Prolonged Services | _____ |
| Preventive Medicine Services | _____ |
| Therapeutic, Prophylactic, or Diagnostic Injections | _____ |
| Psychiatry | _____ |
| Biofeedback | _____ |
| Gastroenterology | _____ |
| Ophthalmology | _____ |
| Otorhinolaryngologic Services | _____ |
| Allergy and Clinical Immunology | _____ |
| Neurology and Neuromuscular Procedures | _____ |
| Chemotherapy Administration | _____ |
| Physical Medicine and Rehabilitation Services | _____ |
| Medical Nutrition Therapy | _____ |
| Home Health Procedures/Services | _____ |

considered under standard practice of medicine and must be provided by a skilled healthcare practitioner. Most payers do not cover services for maintenance therapy or for therapy in which there is no improvement in the patient's condition.

## Modifiers for Evaluation and Management and Medicine Codes

The following modifiers are appropriate for use with Evaluation and Management and Medicine CPT® codes. This is not an exhaustive list of modifiers, only the most commonly used.

*Evaluation and Management:*

-21    Prolonged Evaluation And Management Services.

-24    Unrelated Evaluation And Management Service By The Same Physician During A Postoperative Period.

-25    Significant, Separately Identifiable Evaluation And Management Service By The Same Physician On The Same Day Of The Procedure Or Other Service. This modifier indicates that a completely separate visit was performed by the same provider.

**Example:** A patient visits the doctor for an earache. On the way home he is involved in a car accident. He returns to the same doctor for treatment of a broken arm sustained in the car accident.

-32    Mandated Services.

-52    Reduced Services. These services were less intensive than the services normally associated with this code. This modifier often warrants a reduction in the payment made to the provider.

# On the Job Now

1. (True or False?) If the diagnosis is for psychiatric care, regardless of the service provided, codes 90801 to 90899 are used. _____

2. What are dialysis services? _____

   _____

3. (True or False?) Custodial care is usually a covered service. _____

4. List the three types of end-stage renal disease treatments.

   1. _____

   2. _____

   3. _____

5. What is biofeedback? _____

6. Consultations are usually provided by a _____

7. (True or False?) In order for psychiatric services to be payable, a clinical psychologist requires a referral from an M.D. _____

8. A Skilled Nursing Care Facility provides this type of care. _____

9. (True or False?) A second opinion physician can be in the same medical group as the surgeon. _____

10. What type of care is usually provided by an MFCC? _____

    _____

-57 Decision for Surgery. This procedure was necessary to determine the need for a subsequent surgical procedure. Depending on the amount of time which lapses between the visit and the subsequent surgery, the visit may be considered as part of the overall surgical procedure. Claims with this modifier often require the addition of a report detailing the circumstances. The report and claim should be forwarded to a claim specialist.

*Medicine:*

-22 Unusual Services.

-26 Professional Component.

-51 Multiple Procedures.

-52 Reduced Services.

-76 Repeat Procedure by Same Physician.

-76 Repeat Procedure by Another Physician.

-90 Reference (outside) Laboratory.

## Practice
# Pitfalls

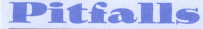

The following are examples of unbundling of medical services:

- Procurement of a rhythm strip in conjunction with an electrocardiogram. The rhythm strip should not be billed separately.

- Procurement of upper extremity (brachial) doppler study in addition to lower extremity doppler study in order to obtain an "anklebrachial index" (ABI). The upper extremity doppler should not be billed separately.

- Procurement of an electrocardiogram as part of a cardiac stress test. The electrocardiogram should not be billed separately.

# X-ray and Laboratory Services

Radiology and laboratory charges may be billed by a physician, an independent laboratory, or a freestanding radiology facility. Here we will discuss some of the basic guidelines used in determining whether billed diagnostic x-ray and laboratory (DXL) services are covered. We will also cover the guidelines for processing laboratory and radiology charges.

**Laboratory examinations** consist of the analyzing of body substances to determine their chemical or tissue make-up. Body fluids or tissues are collected and are either run through analyzing machines or looked at under a microscope to identify any abnormal substances or tissues.

There are basically two types of x-ray and laboratory charges: diagnostic x-ray/lab, and medical management x-ray/lab. **Diagnostic charges** are for initial testing to confirm a diagnosis or to rule out other diagnoses. **Medical management** x-ray/lab charges are incurred to control or manage a diagnosis (i.e., monitoring blood glucose levels on a patient with diabetes).

Laboratory tests which are medically necessary are usually covered expenses and may be payable under an x-ray and laboratory benefit. This benefit pays for the x-ray and laboratory test up to the policy maximum necessary to diagnose or manage a condition, as long as the expense is not payable under another Basic Benefit (i.e., inpatient hospital, preadmission testing, accident, etc.). The laboratory benefit is usually not payable for charges incurred in connection with any examination or test that is not necessary or incident to the establishment of a diagnosis for an injury or illness.

The XYZ plan has a Basic Benefit that covers a maximum of $200 per calendar year for x-ray/lab charges.

# Radiology (X-Ray)

The radiology section of the *CPT®* is arranged according to the anatomic position, that is, by body part, starting at the head and moving downward toward the feet. Radiology service codes range from 70010–79999 (**see Table 6–3**). The following subsections appear in the radiology section of the *CPT®*:

## Diagnostic Radiology (70010–76499)

**Diagnostic x-rays** are flat or two-dimensional pictures of a particular body part or organ. **X-rays** are created

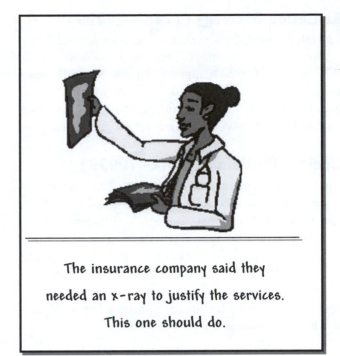

The insurance company said they needed an x-ray to justify the services. This one should do.

| RADIOLOGY CODES | |
|---|---|
| Diagnostic Radiology | 70010 – 76499 |
| Diagnostic Ultrasound | 76506 – 76999 |
| Radiation Oncology | 77261 – 77799 |
| Nuclear Medicine | 78000 – 79999 |

**Table 6–3   Radiology Codes**

by sending low-level radiation through the body and the resulting image is captured on a sheet of film. X-rays are most useful for looking at bones and dense tissue, since softer tissue is not clearly defined.

**CT scans** are made by a process that uses multiple x-ray images to create three-dimensional images of body structures. These scans are used to help identify tumors and cancers located in an organ. CT scans are much more definitive than x-rays.

## Diagnostic Ultrasound (76506–76999)

**Ultrasonography** provides a more definitive type of picture than x-rays. Instead of using radiation, sound waves are bounced off the desired structure to form a picture of the organ. This type of viewing is less potentially damaging than x-rays. This is why ultrasound scanning can be used during pregnancy, whereas x-rays cannot.

## Radiation Oncology (77261–77799)

**Radiation oncology** is the use of radiation to treat a condition. This treatment is used in conjunction with chemotherapy to treat malignant cancers. Normally, radiation therapy is composed of multiple treatments and does not include a "picture" of the body part. It is done for treatment purposes only, not for diagnostic reasons.

## Nuclear Medicine (78000–79999)

**Nuclear medicine** combines the use of radioactive elements and x-rays to image an organ or body part. Certain radioactive elements collect in different organs. The purpose of this type of treatment is to determine whether an organ is working effectively or to see whether it is enlarged. A radioactive element is injected into the patient, and then pictures are taken of the organ at specified intervals to see how, where, and how much of the element collects in a specific organ.

## Modifiers for Radiology (X-Ray) Codes

The following modifiers are appropriate for use with Radiology (X-Ray) CPT® codes. This is not an exhaustive list of modifiers, only the most commonly used.

-22 Unusual Services.
-25 Professional Component.
-32 Mandated Services.
-51 Multiple Procedures.
-52 Reduced Services.
-76 Repeat Procedure By The Same Physician.
-77 Repeat Procedure By Another Physician.
-90 Reference (Outside) Laboratory.
-Lt Left Side of Body.
-Rt Right Side of Body.

## Pathology (Lab)

For laboratory charges, it is important to establish whether the tests are being done as part of a routine check-up or because the patient has symptoms that are being diagnosed. Also, the testing must be appropriate for the reported symptoms. Thus, some tests would be routine for some diagnoses but not for others. This type of discrimination is learned through experience and time. Pathology services range from code 80048 to 89356 in the *CPT*® (**see Table 6–4**).

The subsections of the laboratory portion of the *CPT*® are as follows:

### Practice
# Pitfalls

The following are examples of unbundling of radiology services:

- CPT® code 72110 (Radiologic examination, spine, lumbosacral; minimum of four views) was billed with CPT® code 72114 (Radiologic examination, spine, lumbosacral; complete, including bending views.) However, reimbursement of services for CPT® 72110 is included in the reimbursement of 72114.

- The 3D simulation CPT® code 77295 "bundles" or includes the complex isodose plan CPT® code 77315, which means that it should NOT be billed in addition to the 77295 code.

## Organ or Disease Oriented Panels (80048–80076)

**Panel tests** are composed of multiple tests that are combined and run from one specimen. These tests can be requested from one or two specimens and cost substantially less than several tests ordered separately from separate specimens. These services are very sophisticated, highly computerized, and usually very reliable. CPT® codes 80048–80076 refer to various types of panel tests. The number of tests performed determines which code to use. Providers are allowed to

| PATHOLOGY CODES | |
| --- | --- |
| Organ or Disease Oriented Panels | 80048 – 80076 |
| Drug Testing | 80100 – 80103 |
| Therapeutic Drug Assays | 80150 – 80299 |
| Evocative/Suppression Testing | 80400 – 80440 |
| Consultations (Clinical Pathology) | 80500 – 80502 |
| Urinalysis | 81000 – 81099 |
| Chemistry | 82000 – 84999 |
| Hematology and Coagulation | 85002 – 85999 |
| Immunology | 86000 – 86849 |
| Transfusion Medicine | 86850 – 86999 |
| Microbiology | 87001 – 87999 |
| Anatomic Pathology | 88000 – 88099 |
| Cytopathology | 88104 – 88199 |
| Cytogenetic Studies | 88230 – 88299 |
| Surgical Pathology | 88300 – 88399 |
| Transcutaneous Procedures | 88400 |
| Other Procedures | 89049 – 89240 |
| Reproductive Medicine Procedures | 89250 – 89356 |

**Table 6–4** Pathology Codes

bill for the collection of the specimen, a venipuncture if the specimen is blood, and the handling charge for packaging the specimen.

## Drug Testing (80100-80103)

These codes are used to bill for the testing of bodily fluids to identify a specific class of drugs (i.e. amphetamines). It is important to check the diagnosis when processing these types of claims, as overdoses may fall into the category of accidents (which may have additional benefits), or attempted suicide or self-inflicted injury (for which benefits may be reduced or denied).

## Therapeutic Drug Assays (80150-80299)

These codes are used to bill for monitoring the therapeutic levels of a specific drug (i.e., drug prescribed by a physician).

## Evocative/Suppression Testing (80400-80440)

These codes are used to report panel tests which help providers determine if the patient has a condition creating too little or an excess of hormones or chemicals released by the body. These tests will often confirm or rule out a diagnosis.

## Consultations (Clinical Pathology) (80500-80502)

These codes are used to report consultations or evaluation of a patient's condition using clinical results (lab tests).

## Urinalysis (81000-81099)

Analysis of the urine can provide a wide range of information for the provider. This is one of the most common laboratory tests performed.

## Chemistry (82000-84999)

This section lists the codes that are used to bill for the testing of a specific substance within the patient's body (i.e., a chemical, vitamin, mineral, or hormone). The results of these tests can often help to confirm or deny a diagnosis, or to provide information regarding a patient's condition or behavior.

## Hematology & Coagulation (85002-85999)

These codes are used to report the testing of blood for its components (i.e., hemoglobin count). These tests

can allow a provider to track a patient's condition and to determine if there are any possible contraindications for surgery (i.e., slow blood clotting time).

## Immunology (86000-86849)

These codes are used to report tests done on body fluids to determine prior immune responses (i.e., check for antibodies to fight a specific disease). These tests can help a provider determine if a disease is currently present in a patient's body, or if the patient has been exposed to a disease.

## Transfusion Medicine (86850-86999)

These codes are used to bill for tests performed prior to a transfusion or other procedures when a patient may be given fluids or cells from a donor (i.e., blood typing).

## Microbiology (87001-87999)

Microbiology is the study of microorganisms. These codes report the culture of microorganisms to determine their presence in the human body.

## Anatomic Pathology (88000-88099)

These codes are used to bill for examinations done on a deceased person to assist in determining the cause of death.

## Cytopathology (88104-88199)

Cytopathology is the study of changes in a cell, or the ability of an agent (i.e., virus, bacteria) to destroy a cell. These codes are used to bill for cells removed from a person through smears (i.e. Pap smear), scrapings, or other forms of cell collection.

## Cytogenetic Studies (88230-88299)

Cytogenic refers to the production of cells. These codes report procedures associated with the collection or growing of cells within the lab (i.e., growing a skin graft for a burn patient).

## Surgical Pathology (88300-88399)

The codes in this section report tests done in preparation for or during surgery.

## Transcutaneous Procedures (88400)

The one code in this section is used to report transcutaneous bilirubin (bilirubin secreted through the skin).

## Other Procedures (89049–89240)

This section lists lab procedures that did not fit under any of the other headings.

## Reproductive Medicine Procedures (89250–89356)

The codes in this section report services associated with reproductive procedures (i.e., cryopreservation of embryos and sperm, in vitro fertilization, etc.)

## Papanicolaou (PAP) Smear

A **Papanicolaou or "Pap smear"** is a diagnostic laboratory test for detecting the absence or presence of infection, viruses, trauma, or cancer. The expense for a Pap smear is usually covered when one of the following six conditions exists:

1. The result of the Pap smear is abnormal.
2. Cancer of the cervix, uterus, or vagina has been present or is presently being treated.

## Practice Pitfalls

Following are some general guidelines regarding the processing of DXL claims.

### Automated Laboratory Charge

Automated laboratories offer their services primarily to doctor's offices. Usually, the doctor's office is furnished with all the necessary supplies for securing samples of blood and urine and lab sheets indicating which tests are to be performed on which specimens. Lab reports are usually received from the laboratory within approximately three days. The doctor is usually billed monthly for this service.

### Unbundling

Some providers will unbundle by billing separately for each test performed even though all the tests came from the same specimen and were done simultaneously. If the claim was processed as billed, the provider would be paid significantly more money for doing nothing additional. When a bill is received "unbundled," the examiner needs to rebundle it. An example of unbundling is shown in **Table 6–5**.

In **Table 6–5**, all the billed charges should be combined and coded under one panel code. Benefits would then be determined based on the one code.

## Practice Pitfalls

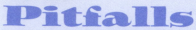

One of the most common places to find unbundling of CPT® codes is in the area of laboratory procedures.

The following are examples of unbundling of laboratory services:

CPT® code 80058 (TORCH antibody panel) includes the following tests:

CPT® code 86644: Antibody – cytomegalovirus
CPT® code 86694: Antibody – herpes simplex
CPT® code 86762: Antibody – rubella
CPT® code 86777: Antibody – toxoplasma

When all four tests are ordered and medically necessary, the panel test must be billed in place of the individual tests.

Some other laboratory codes that may also be subject to unbundling include:

- General Health Panel (80050).
- Electrolyte Panel (80051).
- Lipid Panel (80061).
- Renal Function Panel (80069).

It is also important to review emergency room charges, to be sure that services and supplies that are supposed to be included in the basic emergency room or trauma charge are not billed out separately.

| Bill from Doctor | CPT® Code | Charge | Coding by Examiner | Charge |
|---|---|---|---|---|
| Calcium | 82310 | $20.00 | 80048 | $95.00 |
| CO$_2$ | 82374 | 15.00 | | |
| Chloride | 82435 | 25.00 | | |
| Creatinine | 82565 | 15.00 | | |
| Glucose | 82947 | 10.00 | | |
| Potassium | 84132 | 15.00 | | |
| Sodium | 84295 | 15.00 | | |
| BUN | 84520 | 30.00 | | |
| | | $145.00 | | $95.00 |

**Table 6–5  Unbundling**

3. The patient complains of female reproductive problems.
4. The results of a Pap smear taken in the last 12 months were abnormal.

5. Signs or symptoms are present which, in the physician's opinion, are reasonably related to a gynecologic disorder.

6. The physical examination indicates any abnormal findings of the vagina, cervix, uterus, ovaries, or adnexa.

Usually, routine Pap smears performed in conjunction with a routine physical examination are not covered unless the contract specifically indicates coverage, or the state mandates coverage.

## Component Charges

Whenever a lab or an x-ray test is performed, two distinct services are actually performed:

1. The first service is the taking of the specimen or x-ray. This charge should include the expense for the personnel performing the test and the cost of the necessary equipment. This is called the **technical component**.

2. The second service is the interpretation or the reading of the results of the test. This is called the **professional component** and is denoted by adding modifier -26 to the CPT® code.

An independent pathologist or radiologist often bills separately for the interpretation of the report. This interpretation-only charge is a professional component (PC) fee. To figure the cost of an x-ray or lab test, the PC charge (if billed separately) needs to be added to the base or technical component charge (TC—the charge for performing the test). Sometimes, both the TC charge and the PC charge are billed by the same provider but are broken out separately (not uncommon on hospital bills). When coding the claim, the two charges should be combined and coded as one charge. If the professional component and the technical component are performed by different providers, they are not to be combined and coded as a single expense. In such a case, these separate charges should be coded and paid separately.

A professional component's value ranges from 25% to 40% of the UCR value of the actual test. The technical component's value ranges from 60% to 75% of the UCR value of the test. (For training purposes, contracts that do not state a professional component percentage should be computed at 40% of UCR.)

## Modifiers for Pathology (Lab) Codes

The following modifiers are appropriate for use with Pathology (Lab) CPT® codes. This is not an exhaustive list of modifiers, only the most commonly used.

-22   Unusual Services.

-26   Professional Component.

-32   Mandated Services.

-52   Reduced Services.

-90   Reference (Outside) Laboratory.

# On the Job Now

**Directions:** Answer the following questions without looking back at the material just covered. Write your answers in the space provided.

1. What two distinct services are actually performed whenever a lab or an x-ray test is performed?

   1. _____

   2. _____

2. Define the two services that are performed.

   1. _____

   _____

   2. _____

   _____

# Hospital Services

**Hospital services** are those services performed in a hospital setting. The term is used generically to refer to charges billed by a hospital, urgent care center, surgi-center, alternative birthing center, or similar institution. This chapter deals with the various types of facilities available, their billing formats, and general handling guidelines.

The term "hospital" means an institution that meets most of the following:

1. It mainly provides medical treatment to inpatients.
2. It provides treatment only by or under a staff of physicians.
3. It provides care by registered nurses 24 hours per day.
4. It maintains facilities for diagnosis.
5. It maintains a daily medical record for each patient.
6. It complies with all licensing and other legal requirements.
7. It maintains permanent facilities for surgery.

Most carriers have a file of established hospitals, surgi-centers, skilled nursing facilities, or birthing facilities that are licensed to treat patients in the state where they practice business. Occasionally, a new facility opens and, when claims are received, the information must be requested and verified to determine whether the facility is eligible for payment.

Hospital services are covered under the hospital benefits portion of the contract. Whether the contract is a Basic/Major Medical plan or a Comprehensive Major Medical plan, hospital charges are usually a covered benefit. The following are typical hospital expenses:

- The daily room and board charge of a hospital.
- The charges for outpatient emergency treatment of illness and injuries.
- The charge for outpatient surgery.
- The charges for medical services and supplies during confinement, excluding private duty nursing.
- The charge for administration of anesthesia.
- The ambulance care if billed through the hospital.
- The charges for lab tests and other services performed by an outside facility at the hospital's request.

# UB-92 Billing Form

A review of the UB-92 is necessary before processing to determine whether inpatient or outpatient benefits apply. An inpatient billing will usually have the following: a room and board charge and the statement from and to dates will correspond with the number of room and board days billed. Outpatient bills will usually have the following: an indicator such as 131 in field locator four, the statement from and to dates are the same, the admission and discharge dates are the same, and there is no charge for room and board. Some hospitals do not put the discharge time on the outpatient bill; however, you may want to request this information if the billing appears excessive or if it appears that the patient might have stayed overnight in an extended stay or observation room.

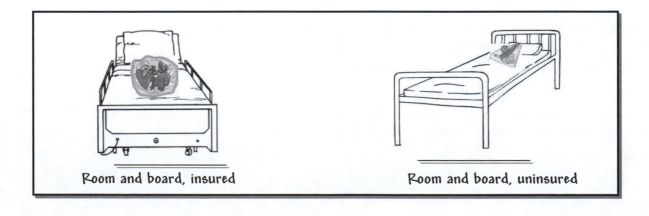

Room and board, insured          Room and board, uninsured

## Inpatient Hospital Claims

On inpatient hospital claims, the provider of service is a facility that provides inpatient care. This may be a hospital, an acute care facility, a skilled nursing facility, a custodial care facility, or a similar facility.

For **inpatient care**, the patient must be admitted into the hospital and stay for a period of time, usually a minimum of 24 hours. There must be a room and board charge. A hospital room and board charge is similar to that for staying in a hotel. The day entered is paid but not the day discharged, as long as the discharge time is before the required checkout time. The UB-92 form should always indicate admission and discharge dates.

When coding inpatient hospital claims, the *CPT®* or *RVS* books are not used unless the billing has itemized some charges according to valid CPT®/RVS codes. Each payer has their own coding guidelines. Therefore, before a claim can be coded for processing, the payer-specific codes must be obtained. Most payers break up the bills according to:

- Room and board charges.
- Ancillary charges.
- Take-home prescriptions.
- Professional fees for exams, surgery, etc.

Providers of service use revenue codes in field locator 42 of the UB-92 form to indicate or identify the specific accommodation, ancillary service, or billing calculation.

### Room and Board

Hospitals have a variety of rooms available which include, but are not limited to:

- **Private**—A single-occupancy room. The extra cost for a private room is not covered by most plans unless the room was necessary due to the patient's illness (i.e., highly contagious disorder).

- **Semiprivate**—A double-occupancy room. Most plans cover the cost of a semiprivate room. The cost may vary based on the type of floor on which the room is located. That is, a semiprivate room in a burn ward may cost more than a semiprivate room in a maternity ward because of the increased level of care required.

- **Ward**—A room with three or more beds. A ward is also covered by most plans. Aside from county hospitals, most facilities no longer offer this type of room.

- **Nursery**—A large room for newborn babies. Twenty or 30 babies may be in a nursery.

- **Specialized Units**—Areas in which special monitoring equipment and a higher ratio of nurses to patients are required. These units are established for extremely ill or terminal patients with different illnesses or injuries that require more acute, intensive care. Specialized units tend to be considerably more expensive than other units. This type of room may cost $1,000 or more per day. Examples are the Intensive Care Unit (ICU), Coronary Care Unit (CCU), and Definitive Observation Unit (DOU).

**Note:** When calculating claim benefits, the normal UCR for ICU rooms is three times the semiprivate room rate.

**Telemetry charges** (specialized observation equipment) may be billed separately from the base room and board amount. In addition, nursing charges may also be billed separately. If so, the telemetry charges and nursing charges should be combined with the base room and board amount to obtain the actual room and board charge.

To code the room and board amount, the number of days in the hospital is determined by counting the day of admission but not the day of discharge. If there is a charge for the day of discharge, the facility will need to be contacted to determine why the last day is being charged. Usually, the charge will be for a late discharge. In this case, the late discharge is covered if it was caused or ordered by the attending physician. A late discharge for the patient's convenience, however, is not usually a covered expense.

Each type of room accommodation is coded on a separate line, and the quantity (number of days) applies to that type of room only. In addition, if either the type of room (semiprivate, private, or other) or the per-day charges are different, even if the room type is the same, separate lines of coding are required. For instance, the following claim is received:

| 5/1/CCYY–5/2/CCYY | Semiprivate $650 per day |
| 5/3/CCYY–5/4/CCYY | Semiprivate $675 per day |

In this case, the two different semiprivate room rates must be coded on two different lines, with the number of services shown on each line as two (unless 5/4 is the discharge date). If the charge per day was the same for all of the semiprivate rooms, only one line of coding would be required with the number of services as four.

Check revenue code ranges 110–179 and 200–219 on the UB-92 for room and board expenses.

## Ancillary Expenses

**Ancillary expenses** are miscellaneous services or supplies that are provided by the hospital on an inpatient or outpatient basis, which are necessary for the medical care or treatment of an individual. The most common charges include x-rays, lab fees, pharmacy, med-surgical supplies, operating room expenses, surgery room supplies, recovery room time, anesthesia supplies, occupational therapy, and inhalation therapy. All these expenses can be combined under a single line of coding for ancillary expenses. The only items that may be separated and coded on separate lines are charges for personal items, noncovered items, doctor's emergency room examination charges, other professional exam charges, or other expenses that may be limited by the plan. This does not include professional component charges (unless specified by the plan).

## Take-Home Prescriptions

Often doctors in a hospital setting prescribe **take-home prescriptions**, or medications to be taken after the patient is released from the hospital. These medications may be dispensed by the hospital pharmacy and the charges included on the hospital bill. The medications are often covered under Major Medical benefits rather than standard hospital benefits. For this reason, these items are usually billed and coded separately, since they are not considered to be hospital expenses and may be subject to other plan provisions. Sometimes the plan has a separate payer for prescriptions, in which case the take-home drugs should be denied.

## Professional Fees

Bills for doctors, anesthesiologists, technicians, and other hospital professionals are often included on the hospital bill rather than billed separately on a CMS-1500. These bills are broken out from the regular hospital bill and paid under the normal plan provisions as if they had been billed on a CMS-1500. Therefore, it is important to go through the itemized billing and determine whether the charges were for materials, equipment, and overhead (rendered by the hospital), or for professional services (rendered by a provider).

## Personal Items

**Personal items** are those items that are primarily for the comfort of the patient and are not medically neces-

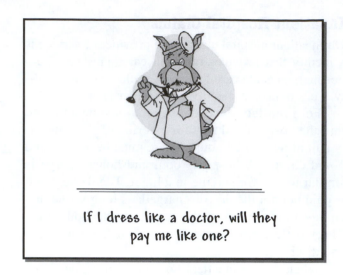

If I dress like a doctor, will they pay me like one?

sary. The following items are considered to be personal items and are not usually covered by a benefit plan. These charges may need to be coded separately, or they may be combined with other ancillary charges and then denied with an appropriate explanation indicating that they are not covered under the plan. Handling procedures vary from payer to payer. Personal items can include:

- Barber expenses.
- Personal hygiene kit.
- Videotaping of birth.
- Birth certificate, photos.
- Cot rental.
- Room transfer requested.
- Lotion.
- Television.
- Telephone.
- Toothbrush, toothpaste.
- Guest trays.
- Mouthwash.
- Gift shop expenses.
- Slippers.

Most hospitals automatically issue an admission kit to incoming patients. An admission kit usually includes an emesis basin, carafe, cup, lotion, tissue, and mouthwash. Some plans administratively allow for one kit. Additional kits are not covered. This type of kit may also be called a maternity kit, Ob-Gyn kit, hygiene kit, patient comfort kit, and other names. Therefore, if items such as mouthwash and toothpaste are billed separately in addition to a kit, they are not usually considered covered charges. (Even if a kit is not billed, these types of charges are not usually allow-able.) It is important to consider if there is a medical necessity for an item prior to denying it. For example, the hospital bill may list a razor. If the patient was scheduled for surgery and the nurse shaved the opera-tive area, the razor would be considered medically necessary.

## Outpatient Hospital Claims

The **outpatient** provider of service is a hospital facili-ty (the title may be Hospital, Medical Center, Surgi-center, or Birthing Center) in which there are no room and board charges. Commonly, "come-and-go" or out-patient surgery is performed in the outpatient depart-ment because an inpatient admission is not medically necessary. An outpatient hospital facility may have two departments:

1. The Emergency Room, and
2. Outpatient Clinics.

There may be facility charges such as emergency room usage fees, examination room usage charges, op-erating room expenses, and recovery room expenses. In an outpatient setting, ancillary expenses include everything except professional fees for examinations, surgery, and other professional services. Clinic charges should be treated as an office visit as far as coding for the physician. The actual facility usage fee is not coded with or considered a professional fee. It is coded sepa-rately.

Other commonly submitted outpatient charges may be for lab or x-ray services, pharmacy, or durable medical equipment.

## Miscellaneous Facilities

Many other types of treatment centers may be classi-fied as facilities. Usually, they are designed to handle specialized treatment programs such as psychiatric care, alcoholism, and emergency care. The following is a sampling of other types of facilities in existence.

### Day Care/Night Care Centers

As the name implies, **day care centers** provide treat-ment during the daylight hours with the patient being released at night. **Night care centers** allow the patient to pursue a normal routine during the day such as working, and be treated at the center and maintained there overnight. Generally, these types of centers are for treatment of mental or nervous disorders.

A great disparity is seen in the handling of these claims from payer to payer. Usually, the following is required by the examiner to determine whether the treatment or the facility is eligible for benefits. A com-plete review of the facility must be made including:

- Staffing—the type of licensing required for the staff.
- Type of billing—how the bills are broken down, whether they are inclusive, itemized, and so on.
- Type of state or federal licensing the facility has.
- The facility's primary purpose (custodial care, active treatment, or other).
- A detailed description of the type of treatment including length of each treatment, licensing of person actually performing the treatment, ancillary services, and other pertinent data.

Often, senior examiners may handle day care claims to ensure that the proper correspondence is prepared and mailed. They also review the documentation when a reply is received. Before any benefits are denied, all plan provisions and limitations must be verified.

### Urgent Care Centers

An **urgent care center** is a facility that follows profes-sionally recognized standards to provide urgent or emergency treatment. Many plans have specialized benefits to handle this type of center. An urgent care center generally meets these eight requirements:

1. Mainly provides urgent or emergency medical treatment for acute conditions.
2. Does not provide services or accommodations for overnight stays.
3. Is open to receive patients every day of the calendar year.
4. Has a physician trained in emergency medicine, nurses, and other supporting personnel specially trained in emergency care on duty at all times.
5. Has x-ray and laboratory diagnostic facilities, emergency equipment, trays, and supplies available for use in life-threatening events.
6. Has a written agreement with a local acute care inpatient facility for the immediate transfer of patients who require more intensive care than can be furnished at an outpatient facility, has written guidelines for stabilizing and transporting such

patients, and has immediate and reliable direct communication channels with the acute care facility.

7. Complies with all state and federal licensing and other legal requirements.

8. Is not the office or clinic of any physician.

Generally, a medical emergency exists when:

- Severe symptoms occur. The symptoms must be severe enough to cause a person to seek immediate medical aid regardless of the hour of the day or night.

- The severe symptoms must occur suddenly and unexpectedly. A chronic condition with sub-acute symptoms that have existed over a period of time usually does not qualify as a medical emergency. However, symptoms that become severe enough to require immediate medical aid may qualify.

- Immediate care was secured. Usually, a medical emergency would not be considered to exist if medical care was not received immediately after the appearance of acute symptoms. A telephone call to a doctor does not fulfill this requirement if the actual examination and treatment are deferred until the next day.

The administration of the urgent care benefit varies greatly. Therefore, refer to the plan provisions prior to taking any action on such claims.

Some patients will seek urgent care treatment for nonemergency reasons (i.e., the patient is suffering from flu symptoms and doesn't want to take time off to see a doctor). Some payers will deny or reduce payment on these claims based on the reasoning that the level of care obtained was not consistent with the situation.

## Surgi-centers

**Ambulatory surgical centers (Surgi-centers)** are equipped to allow for the performance of surgery on an outpatient basis. These centers may be freestanding or attached to a major acute care facility. Surgi-centers provide financial savings by eliminating the need for admission into an inpatient facility. An ambulatory surgical facility is a specialized facility that meets all eight of the professionally recognized standards indicated below:

1. Provides a setting for outpatient surgeries.

2. Does not provide services or accommodations for overnight stays.

3. Has at least two operating rooms and one recovery room; all the medical equipment needed to support the surgery being performed; x-ray and laboratory diagnostic facilities; and emergency equipment, trays, and supplies for use in life-threatening events.

4. Has a medical staff that is supervised full-time by a physician including a registered nurse when patients are in the facility.

5. Maintains a medical record for each patient.

6. Has a written agreement with a local acute care facility for the immediate transfer of patients who require greater care than can be provided on an outpatient basis.

7. Complies with all state and federal licensing and other legal requirements.

8. Is not an office or clinic for any physician.

Usually, plans provide benefits on a global basis, covering the facility room usage charge, supplies (i.e., anesthesia gases, medications, trays) on the same basis as inpatient hospital services. However, as with other benefits, coverage provisions vary greatly.

## Alternative Birthing Centers

**Alternative birthing centers (ABCs)** are outpatient care centers that provide special rooms for routine deliveries. As a rule, these centers provide quiet, nontraditional types of home-style rooms which are designed to allow the parents to be together and participate in the birthing experience.

Often, a nurse practitioner rather than a physician is in attendance. The mother normally goes home within five to 12 hours after the delivery. As with other types of outpatient facilities, the following six or similar requirements are necessary for a facility to qualify as a birthing center:

1. Does not provide services or accommodations for overnight stays.

2. Has a medical staff that is supervised full-time by a physician. A registered nurse is also in attendance when patients are in the facility.

3. Maintains a medical record for each patient.

4. Has a written agreement with a local acute care facility for the immediate transfer of patients who require greater care than can be provided on an outpatient basis.

**5.** Complies with all state and federal licensing and other legal requirements.

**6.** Is not an office or clinic for any physician.

Most confinements at an ABC should not exceed a 24-hour period without the transfer to an acute care facility. If the stay exceeds 24 hours, charges should be referred for investigation as to the medical necessity of the continued stay.

## Rehabilitation Facilities

**Rehabilitation facilities** specialize in long-term, post-sickness, or post-injury care. Rehabilitative treatment rather than active medical care is provided. This treatment is designed to return a patient to a normal or more normal state. Rehabilitative care is designed for those who are left paralyzed, deformed, handicapped, or otherwise not totally functional as a result of an accident, injury, or illness such as a stroke or spinal cord injury.

Although care at a rehabilitation facility is more aggressive than that provided in a convalescent facility, this type of care is generally very similar to convalescent care.

Many plans provide for some type of rehabilitative care. The limitations are usually based on a point at which progress ceases and the condition or status of the patient is stabilized. However, some plans do not provide any benefits for rehabilitative treatment.

## Convalescent Hospitals

**Convalescent facilities** are usually considered to be midrange facilities which provide nonacute care for persons recovering from an acute illness or injury. Usually, admission into a convalescent facility must commence within a specified number of days following a discharge from an acute care facility. The care provided must be active treatment, not custodial care.

The institution generally must meet all seven of the following requirements to be considered an eligible convalescent facility:

**1.** Is primarily engaged in providing skilled nursing care to sick or injured persons as inpatients under 24-hour supervision of a physician or registered nurse.

**2.** Has on duty at all times a registered nurse, licensed vocational nurse, or skilled practical nurse. A registered nurse must be on duty at least eight hours a day.

**3.** Is not, other than incidentally, a place for drug addicts, alcoholics, mentally ill persons, or senile or mentally deficient persons.

**4.** Maintains a medical record for each patient.

**5.** Has a written agreement with a local acute care facility for the immediate transfer of patients who require greater care than can be provided in a nonacute care facility.

**6.** Complies with all state and federal licensing and other legal requirements.

**7.** Is not an office or clinic for any physician.

Many plans provide very limited convalescent care benefits. However, always verify that the care being provided is not custodial. Some rehabilitative services may be provided and may be billed separately or included on a global basis (no breakdown).

## Nursing Homes

**Nursing homes** specialize in custodial care, that is, care that is primarily for the purpose of meeting the personal needs of the patient and that could be provided by personnel without professional skills or training. Custodial care may include assistance with walking, bathing, dressing, eating, and other activities. Most plans do not provide custodial care coverage or, if they do, payment is limited. If there is a question whether or not care is custodial, copies of the provider's nursing notes and admission or discharge summary should be requested.

## Hospice Care

**Hospice care** is a healthcare program providing coordinated services in a home setting. Sometimes care is provided in the patient's home by visiting specialists and sometimes patients are admitted to a hospice facility. Usually, such care is provided only for persons suffering from a terminal condition, generally with a life expectancy of six months or less. The hospice concept is based on the following principles:

- The beneficiaries of the program are both the terminally ill person and his or her family.
- An interdisciplinary team is required to serve the patient, including nurses, social workers, psychologists, clergy, volunteers, and other professionals.
- The alleviation of pain and suffering is emphasized rather than the treatment of the illness.
- Support is provided for all family members to help offset emotional pain.

Hospice care is billed in a variety of methods. If the patient is in a hospice facility, the facility will submit a single bill for all charges. If the patient is receiving treatment in their own home, the billing may be provided by a hospice agency which is then responsible for paying other providers. Another method may be that of separate bills from the various providers. Usually, such services include the rental of beds, commodes, and other equipment, along with various medications and supplies required to care for a terminally ill person. For hospice care to be covered, the contract usually specifies such benefits.

# On the Job Now

**Directions:** Answer the following questions without looking back at the material just covered. Write your answers in the space provided.

1. Define hospital services. _____

_____

2. What type of claim form is used to bill for hospital services? _____

3. Name the two types of outpatient hospital facility departments.

1. _____

2. _____

4. What is the difference between an inpatient and an outpatient provider service?

_____

_____

5. Name the eight examples given as miscellaneous facilities that use the UB-92 Billing Form to file claims.

1. _____

2. _____

3. _____

4. _____

5. _____

6. _____

7. _____

8. _____

6. Name the four categories of hospital charges that most payers use.

1. _____

2. _____

3. _____

4. _____

# Ambulance Services

**Ambulance expenses** are charges billed for transporting an injured or ill person to a medical facility. Ambulance services are not considered professional or hospital services.

Following are four types of ambulance services that are in common use:

1. Air Ambulance
2. Paramedics
3. Mobile Intensive Care Unit
4. Van Transportation Unit

When ambulance services occur and charges are received, an investigation to determine whether the charges are eligible for coverage under the insured plan must be undertaken. Under most plans, charges must be from a professional ambulance service; private automobiles, taxicabs, or similar vehicles are usually not covered.

The plan provisions will indicate which limitations apply. Major Medical plans usually designate a maximum allowable/payable amount for each trip based on usual and customary guidelines. Expenses commonly billed by an ambulance service include:

- Base call charge. This is the amount automatically charged for the ambulance to respond to a call even if the patient is not subsequently transported.
- Oxygen and oxygen supplies.
- Mileage.
- Linens.
- Emergency response charge. This is an extra expense in addition to the base charge, which may be added if the patient's condition is severe enough that resuscitation efforts or other types of stabilization measures are required.
- Paramedic response charge. If paramedics rather than emergency medical technicians (EMTs) are used, an extra expense may be added.

## Air Ambulance

An **air ambulance** is a helicopter or other flight vehicle used to transport severely injured or ill persons to a hospital. Air medical transport may be covered if:

1. The facility in the area where the patient is injured cannot manage the patient's condition and it is medically necessary to transfer the patient by air to another facility more equipped to treat the patient, or

## Practice Pitfalls

Benefits are usually payable for transfer to another hospital when medically necessary. For example, if one hospital does not have the facilities to treat the patient's medical condition, the patient may be transferred to the closest hospital with appropriate facilities.

An ambulance expense is covered under Major Medical, basic ambulance, and basic hospital benefits under the following conditions:

1. The ambulance must be medically necessary and not for the patient's convenience.
2. Transportation is provided by a professional ambulance/paramedic service.
3. Transportation is to the nearest facility capable of treating the patient.
4. Transportation is provided from one facility to another when the necessary treatment cannot be obtained from the first hospital.
5. Transportation to home from a facility is provided if the patient is unable to travel in an upright position. Exceptions such as this vary by plan, so refer to the plan provisions before processing.
6. Charges for ambulance services are covered when either emergency room or inpatient hospital charges are also billed. An exception would be in the case of an insured that is dead on arrival at the hospital.
7. Transportation to a facility if the claimant is dead on arrival, even though no treatment or charges are incurred at the facility.

Basic benefits usually designate a maximum allowable/payable amount for:

1. Each trip to and from a facility.
2. All trips made during a period of disability.
3. All expenses incurred during a calendar year.

2. Ground transport time would be prolonged, and thus compromise the patient's medical status.

Coverage is limited to the regular air ambulance charge for transportation to the nearest facility in the area that can handle the case.

Under a Basic plan, all trip or per disability limitations apply. A few Basic plans may have a special allowance designated to cover air medical transport. However, many plans do not cover this type of service, regardless of the reason required. The cost of air ambulance ranges upward from a base charge of about $1,200 and is usually based on an hourly rate.

When a person becomes ill while traveling, he or she may want to be transferred to a hospital near home or be treated by a specific specialist in another city, even though the city where he or she is located has qualified specialists in the field. In these instances, ambulance expenses are not covered, regardless of whether an air ambulance or a conventional ambulance is used. This is because the transportation is not considered "medically necessary."

Charges for commercial or private airplane transportation, regardless of the reason required, are usually not covered.

## Paramedics

**Paramedics** are specially trained emergency medical personnel who render emergency treatment at the scene of the injury or illness. They are trained in advanced life support, whereas **Emergency Medical Technicians (EMTs)** are trained in basic life support. There are significant differences in educational and certification requirements of a paramedic compared with those of an EMT. Consequently, when a paramedic is required, an additional fee is usually charged.

Paramedic fees may be covered under a Basic ambulance benefit or may be strictly allowable under Major Medical. The plan provisions should stipulate the handling of this expense.

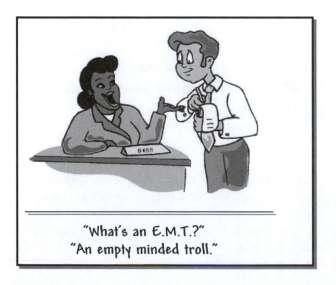

"What's an E.M.T.?"
"An empty minded troll."

## Mobile Intensive Care Unit

A **mobile intensive care unit** is a life support vehicle equipped to provide care to critically ill patients who require transportation to a hospital or from one hospital to another. It is designed to serve as an extension of an intensive care unit at a hospital.

The staffing of this unit usually involves a registered nurse and several other allied health professionals. The fees are in the same range as that for an air ambulance. Such charges may be covered if they are determined to be medically necessary in lieu of regular ambulance services.

## Van Transportation Unit

Many companies provide nonemergency transportation of the disabled to doctors' offices or hospital facilities. **Van transportation units** are specially equipped to handle wheelchairs and patients who are unable to get in and out of a regular vehicle. As a rule, it is required that the patient be able to sit in an upright position. The driver may have very basic medical training, such as cardiopulmonary resuscitation (CPR), but is generally not able or equipped to handle acute patients. This type of transportation is not covered by most plans because it is not considered medically necessary.

# Durable Medical Equipment (DME) Billing Procedures

**Durable medical equipment (DME)** is an item that can be used for an extended period of time without significant deterioration (i.e., it can stand repeated use). Therefore, an item that can be rented and returned for re-use would meet the requirement for durability. Medical supplies of a disposable nature, such as incontinence pads and surgical stockings, would not qualify as durable. (However, these items may be covered under the plan as medical supplies.)

**Medically oriented equipment** is primarily and customarily used for medical purposes (i.e., it is designed to fulfill a medical need). Therefore, it is generally not useful in the absence of an illness or injury. For example, an air conditioner may be used in the case of a heart patient to lower room temperature and reduce fluid loss. However, since the primary and customary use is nonmedical in nature, an air conditioner cannot be considered medical equipment. If the item could be used in a regular manner in the absence of a diagnosis, it is probably nonmedical in nature.

Most plans allow for the purchase or temporary rental of equipment and supplies when prescribed by a physician. However, certain requirements must be satisfied before authorizing payment.

Basically, three tests must be applied to items billed as DME in determining whether or not the items may be covered under a plan:

1. Does the item satisfy the definition of DME?
2. Is the item reasonable and necessary for the treatment of an illness or injury or for improvement of the functioning of a malformed body part?
3. Is the item prescribed for use in the patient's home?

Only when all three conditions are met will the item be covered by the plan.

## Evaluating Reasonable and Necessary

An item may meet the definition of DME and yet not be covered by the plan. Two things to be considered are:

1. **Reasonableness.** This evaluates the soundness and practicality of the DME approach to therapy, including such factors as:
   a. Is the need for the unit based on failures of other less costly approaches?
   b. Have more conservative means been attempted?
   c. What benefits will be derived from the unit?
   d. Do the benefits justify the expense?
2. **Necessity.** Equipment is necessary when it is expected to make a meaningful contribution to the treatment of the patient's illness or injury or to the improvement of the functioning of a malformed body part. Physicians tend to prescribe equipment based on a variety of reasons including:
   a. Familiarity. The physician is familiar with a particular piece of equipment. Other less expensive, more effective means of treatment or equipment may be available.
   b. Current popularity. As with clothing fashions, treatment and equipment popularity runs in cycles. Patients may even request the use of some pieces of equipment because it is hyped by the news media or some other medium. The particular equipment may not be the best or least expensive treatment available.

   c. Monetarily beneficial. Some equipment suppliers provide monetary inducements to physicians who use their equipment. Therefore, some physicians may routinely prescribe certain equipment based on this factor.

Even with a physician's prescription, it may be necessary to refer the claim to a consultant for review prior to payment or approval for purchase.

## DME for Patient's Home Use

For DME to be purchased or temporarily rented, the equipment must be prescribed for use in the home. Therefore, any facility that meets at least the minimum requirements of the definition of a hospital or skilled nursing facility is usually excluded from consideration.

A patient's home can be considered, but is not limited to:

- His or her own home, apartment, or dwelling.
- A relative's home.
- A home for the elderly.
- A nursing home.

## Practice Pitfalls

All claims for DME should be documented with the following information:

1. A description of the equipment prescribed by the physician. If the item is a commonly used item, a detailed description may not be necessary. However, with new equipment, it is important to try to obtain a marketing or manufacturer's brochure that indicates how the item is constructed and how it functions.
2. A statement of the medical necessity of the equipment. This should be in the form of a prescription showing the imprinted name, address, and telephone number of the prescribing physician. The related diagnosis should also be indicated.
3. An indication as to whether the item is to be rented or purchased and the rental or purchase price.
4. The estimated length of time that the equipment will be needed. This information will aid in the analysis of whether a rental or a purchase is more economical.
5. An indication as to where the equipment will be used and for how long.

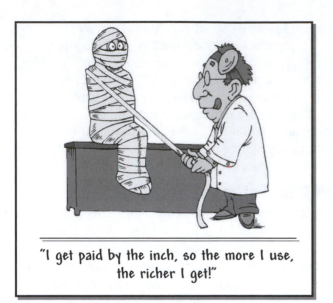

"I get paid by the inch, so the more I use, the richer I get!"

## Rental Versus Purchasing Determinations

The following four steps will assist in determining the most cost-efficient means of reimbursement.

1. Determine the period of time in months for which the item will be medically required from the information provided by the attending physician.

2. Multiply the number of months by the monthly rental fee. (This must be obtained from the supplier. Do not include the costs of perishable supplies, batteries, electrodes, and other items).

    Estimated length of use in months × monthly rental fee = total estimated equipment rental fee.

3. Request the supplier's purchase price for the equipment. Compare the purchase price to the calculated total estimated rental fee obtained in step #2.

4. If the total estimated rental fee is less than or equal to the purchase price, allow for the rental. If the rental fee is greater than the purchase price, rental is allowed up to but not exceeding the purchase price. Purchase of the item is not required. However, both the member and the supplier need to be notified that an expense that is higher than the purchase price will not be allowed under the plan.

## Repairs, Replacement, and Delivery

Repairs are covered when necessary to make the equipment functional. If the expense for repairs exceeds the estimated cost of purchasing or renting new equipment for the remaining period of medical need, payment is limited to the lower amount. Verify manufacturer's warranties before payment of repair fees.

Replacements are usually covered in cases of irreparable damage or wear or when the patient's physical condition has changed. Replacements due to wear or changes in the patient's physical condition must be supported by a current physician's order. Replacements due to loss may or may not be covered, depending on the circumstances. Usually, replacement is not covered when disrepair or loss results from a patient's carelessness. Other reasons for repair or replacement may be covered based on the plan provisions.

Charges for delivery of the DME and oxygen are usually covered.

# On the Job Now

**Directions:** Answer the following questions without looking back at the material just covered. Write your answers in the space provided.

1. What are the three tests (questions) that must be applied to items billed as DME in determining whether or not the items may be covered under a plan?

    1. _____

    2. _____

    3. _____

2. Will a plan cover a billed DME if two out of the three conditions are met? _____

## Types of Durable Medical Equipment (DME)

### Oxygen

Many plans cover the use of oxygen under DME benefits. Even though the oxygen itself is not durable, the canister in which the oxygen is contained and transported is durable, and it therefore falls under the category of DME.

Remember that these are general guidelines only. The specific guidelines may vary from payer to payer.

### Prosthetic Devices

**Prosthetic devices** are designed to replace a missing body part or to restore some function to a paralyzed body part.

Prosthetic devices include the making and application of an artificial part medically necessary to replace a lost or impaired body part or function, such as an artificial arm or leg, obturator, or urinary collection and retention systems.

Covered expenses associated with prosthetics include:

- Shipping and handling as part of the purchase price.
- Temporary postoperative prostheses.
- Replacement charges when replacement is due to a change in the patient's physical condition. (Children often need replacement prostheses every six to 12 months depending on their growth rate and other factors.) Replacement is not covered for wear and tear.

### Medical/Surgical Supplies

Perishable medical/surgical supplies may be covered under the plan if the items can be used only by the patient and are medically necessary in the treatment of the illness or injury. Medical and surgical supplies include:

1. Disposable, nondurable supplies and accessories required to operate medical equipment or prosthetic devices.
2. Necessary drugs and biological items put directly into equipment (such as nonprescription nutrients).
3. Initial and replacement accessories essential for operating medical equipment.
4. Supplies furnished and charged by a hospital, surgical center, or physician as part of active therapy, such as ace bandage, cast, or cervical collar.

Do not include items or supplies that could be used by the patient or a member of the patient's family for purposes other than medical care.

Questionable items should be referred to your supervisor or other designated person with the following information:

- Patient's diagnosis.
- Prescription from attending physician.
- Product description, literature, and prices.

See Appendix C for a list of DME coverage guidelines. This list is provided as a guide only. Actual administration may vary from company to company.

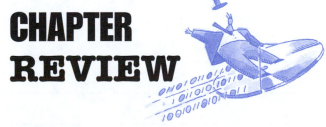

# CHAPTER REVIEW

### Summary

- Physician's services include a wide array of services from treating a patient in the office to providing services in an emergency room setting or at a skilled nursing facility.
- Physician's services charges may be billed by a variety of practitioners.

- It is important to learn to identify the covered providers, and use these guidelines to determine whether the charges billed are covered services.
- X-ray and laboratory services are essential in determining the patient's problems, ruling out conditions, and managing illnesses or injuries. It is now possible to perform certain tests in the privacy of one's home (i.e., pregnancy and glucose level tests).
- There are rules and guidelines used to process charges received for laboratory and radiology services.
- These guidelines should enable you to identify covered services and determine the correct processing procedures for these services.

- Hospitals provide a sterile environment to have medically necessary services and treatments, surgical or otherwise. They also provide a controlled environment in which to recover.
- Most plans and payers have specific handling guidelines that should be checked before processing.
- Ambulance expenses are expenses that are incurred to transfer an injured or sick person to a medical facility. These expenses are not considered professional or hospital services.
- Charges for an ambulance, air ambulance, paramedics or a mobile intensive care unit are often payable under Basic or Major Medical if services are considered medically necessary.
- Durable medical equipment includes medical-surgical equipment that can stand repeated use, is not useful in the absence of illness or injury, and is prescribed by a physician. In addition, the item must be necessary and reasonable for the treatment of the illness or injury or to replace an injured or lost bodily part or function, and must be appropriate for home use.
- In addition to the cost of the item, charges are also covered for shipping, handling, and postage, which are considered part of the purchase price.
- Necessary repairs to purchased equipment (if the equipment is not covered under warranty) are also covered. However, the cost of repairs is usually not covered for rented equipment.

## Assignments

Complete the Questions for Review.
Complete Exercises 6–1 through 6–16.

## Questions for Review

**Directions:**   Answer the following questions without looking back at the material just covered. Write your answers in the space provided.

1. What is the numeric range of the CPT® laboratory panel codes? _____

2. What are panel tests? _____

_____

3. What is unbundling? _____

_____

_____

4. What are professional and technical components? _____

_____

_____

_____

5. What does modifier -26 denote? _____

_____

6. Name the five varieties of hospital rooms.

   1. _____

   2. _____

3. _____

4. _____

5. _____

7. What are ancillary services? _____

_____

8. List at least three items that may be considered personal items. _____

_____

9. What are urgent care centers? _____

_____

10. What are surgi-centers? _____

_____

11. What does the abbreviation ABC stand for and what is it? _____

_____

12. Name the three different types of benefits that may cover ambulance expenses.

1. _____

2. _____

3. _____

13. The base call charge is _____

_____

14. (True or False?) If a person is injured while on vacation, most plans will pay to have the patient transported to the nearest facility to his or her home, even if there is no other reason for the transfer._____

15. (True or False?) In an emergency, taxicab fees would be covered since the transportation was medically necessary. _____

16. Name the two circumstances in which air ambulance charges may be covered under a plan.

1. _____

2. _____

**17.** With what information should all DME claims be documented?

1. _____

_____

2. _____

_____

3. _____

_____

4. _____

_____

5. _____

_____

**18.** Repairs are covered when necessary to make the equipment _____

**19.** Replacements are usually covered in cases of irreparable damages or because of _____

_____

**20.** _____ are designed to replace a missing body part or to restore function to a paralyzed part.

If you were unable to answer any of these questions, refer back to that section and then fill in the answers.

# Exercise 6-1

**Directions:** Find and circle the words listed below. Words can appear horizontally, vertically, diagonally, forward, or backward.

```
M S S Z S K I C U V I O U T Q S K E A Y P A H O T
M I C E P E I Z H N J G S S E Q R J M G R D O X A
T W S N C T M T C R B Z E C X U G A J O O W G C Q
Y E T C U I K O K D R U I V T C I R O L F Y S Z E
V H L Z E G V N H O G V N C S N R W K O E C W H C
H V A E S L N E G G R S N D T X K M O C S Z P Z F
S I G I M M L Z D E N U Q E L U T M M N S H B G K
C H Y O K E G A S C P I N J J I V X D O I H R S A
Z W M Z O X T Y N U I A S E J D N A D N O E U T O
B T J U L T T R C E N T G R I Y I G W O N I O C N
L O O Z U I V A Y C O H E A U R F Z U I A N A V V
F Y G E L Q N H E C H U L H A N A R J T L P L S F
A U G I H Q J T I N H Y S M T G I V D A S A O N Z
O I C M T B H M B D S A B S C S H H T I E T C E L
U A H M J E Y O T I L U R K E I O B Y D R I I C Y
F V V K R Q V N S E L V V G Z R R R Y A V E N E Y
X S Y A R X O Q H A U D J W E Y V H P R I N A S C
E W P M D M S W N N F G Y E Q S Y I I Z C T P S Q
D Y N I G H T C A R E C E N T E R S C R E C A I L
W T B A I B E N O I T A T L U S N O C E S A P T I
P S X B D O T L O U T P A T I E N T K H S R N Y P
W N H B I V L O D P X D X D U D X C G C J E C M E
F P B J B C Q R K N O S Z S D K R P Y A B G J S M
S E S N E P X E E C N A L U B M A Z L Q H V D A Z
M G B E E Q N Y R A C O F K B X K J W F F U E Y L
```

1. Acupuncture
2. Air Ambulance
3. Ambulance Expenses
4. Consultation
5. Dialysis
6. Facility Services
7. Inpatient Care
8. Maintenance Therapy
9. Miscellaneous Services
10. Necessity
11. Night Care Centers
12. Nursing Homes
13. Outpatient
14. Papanicolaou
15. Professional Services
16. Prosthetic Devices
17. Radiation Oncology
18. Telemetry Charges
19. X-rays

# Exercise 6-2

**Directions:** Complete the crossword puzzle by filling in a word from the keywords that fits each clue.

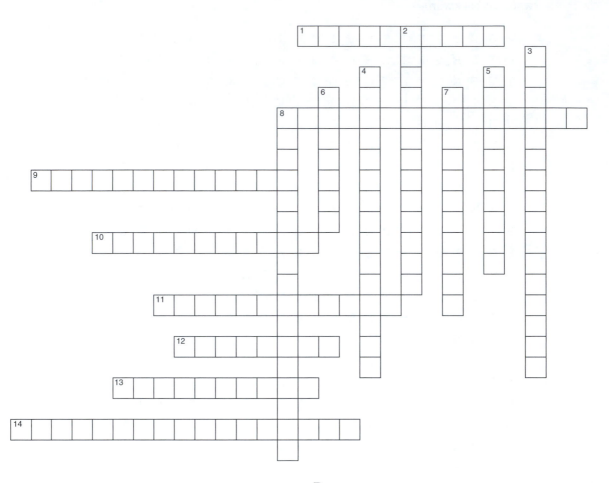

**Across**

1. A retraining of the muscles that control vision.
8. A diagnostic imaging technique that uses sound waves to create images of internal organs.
9. Care that is primarily for the purpose of meeting the personal daily needs of the patient and can be provided by personnel without medical care skills or training.
10. Training an individual to consciously control automatic, internal bodily functions.
11. Facilities that allow for the performance of surgery on an outpatient basis.
12. Charges for DXL services performed on an expedited priority basis.
13. Multiple tests that are combined and run from one specimen.
14. Charges for initial testing to confirm a diagnosis or to rule out other diagnoses.

**Down**

2. Those items that are primarily for the comfort of the patient and are not medically necessary.
3. Services performed in a hospital setting.
4. Flat or two-dimensional pictures of a particular body part or organ.
5. Specially trained emergency medical personnel who render emergency treatment at the scene of the injury or illness.
6. Scans made by a process that uses multiple x-ray images to create three-dimensional images of body structures.
7. A healthcare program providing coordinated services in a home setting.
8. Facilities that provide urgent or emergency treatment.

# Exercise 6-3

**Directions:** Match the following terms with the proper definition by writing the letter of the correct definition in the space next to the term.

1. _____ Alternative Birthing Centers

2. _____ Ambulatory Surgical Centers

3. _____ Ancillary Expenses

4. _____ Convalescent Facilities

5. _____ Day Care Centers

6. _____ Durable Medical Equipment

7. _____ Emergency Medical Technician

8. _____ Laboratory Examinations

9. _____ Medical Management

10. _____ Medically Oriented Equipment

11. _____ Mobile Intensive Care Unit

12. _____ Office or Other Outpatient Visit

13. _____ Professional Component

14. _____ Rehabilitation Facilities

15. _____ Speech Therapy

16. _____ Take-Home Prescriptions

17. _____ Technical Component

18. _____ Van Transportation Units

a. Vehicles specially equipped to handle wheelchairs and patients who are unable to get in and out of a regular vehicle.

b. Collection of a specimen or taking of an x-ray.

c. Medications to be taken after the patient is released from the hospital.

d. Office visits or other encounters between a physician and patient that occur outside a hospital setting.

e. Therapy to correct speech impairments.

f. The reading or interpreting of lab results or x-rays.

g. Specialize in long-term, post sickness, or post-injury care.

h. A life support vehicle equipped to provide care to critically ill patients during transportation to a hospital.

i. The analyzing of body substances to determine their chemical or tissue make-up.

j. A person trained in basic life support.

k. X-ray and laboratory charges that are incurred to control or manage a diagnosis (i.e., monitoring blood glucose levels on a patient with diabetes).

l. Items primarily and customarily used for medical purposes.

m. A center equipped to allow for the performance of surgery on an outpatient basis. These centers may be freestanding or attached to a major acute care facility.

n. Provide treatment during the daylight hours with the patient being released at night.

o. Items that can be used for an extended period of time without significant deterioration.

p. Usually considered to be midrange facilities that provide nonacute care for persons recovering from an acute illness or injury.

q. Miscellaneous services or supplies that are provided by the hospital on an inpatient or outpatient basis, which are necessary for the medical care or treatment of an individual.

r. Outpatient care centers that provide special rooms for routine deliveries.

# Exercises **6-4** through **6-16**

**Directions:** Process on a Payment Worksheet each of the physician, DXL, hospital, ambulance, and DME services claims found on the following pages. Refer to Appendices A, B, and C for contract and additional information.

All insureds are eligible for coverage under their respective plans. There are no beginning financials for members. Amounts paid for each claim throughout this book should be accumulated and carried forward to subsequent claims.

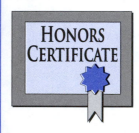

## Honors Certification™

The Honors Certification™ challenge for this chapter consists of a written test of the information contained within this chapter. Additionally, you will be given claims to process using the contracts contained in this book. Each incorrect answer will result in a deduction of up to 5% from your grade. You must achieve a score of 80% or higher to pass this test. If you fail the test on your first attempt, you may retake the test one additional time. The items included in the second test may be different from those in the first test.

PLEASE
DO NOT
STAPLE
IN THIS
AREA

ROVER INSURERS INC
5931 ROLLING ROAD
RONSON CO 81369

APPROVED MOB-0938-0008

□□□ PICA

# HEALTH INSURANCE CLAIM FORM

PICA □□□

| 1. MEDICARE   MEDICAID   CHAMPUS   CHAMPVA   GROUP HEALTH PLAN   FECA BLK LUNG   OTHER | 1a. INSURED'S I.D NUMBER (FOR PROGRAM IN ITEM 1) |
|---|---|
| ☐ (Medicare #)  ☐ (Medicaid #)  ☐ (Sponsor's SSN)  ☐ (VA File #)  ☒ (SSN or ID)  ☐ (SSN)  ☐ (ID) | 999 99 NIN |

| 2. PATIENT'S NAME (Last, First, Middle Initial). | 3. PATIENT'S BIRTH DATE | 4. INSURED'S NAME (Last, First, Middle Initial) |
|---|---|---|
| BOSSY BETTY B | MM 09  DD 19  YY CCYY-47   SEX  M ☐  F ☒ | SAME |

| 5. PATIENT'S ADDRESS (No., Street) | 6. PATIENT'S RELATIONSHIP TO INSURED | 7. INSURED'S ADDRESS (No., Street) |
|---|---|---|
| 7991 BAGEL BLVD | Self ☒  Spouse ☐  Child ☐  Other ☐ | |

| CITY | STATE | 8. PATIENT STATUS | CITY | STATE |
|---|---|---|---|---|
| BARSTOW | NY | Single ☐  Married ☒  Other ☐ | | |

| ZIP CODE | TELEPHONE (Include Area Code) | | ZIP CODE | TELEPHONE (INCLUDE AREA CODE) |
|---|---|---|---|---|
| 81569 | (914) 555 3399 | Employed ☒  Full-Time Student ☐  Part-Time Student ☐ | | |

| 9. OTHER INSURED'S NAME (Last, First, Middle Initial) | 10. IS PATIENT'S CONDITION RELATED TO: | 11. INSURED'S POLICY GROUP OR FECA NUMBER: 21088NIN |
|---|---|---|
| a. OTHER INSURED'S POLICY OR GROUP NUMBER | a. EMPLOYMENT? (CURRENT OR PREVIOUS) ☐ YES  ☒ NO | a. INSURED'S DATE OF BIRTH  MM  DD  YY   SEX  M ☐  F ☐ |
| b. OTHER INSURED'S DATE OF BIRTH  MM  DD  YY   SEX  M ☐  F ☐ | b. AUTO ACCIDENT?   PLACE (State) ☐ YES  ☒ NO | b. EMPLOYER'S NAME OR SCHOOL NAME  NINJA ENTERPRISES |
| c. EMPLOYER'S NAME OR SCHOOL NAME | c. OTHER ACCIDENT? ☐ YES  ☒ NO | c. INSURANCE PLAN NAME OR PROGRAM NAME  ROVER INSURERS INC |
| d. INSURANCE PLAN NAME OR PROGRAM NAME | 10d. RESERVED FOR LOCAL USE | d. IS THERE ANOTHER HEALTH BENEFIT PLAN? ☐ YES  ☒ NO  *if yes,* return to and complete item 9 a-d |

READ BACK OF FORM BEFORE COMPLETING & SIGNING THIS FORM

12. PATIENT'S OR AUTHORIZED PERSON'S SIGNATURE I authorize the release of any medical or other information necessary to process this claim. I also request payment of government benefits either to myself or to the party who accepts assignment below.

SIGNED **SIGNATURE ON FILE**   DATE

13. INSURED'S OR AUTHORIZED PERSON'S SIGNATURE I authorize payment of medical benefits to the undersigned physician or supplier for services described below.

SIGNED **SIGNATURE ON FILE**

| 14. DATE OF CURRENT ◄ ILLNESS (1st symptom) ◄ INJURY (Accident) PREGNANCY (LMP)  MM 02  DD 06  YY | 15. IF PATIENT HAS HAD SAME OR SIMILAR ILLNESS, GIVE FIRST DATE  MM  DD  YY | 16. DATES PATIENT UNABLE TO WORK IN CURRENT OCCUPATION  MM  DD  YY  FROM   TO  MM  DD  YY |
|---|---|---|
| 17. NAME OF REFERRING PHYSICIAN OR OTHER SOURCE | 17a. I.D. NUMBER OF REFERRING PHYSICIAN | 18. HOSPITALIZATION DATES RELATED TO CURRENT SERVICES  FROM  MM 02  DD 06  YY   TO  MM 02  DD 14  YY |
| 19. RESERVED FOR LOCAL USE | | 20. OUTSIDE LAB?  ☐ YES  ☐ NO   $ CHARGES |

21. DIAGNOSIS OR NATURE OF ILLNESS OR INJURY, (RELATE ITEMS 1,2,3, OR 4 TO ITEM 24E BY LINE)

1. 410 . 91   3.
2.   4.

22. MEDICAID RESUBMISSION CODE   ORIGINAL REF. NO.

23. PRIOR AUTHORIZATION NUMBER

| 24. A. DATE(S) OF SERVICE |  |  |  |  |  | B. Place of Service | C. Type of Service | D. PROCEDURES, SERVICES, OR SUPPLIES (Explain Unusual Circumstances) CPT/HCPS \| MODIFIER | E. DIAGNOSIS CODE | F. $ CHARGES | G. DAYS OR UNITS | H. EPSDT Family Plan | I. EMG | J. COB | K. RESERVED FOR LOCAL USE |
|---|---|---|---|---|---|---|---|---|---|---|---|---|---|---|---|
| From MM | DD | YY | To MM | DD | YY | | | | | | | | | | |
| 02 | 06 | YY | 02 | 06 | YY | 23 | | 99285 | 1 | 1600 \| 00 | 1 | | | | |
| 02 | 06 | YY | 02 | 06 | YY | 23 | | 93000 | 1 | 420 \| 00 | 1 | | | | |
| | | | | | | | | | | | | | | | |
| | | | | | | | | | | | | | | | |
| | | | | | | | | | | | | | | | |
| | | | | | | | | | | | | | | | |

| 25. FEDERAL TAX I.D. NUMBER   SSN EIN | 26. PATIENT'S ACCOUNT NO. | 27. ACCEPT ASSIGNMENT? (For govt. claims, see back) | 28. TOTAL CHARGE | 29. AMOUNT PAID | 30. BALANCE DUE |
|---|---|---|---|---|---|
| 90-9999779   ☐ ☒ | 001   939 | ☐ YES  ☒ NO | $ 2020 \| 00 | $ 0 \| 00 | $ 2020 \| 00 |

| 31. SIGNATURE OF PHYSICIAN OR SUPPLIER INCLUDING DEGREES OR CREDENTIALS (I certify that the statements on the reverse apply to this bill and are made a part thereof.)  SIGNED *Gal Bladder MD* DATE 02/08/YY | 32. NAME AND ADDRESS OF FACILITY WHERE SERVICES WERE RENDERED (If other than home or office)  HEADACHE HOSPITAL 2000 HAZARD STREET HELP NY 12899 | 33. PHYSICIAN'S, SUPPLIERS BILLING NAME, ADDRESS, ZIP CODE & PHONE #  GAL BLADDER MD      NETWORK PROVIDER 1990 GATEWAY DRIVE STE 919G GOVERN NY 12899 (914) 555 8899  PIN# GAL001      GRP# |
|---|---|---|

(APPROVED BY AMA COUNCIL ON MEDICAL SERVICE 8/88)   **PLEASE PRINT OR TYPE**   FORM CMS-1500   (12-90) FORM OWCP-1500   FORM RRB-1500 FORM AMA-OP050591

**Exercise 6–4**

PLEASE DO NOT STAPLE IN THIS AREA

WINTER INSURANCE CO
9763 WESTERN WAY
WHITTIER CO 82963

APPROVED MOB-0938-0008

□□□ PICA

# HEALTH INSURANCE CLAIM FORM

PICA □□□

| 1. MEDICARE | MEDICAID | CHAMPUS | CHAMPVA | GROUP HEALTH PLAN | FECA BLK LUNG | OTHER | 1a. INSURED'S I.D NUMBER (FOR PROGRAM IN ITEM 1) |
|---|---|---|---|---|---|---|---|
| ☐ (Medicare #) | ☐ (Medicaid #) | ☐ (Sponsor's SSN) | ☐ (VA File #) | ☒ (SSN or ID) | ☐ (SSN) | ☐ (ID) | 444 44 ABC |

**2. PATIENT'S NAME (Last, First, Middle Initial).**
DINGBAT DANNY D

**3. PATIENT'S BIRTH DATE**
MM 04 DD 24 YY CCYY-10    SEX M ☒  F ☐

**4. INSURED'S NAME (Last, First, Middle Initial)**
DINGBAT DANA D

**5. PATIENT'S ADDRESS (No., Street)**
404 DOORWAY DRIVE

**6. PATIENT'S RELATIONSHIP TO INSURED**
Self ☐   Spouse ☐   Child ☒   Other ☐

**7. INSURED'S ADDRESS (No., Street)**
SAME

**CITY** DENVER   **STATE** ND

**8. PATIENT STATUS**
Single ☒   Married ☐   Other ☐
Employed ☐   Full-Time Student ☒   Part-Time Student ☐

**CITY**   **STATE**

**ZIP CODE** 58444   **TELEPHONE (Include Area Code)** (701) 555 3344

**ZIP CODE**   **TELEPHONE (INCLUDE AREA CODE)**

**9. OTHER INSURED'S NAME (Last, First, Middle Initial)**

**10. IS PATIENT'S CONDITION RELATED TO:**

**11. INSURED'S POLICY GROUP OR FECA NUMBER:**
36928ABC

**a. OTHER INSURED'S POLICY OR GROUP NUMBER**

**a. EMPLOYMENT? (CURRENT OR PREVIOUS)**
☐ YES   ☒ NO

**a. INSURED'S DATE OF BIRTH**
MM 04 DD 04 YY CCYY-37    SEX M ☐  F ☒

**b. OTHER INSURED'S DATE OF BIRTH**
MM DD YY    SEX M ☐  F ☐

**b. AUTO ACCIDENT?**   PLACE (State)
☐ YES   ☒ NO

**b. EMPLOYER'S NAME OR SCHOOL NAME**
ABC CORPORATION

**c. EMPLOYER'S NAME OR SCHOOL NAME**

**c. OTHER ACCIDENT?**
☒ YES   ☐ NO

**c. INSURANCE PLAN NAME OR PROGRAM NAME**
WINTER INSURANCE COMPANY

**d. INSURANCE PLAN NAME OR PROGRAM NAME**

**10d. RESERVED FOR LOCAL USE**

**d. IS THERE ANOTHER HEALTH BENEFIT PLAN?**
☐ YES   ☒ NO   *if yes, return to and complete item 9 a-d*

READ BACK OF FORM BEFORE COMPLETING & SIGNING THIS FORM

**12. PATIENT'S OR AUTHORIZED PERSON'S SIGNATURE** I authorize the release of any medical or other information necessary to process this claim. I also request payment of government benefits either to myself or to the party who accepts assignment below.

SIGNED SIGNATURE ON FILE   DATE

**13. INSURED'S OR AUTHORIZED PERSON'S SIGNATURE** I authorize payment of medical benefits to the undersigned physician or supplier for services described below.

SIGNED SIGNATURE ON FILE

**14. DATE OF CURRENT:** ◄ ILLNESS (1st symptom) INJURY (Accident) PREGNANCY (LMP)
MM 01 DD 26 YY

**15. IF PATIENT HAS HAD SAME OR SIMILAR ILLNESS, GIVE FIRST DATE** MM DD YY

**16. DATES PATIENT UNABLE TO WORK IN CURRENT OCCUPATION**
FROM MM DD YY   TO MM DD YY

**17. NAME OF REFERRING PHYSICIAN OR OTHER SOURCE**

**17a. I.D. NUMBER OF REFERRING PHYSICIAN**

**18. HOSPITALIZATION DATES RELATED TO CURRENT SERVICES**
FROM MM 01 DD 26 YY YY   TO MM 02 DD 10 YY YY

**19. RESERVED FOR LOCAL USE**

**20. OUTSIDE LAB?**   $ CHARGES
☐ YES   ☐ NO

**21. DIAGNOSIS OR NATURE OF ILLNESS OR INJURY, (RELATE ITEMS 1,2,3, OR 4 TO ITEM 24E BY LINE)**

1. 807 . 01
2. 823 . 32
3. 800 . 40
4. E884 . 9

**22. MEDICAID RESUBMISSION CODE**   ORIGINAL REF. NO.

**23. PRIOR AUTHORIZATION NUMBER**

| 24. A DATE(S) OF SERVICE From MM DD YY   To MM DD YY | B Place of Service | C Type of Service | D PROCEDURES, SERVICES, OR SUPPLIES (Explain Unusual Circumstances) CPT/HCPS \| MODIFIER | E DIAGNOSIS CODE | F $ CHARGES | G DAYS OR UNITS | H EPSDT Family Plan | I EMG | J COB | K RESERVED FOR LOCAL USE |
|---|---|---|---|---|---|---|---|---|---|---|
| 01 26 YY 01 26 YY | 23 | 1 | 99285 | 1 2 3 4 | 882 00 | 1 | | | | |
| | | | | | | | | | | |
| | | | | | | | | | | |
| | | | | | | | | | | |
| | | | | | | | | | | |
| | | | | | | | | | | |

**25. FEDERAL TAX I.D. NUMBER** SSN EIN
70-9899774   ☐ ☒

**26. PATIENT'S ACCOUNT NO.**
001   434

**27. ACCEPT ASSIGNMENT?** (For govt. claims, see back)
☒ YES   ☐ NO

**28. TOTAL CHARGE**
$ 882 00

**29. AMOUNT PAID**
$ 0 00

**30. BALANCE DUE**
$ 882 00

**31. SIGNATURE OF PHYSICIAN OR SUPPLIER INCLUDING DEGREES OR CREDENTIALS** (I certify that the statements on the reverse apply to this bill and are made a part thereof.)
SIGNED Art Terry MD DATE 02/10/YY

**32. NAME AND ADDRESS OF FACILITY WHERE SERVICES WERE RENDERED (If other than home or office)**
HACKIM HOSPITAL
1000 HIDE STREET
HUSHTOWN ND 58444

**33. PHYSICIAN'S, SUPPLIERS BILLING NAME, ADDRESS, ZIP CODE & PHONE #**
ART TERRY MD
4567 DOVER DRIVE STE 404D
DOLTER ND 58444
(701) 555 0044
PIN# C43101   GRP#

(APPROVED BY AMA COUNCIL ON MEDICAL SERVICE 8/88)   **PLEASE PRINT OR TYPE**
FORM CMS-1500 (12-90)
FORM OWCP-1500   FORM RRB-1500
FORM AMA-OP050591

**Exercise 6–5**

PLEASE
DO NOT
STAPLE
IN THIS
AREA

BALL INSURANCE CARRIERS
3895 BUBBLE BLVD STE 283
BOXWOOD CO 85926

APPROVED MOB-0938-0008

□□□ PICA

## HEALTH INSURANCE CLAIM FORM

PICA □□□

| 1. | MEDICARE | MEDICAID | CHAMPUS | CHAMPVA | GROUP HEALTH PLAN | FECA BLK LUNG | OTHER | 1a. INSURED'S I.D NUMBER (FOR PROGRAM IN ITEM 1) |
|---|---|---|---|---|---|---|---|---|
| | ☐ (Medicare #) | ☐ (Medicaid #) | ☐ (Sponsor's SSN) | ☐ (VA File #) | ☒ (SSN or ID) | ☐ (SSN) | ☐ (ID) | 555 55 XYZ |

2. PATIENT'S NAME (Last, First, Middle Initial).
PATIENT PATTY P

3. PATIENT'S BIRTH DATE
MM 05  DD 15  YY CCYY-35   SEX M ☐  F ☒

4. INSURED'S NAME (Last, First, Middle Initial)
SAME

5. PATIENT'S ADDRESS (No., Street)
655 PAIN LANE

6. PATIENT'S RELATIONSHIP TO INSURED
Self ☒   Spouse ☐   Child ☐   Other ☐

7. INSURED'S ADDRESS (No., Street)

CITY
PEN

STATE
PA

8. PATIENT STATUS
Single ☒   Married ☐   Other ☐
Employed ☒   Full-Time Student ☐   Part-Time Student ☐

CITY

STATE

ZIP CODE
15522

TELEPHONE (Include Area Code)
(878) 555 3355

ZIP CODE

TELEPHONE (INCLUDE AREA CODE)

9. OTHER INSURED'S NAME (Last, First, Middle Initial)

10. IS PATIENT'S CONDITION RELATED TO:

11. INSURED'S POLICY GROUP OR FECA NUMBER:
62958XYZ

a. OTHER INSURED'S POLICY OR GROUP NUMBER

a. EMPLOYMENT? (CURRENT OR PREVIOUS)
☐ YES   ☒ NO

a. INSURED'S DATE OF BIRTH
MM  DD  YY   SEX M ☐   F ☐

b. OTHER INSURED'S DATE OF BIRTH
MM  DD  YY   SEX M ☐   F ☐

b. AUTO ACCIDENT?   PLACE (State)
☐ YES   ☒ NO

b. EMPLOYER'S NAME OR SCHOOL NAME
XYZ CORPORATION

c. EMPLOYER'S NAME OR SCHOOL NAME

c. OTHER ACCIDENT?
☐ YES   ☒ NO

c. INSURANCE PLAN NAME OR PROGRAM NAME
BALL INSURANCE CARRIERS

d. INSURANCE PLAN NAME OR PROGRAM NAME

10d. RESERVED FOR LOCAL USE

d. IS THERE ANOTHER HEALTH BENEFIT PLAN?
☐ YES   ☒ NO   *if yes*, return to and complete item 9 a-d

READ BACK OF FORM BEFORE COMPLETING & SIGNING THIS FORM

12. PATIENT'S OR AUTHORIZED PERSON'S SIGNATURE I authorize the release of any medical or other information necessary to process this claim. I also request payment of government benefits either to myself or to the party who accepts assignment below.

SIGNED **SIGNATURE ON FILE**   DATE

13. INSURED'S OR AUTHORIZED PERSON'S SIGNATURE I authorize payment of medical benefits to the undersigned physician or supplier for services described below.

SIGNED **SIGNATURE ON FILE**

14. DATE OF CURRENT: ◄ ILLNESS (1st symptom) ◄ INJURY (Accident) PREGNANCY (LMP)
MM 02  DD 02  YY YY

15. IF PATIENT HAS HAD SAME OR SIMILAR ILLNESS, GIVE FIRST DATE   MM  DD  YY

16. DATES PATIENT UNABLE TO WORK IN CURRENT OCCUPATION
FROM MM  DD  YY   TO MM  DD  YY

17. NAME OF REFERRING PHYSICIAN OR OTHER SOURCE

17a. I.D. NUMBER OF REFERRING PHYSICIAN

18. HOSPITALIZATION DATES RELATED TO CURRENT SERVICES
FROM MM  DD  YY   TO MM  DD  YY

19. RESERVED FOR LOCAL USE

20. OUTSIDE LAB?   $ CHARGES
☐ YES   ☐ NO

21. DIAGNOSIS OR NATURE OF ILLNESS OR INJURY, (RELATE ITEMS 1,2,3, OR 4 TO ITEM 24E BY LINE)

1. 233 . 0
2.
3.
4.

22. MEDICAID RESUBMISSION
CODE   ORIGINAL REF. NO.

23. PRIOR AUTHORIZATION NUMBER

| 24. A DATE(S) OF SERVICE | | | | | | B Place of Service | C Type of Service | D PROCEDURES, SERVICES, OR SUPPLIES (Explain Unusual Circumstances) CPT/HCPS | MODIFIER | E DIAGNOSIS CODE | F $ CHARGES | | G DAYS OR UNITS | H EPSDT Family Plan | I EMG | J COB | K RESERVED FOR LOCAL USE |
|---|---|---|---|---|---|---|---|---|---|---|---|---|---|---|---|---|---|
| From MM DD YY | | | To MM DD YY | | | | | | | | | | | | | | |
| 02 | 02 | YY | 02 | 04 | YY | 11 | 1 | 99213 | | 1 | 330 | 00 | 1 | | | | |
| | | | | | | | | | | | | | | | | | |
| | | | | | | | | | | | | | | | | | |
| | | | | | | | | | | | | | | | | | |
| | | | | | | | | | | | | | | | | | |
| | | | | | | | | | | | | | | | | | |

25. FEDERAL TAX I.D. NUMBER   SSN EIN
70-4785959   ☐ ☒

26. PATIENT'S ACCOUNT NO.
0425501   535

27. ACCEPT ASSIGNMENT? (For govt. claims, see back)
☐ YES   ☒ NO

28. TOTAL CHARGE
$ 330 | 00

29. AMOUNT PAID
$ 150 | 00

30. BALANCE DUE
$ 180 | 00

31. SIGNATURE OF PHYSICIAN OR SUPPLIER INCLUDING DEGREES OR CREDENTIALS (I certify that the statements on the reverse apply to this bill and are made a part thereof.)

SIGNED *Amber U Lance MD*   DATE 02/10/YY

32. NAME AND ADDRESS OF FACILITY WHERE SERVICES WERE RENDERED (If other than home or office)

33. PHYSICIAN'S, SUPPLIERS BILLING NAME, ADDRESS, ZIP CODE & PHONE #
AMBER U LANCE MD
5005 ANSWER STREET STE 5123A
AGE PA 15522
(878) 555 3155
PIN# E99699   GRP#

(APPROVED BY AMA COUNCIL ON MEDICAL SERVICE 8/88)

**PLEASE PRINT OR TYPE**

FORM CMS-1500   (12-90)
FORM OWCP-1500   FORM RRB-1500
FORM AMA-OP050591

**Exercise 6–6**

PLEASE DO NOT STAPLE IN THIS AREA

ROVER INSURERS INC
5931 ROLLING ROAD
RONSON CO 81369

APPROVED MOB-0938-0008

□□□ PICA

# HEALTH INSURANCE CLAIM FORM

PICA □□□

| 1. | MEDICARE ☐ (Medicare #) | MEDICAID ☐ (Medicaid #) | CHAMPUS ☐ (Sponsor's SSN) | CHAMPVA ☐ (VA File #) | GROUP HEALTH PLAN ☒ (SSN or ID) | FECA BLK LUNG ☐ (SSN) | OTHER ☐ (ID) | 1a. INSURED'S I.D NUMBER (FOR PROGRAM IN ITEM 1) 999 99 NIN |

2. PATIENT'S NAME (Last, First, Middle Initial).
BOSSY BETTY B

3. PATIENT'S BIRTH DATE  MM 09  DD 19  YY CCYY-47   SEX  M ☐  F ☒

4. INSURED'S NAME (Last, First, Middle Initial)
SAME

5. PATIENT'S ADDRESS (No., Street)
7991 BAGEL BLVD

CITY BARSTOW   STATE NY

ZIP CODE 10012   TELEPHONE (Include Area Code) (914) 555 3399

6. PATIENT'S RELATIONSHIP TO INSURED
Self ☒  Spouse ☐  Child ☐  Other ☐

7. INSURED'S ADDRESS (No., Street)

CITY   STATE

ZIP CODE   TELEPHONE (INCLUDE AREA CODE)

8. PATIENT STATUS
Single ☐  Married ☒  Other ☐
Employed ☒  Full-Time Student ☐  Part-Time Student ☐

9. OTHER INSURED'S NAME (Last, First, Middle Initial)

a. OTHER INSURED'S POLICY OR GROUP NUMBER

b. OTHER INSURED'S DATE OF BIRTH  MM  DD  YY   SEX  M ☐  F ☐

c. EMPLOYER'S NAME OR SCHOOL NAME

d. INSURANCE PLAN NAME OR PROGRAM NAME

10. IS PATIENT'S CONDITION RELATED TO:

a. EMPLOYMENT? (CURRENT OR PREVIOUS)  YES ☐  NO ☒

b. AUTO ACCIDENT?  YES ☐  NO ☒   PLACE (State) |_____|

c. OTHER ACCIDENT?  YES ☐  NO ☒

10d. RESERVED FOR LOCAL USE

11. INSURED'S POLICY GROUP OR FECA NUMBER:
21088NIN

a. INSURED'S DATE OF BIRTH  MM  DD  YY   SEX  M ☐  F ☐

b. EMPLOYER'S NAME OR SCHOOL NAME
NINJA ENTERPRISES

c. INSURANCE PLAN NAME OR PROGRAM NAME
ROVER INSURERS INC

d. IS THERE ANOTHER HEALTH BENEFIT PLAN?  YES ☐  NO ☒   *if yes*, return to and complete item 9 a-d

READ BACK OF FORM BEFORE COMPLETING & SIGNING THIS FORM

12. PATIENT'S OR AUTHORIZED PERSON'S SIGNATURE I authorize the release of any medical or other information necessary to process this claim. I also request payment of government benefits either to myself or to the party who accepts assignment below.

SIGNED SIGNATURE ON FILE   DATE _____

13. INSURED'S OR AUTHORIZED PERSON'S SIGNATURE I authorize payment of medical benefits to the undersigned physician or supplier for services described below.

SIGNED SIGNATURE ON FILE

14. DATE OF CURRENT: ◄ ILLNESS (1st symptom) / INJURY (Accident) / PREGNANCY (LMP)  MM 02  DD 06  YY YY

15. IF PATIENT HAS HAD SAME OR SIMILAR ILLNESS, GIVE FIRST DATE  MM  DD  YY

16. DATES PATIENT UNABLE TO WORK IN CURRENT OCCUPATION  FROM MM DD YY  TO MM DD YY

17. NAME OF REFERRING PHYSICIAN OR OTHER SOURCE

17a. I.D. NUMBER OF REFERRING PHYSICIAN

18. HOSPITALIZATION DATES RELATED TO CURRENT SERVICES  FROM MM 02 DD 06 YY YY  TO MM 02 DD 14 YY YY

19. RESERVED FOR LOCAL USE

20. OUTSIDE LAB?  YES ☐  NO ☐   $ CHARGES

21. DIAGNOSIS OR NATURE OF ILLNESS OR INJURY, (RELATE ITEMS 1,2,3, OR 4 TO ITEM 24E BY LINE)

1. | 410 . 91
2. | . |
3. | . |
4. | . |

22. MEDICAID RESUBMISSION CODE   ORIGINAL REF. NO.

23. PRIOR AUTHORIZATION NUMBER

| 24. A DATE(S) OF SERVICE From MM DD YY | To MM DD YY | B Place of Service | C Type of Service | D PROCEDURES, SERVICES, OR SUPPLIES (Explain Unusual Circumstances) CPT/HCPS | MODIFIER | E DIAGNOSIS CODE | F $ CHARGES | G DAYS OR UNITS | H EPSDT Family Plan | I EMG | J COB | K RESERVED FOR LOCAL USE |
|---|---|---|---|---|---|---|---|---|---|---|---|---|
| 02 06 YY | 02 06 YY | 21 | | 93000 | | 1 | 340 00 | 1 | | | | |
| 02 06 YY | 02 06 YY | 21 | | 93545 | | 1 | 770 00 | 1 | | | | |
| 02 06 YY | 02 06 YY | 21 | | 85025 | | 1 | 40 00 | 1 | | | | |
| 02 06 YY | 02 06 YY | 21 | | 86901 | | 1 | 45 00 | 1 | | | | |
| 02 06 YY | 02 06 YY | 21 | | 85610 | | 1 | 30 00 | 1 | | | | |

25. FEDERAL TAX I.D. NUMBER  70-8989779   SSN ☐  EIN ☒

26. PATIENT'S ACCOUNT NO. 001   939

27. ACCEPT ASSIGNMENT? (For govt. claims, see back)  YES ☒  NO ☐

28. TOTAL CHARGE  $ 1225 00

29. AMOUNT PAID  $ 0 00

30. BALANCE DUE  $ 1225 00

31. SIGNATURE OF PHYSICIAN OR SUPPLIER INCLUDING DEGREES OR CREDENTIALS (I certify that the statements on the reverse apply to this bill and are made a part thereof.)

SIGNED *Daniel Drawblood MD*  DATE 02/12/YY

32. NAME AND ADDRESS OF FACILITY WHERE SERVICES WERE RENDERED (If other than home or office)
HEADACHE HOSPITAL
2000 HAZARD STREET
HELP NY 12899

33. PHYSICIAN'S, SUPPLIERS BILLING NAME, ADDRESS, ZIP CODE & PHONE #
DANIEL DRAWBLOOD MD   NETWORK PROVIDER
HEADACHE HOSPITAL
2000 HAZARD STREET
HELP NY 12899
(914) 555 8899
PIN# F67267   GRP#

(APPROVED BY AMA COUNCIL ON MEDICAL SERVICE 8/88)   **PLEASE PRINT OR TYPE**

FORM CMS-1500 (12-90)
FORM OWCP-1500   FORM RRB-1500
FORM AMA-OP050591

**Exercise 6–7**

PLEASE
DO NOT
STAPLE
IN THIS
AREA

WINTER INSURANCE CO
9763 WESTERN WAY
WHITTIER CO  82963

APPROVED MOB-0938-0008

□□□ PICA

# HEALTH INSURANCE CLAIM FORM

PICA □□□

| 1. | MEDICARE | MEDICAID | CHAMPUS | CHAMPVA | GROUP HEALTH PLAN | FECA BLK LUNG | OTHER | 1a. INSURED'S I.D NUMBER (FOR PROGRAM IN ITEM 1) |
|---|---|---|---|---|---|---|---|---|

☐ (Medicare #)  ☐ (Medicaid #)  ☐ (Sponsor's SSN)  ☐ (VA File #)  ☒ (SSN or ID)  ☐ (SSN)  ☐ (ID)

444 44 ABC

| 2. PATIENT'S NAME (Last, First, Middle Initial). | 3. PATIENT'S BIRTH DATE | | | SEX | 4. INSURED'S NAME (Last, First, Middle Initial) |
|---|---|---|---|---|---|

DINGBAT DANNY D

MM 04  DD 24  YY CCYY-10   M ☒  F ☐

DINGBAT DANA D

| 5. PATIENT'S ADDRESS (No., Street) | 6. PATIENT'S RELATIONSHIP TO INSURED | 7. INSURED'S ADDRESS (No., Street) |
|---|---|---|

404 DOORWAY DRIVE

Self ☐   Spouse ☐   Child ☒   Other ☐

SAME

| CITY | STATE | 8. PATIENT STATUS | CITY | STATE |
|---|---|---|---|---|

DENVER    ND

Single ☒   Married ☐   Other ☐

| ZIP CODE | TELEPHONE (Include Area Code) | | ZIP CODE | TELEPHONE (INCLUDE AREA CODE) |
|---|---|---|---|---|

58444    (701) 555 3344

Employed ☐   Full-Time Student ☒   Part-Time Student ☐

| 9. OTHER INSURED'S NAME (Last, First, Middle Initial) | 10. IS PATIENT'S CONDITION RELATED TO: | 11. INSURED'S POLICY GROUP OR FECA NUMBER: |
|---|---|---|

36928ABC

| a. OTHER INSURED'S POLICY OR GROUP NUMBER | a. EMPLOYMENT? (CURRENT OR PREVIOUS) | a. INSURED'S DATE OF BIRTH | SEX |
|---|---|---|---|

☐ YES   ☒ NO

MM 04  DD 04  YY CCYY-37   M ☐  F ☒

| b. OTHER INSURED'S DATE OF BIRTH | | | SEX | b. AUTO ACCIDENT?   PLACE (State) | b. EMPLOYER'S NAME OR SCHOOL NAME |
|---|---|---|---|---|---|

MM  DD  YY    M ☐  F ☐

☐ YES   ☒ NO

ABC CORPORATION

| c. EMPLOYER'S NAME OR SCHOOL NAME | c. OTHER ACCIDENT? | c. INSURANCE PLAN NAME OR PROGRAM NAME |
|---|---|---|

☒ YES   ☐ NO

WINTER INSURANCE COMPANY

| d. INSURANCE PLAN NAME OR PROGRAM NAME | 10d. RESERVED FOR LOCAL USE | d. IS THERE ANOTHER HEALTH BENEFIT PLAN? |
|---|---|---|

☐ YES   ☒ NO   if yes, return to and complete item 9 a-d

READ BACK OF FORM BEFORE COMPLETING & SIGNING THIS FORM

12. PATIENT'S OR AUTHORIZED PERSON'S SIGNATURE I authorize the release of any medical or other information necessary to process this claim. I also request payment of government benefits either to myself or to the party who accepts assignment below.

SIGNED  SIGNATURE ON FILE          DATE

13. INSURED'S OR AUTHORIZED PERSON'S SIGNATURE I authorize payment of medical benefits to the undersigned physician or supplier for services described below.

SIGNED  SIGNATURE ON FILE

| 14. DATE OF CURRENT: ◄ ILLNESS (1st symptom) ◄ INJURY (Accident) PREGNANCY (LMP) | 15. IF PATIENT HAS HAD SAME OR SIMILAR ILLNESS, GIVE FIRST DATE MM DD YY | 16. DATES PATIENT UNABLE TO WORK IN CURRENT OCCUPATION |
|---|---|---|

MM 01  DD 26  YY YY

FROM  MM DD YY    TO  MM DD YY

| 17. NAME OF REFERRING PHYSICIAN OR OTHER SOURCE | 17a. I.D. NUMBER OF REFERRING PHYSICIAN | 18. HOSPITALIZATION DATES RELATED TO CURRENT SERVICES |
|---|---|---|

FROM  01 26 YY    TO  02 08 YY

| 19. RESERVED FOR LOCAL USE | 20. OUTSIDE LAB?   $ CHARGES |
|---|---|

☐ YES   ☐ NO

21. DIAGNOSIS OR NATURE OF ILLNESS OR INJURY, (RELATE ITEMS 1,2,3, OR 4 TO ITEM 24E BY LINE)

22. MEDICAID RESUBMISSION CODE   ORIGINAL REF. NO.

1. |  807 . 01     3. |  800 . 40

2. |  823 . 32     4. |  E884 . 9

23. PRIOR AUTHORIZATION NUMBER

| 24. A. DATE(S) OF SERVICE From | | | To | | | B. Place of Service | C. Type of Service | D. PROCEDURES, SERVICES, OR SUPPLIES (Explain Unusual Circumstances) CPT/HCPS | MODIFIER | E. DIAGNOSIS CODE | F. $ CHARGES | G. DAYS OR UNITS | H. EPSDT Family Plan | I. EMG | J. COB | K. RESERVED FOR LOCAL USE |
|---|---|---|---|---|---|---|---|---|---|---|---|---|---|---|---|---|
| MM | DD | YY | MM | DD | YY | | | | | | | | | | | |
| 01 | 26 | YY | 01 | 26 | YY | 21 | 1 | 70260 | Technical Component | 3 4 | 70 00 | 1 | | | | |
| 01 | 26 | YY | 01 | 26 | YY | 21 | 1 | 71020 | Technical Component | 1 4 | 55 00 | 1 | | | | |
| 01 | 26 | YY | 01 | 26 | YY | 21 | 1 | 73550 | Technical Component | 2 4 | 80 00 | 2 | | | | |
| 01 | 26 | YY | 01 | 26 | YY | 21 | 1 | 73590 | Technical Component | 2 4 | 100 00 | 2 | | | | |
| 01 | 26 | YY | 01 | 26 | YY | 21 | 1 | 70450 | Technical Component | 3 4 | 325 00 | 1 | | | | |
| 01 | 26 | YY | 01 | 26 | YY | 21 | 1 | 73718 | Technical Component | 2 4 | 770 00 | 1 | | | | |

| 25. FEDERAL TAX I.D. NUMBER  SSN EIN | 26. PATIENT'S ACCOUNT NO. | 27. ACCEPT ASSIGNMENT? (For govt. claims, see back) | 28. TOTAL CHARGE | 29. AMOUNT PAID | 30. BALANCE DUE |
|---|---|---|---|---|---|

70-8989898   ☐ ☒

001   434

☒ YES   ☐ NO

$ 1400 00   $ 0 00   $ 1400 00

| 31. SIGNATURE OF PHYSICIAN OR SUPPLIER INCLUDING DEGREES OR CREDENTIALS (I certify that the statements on the reverse apply to this bill and are made a part thereof.) | 32. NAME AND ADDRESS OF FACILITY WHERE SERVICES WERE RENDERED (If other than home or office) | 33. PHYSICIAN'S, SUPPLIERS BILLING NAME, ADDRESS, ZIP CODE & PHONE # |
|---|---|---|

HACKIM HOSPITAL
1000 HIDE STREET
HUSHTOWN ND 58444

RITA X RAY MD
HACKIM HOSPITAL
1000 HIDE STREET
HUSHTOWN ND 58444
(710) 555 4004

SIGNED  Rita X Ray MD  DATE 02/08/YY

PIN#  G88888     GRP#

(APPROVED BY AMA COUNCIL ON MEDICAL SERVICE 8/88)

PLEASE PRINT OR TYPE

FORM CMS-1500  (12-90)
FORM OWCP-1500    FORM RRB-1500
FORM AMA-OP050591

**Exercise 6–8**

BALL INSURANCE CARRIERS
3895 BUBBLE BLVD STE 283
BOXWOOD CO 85926

APPROVED MOB-0938-0008

## HEALTH INSURANCE CLAIM FORM

PICA □□□

| 1. | MEDICARE | MEDICAID | CHAMPUS | CHAMPVA | GROUP HEALTH PLAN | FECA BLK LUNG | OTHER | 1a. INSURED'S I.D NUMBER (FOR PROGRAM IN ITEM 1) |
|---|---|---|---|---|---|---|---|---|
| | □ (Medicare #) | □ (Medicaid #) | □ (Sponsor's SSN) | □ (VA File #) | ☒ (SSN or ID) | □ (SSN) | □ (ID) | 555 55 XYZ |

| 2. PATIENT'S NAME (Last, First, Middle Initial). | 3. PATIENT'S BIRTH DATE | 4. INSURED'S NAME (Last, First, Middle Initial) |
|---|---|---|
| PATIENT PATTY P | MM 05 DD 15 YY CCYY-35 M □ F ☒ | SAME |

| 5. PATIENT'S ADDRESS (No., Street) | 6. PATIENT'S RELATIONSHIP TO INSURED | 7. INSURED'S ADDRESS (No., Street) |
|---|---|---|
| 655 PAIN LANE | Self ☒ Spouse □ Child □ Other □ | |

| CITY | STATE | 8. PATIENT STATUS | CITY | STATE |
|---|---|---|---|---|
| PEN | PA | Single ☒ Married □ Other □ | | |
| ZIP CODE 15522 | TELEPHONE (Include Area Code) (878) 555 3355 | Employed ☒ Full-Time Student □ Part-Time Student □ | ZIP CODE | TELEPHONE (INCLUDE AREA CODE) |

| 9. OTHER INSURED'S NAME (Last, First, Middle Initial) | 10. IS PATIENT'S CONDITION RELATED TO: | 11. INSURED'S POLICY GROUP OR FECA NUMBER: 62958XYZ |
|---|---|---|
| a. OTHER INSURED'S POLICY OR GROUP NUMBER | a. EMPLOYMENT? (CURRENT OR PREVIOUS) □ YES ☒ NO | a. INSURED'S DATE OF BIRTH MM DD YY SEX M □ F □ |
| b. OTHER INSURED'S DATE OF BIRTH MM DD YY SEX M □ F □ | b. AUTO ACCIDENT? PLACE (State) □ YES ☒ NO | b. EMPLOYER'S NAME OR SCHOOL NAME XYZ CORPORATION |
| c. EMPLOYER'S NAME OR SCHOOL NAME | c. OTHER ACCIDENT? □ YES ☒ NO | c. INSURANCE PLAN NAME OR PROGRAM NAME BALL INSURANCE CARRIERS |
| d. INSURANCE PLAN NAME OR PROGRAM NAME | 10d. RESERVED FOR LOCAL USE | d. IS THERE ANOTHER HEALTH BENEFIT PLAN? □ YES ☒ NO if yes, return to and complete item 9 a-d |

READ BACK OF FORM BEFORE COMPLETING & SIGNING THIS FORM

12. PATIENT'S OR AUTHORIZED PERSON'S SIGNATURE I authorize the release of any medical or other information necessary to process this claim. I also request payment of government benefits either to myself or to the party who accepts assignment below.

SIGNED **SIGNATURE ON FILE**          DATE

13. INSURED'S OR AUTHORIZED PERSON'S SIGNATURE I authorize payment of medical benefits to the undersigned physician or supplier for services described below.

SIGNED **SIGNATURE ON FILE**

| 14. DATE OF CURRENT: MM 02 DD 16 YY YY ◄ ILLNESS (1st symptom) INJURY (Accident) PREGNANCY (LMP) | 15. IF PATIENT HAS HAD SAME OR SIMILAR ILLNESS. GIVE FIRST DATE MM DD YY | 16. DATES PATIENT UNABLE TO WORK IN CURRENT OCCUPATION MM DD YY MM DD YY FROM TO |
|---|---|---|
| 17. NAME OF REFERRING PHYSICIAN OR OTHER SOURCE | 17a. I.D. NUMBER OF REFERRING PHYSICIAN | 18. HOSPITALIZATION DATES RELATED TO CURRENT SERVICES MM DD YY MM DD YY FROM 02 16 YY TO 02 16 YY |
| 19. RESERVED FOR LOCAL USE | | 20. OUTSIDE LAB? □ YES □ NO $ CHARGES |

| 21. DIAGNOSIS OR NATURE OF ILLNESS OR INJURY, (RELATE ITEMS 1,2,3, OR 4 TO ITEM 24E BY LINE) | 22. MEDICAID RESUBMISSION CODE ORIGINAL REF. NO. |
|---|---|
| 1. 233 . 0          3. ____ . ____ | 23. PRIOR AUTHORIZATION NUMBER |
| 2. ____ . ____       4. ____ . ____ | |

| 24. A DATE(S) OF SERVICE | | B Place of Service | C Type of Service | D PROCEDURES, SERVICES, OR SUPPLIES (Explain Unusual Circumstances) CPT/HCPS | MODIFIER | E DIAGNOSIS CODE | F $ CHARGES | G DAYS OR UNITS | H EPSDT Family Plan | I EMG | J COB | K RESERVED FOR LOCAL USE |
|---|---|---|---|---|---|---|---|---|---|---|---|---|
| From MM DD YY | To MM DD YY | | | | | | | | | | | |
| 02 16 YY | 02 16 YY | 11 | 1 | 76092 | | 1 | 165 00 | 1 | | | | |
| | | | | | | | | | | | | |
| | | | | | | | | | | | | |
| | | | | | | | | | | | | |
| | | | | | | | | | | | | |
| | | | | | | | | | | | | |

| 25. FEDERAL TAX I.D. NUMBER SSN EIN | 26. PATIENT'S ACCOUNT NO. | 27. ACCEPT ASSIGNMENT? (For govt. claims, see back) | 28. TOTAL CHARGE | 29. AMOUNT PAID | 30. BALANCE DUE |
|---|---|---|---|---|---|
| 70-4231234 □ ☒ | 001 535 | ☒ YES □ NO | $ 165 00 | $ 0 00 | $ 165 00 |

| 31. SIGNATURE OF PHYSICIAN OR SUPPLIER INCLUDING DEGREES OR CREDENTIALS (I certify that the statements on the reverse apply to this bill and are made a part thereof.) | 32. NAME AND ADDRESS OF FACILITY WHERE SERVICES WERE RENDERED (If other than home or office) | 33. PHYSICIAN'S, SUPPLIERS BILLING NAME, ADDRESS, ZIP CODE & PHONE # |
|---|---|---|
| SIGNED *Irene N Jection MD* DATE 02/11/YY | HELPER HOSPITAL 25450 HAMMER AVE HUMMER TOWN PA 15522 | IRENE N JECTION MD HELPER HOSPITAL 25450 HAMMER AVE HUMMER TOWN PA 15522 (878) 555 6455 PIN# H37841       GRP# |

(APPROVED BY AMA COUNCIL ON MEDICAL SERVICE 8/88)          **PLEASE PRINT OR TYPE**          FORM CMS-1500 (12-90)
FORM OWCP-1500          FORM RRB-1500
FORM AMA-OP050591

**Exercise 6–9**

APPROVED OMB NO. 0938-0279

ST-1843 1PLY UB-92

| | | | |
|---|---|---|---|
| HEADACHE HOSPITAL | 2 | 3 PATIENT CONTROL NO. | 4 TYPE OF BILL |
| 2000 HAZARD STREET | | 7654321 | 111 |
| HELP NY 12899 | 5 FED. TAX NO. 70-5555555 | 6 STATEMENT COVERS PERIOD FROM 0206YY THROUGH 0214YY | 7 COV D. 08 | 8 N-C D. 0 | 9 C-I D. | 10 L-R D. | 11 |

| 12 PATIENT NAME | 13 PATIENT ADDRESS |
|---|---|
| BOSSY BETTY B | 7991 BAGEL BLVD BARSTOW NY 10012 |

| 14 BIRTHDATE | 15 SEX | 16 MS | 17 DATE ADMISSION | 18 HR | 19 TYPE | 20 SRC | 21 D HR | 22 STAT | 23 MEDICAL RECORD NO. | CONDITION CODES 24 25 26 27 28 29 30 | 31 |
|---|---|---|---|---|---|---|---|---|---|---|---|
| 0919CCYY-47 | F | M | 0206YY | 10 | 1 | 7 | 13 | 01 | | | |

| 32 OCCURRENCE CODE DATE | 33 OCCURRENCE CODE DATE | 34 OCCURRENCE CODE DATE | 35 OCCURRENCE CODE DATE | 36 OCCURRENCE SPAN CODE FROM THROUGH | 37 |
|---|---|---|---|---|---|
| a | | | | | A B C |
| b | | | | | |

38
BETTY B BOSSY
7991 BAGEL BLVD
BARSTOW NY 10012

| 39 CODE | VALUE CODES AMOUNT | 40 CODE | VALUE CODES AMOUNT | 41 CODE | VALUE CODES AMOUNT | |
|---|---|---|---|---|---|---|
| a 01 | 360 00 | | | | | a |
| b | | | | | | b |
| c | | | | | | c |
| d | | | | | | d |

| 42 REV. CD. | 43 DESCRIPTION | 44 HCPCS / RATES | 45 SERV. DATE | 46 SERV. UNITS | 47 TOTAL CHARGES | 48 NON-COVERED CHARGES | 49 | |
|---|---|---|---|---|---|---|---|---|
| 1 | 130 | ROOM-BOARD/3 & 4 BED | 395.00 | | 8 | 3160 00 | | 1 |
| 2 | 250 | PHARMACY | | | 108 | 3416 00 | | 2 |
| 3 | 260 | IV THERAPY | | | 4 | 1400 00 | | 3 |
| 4 | 270 | MED-SUR SUPPLIES | | | 4 | 1125 00 | | 4 |
| 5 | 300 | LABORATORY | | | 1 | 772 00 | | 5 |
| 6 | 410 | RESPIRATORY SVC | | | 9 | 294 00 | | 6 |
| 7 | 730 | EKG/ECG | | | 1 | 79 00 | | 7 |
| 23 | 001 | TOTAL CHARGES | | | | 10246 00 | | 23 |

| 50 PAYER | 51 PROVIDER NO | 52 REL INFO | 53 ASG BEN | 54 PRIOR PAYMENTS | 55 EST. AMOUNT DUE | 56 | |
|---|---|---|---|---|---|---|---|
| A ROVER INSURERS INC | | Y | Y | 0 00 | 10246 00 | | A |
| B | | | | | | | B |
| C | | | | | | | C |

57                                    DUE FROM PATIENT ▶

| 58 INSURED'S NAME | 59 P. REL | 60 CERT. - SSN - HIC. - ID NO. | 61 GROUP NAME | 62 INSURANCE GROUP NO. | |
|---|---|---|---|---|---|
| A BETTY B BOSSY | 18 | 999 99 NIN | | 21088NIN | A |
| B | | | | | B |
| C | | | | | C |

| 63 TREATMENT AUTHORIZATION CODES | 64 ESC | 65 EMPLOYER NAME | 66 EMPLOYER LOCATION | |
|---|---|---|---|---|
| A | 1 | NINJA ENTERPRISES | 1234 NOCKOUT ROAD NEWTON NM 88012 | A |
| B | | | | B |
| C | | | | C |

| 67 PRIN. DIAG. CD. | 68 CODE | 69 CODE | 70 CODE | OTHER DIAG. CODES 71 CODE 72 CODE | 73 CODE | 74 CODE | 75 CODE | 76 ADM. DIAG. CD. | 77 E-CODE | 78 |
|---|---|---|---|---|---|---|---|---|---|---|
| 410.91 | | | | | | | | | | |

| 79 P.C. | 80 PRINCIPAL PROCEDURE CODE DATE | 81 OTHER PROCEDURE CODE DATE | OTHER PROCEDURE CODE DATE | 82 ATTENDING PHYS. ID A21212 |
|---|---|---|---|---|
| | | A | B | ABE DOMIN MD |
| | OTHER PROCEDURE CODE DATE C | OTHER PROCEDURE CODE DATE D | OTHER PROCEDURE CODE DATE E | 83 OTHER PHYS. ID |

| 84 REMARKS | 85 PROVIDER REPRESENTATIVE | 86 DATE |
|---|---|---|
| a NETWORK PROVIDER | X  Betty Biller | 02/16/YY |
| Precertification received | | |

UB-92 HCFA-1450          OCR/ORIGINAL          I CERTIFY THE CERTIFICATIONS ON THE REVERSE APPLY TO THIS BILL AND ARE MADE A PART HEREOF.

**Exercise 6–10**

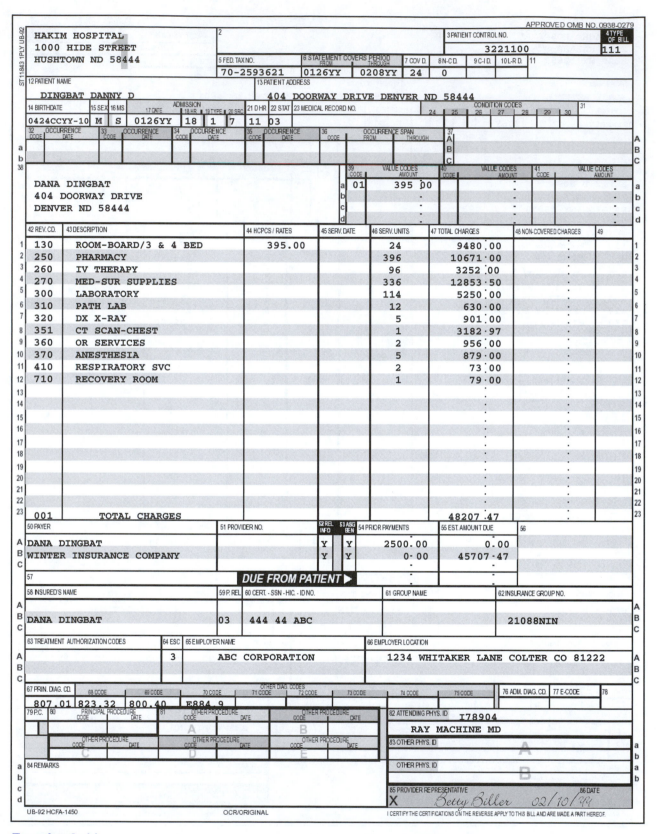

**Exercise 6–11**

APPROVED OMB NO. 0938-0279

| | | | | |
|---|---|---|---|---|
| HELPER HOSPITAL<br>25450 HAMMER AVE<br>HUMMER TOWN PA 15522 | 2 | | 3 PATIENT CONTROL NO.<br>9876543 | 4 TYPE OF BILL<br>131 |

| 5 FED. TAX NO. | 6 STATEMENT COVERS PERIOD FROM | THROUGH | 7 COV D. | 8 N-C D. | 9 C-I D. | 10 L-R D. | 11 |
|---|---|---|---|---|---|---|---|
| 70-5621347 | 0216YY | 0216YY | 0 | 0 | | | |

**12 PATIENT NAME**　PATIENT PATTY P

**13 PATIENT ADDRESS**　655 PAIN LANE PEN PA 15522

| 14 BIRTHDATE | 15 SEX | 16 MS | 17 DATE | ADMISSION 18 HR. | 19 TYPE | 20 SRC | 21 D HR | 22 STAT | 23 MEDICAL RECORD NO. | | CONDITION CODES 24 25 26 27 28 29 30 | 31 |
|---|---|---|---|---|---|---|---|---|---|---|---|---|
| 0515CCYY-35 | F | S | 0216YY | 07 | 3 | 1 | 17 | 01 | | | | |

| 32 OCCURRENCE CODE DATE | 33 OCCURRENCE CODE DATE | 34 OCCURRENCE CODE DATE | 35 OCCURRENCE CODE DATE | 36 OCCURRENCE SPAN CODE FROM THROUGH | 37 A B C |
|---|---|---|---|---|---|

38　PATTY P PATIENT<br>655 PAIN LANE<br>PEN PA 15522

| | 39 CODE | VALUE CODES AMOUNT | 40 CODE | VALUE CODES AMOUNT | 41 CODE | VALUE CODES AMOUNT | |
|---|---|---|---|---|---|---|---|
| a | | | | | | | a |
| b | | | | | | | b |
| c | | | | | | | c |
| d | | | | | | | d |

| | 42 REV. CD. | 43 DESCRIPTION | 44 HCPCS / RATES | 45 SERV. DATE | 46 SERV. UNITS | 47 TOTAL CHARGES | 48 NON-COVERED CHARGES | 49 | |
|---|---|---|---|---|---|---|---|---|---|
| 1 | 250 | PHARMACY | | | 8 | 360 90 | | | 1 |
| 2 | 270 | MED-SUR SUPPLIES | | | 23 | 628 50 | | | 2 |
| 3 | 300 | LABORATORY | | | 3 | 146 90 | | | 3 |
| 4 | 360 | OR SERVICES | | | 6 | 1407 60 | | | 4 |
| 5 | 370 | ANESTHESIA | | | 1 | 299 75 | | | 5 |
| 6 | 410 | RESPIRATORY SVC | | | 1 | 12 35 | | | 6 |
| 23 | 001 | TOTAL CHARGES | | | | 2856 00 | | | 23 |

| 50 PAYER | 51 PROVIDER NO. | 52 REL INFO | 53 ASG BEN | 54 PRIOR PAYMENTS | 55 EST AMOUNT DUE | 56 | |
|---|---|---|---|---|---|---|---|
| A | BALL INSURANCE CARRIERS | | Y | Y | 500 00 | 2356 00 | |
| B | | | | | | | |
| C | | | | | | | |

57　**DUE FROM PATIENT ▶**

| 58 INSURED'S NAME | 59 P. REL | 60 CERT. - SSN - HIC. - ID NO. | 61 GROUP NAME | 62 INSURANCE GROUP NO. | |
|---|---|---|---|---|---|
| A | | | | | A |
| B PATTY P PATIENT | 01 | 555 55 XYZ | | 62958XYZ | B |
| C | | | | | C |

| 63 TREATMENT AUTHORIZATION CODES | 64 ESC | 65 EMPLOYER NAME | 66 EMPLOYER LOCATION | |
|---|---|---|---|---|
| A | | | | A |
| B | 1 | XYZ CORPORATION | 9817 BOBCAT BLVD BASTION CO 81319 | B |
| C | | | | C |

| 67 PRIN. DIAG. CD. | 68 CODE | 69 CODE | 70 CODE | OTHER DIAG. CODES 71 CODE 72 CODE | 73 CODE | 74 CODE | 75 CODE | 76 ADM. DIAG. CD. | 77 E-CODE | 78 |
|---|---|---|---|---|---|---|---|---|---|---|
| 233.0 | | | | | | | | | | |

| 79 P.C. | 80 PRINCIPAL PROCEDURE CODE DATE | 81 OTHER PROCEDURE CODE DATE | OTHER PROCEDURE CODE DATE | 82 ATTENDING PHYS. ID　J48748<br>SAM A PILLER MD | |
|---|---|---|---|---|---|
| | | A | B | 83 OTHER PHYS. ID　A | a |
| | OTHER PROCEDURE CODE DATE　C | OTHER PROCEDURE CODE DATE　D | OTHER PROCEDURE CODE DATE　E | OTHER PHYS. ID　B | b |

| 84 REMARKS | 85 PROVIDER REPRESENTATIVE<br>X　*Betty Biller* | 86 DATE<br>02/19/YY |
|---|---|---|

UB-92 HCFA-1450　　　　OCR/ORIGINAL　　　　I CERTIFY THE CERTIFICATIONS ON THE REVERSE APPLY TO THIS BILL AND ARE MADE A PART HEREOF.

ST1 1843 1PLY UB-92

**Exercise 6–12**

PLEASE
DO NOT
STAPLE
IN THIS
AREA

ROVER INSURERS INC
5931 ROLLING ROAD
RONSON CO 81369

APPROVED MOB-0938-0008

□□□ PICA

# HEALTH INSURANCE CLAIM FORM

PICA □□□

| 1. | MEDICARE | MEDICAID | CHAMPUS | CHAMPVA | GROUP HEALTH PLAN | FECA BLK LUNG | OTHER | 1a. INSURED'S I.D NUMBER (FOR PROGRAM IN ITEM 1) |
|---|---|---|---|---|---|---|---|---|

☐ (Medicare #) ☐ (Medicaid #) ☐ (Sponsor's SSN) ☐ (VA File #) ☒ (SSN or ID) ☐ (SSN) ☐ (ID)

999 99 NIN

2. PATIENT'S NAME (Last, First, Middle Initial).

BOSSY BETTY B

3. PATIENT'S BIRTH DATE
MM 09 | DD 19 | YY CCYY-47    SEX  M ☐  F ☒

4. INSURED'S NAME (Last, First, Middle Initial)

SAME

5. PATIENT'S ADDRESS (No., Street)

7991 BAGEL BLVD

6. PATIENT'S RELATIONSHIP TO INSURED
Self ☒  Spouse ☐  Child ☐  Other ☐

7. INSURED'S ADDRESS (No., Street)

CITY
BARSTOW
STATE NY

8. PATIENT STATUS
Single ☐  Married ☒  Other ☐
Employed ☒  Full-Time Student ☐  Part-Time Student ☐

CITY
STATE

ZIP CODE
10012
TELEPHONE (Include Area Code)
(914) 555 3399

ZIP CODE
TELEPHONE (INCLUDE AREA CODE)

9. OTHER INSURED'S NAME (Last, First, Middle Initial)

10. IS PATIENT'S CONDITION RELATED TO:

11. INSURED'S POLICY GROUP OR FECA NUMBER:

21088NIN

a. OTHER INSURED'S POLICY OR GROUP NUMBER

a. EMPLOYMENT? (CURRENT OR PREVIOUS)
☐ YES  ☒ NO

a. INSURED'S DATE OF BIRTH
MM | DD | YY    SEX  M ☐  F ☐

b. OTHER INSURED'S DATE OF BIRTH
MM | DD | YY    SEX  M ☐  F ☐

b. AUTO ACCIDENT?    PLACE (State)
☐ YES  ☒ NO

b. EMPLOYER'S NAME OR SCHOOL NAME

NINJA ENTERPRISES

c. EMPLOYER'S NAME OR SCHOOL NAME

c. OTHER ACCIDENT?
☐ YES  ☒ NO

c. INSURANCE PLAN NAME OR PROGRAM NAME

ROVER INSURERS INC

d. INSURANCE PLAN NAME OR PROGRAM NAME

10d. RESERVED FOR LOCAL USE

d. IS THERE ANOTHER HEALTH BENEFIT PLAN?
☐ YES  ☒ NO    *if yes*, return to and complete item 9 a-d

READ BACK OF FORM BEFORE COMPLETING & SIGNING THIS FORM

12. PATIENT'S OR AUTHORIZED PERSON'S SIGNATURE I authorize the release of any medical or other information necessary to process this claim. I also request payment of government benefits either to myself or to the party who accepts assignment below.

SIGNED  SIGNATURE ON FILE    DATE

13. INSURED'S OR AUTHORIZED PERSON'S SIGNATURE I authorize payment of medical benefits to the undersigned physician or supplier for services described below.

SIGNED  SIGNATURE ON FILE

14. DATE OF CURRENT:  ◄  ILLNESS (1st symptom)    INJURY (Accident)    PREGNANCY (LMP)
MM 02 | DD 06 | YY YY

15. IF PATIENT HAS HAD SAME OR SIMILAR ILLNESS. GIVE FIRST DATE  MM | DD | YY

16. DATES PATIENT UNABLE TO WORK IN CURRENT OCCUPATION
MM | DD | YY    MM | DD | YY
FROM    TO

17. NAME OF REFERRING PHYSICIAN OR OTHER SOURCE

17a. I.D. NUMBER OF REFERRING PHYSICIAN

18. HOSPITALIZATION DATES RELATED TO CURRENT SERVICES
MM | DD | YY    MM | DD | YY
FROM    TO

19. RESERVED FOR LOCAL USE

20. OUTSIDE LAB?    $ CHARGES
☐ YES  ☐ NO

21. DIAGNOSIS OR NATURE OF ILLNESS OR INJURY, (RELATE ITEMS 1,2,3, OR 4 TO ITEM 24E BY LINE)

1. | 786 . 50
2. | . 
3. | . 
4. | . 

22. MEDICAID RESUBMISSION CODE    ORIGINAL REF. NO.

23. PRIOR AUTHORIZATION NUMBER

| 24. | A DATE(S) OF SERVICE | | | | | B Place of Service | C Type of Service | D PROCEDURES, SERVICES, OR SUPPLIES (Explain Unusual Circumstances) CPT/HCPS | MODIFIER | E DIAGNOSIS CODE | F $ CHARGES | G DAYS OR UNITS | H EPSDT Family Plan | I EMG | J COB | K RESERVED FOR LOCAL USE |
|---|---|---|---|---|---|---|---|---|---|---|---|---|---|---|---|---|---|
| | From MM DD YY | | | To MM DD YY | | | | | | | | | | | | |
| | 02 | 06 | YY | 02 | 06 | YY | 41 | 1 | A0433 | | 1 | 610 00 | 1 | | Y | | |

25. FEDERAL TAX I.D. NUMBER    SSN EIN
70-8888779    ☐ ☒

26. PATIENT'S ACCOUNT NO.
001    939

27. ACCEPT ASSIGNMENT? (For govt. claims, see back)
☒ YES  ☐ NO

28. TOTAL CHARGE
$ 610 00

29. AMOUNT PAID
$ 0 00

30. BALANCE DUE
$ 610 00

31. SIGNATURE OF PHYSICIAN OR SUPPLIER INCLUDING DEGREES OR CREDENTIALS (I certify that the statements on the reverse apply to this bill and are made a part thereof.)

SIGNED  Nita Ring  DATE 02/21/YY

32. NAME AND ADDRESS OF FACILITY WHERE SERVICES WERE RENDERED (If other than home or office)

HEADACHE HOSPITAL
2000 HAZARD STREET
HELP NY 12899

33. PHYSICIAN'S, SUPPLIERS BILLING NAME, ADDRESS, ZIP CODE & PHONE #

AWESOME AMBULANCE SERVICE    NETWORK PROVIDER
909 ANDY AVENUE
ANNSTOWN NY 12899
(914) 555 9876

PIN#  A95911    GRP#

(APPROVED BY AMA COUNCIL ON MEDICAL SERVICE 8/88)

**PLEASE PRINT OR TYPE**

FORM CMS-1500  (12-90)
FORM OWCP-1500    FORM RRB-1500
FORM AMA-OP050591

**Exercise 6–13**

PLEASE
DO NOT
STAPLE
IN THIS
AREA

□□□ PICA

WINTER INSURANCE CO
9763 WESTERN WAY
WHITTIER CO 82963

APPROVED MOB-0938-0008

## HEALTH INSURANCE CLAIM FORM

PICA □□□

| 1. | MEDICARE | MEDICAID | CHAMPUS | CHAMPVA | GROUP HEALTH PLAN | FECA BLK LUNG | OTHER | 1a. INSURED'S I.D NUMBER (FOR PROGRAM IN ITEM 1) |
|---|---|---|---|---|---|---|---|---|
| | ☐ (Medicare #) | ☐ (Medicaid #) | ☐ (Sponsor's SSN) | ☐ (VA File #) | ☒ (SSN or ID) | ☐ (SSN) | ☐ (ID) | 444 44 ABC |

| 2. PATIENT'S NAME (Last, First, Middle Initial). | 3. PATIENT'S BIRTH DATE | 4. INSURED'S NAME (Last, First, Middle Initial) |
|---|---|---|
| DINGBAT DANNY D | MM 04 DD 24 YY CCYY-10  SEX M ☒ F ☐ | DINGBAT DANA D |

| 5. PATIENT'S ADDRESS (No., Street) | 6. PATIENT'S RELATIONSHIP TO INSURED | 7. INSURED'S ADDRESS (No., Street) |
|---|---|---|
| 404 DOORWAY DRIVE | Self ☐  Spouse ☐  Child ☒  Other ☐ | SAME |

| CITY | STATE | 8. PATIENT STATUS | CITY | STATE |
|---|---|---|---|---|
| DENVER | ND | Single ☒  Married ☐  Other ☐ | | |
| ZIP CODE | TELEPHONE (Include Area Code) | Employed ☐  Full-Time ☒  Part-Time ☐ Student   Student | ZIP CODE | TELEPHONE (INCLUDE AREA CODE) |
| 58444 | (701) 555 3344 | | | |

| 9. OTHER INSURED'S NAME (Last, First, Middle Initial) | 10. IS PATIENT'S CONDITION RELATED TO: | 11. INSURED'S POLICY GROUP OR FECA NUMBER: |
|---|---|---|
| | | 36928ABC |
| a. OTHER INSURED'S POLICY OR GROUP NUMBER | a. EMPLOYMENT? (CURRENT OR PREVIOUS)  ☐ YES  ☒ NO | a. INSURED'S DATE OF BIRTH  MM 04 DD 04 YY CCYY -37  SEX M ☐ F ☒ |
| b. OTHER INSURED'S DATE OF BIRTH  MM DD YY  SEX M ☐ F ☐ | b. AUTO ACCIDENT?  PLACE (State)  ☐ YES  ☒ NO | b. EMPLOYER'S NAME OR SCHOOL NAME  ABC CORPORATION |
| c. EMPLOYER'S NAME OR SCHOOL NAME | c. OTHER ACCIDENT?  ☒ YES  ☐ NO | c. INSURANCE PLAN NAME OR PROGRAM NAME  WINTER INSURANCE COMPANY |
| d. INSURANCE PLAN NAME OR PROGRAM NAME | 10d. RESERVED FOR LOCAL USE | d. IS THERE ANOTHER HEALTH BENEFIT PLAN?  ☐ YES  ☒ NO  *if yes*, return to and complete item 9 a-d |

READ BACK OF FORM BEFORE COMPLETING & SIGNING THIS FORM

| 12. PATIENT'S OR AUTHORIZED PERSON'S SIGNATURE I authorize the release of any medical or other information necessary to process this claim. I also request payment of government benefits either to myself or to the party who accepts assignment below. | 13. INSURED'S OR AUTHORIZED PERSON'S SIGNATURE I authorize payment of medical benefits to the undersigned physician or supplier for services described below. |
|---|---|
| SIGNED SIGNATURE ON FILE       DATE | SIGNED SIGNATURE ON FILE |

| 14. DATE OF CURRENT:  ◄ ILLNESS (1st symptom)  ◄ INJURY (Accident)  PREGNANCY (LMP) | 15. IF PATIENT HAS HAD SAME OR SIMILAR ILLNESS. GIVE FIRST DATE  MM DD YY | 16. DATES PATIENT UNABLE TO WORK IN CURRENT OCCUPATION  MM DD YY   MM DD YY |
|---|---|---|
| MM 01 DD 26 YY | | FROM       TO |

| 17. NAME OF REFERRING PHYSICIAN OR OTHER SOURCE | 17a. I.D. NUMBER OF REFERRING PHYSICIAN | 18. HOSPITALIZATION DATES RELATED TO CURRENT SERVICES  MM DD YY   MM DD YY |
|---|---|---|
| | | FROM 01 26 YY  TO |

| 19. RESERVED FOR LOCAL USE | 20. OUTSIDE LAB?  ☐ YES  ☐ NO       $ CHARGES |
|---|---|

| 21. DIAGNOSIS OR NATURE OF ILLNESS OR INJURY, (RELATE ITEMS 1,2,3, OR 4 TO ITEM 24E BY LINE) | 22. MEDICAID RESUBMISSION  CODE       ORIGINAL REF. NO. |
|---|---|
| 1. 959 . 01       3. E884 . 9 | 23. PRIOR AUTHORIZATION NUMBER |
| 2. 823 . 32       4. E885 . 2 | |

| 24. A. DATE(S) OF SERVICE | | | | | B. Place of Service | C. Type of Service | D. PROCEDURES, SERVICES, OR SUPPLIES (Explain Unusual Circumstances) CPT/HCPS   MODIFIER | E. DIAGNOSIS CODE | F. $ CHARGES | G. DAYS OR UNITS | H. EPSDT Family Plan | I. EMG | J. COB | K. RESERVED FOR LOCAL USE |
|---|---|---|---|---|---|---|---|---|---|---|---|---|---|---|---|
| From MM | DD | YY | To MM | DD | YY | | | | | | | | | | |
| 01 | 26 | YY | 01 | 26 | YY | 41 | 1 | A0427 | 1 2 3 4 | 535 00 | 1 | | Y | | |
| | | | | | | | | | | | | | | | |
| | | | | | | | | | | | | | | | |
| | | | | | | | | | | | | | | | |
| | | | | | | | | | | | | | | | |

| 25. FEDERAL TAX I.D. NUMBER     SSN EIN | 26. PATIENT'S ACCOUNT NO. | 27. ACCEPT ASSIGNMENT? (For govt. claims, see back) | 28. TOTAL CHARGE | 29. AMOUNT PAID | 30. BALANCE DUE |
|---|---|---|---|---|---|
| 70-8888797   ☐ ☒ | DANDI001   434 | ☒ YES  ☐ NO | $ 535 00 | $ 0 00 | $ 535 00 |

| 31. SIGNATURE OF PHYSICIAN OR SUPPLIER INCLUDING DEGREES OR CREDENTIALS (I certify that the statements on the reverse apply to this bill and are made a part thereof.) | 32. NAME AND ADDRESS OF FACILITY WHERE SERVICES WERE RENDERED (If other than home or office) | 33. PHYSICIAN'S, SUPPLIERS BILLING NAME, ADDRESS, ZIP CODE & PHONE # |
|---|---|---|
| SIGNED *Cy Rem*   DATE *02/11/YY* | | ANSWER AMBULANCE SERVICE  1140 ANY WAY  AMBLER ND 5844  (701) 555 4532 |
| | | PIN# A42242       GRP# |

(APPROVED BY AMA COUNCIL ON MEDICAL SERVICE 8/88)

**PLEASE PRINT OR TYPE**

FORM CMS-1500   (12-90)
FORM OWCP-1500     FORM RRB-1500
FORM AMA-OP050591

**Exercise 6–14**

PLEASE
DO NOT
STAPLE
IN THIS
AREA

ROVER INSURERS INC
5931 ROLLING ROAD
RONSON CO 81369

APPROVED MOB-0938-0008

□□□ PICA

## HEALTH INSURANCE CLAIM FORM

PICA □□□

| 1. | MEDICARE | MEDICAID | CHAMPUS | CHAMPVA | GROUP HEALTH PLAN | FECA BLK LUNG | OTHER | 1a. INSURED'S I.D NUMBER (FOR PROGRAM IN ITEM 1) |
|---|---|---|---|---|---|---|---|---|
| | ☐ (Medicare #) | ☐ (Medicaid #) | ☐ (Sponsor's SSN) | ☐ (VA File #) | ☒ (SSN or ID) | ☐ (SSN) | ☐ (ID) | 999 99 NIN |

2. PATIENT'S NAME (Last, First, Middle Initial).
BOSSY BETTY B

3. PATIENT'S BIRTH DATE
MM 09 | DD 19 | YY CCYY-47    SEX M ☐  F ☒

4. INSURED'S NAME (Last, First, Middle Initial)
SAME

5. PATIENT'S ADDRESS (No., Street)
7991 BAGEL BLVD

6. PATIENT'S RELATIONSHIP TO INSURED
Self ☒  Spouse ☐  Child ☐  Other ☐

7. INSURED'S ADDRESS (No., Street)

CITY
BARSTOW          STATE NY

8. PATIENT STATUS
Single ☐  Married ☒  Other ☐
Employed ☒  Full-Time Student ☐  Part-Time Student ☐

CITY          STATE

ZIP CODE 10012   TELEPHONE (Include Area Code) (914) 555 3399

ZIP CODE   TELEPHONE (INCLUDE AREA CODE)

9. OTHER INSURED'S NAME (Last, First, Middle Initial)

10. IS PATIENT'S CONDITION RELATED TO:

11. INSURED'S POLICY GROUP OR FECA NUMBER:
21088NIN

a. OTHER INSURED'S POLICY OR GROUP NUMBER

a. EMPLOYMENT? (CURRENT OR PREVIOUS)
☐ YES  ☒ NO

a. INSURED'S DATE OF BIRTH
MM | DD | YY    SEX M ☐  F ☐

b. OTHER INSURED'S DATE OF BIRTH
MM | DD | YY    SEX M ☐  F ☐

b. AUTO ACCIDENT?   PLACE (State)
☐ YES  ☒ NO |___|

b. EMPLOYER'S NAME OR SCHOOL NAME
NINJA ENTERPRISES

c. EMPLOYER'S NAME OR SCHOOL NAME

c. OTHER ACCIDENT?
☐ YES  ☒ NO

c. INSURANCE PLAN NAME OR PROGRAM NAME
ROVER INSURERS INC

d. INSURANCE PLAN NAME OR PROGRAM NAME

10d. RESERVED FOR LOCAL USE

d. IS THERE ANOTHER HEALTH BENEFIT PLAN?
☐ YES  ☒ NO   *if yes, return to and complete item 9 a-d*

READ BACK OF FORM BEFORE COMPLETING & SIGNING THIS FORM
12. PATIENT'S OR AUTHORIZED PERSON'S SIGNATURE I authorize the release of any medical or other information necessary to process this claim. I also request payment of government benefits either to myself or to the party who accepts assignment below.

SIGNED SIGNATURE ON FILE          DATE

13. INSURED'S OR AUTHORIZED PERSON'S SIGNATURE I authorize payment of medical benefits to the undersigned physician or supplier for services described below.

SIGNED SIGNATURE ON FILE

14. DATE OF CURRENT: ◄ ILLNESS (1st symptom) ◄ INJURY (Accident) PREGNANCY (LMP)
MM 02 | DD 06 | YY YY

15. IF PATIENT HAS HAD SAME OR SIMILAR ILLNESS, GIVE FIRST DATE   MM | DD | YY

16. DATES PATIENT UNABLE TO WORK IN CURRENT OCCUPATION
MM | DD | YY   FROM        TO        MM | DD | YY

17. NAME OF REFERRING PHYSICIAN OR OTHER SOURCE

17a. I.D. NUMBER OF REFERRING PHYSICIAN

18. HOSPITALIZATION DATES RELATED TO CURRENT SERVICES
MM DD YY   FROM 02 06 YY   TO 02 14 YY

19. RESERVED FOR LOCAL USE

20. OUTSIDE LAB?   $ CHARGES
☐ YES  ☐ NO

21. DIAGNOSIS OR NATURE OF ILLNESS OR INJURY, (RELATE ITEMS 1,2,3, OR 4 TO ITEM 24E BY LINE)

1. | 410 . 91
2. | .
3. | .
4. | .

22. MEDICAID RESUBMISSION CODE | ORIGINAL REF. NO.

23. PRIOR AUTHORIZATION NUMBER

| 24. A DATE(S) OF SERVICE | | | | | | | B Place of Service | C Type of Service | D PROCEDURES, SERVICES, OR SUPPLIES (Explain Unusual Circumstances) CPT/HCPS | MODIFIER | E DIAGNOSIS CODE | F $ CHARGES | G DAYS OR UNITS | H EPSDT Family Plan | I EMG | J COB | K RESERVED FOR LOCAL USE |
|---|---|---|---|---|---|---|---|---|---|---|---|---|---|---|---|---|---|
| From MM | DD | YY | To MM | DD | YY | | | | | | | | | | | | |
| 02 | 06 | YY | 02 | 06 | YY | 99 | 1 | E0617 | | 1 | 2275 \| 00 | 1 | | | | |
| | | | | | | | | | | | | | | | | |
| | | | | | | | | | | | | | | | | |
| | | | | | | | | | | | | | | | | |
| | | | | | | | | | | | | | | | | |
| | | | | | | | | | | | | | | | | |

25. FEDERAL TAX I.D. NUMBER   SSN EIN
70-0013779   ☐ ☒

26. PATIENT'S ACCOUNT NO.
BETBS001   939

27. ACCEPT ASSIGNMENT? (For govt. claims, see back)
☒ YES  ☐ NO

28. TOTAL CHARGE
$ 2275 | 00

29. AMOUNT PAID
$ 0 | 00

30. BALANCE DUE
$ 2275 | 00

31. SIGNATURE OF PHYSICIAN OR SUPPLIER INCLUDING DEGREES OR CREDENTIALS (I certify that the statements on the reverse apply to this bill and are made a part thereof.)

SIGNED *Trina Ment*  DATE 02/19/YY

32. NAME AND ADDRESS OF FACILITY WHERE SERVICES WERE RENDERED (If other than home or office)
HEADACHE HOSPITAL
2000 HAZARD STREET
HELP NY 12899

33. PHYSICIAN'S, SUPPLIERS BILLING NAME, ADDRESS, ZIP CODE & PHONE #
MISSING MEDICAL EQUIPMENT
88 MAD ROAD
MILES NY 12899
(914) 555 0509
PIN# M10359   |   GRP#

(APPROVED BY AMA COUNCIL ON MEDICAL SERVICE 8/88)   **PLEASE PRINT OR TYPE**

FORM CMS-1500   (12-90)
FORM OWCP-1500   FORM RRB-1500
FORM AMA-OP050591

**Exercise 6–15**

PLEASE
DO NOT
STAPLE
IN THIS
AREA

WINTER INSURANCE CO
9763 WESTERN WAY
WHITTIER CO 82963

APPROVED MOB-0938-0008

□□□ PICA

# HEALTH INSURANCE CLAIM FORM

PICA □□□

| 1. MEDICARE  MEDICAID  CHAMPUS  CHAMPVA  GROUP HEALTH PLAN  FECA BLK LUNG  OTHER | 1a. INSURED'S I.D NUMBER (FOR PROGRAM IN ITEM 1) |
|---|---|
| ☐ (Medicare #) ☐ (Medicaid #) ☐ (Sponsor's SSN) ☐ (VA File #) ☒ (SSN or ID) ☐ (SSN) ☐ (ID) | 444 44 ABC |

| 2. PATIENT'S NAME (Last, First, Middle Initial). | 3. PATIENT'S BIRTH DATE  SEX | 4. INSURED'S NAME (Last, First, Middle Initial) |
|---|---|---|
| DINGBAT DANNY D | MM 04  DD 24  YY CCYY -10  M ☒  F ☐ | DINGBAT DANA D |

| 5. PATIENT'S ADDRESS (No., Street) | 6. PATIENT'S RELATIONSHIP TO INSURED | 7. INSURED'S ADDRESS (No., Street) |
|---|---|---|
| 404 DOORWAY DRIVE | Self ☐  Spouse ☐  Child ☒  Other ☐ | SAME |

| CITY | STATE | 8. PATIENT STATUS | CITY | STATE |
|---|---|---|---|---|
| DENVER | ND | Single ☒  Married ☐  Other ☐ | | |

| ZIP CODE | TELEPHONE (Include Area Code) | | ZIP CODE | TELEPHONE (INCLUDE AREA CODE) |
|---|---|---|---|---|
| 58444 | (701) 555 3344 | Employed ☐  Full-Time Student ☒  Part-Time Student ☐ | | |

| 9. OTHER INSURED'S NAME (Last, First, Middle Initial) | 10. IS PATIENT'S CONDITION RELATED TO: | 11. INSURED'S POLICY GROUP OR FECA NUMBER: |
|---|---|---|
| | | 36928ABC |

| a. OTHER INSURED'S POLICY OR GROUP NUMBER | a. EMPLOYMENT? (CURRENT OR PREVIOUS)  ☐ YES  ☒ NO | a. INSURED'S DATE OF BIRTH  MM 04  DD 04  YY CCYY -37  SEX  M ☐  F ☒ |
|---|---|---|

| b. OTHER INSURED'S DATE OF BIRTH  MM  DD  YY  SEX  M ☐  F ☐ | b. AUTO ACCIDENT?  PLACE (State)  ☐ YES  ☒ NO | b. EMPLOYER'S NAME OR SCHOOL NAME  ABC CORPORATION |
|---|---|---|

| c. EMPLOYER'S NAME OR SCHOOL NAME | c. OTHER ACCIDENT?  ☒ YES  ☐ NO | c. INSURANCE PLAN NAME OR PROGRAM NAME  WINTER INSURANCE COMPANY |
|---|---|---|

| d. INSURANCE PLAN NAME OR PROGRAM NAME | 10d. RESERVED FOR LOCAL USE | d. IS THERE ANOTHER HEALTH BENEFIT PLAN?  ☐ YES  ☒ NO  *if yes,* return to and complete item 9 a-d |
|---|---|---|

READ BACK OF FORM BEFORE COMPLETING & SIGNING THIS FORM

12. PATIENT'S OR AUTHORIZED PERSON'S SIGNATURE I authorize the release of any medical or other information necessary to process this claim. I also request payment of government benefits either to myself or to the party who accepts assignment below.

SIGNED SIGNATURE ON FILE          DATE

13. INSURED'S OR AUTHORIZED PERSON'S SIGNATURE I authorize payment of medical benefits to the undersigned physician or supplier for services described below.

SIGNED SIGNATURE ON FILE

| 14. DATE OF CURRENT: ◄ ILLNESS (1st symptom) ◄ INJURY (Accident) PREGNANCY (LMP)  MM 01  DD 26  YY | 15. IF PATIENT HAS HAD SAME OR SIMILAR ILLNESS, GIVE FIRST DATE  MM  DD  YY | 16. DATES PATIENT UNABLE TO WORK IN CURRENT OCCUPATION  MM  DD  YY  MM  DD  YY  FROM  TO |
|---|---|---|

| 17. NAME OF REFERRING PHYSICIAN OR OTHER SOURCE | 17a. I.D. NUMBER OF REFERRING PHYSICIAN | 18. HOSPITALIZATION DATES RELATED TO CURRENT SERVICES  MM  DD  YY  MM  DD  YY  FROM  TO |
|---|---|---|

| 19. RESERVED FOR LOCAL USE | 20. OUTSIDE LAB?  CHARGES $  ☐ YES  ☐ NO |
|---|---|

21. DIAGNOSIS OR NATURE OF ILLNESS OR INJURY, (RELATE ITEMS 1,2,3, OR 4 TO ITEM 24E BY LINE)

1. 823 .32
2.
3.
4.

22. MEDICAID RESUBMISSION CODE          ORIGINAL REF. NO.

23. PRIOR AUTHORIZATION NUMBER

| 24. A DATE(S) OF SERVICE | | | B Place of Service | C Type of Service | D PROCEDURES, SERVICES, OR SUPPLIES (Explain Unusual Circumstances)  CPT/HCPS | MODIFIER | E DIAGNOSIS CODE | F $ CHARGES | G DAYS OR UNITS | H EPSDT Family Plan | I EM G | J COB | K RESERVED FOR LOCAL USE |
|---|---|---|---|---|---|---|---|---|---|---|---|---|---|
| From MM DD YY | To MM DD YY | | | | | | | | | | | | |
| 02 08 YY | 02 08 YY | | 99 | 1 | E0114 | | 1 | 121 00 | 1 | | | | |
| 02 08 YY | 02 08 YY | | 99 | 1 | L2126 | | 1 | 200 00 | 1 | | | | |
| 02 08 YY | 02 08 YY | | 99 | 1 | E0144 | | 1 | 160 00 | 1 | | | | |
| | | | | | | | | | | | | | |
| | | | | | | | | | | | | | |
| | | | | | | | | | | | | | |

| 25. FEDERAL TAX I.D. NUMBER  SSN  EIN | 26. PATIENT'S ACCOUNT NO. | 27. ACCEPT ASSIGNMENT? (For govt. claims, see back) | 28. TOTAL CHARGE | 29. AMOUNT PAID | 30. BALANCE DUE |
|---|---|---|---|---|---|
| 70-0012774  ☐ ☒ | 001 434 | ☐ YES  ☒ NO | $ 481 00 | $ 0 00 | $ 481 00 |

| 31. SIGNATURE OF PHYSICIAN OR SUPPLIER INCLUDING DEGREES OR CREDENTIALS (I certify that the statements on the reverse apply to this bill and are made a part thereof.)  SIGNED *Missy Maker*  DATE 02/20/YY | 32. NAME AND ADDRESS OF FACILITY WHERE SERVICES WERE RENDERED (If other than home or office) | 33. PHYSICIAN'S, SUPPLIERS BILLING NAME, ADDRESS, ZIP CODE & PHONE #  MIRACLE MEDICAL EQUIPMENT  44 MALL BLVD  MANNER ND 58441  (701) 555 1341  PIN# M01234  GRP# |
|---|---|---|

(APPROVED BY AMA COUNCIL ON MEDICAL SERVICE 8/88)          **PLEASE PRINT OR TYPE**          FORM CMS-1500 (12-90)
FORM OWCP-1500  FORM RRB-1500
FORM AMA-OP050591

**Exercise 6–16**

# 7

# Surgery

# and Anesthesia Claims

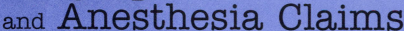

## After completion of this chapter
**you will be able to:**

- Define surgery and list the four general classifications of surgery.

- Process surgery claims.

- Identify and explain the general guidelines that relate to processing surgery claims.

- Identify possible cosmetic procedures.

- Define pre and postoperative care and determine when it is included with surgery.

- Apply surgical guidelines as they relate to maternity and cosmetic procedures.

- Identify and explain the general guidelines that relate to processing obesity surgery, assistant surgery, multiple surgery, and cosurgery claims.

- List and explain the general guidelines regarding podiatric procedures.

- Identify the guidelines for proper surgical coding of podiatric services.

- Identify common foot conditions and treatment procedures.

- Process podiatric surgery claims.

- Explain the role of assistant surgeons in podiatric surgeries.

- Define and explain the four methods of anesthesia administration.

- Identify codes which fall within the anesthesia range of the CPT®.

- Calculate anesthesia benefits using both basic and time units.

- Identify anesthesia modifiers.

- Identify qualifying circumstances of anesthesia.

- Explain processing guidelines for epidural anesthesia.

# Keywords and concepts

## you will learn in this chapter:

- Abortion
- Anesthesia
- Arthroplasty
- Assistant Surgeon
- Bilateral Procedures
- Block Procedures
- Bone Spur
- Bunion
- By Report (BR)
- Capsulotomy
- Chromosomal Analysis
- Cosmetic Procedure
- Cosmetic Surgery
- Cosurgeons
- Diagnostic Procedures
- Dorsal Osteotomy
- Dwyer Procedure
- Endogenous Obesity
- Epidural Anesthesia
- Exogenous Obesity
- False Nail
- Flat Feet
- Follow-up Days

- Ganglions
- General Anesthesia
- Global Approach
- Hammertoes
- Heel Spur
- High-arched Feet
- Hospital Staff Anesthesiologist
- Hypnosis
- In Vitro Fertilization
- Incidental Procedure
- Independent Anesthesiologist
- Infusion Pump
- Ingrown Toenail
- Intractable Pain
- Intravenous (IV) Sedation
- In Utero Fetal Surgery
- Joints
- Ligaments
- Local Anesthesia
- Matrixectomy
- Metatarsal Plantar Callus
- Monitored Anesthesia Care (MAC)

- Multiple Procedures
- Nerve Block Anesthesia
- Neuroma
- Optional Modifiers
- Orthosis
- Orthotic Devices
- Physical Status Modifiers
- Podiatry
- Positional Bunion
- Reconstruction
- Regional Anesthesia
- Saddle Block
- Serial Surgery
- Spinal Anesthesia
- Structural Bunion
- Surgery
- Tenotomy
- Therapeutic Procedures
- Topical Anesthesia
- Unusual Services
- Warts

**Surgery** is defined as the branch of medicine that treats diseases, injuries, and deformities through operative or invasive methods. Although surgery usually involves cutting, cutting does not have to be involved for a procedure to be considered surgical. The surgical concept is anything that involves removing, altering, repairing, entering, or the carrying out of any other invasion of the body. Therefore, insertion of a tube into a person's throat does not involve cutting but is considered surgical in nature because it invades the body. There are also many laser procedures that are considered surgical.

Most benefit plans cover only surgeries that are necessitated by disease or injury. In other words, the procedure must be considered medically necessary to repair or improve function or diagnose an illness. In addition, because a procedure is listed in the surgery section of the *CPT®* does not mean that the procedure is allowable under a benefit plan, nor does it mean that it will necessarily be coded as a surgical procedure. The coding of procedures varies from company to company.

## Surgical Procedures

In general, surgical procedures can be classified as one of the following types:

- Diagnostic.
- Therapeutic.
- Reconstructive.
- Cosmetic.

**Diagnostic procedures** are procedures performed to determine the presence of disease or the cause of the patient's symptoms. One of the most commonly used forms of diagnostic surgery is the endoscopic procedure. This type of procedure involves making a small incision on the exterior part of the patient's body in the area near the organ or space being examined. Then, a very small instrument, called a scope, is inserted through the incision into the body cavity. The surgeon can then look through the scope and see the interior of the examination area. If desired, pictures or a video may be taken of the area. Examples of diagnostic procedures include bronchoscopy (31622), gastroscopy (43234), and sigmoidoscopy (45330).

**Therapeutic procedures** are performed to remove or correct the functioning of a body part that is diseased or injured. Failure to perform a therapeutic procedure could result in either the patient's loss of life or a progressive functional decline.

A removal, repair, or manipulation may be involved in the correction of the abnormally functioning organ. Some cutting is usually required. However, with continual medical advances, more and more procedures are being performed without cutting or with minimal incisions. Examples of therapeutic procedures are liver transplant (47135), craniectomy (removal of tumor of the brain) (61510), and appendectomy (44950).

**Reconstruction** is performed to rebuild or aesthetically restore a part of the body that was damaged or defective as a result of an illness or injury. Reconstruction is necessary to return the body to its normal or near-normal appearance and may or may not affect the functioning of the organ/area. Even though reconstruction may be necessary for purely cosmetic reasons, it is considered eligible under most plans as long as it is necessitated as a result of a disease or injury occurring while the claimant was covered under the plan. If the injury or illness occurred prior to the date that the claimant was covered under the plan, the repair may be considered cosmetic, not reconstructive. Examples of reconstructive procedures are rhinoplasty (surgical correction of the external appearance of the nose; 30400–30462) and breast augmentation/reconstruction (after mastectomy resulting from breast cancer; 19324–19499).

**Cosmetic procedures** are those procedures performed solely to improve the appearance of a body part and are not usually covered by benefit plans. If the procedure is functional in nature, cosmetic exclusions do not apply. For example, a scar revision is performed as a result of a contracture of a scar received in an accident. The release of the contracture is considered functional in nature, although the appearance of the scar might also be significantly improved.

Situations may arise in which it is difficult to ascertain whether a procedure should be considered cosmetic or reconstructive. In these instances, a professional opinion is required.

# Surgery and the *CPT*®

For all procedures in the surgical section, codes are listed by body system (i.e., integumentary, digestive, etc.); then in body part order from the head downward. Surgery CPT® codes range from 10040–69990 (**see Table 7–1**). The following list provides an introduction to each section, along with any special handling required for that section.

## Integumentary System (10040–19499)

These codes are used to bill for procedures done on the integumentary system or skin.

### Lesions

Lesions are coded according to the overall size of the lesion removed (not necessarily the size sent for biopsy). If a lesion's measurements are covered by several size ranges (i.e., a lesion that is 3 cm × 2 cm × 1 cm deep), the highest measurement should be used (i.e., 3 cm).

### Repairs

As with lesions, repairs are coded according to the length of the wound being repaired. However, there is an additional consideration for the depth and complexity of the wound. If multiple wounds are closed during the same operative session within a specific region (i.e., head), the total length of the repaired wounds should be added together and one code used for all repairs.

## Skin grafts

Skin grafts should be coded according to the size of the recipient area, not the donor area. The skin graft should be coded separately from the closure (repair) of the donor site.

## Musculoskeletal System (20000–29999)

These codes are used to bill for procedures done on the muscles and bones of the body. In this section the term "complicated" means that there was infection, delayed treatment, or the surgery took an extraordinary amount of time. Complicated codes often require that the claim and an operating report be sent for medical review.

Repair of the wound site is an integral part of musculoskeletal surgery and should not be reported separately.

## Bone, cartilage, and fascia grafts

The codes for bone, cartilage and fascia grafts include the acquiring of the donor graft. If a different physician acquires the grafts, that additional physician should bill using modifier -80 (assistant surgeon).

## Respiratory System (30000–32999)

These codes are used to bill for procedures done on the organs of the respiratory system.

## Cardiovascular System (33010–37799)

These codes are used to bill for invasive procedures on the heart, veins, and arteries. Codes for minor procedures involving the veins and arteries (i.e., injection), and cardiac catheterization are not included. These procedures are found in the Medicine section (see the Physician's, Clinical, and Hospital Services Claims chapter for more information).

## Pacemaker Replacement

When a physician bills for the replacement of a pacemaker, two procedures are allowed: one for the removal of the old battery/pulse generator, and another for the insertion of the new battery/pulse generator.

## Hemic and Lymphatic Systems (38100–38999)

These codes are used to bill for procedures of the spleen and lymph nodes, as well as bone marrow transplants.

## Bone Marrow/Stem Cell Transplants

Codes in this section (38207–38215) may be reported once a day, regardless of the number of cells being transplanted during any given session.

## Mediastinum and Diaphragm (39000–39599)

These codes are used to bill for procedures of the mediastinum and diaphragm.

## Digestive System (40490–49999)

These codes are used to bill for procedures performed on all the organs of the digestive system, from the lips (mouth) down to the anus.

## Endoscopies

The appropriate code for endoscopies is determined by the organs the endoscope is passed through. An endoscope which is only passed into the esophagus would receive one code, while an endoscope passed through the esophagus to the duodenum would receive a different code.

## Appendectomies

The reason for an appendectomy must be documented (i.e., appendicitis). If an appropriate diagnosis code is not given (one which requires an appendectomy), and the appendectomy is performed in conjunction with another surgery, the appendectomy should be considered incidental to the other surgery performed.

## Hernia Repair

The age of the patient is one of the prevailing factors in choosing the correct code for a hernia repair. Claims examiners should be sure that the age of the patient matches the code given.

## Urinary System (50010–53899)

These codes are used to bill for procedures performed on the kidneys, ureters, bladder, urethra, and include prostate resections. This section often combines several procedures together under one code. If an included procedure requires significant additional time or effort, modifier -22 (unusual circumstances) should be used. Reporting of this modifier requires the submission of an operative report so the claim may be sent for review.

## Male Genital System (54000-55899)

These codes are used to bill for procedures performed on the male genital system, including all male reproductive organs.

## Intersex Surgery (55970-55980)

These codes are used to bill for procedures performed to transform a patient from one gender to another. These procedures are often excluded by most health plans.

## Female Genital System (56405-58999)

These codes are used to bill for procedures performed on the female genital system, including all female reproductive organs. However, maternity care is covered under the following subsection.

### Pelvic Examinations

Pelvic examinations should not be coded separately when another pelvic region procedure is performed. D&C is considered to be an integral part of a pelvic exam; therefore, it is also not coded separately when another pelvic region procedure is performed.

### Laporoscopy/Hystoroscopy

The codes in this section often combine several procedures under one code. If an included procedure requires significant additional time or effort, modifier -22 (unusual circumstances) should be used. Reporting of this modifier requires the addition of the operating report so the claim may be sent for review.

## Maternity Care and Delivery (59000-59899)

See the following section regarding maternity care.

## Endocrine System (60000-60699)

These codes are used to bill for procedures on the thymus, adrenal glands, thyroid and parathyroid. Pituitary glands and pineal glands are included in the Nervous System codes.

## Nervous System (61000-64999)

These codes are used to bill for procedures on the organs of the nervous system, including the nerves, brain, and spinal cord. Procedures on the pituitary glands and pineal glands are also included in this section since they are both located in the brain.

## Eye and Ocular Adnexa (65091-68899)

These codes are used to bill for surgical procedures on the eye and ocular adnexa. Diagnostic procedures for the eye and ocular adnexa are reported using the Medicine section of the *CPT*®. Procedures performed only on the eyelid are coded using the surgical codes in the integumentary system.

### Cataract Surgery

Any injections performed during cataract surgery are considered to be an integral part of the procedure and are not allowed separately.

## Auditory System (69000-69979)

These codes are used to bill for procedures performed on the organs of the auditory (hearing) system. This section includes surgical procedures only. Diagnostic procedures are reported using the Medicine section of the *CPT*®. Repairs to the outer ear are included in the surgery codes for the integumentary system.

## Operating Microscope (69990)

This code is used to bill for the use of an operating microscope during a surgical procedure. It is reported in addition to the actual surgical procedure being performed.

| SURGERY CODES | |
|---|---|
| Integumentary System | 10040 – 19499 |
| Musculoskeletal System | 20000 – 29999 |
| Respiratory System | 30000 – 32999 |
| Cardiovascular System | 33010 – 37799 |
| Hemic and Lymphatic System | 38100 – 38999 |
| Mediastinum and Diaphragm | 39000 – 39599 |
| Digestive System | 40490 – 49999 |
| Urinary System | 50010 – 53899 |
| Male Genital System | 54000 – 55899 |
| Intersex Surgery | 55970 – 55980 |
| Female Genital System | 56405 – 58999 |
| Maternity Care and Delivery | 59000 – 59899 |
| Endocrine System | 60000 – 60699 |
| Nervous System | 61000 – 64999 |
| Eye and Ocular Adnexa | 65091 – 68899 |
| Auditory System | 69000 – 69979 |
| Operating Microscope | 69990 |

**Table 7–1** **Surgery Codes**

# On the Job Now

**Directions:** Write the codes for each section and the procedures that are listed under each section in the space provided.

| Section | Codes | Procedures |
|---|---|---|
| Integumentary System | _____ | _____ |
| Musculoskeletal System | _____ | _____ |
| Cardiovascular System | _____ | _____ |
| Hemic and Lymphatic Systems | _____ | _____ |
| Digestive System | _____ | _____ |
| Female Genital System | _____ | _____ |
| Eye and Ocular Adnexa | _____ | _____ |

## General Guidelines

The following guidelines will assist you in the processing of surgery claims.

### Surgery in a Physician's Office

Claims for surgery performed in a physician's office are often itemized for each charge incurred; such as the surgery, local anesthesia, medication, surgical trays, and dressings.

Generally, the charge by the physician for surgery should include performing the surgical procedure, administering local anesthetic (if required), and all routine follow-up care. The charge for surgery always includes:

- The immediate preoperative visit.
- The surgical procedure.
- Local anesthesia (i.e., topical, digital block).
- Routine follow-up care (visits) provided within the follow-up days listed in the *RVS*.

Non-routine follow-up visits due to complications or other reasons may be billed and considered separately from the original surgical charge. Medical supplies, medications, x-rays, facility fees, and other services are usually considered separately.

## Preoperative Care

The immediate preoperative visit in the hospital or elsewhere is generally necessary to examine the patient, complete the hospital records, and initiate the treatment program. Charges for these procedures are included in the surgical allowance. However, a separate allowance may be warranted for preoperative services in the following circumstances:

1. When the preoperative visit is the initial visit (i.e., in an emergency room), and prolonged detention or evaluation is required to prepare the patient or to establish the need for the surgery.

2. When the preoperative visit is a consultation. Be sure the physician has not "up coded" a preoperative visit to increase benefits. An example is a surgeon billing for a consultation prior to surgery when in fact the visit was a simple preoperative visit.

3. When procedures that are not usually part of the basic surgical procedure (i.e., bronchoscopy prior to chest surgery) are provided during the immediate preoperative period.

4. When a procedure could normally be performed in the office, but under certain circumstances requires hospitalization (i.e., patient's age, condition. See modifier code -22 in the CPT®).

## Follow-Up Days

**Follow-up days** are days immediately following a surgical procedure in which a doctor must monitor a patient's condition for that particular procedure. The *RVS* lists unit values for surgical procedures that include the surgery, local anesthesia, and the normal, uncomplicated follow-up care associated with the procedure for the time period indicated in the section titled Follow-up Days. Complications or other circumstances requiring additional or unusual services concurrent with the procedure or procedures, or during the listed period of normal follow-up care, may warrant additional charges on a fee-for-service basis. However, unless the physician specifically indicates unusual circumstances, it should be assumed that the follow-up care is routine. Regardless of how the physician bills, all visits occurring within the listed follow-up days should be combined with the surgical charge. The following are categories of follow-up care:

1. Follow-up care for diagnostic procedures (i.e., endoscopy, injection procedures for radiology) includes only care that is related to recovery from the diagnostic procedure itself. Care of the underlying condition for which the diagnostic procedure was performed or other accompanying conditions is not included and may be charged separately in accordance with the services rendered.

2. Follow-up care for therapeutic procedures generally includes all normal postoperative care. Complications, exacerbations, recurrence, or the presence of other diseases or injuries requiring additional services concurrent with the surgical procedure(s) or during the indicated period of normal follow-up care may warrant additional charges coded and allowable separately.

3. When additional surgical procedure(s) are carried out within the listed period of follow-up care for a previous surgery, the follow-up periods will run concurrently through their normal termination.

Charges for routine follow-up care should be combined with the surgical charge and the total compared with the UCR fee for the procedure performed. Some plans follow this approach while others deny the visit as being within the follow-up period, if they are billed separately.

**Example:** Procedure: 40808, biopsy, 10 follow-up days

| Description | Date | CPT® Code | Charge |
|---|---|---|---|
| Office Visit | 4/1/CCYY | 99213 | $ 25 |
| Surgery | 4/3/CCYY | 40808 | 350 |
| Follow up Hospital Visit | 4/4/CCYY | 99221 | 25 |
| Follow up Hospital Visit | 4/5/CCYY | 99231 | 25 |
| Follow up Office Visit | 4/10/CCYY | 99213 | 30 |
| | | | $455 |

Based on administrative practices, the preoperative visit may or may not be considered part of the surgical charge. In the example, and unless you are told otherwise, assume that the preoperative visit is part of the surgery charge. Therefore, $455 would be compared against the plan's UCR limitation for the surgery.

## By Report Procedures

Some procedures are so unusual or variable that it is impossible to determine a standard UCR or unit value allowance. These procedures are called **By Report (BR)** procedures. The *RVS* may refer to these procedures as Relative Value Not Established (RNE). BR and RNE procedures need to be referred to a professional review unit, a supervisor, or a consultant for review to determine the allowance. For proper review, a copy of the operative report is required. The anesthesia record may also be needed. If the operative report is not submitted with the claim, the claim should be pended and a copy requested before referral.

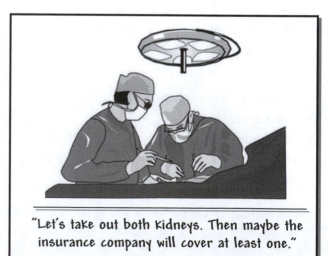

"Let's take out both kidneys. Then maybe the insurance company will cover at least one."

## Multiple or Bilateral Procedures

**Multiple procedures** are more than one surgical procedure performed during the same operative session. These surgeries are denoted by adding modifier -51 to the CPT® code. **Bilateral procedures** are surgeries that involve a pair of similar body parts (i.e., breasts, eyes). There are two main types of multiple or bilateral procedures: same time, different operative field and same time, same operative field.

### Same Time, Different Operative Field

When more than one surgery is performed during the same operative session but through a different orifice (opening) or incision or in a different operative field, 100% of the UCR is allowable for the major procedure, and 50% of the UCR (or actual charge, whichever is less) is allowed for the second procedure. 25% of UCR (or actual charge, whichever is less) is allowed for each additional procedure. Some insurance carriers, however, do not apply the 25% rule, allowing 100% for the primary procedure and 50% thereafter. Bilateral procedures have the same rules as multiple procedures performed through different incisions. Multiply the UCR allowance for the single procedure by 150% or 1.5. If there is an established bilateral CPT® code, that code would be allowable at 100% only because the units have already been assigned at 150% of the unit value for the single procedure. There are two ways to identify a bilateral procedure. The provider will list the CPT® and use modifier -50 to denote a bilateral procedure. Sometimes the provider will identify LT (left) or RT (right) next to each procedure. When in doubt, obtain an operative report.

### Same Time, Same Operative Field

When multiple procedures are performed during the same operative session through the same incision, orifice, or operative field, the additional procedures are usually considered to be incidental.

An **incidental procedure** is one that does not add significant time or complexity to the operative session. In such a case, the allowed amount will be that of the major procedure only.

However, if the additional procedures are not incidental, the rules for handling multiple procedures previously explained would apply. That is, the major procedure would be considered at 100% of UCR and the lesser at 50%.

**Example:** The following bill is received from the provider:

|  | Billed Amount | UCR |
|---|---|---|
| Tonsillectomy (42821) | $600 | $600 |
| Eustachian tube inflation (69400) | 300 | 200 |

Following the rules previously indicated, 100% of the major procedure plus 50% of the lesser procedure would be allowed. Therefore, the allowed amount in this example would be:

| | |
|---|---|
| 100% of $600 | $600 |
| +50% of $200 | $100 |
| Total Allowance | $700 |
| | |
| Total Billed Amount | $900 |
| Less Allowed Amount | −$700 |
| Member's Responsibility | $200 |

## Practice

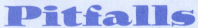
Pitfalls

The following are examples of incidental surgical procedures:

- The removal of an asymptomatic appendix is considered an incidental procedure when performed during hysterectomy surgery. Integral procedures are those procedures performed as part of a more complex primary procedure.

- A patient undergoes a transurethral incision of the prostate (CPT® code 52000), the cystourethroscopy is considered integral to the performance of the prostate procedure.

- Removal of a cerumen impaction prior to myringotomy. The cerumen impaction is precluding access to the tympanic membrane and its removal is necessary for the successful completion of the myringotomy. Thus, the cerumen impaction should not be billed separately.

- Lysis of adhesions and exploratory laparotomy billed with colon resection or other abdominal surgery. These procedures represent gaining access to the organ in question and should not be billed separately.

## Gender Designated Surgery

Certain CPT® codes are designated for male or female. Ensure that the submitted code designation accurately reflects the gender of the patient.

- An example is CPT® code 53210 for total urethrectomy including cystostomy in a female, as opposed to CPT® code 53215 for the male.

## Global UCR

It is important to look at the total billing so as not to penalize the claimant for the way the physician bills. Thus, the total amount allowed for UCR is used, even if the physician misallocates the billing for the procedures.

**Example:** If the same procedures as above were billed in the following way:

|  | Billed Amount | UCR |
|---|---|---|
| Tonsillectomy (42821) | $300 | $600 |
| Eustachian tube inflation (69400) | +600 | +100 |
| Total Billed Amount | $900 | $700 |

Normal UCR would be:

| | |
|---|---|
| 1st procedure – 100% of $600 up to the actual charge amount | $300 |
| 2nd procedure – 50% of $200 or the actual charge, whichever is less | +100 |
| Total Allowance | $400 |

By referring to the *RVS*, you can determine that the major procedure is the tonsillectomy, which allows 16.39 units, whereas eustachian tube inflation allows only 1.39 units. However, the physician billed the tonsillectomy as the minor procedure.

As shown, this calculation would be financially detrimental to the claimant solely because the physician's office did not properly allocate the expenses. Therefore, nearly all multiple surgery claims are calculated using a "**global approach**." In a global approach, the total billed amount should be compared with the total UCR amount. In our example, the total UCR amount is $700 versus the total billed amount of $900. The objective is to deny amounts in excess of the global UCR.

**Example:** If the same procedures as above were billed in the following way:

|  | Billed Amount | UCR |
|---|---|---|
| Tonsillectomy (42821) | $300 | $600 |
| Eustachian tube inflation (69400) | +600 | +100 |
| Total Billed Amount | $900 | $700 |

Global UCR would be:

| | |
|---|---|
| Major procedure UCR – Tonsillectomy | $600 |
| Minor procedure UCR – Eustachian tube inflation | +100 |
| Total Global Allowance | $700 |

Some insurance companies use CMS guidelines. When multiple surgeries are performed and the additional procedures are not incidental, CMS guidelines are as follows:

Major procedure: 100% of UCR or the billed amount, whichever is less.

2nd through 5th procedure: 50% of UCR or billed amount, whichever is less.

Multiple procedures (more than two) are often referred to consultants or professional review departments, which consist of medical doctors and nurses, for analysis before payment. The consultants or review department may give alternative instructions based on the actual operative report.

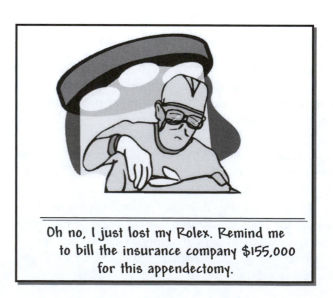

Oh no, I just lost my Rolex. Remind me to bill the insurance company $155,000 for this appendectomy.

## Block Procedures

**Block procedures** are multiple surgical procedures performed during the same operative session, in the same operative area. The objective of these codes is to handle multiple repetitions of the same service. A block procedure consists of a primary code and subsequent modifying codes.

### Example:

11100   is for biopsy of skin, subcutaneous tissue or mucous membrane, single lesion.

11101   is for each separate/additional lesion.

Therefore, if a bill was received for the removal of five lesions, the total allowance would be based on the following unit factors:

| | |
|---|---|
| 1.24 | Units for the lesion |
| <u>2.60</u> | Units total for lesions 2, 3, 4, and 5 $(4 \times .65)$ |
| 3.84 | Total units allowed |

For another example of a block procedure or add-ons, refer to Moh's surgery in the *CPT*®. The *CPT*® is now a great source for identifying add-ons and procedures exempt from the multiple surgery rule. Usually you will see either a "+" or O next to the CPT® code, indicating the procedure is not subject to multiple surgery reduction.

## Unbundling

As briefly discussed in the Physician's, Clinical, and Hospital Services Claims chapter, some physicians practice what is known as "unbundling." The surgeon is considered to have "unbundled" when he bills separately for procedures that are a part of the major procedure. For example, a hysterectomy can be performed with or without the removal of the ovaries and/or the fallopian tubes. Therefore, a physician billing for a hysterectomy and removal of the ovaries has unbundled the surgery. The maximum allowance is the UCR for the hysterectomy. An extreme example is a surgeon billing for the removal of a gallbladder and also billing for the repair of an open wound. Of course the repair is not covered, as it is inherently part of the gallbladder surgery. Care in processing multiple surgeries should be taken to ensure that there is no unbundling and that the minor procedures are reduced accordingly.

## Maternity Expenses

Most plans provide coverage for maternity-related expenses on the same basis as any other illness. The services normally provided in maternity cases include all routine, antepartum care (prior to delivery), delivery, and all routine, postpartum care (after delivery). The maternity CPT® codes are based on this premise unless the specific code indicates otherwise. Therefore, if a physician itemizes charges for different segments, the charges should be combined and lumped together under the single appropriate code. This would apply unless the patient sees different doctors for antepartum care and for delivery or for any other combination. In such a case the benefits would be allowed in a way to compensate the physicians appropriately for their services.

### Antepartum care (prenatal) includes:
- Initial and subsequent history.
- Physician's exams, usually one per month for the first eight months, then weekly during the 9th month.
- Weight, blood pressure, and urinalysis (monthly or weekly).
- Fetal heart tones.
- Maternity counseling on food requirements, vitamins, and related items.

### Delivery includes:
- Vaginal delivery (with or without episiotomy, forceps, or breech delivery).
- Cesarean delivery.

### Postpartum care (after delivery) includes:
- Postdelivery hospital visits.
- Postdelivery office visits (usually one or two routine check-ups) during the first six weeks following delivery.

## Maternity Billing Procedures

Maternity cases are usually billed in a unique manner. Some physicians require full payment from the patient before the delivery date. Conversely, most benefit plans will not process the claim for any benefits until after the delivery. Therefore, the patient often has a substantial, initial out-of-pocket expense. The following are some of the more common maternity billing procedures:

1. **Lump sum billings:**  When a lump sum charge (a single, all-encompassing charge) is made for total

obstetric care, the charge should be coded and processed under the appropriate CPT®/RVS code for total obstetric care.

2. **Itemized billings after delivery:** When charges for antepartum care, delivery, and postpartum care are itemized by the physician, the charges should be combined into one charge and processed under the CPT® code for total obstetric care. Charges for routine ultrasonography may or may not be covered by the plan. Usually, these charges are considered and coded separately from obstetric care. Charges for lab studies, especially urinalysis, are usually considered part of the complete care unless the physician indicates medical necessity for services beyond routine care. (Routine lab expenses may be coded and allowed separately. This varies by payer.)

3. **Predelivery billings:** When a physician bills for the total obstetric care prior to delivery (based on monthly installments, for example, 80% of the charge by the 7th month), the plan may deny the claim and ask the doctor to rebill after delivery. Other plans may consider payment on the part of the services that have been provided as of the date of the billing. Clarification needs to be requested.

4. **Two or more physicians (unrelated, not in the same medical group):** If two or more physicians are involved in the total obstetric care of a patient (usually one performs the delivery and the other provides the antepartum or postpartum care), each physician's charge should be processed separately for the services rendered. CPT® code 59409 is for a vaginal delivery only. For antepartum care only (up to three office visits), use the appropriate office visit code range of 99201–99205 for the initial visit and 99211–99215 for subsequent visits. Antepartum care beyond three visits should be billed using CPT® code 59425 or 59426. 59430 is for postpartum care only.

## Other Maternity-Related Procedures

The following are other types of maternity claims that you may encounter:

1. **Artificial insemination** is the introduction of semen into the vagina or cervix by artificial means. Some plans consider this a covered expense, and some do not since it is not for the treatment of a disease or injury.

2. **Amniocentesis/chromosomal analysis** is the transabdominal perforation of the uterus for the

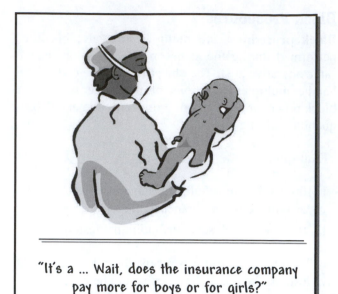

"It's a ... Wait, does the insurance company pay more for boys or for girls?"

purpose of withdrawing amniotic fluid surrounding the fetus. The chromosomal analysis is the diagnostic study performed on the fluid to study the number and structure of the chromosomes to determine whether any abnormalities are present.

An amniocentesis/chromosomal analysis is performed:

- To identify genetic defects of the fetus.
- To determine whether the fetus has attained an adequate state of gestation.
- To determine the sex of the fetus.

Charges for amniocentesis and chromosomal analysis are usually covered if the attending physician can demonstrate the medical necessity of testing for the patient, such as a family history of specific genetic defects, or a maternal age of greater than 35 years. The use of these tests to determine fetal sex alone is not covered by most plans.

**In utero fetal surgery** has made it possible to perform surgery on a fetus while it is in the mother's womb; and also to remove the fetus from the womb, perform surgery, and return it back to the womb, with the pregnancy continuing to term. If the surgery is covered, it is often covered as the mother's expense as a complication of pregnancy.

**In vitro fertilization** is the fertilization of the ovum within a test tube. Charges for in vitro fertilization may be covered. Refer to the plan for verification.

**Abortion** is a premature expulsion of an embryo or nonviable fetus. There are three different types of abortions:

# On the Job Now

**Directions:** Answer the following questions without looking back at the material just covered. Write your answers in the space provided.

1. What would be the reason that maternity charges not be combined and lumped together under the single appropriate code? _____

   _____

2. List the four common maternity billing procedures.

   1. _____

   2. _____

   3. _____

   4. _____

1. A spontaneous abortion occurring naturally.

2. A therapeutic abortion intentionally induced because the life of the mother would be endangered if the pregnancy were allowed to continue to term.

3. An elective abortion intentionally induced to terminate an unwanted pregnancy.

Coverage for abortions varies greatly from plan to plan. Spontaneous and therapeutic abortions are covered by most plans; however, elective abortions are often excluded. In addition, some plans may pay for certain services for spouses but exclude these services for dependent children. Therefore, read the plan document carefully before processing these types of expenses.

## Delivery with Tubal Ligation

Sterilization is a surgical method to achieve permanent infertility. Sterilization procedures include tubal ligations for females and vasectomies for males. It is becoming more common for health plans to cover sterilization procedures.

When the plan provides coverage for sterilization procedures and a tubal ligation is performed during the same operative session as that for a vaginal delivery, the UCR fee (or the actual charge, whichever is less) for the delivery would be allowed at 100% and the sterilization fee would be reduced to 50% of UCR.

When a sterilization procedure is performed during the same hospitalization as that for a vaginal delivery but not in the same operative session, 100% of the fee or UCR would be allowed for each procedure.

When a tubal ligation is performed during the same operative session as that for a cesarean section or intra-abdominal surgery, the C-section should be processed under the appropriate CPT®/RVS code and the tubal under CPT® code 58611. The UCR for both the C-section and the tubal ligation should be allowed at 100% since the relative value for 58611 has already been reduced.

**Vaginal delivery with:**

| | |
|---|---|
| Tubal ligation | 59400–100% |
| During same operative session | 58605–50% |

**Vaginal delivery with:**

| | |
|---|---|
| Tubal ligation | 59400–100% |
| Not during same operative session | 58605–100% |

**C-section delivery with:**

| | |
|---|---|
| Tubal ligation | 59510–100% |
| During same operative session | 58611–50% |

**C-section delivery with:**

| | |
|---|---|
| Tubal ligation | 59510–100% |
| Not during same operative session | 58605–100% |

For those plans that do not cover sterilization, the expense for a tubal ligation, regardless of when it is performed, would be denied as not a covered expense.

# Cosmetic Surgery

**Cosmetic surgery** is a surgical procedure performed solely to improve appearance and is usually not covered by benefit plans.

To properly handle possible cosmetic claims, you must become familiar with the terminology. The following are some of the more common cosmetic procedures and are therefore not usually covered. However, each claim should be investigated and evaluated on an individual basis. The primary intent of each procedure must be established to determine whether the procedure is cosmetic or reconstructive.

Although some procedures are cosmetic in nature, they may also be performed for functional reasons. For instance, a blepharoplasty is the removal of excessive skin and fat from the eyelids. Certainly, removal of excessive skin and fat improves the person's appearance. However, most plans will cover blepharoplasty when the skin overhang is so extensive that it interferes with the patient's peripheral vision.

When the restorative or cosmetic nature of the procedure is not obvious, claim investigation must be initiated with a careful review of the following documents:

- Hospital admission history and physical.
- Operative report.
- Pathology report.
- Preoperative and postoperative photographs.
- A narrative report from a referring physician, if available.

## Preoperative and Postoperative Photographs

Providers routinely take preoperative and postoperative photographs. These photos are sometimes needed to determine whether a surgery was cosmetic in nature.

To request photographs, use a standard request for additional information form letter. The operative report for the procedure should be requested at the same time.

When the operative report and photographs are received, they should be compared with the claim to determine the reason for the surgery. If the surgery appears to be cosmetic in nature, the claim, along with the photographs and any reports, should be forwarded to a consultant for review.

## Possible Cosmetic Procedures

Following is a list of common surgical procedures that may be considered cosmetic in nature. Keep in mind that numerous other procedures and services would

## Practice Pitfalls

Following are three general guidelines regarding cosmetic surgeries:

1. Cosmetic surgery preformed purely for cosmetic reasons is not covered. However, cosmetic surgery after an accident, injury, or surgical procedure may be covered (i.e., breast reconstruction after a mastectomy).

2. When there is an underlying condition, the surgery is not considered cosmetic regardless of the nature of the surgery (i.e., removal of a scar if there is an underlying disease).

3. When processing a surgical claim, determine the primary reason for the surgical procedure. If the treatment is due to injury or disease, the surgery is not considered cosmetic.

fall under a cosmetic heading. This sample list is for training purposes only, and the individual plan guidelines should be consulted prior to processing a surgery claim.

**Blepharoplasty**—Surgical repair of the eyelids. This surgery is performed to correct blepharoptosis, which is a drooping of the upper eyelid. This condition may cause impairment of peripheral vision. The surgery may be of the upper lid only, the lower lid only, or both upper and lower lids. Surgery of both lids requires the use of modifier -50.

When blepharoplasty is performed on the upper lid, the removal of the fat decreases the bulging lid, relieving the patient of a perpetual "tired look" about the eyes and thus imparting a more youthful appearance. The diagnosis most often listed on the claim is blepharochalasis, which means, "acquired atrophy of the skin of the upper eyelid as in aging."

Blepharoplasty may also be preformed for ptosis, which is an abnormal downward displacement of the eyelid due to muscle weakness, eyelid trauma, facial nerve paralysis, or loss of innervation. As this condition worsens, vision is progressively impaired by the tissue obstructing the pupil. The operative report for treatment of functional blepharoptosis will describe structural rearrangement such as palpebral muscle shortening, resection of the part of the upper lid including the tarsal plate, nerve and muscle transplantation, and facial sling.

Vision impairment is the only condition for which an upper lid blepharoplasty would be considered non-cosmetic. The documentation required to assess visual impairment includes at least one of the following:

- Results of a tangent screen examination.
- Results of a confrontation test.
- Results of perimeter testing.

The latter tests measure the patient's peripheral vision and support the medical record and preoperative photos in establishing the functional need for surgery.

Claims received for lower lid blepharoplasty are usually purely cosmetic. The surgery consists of removing the herniated fat pads in the lower lid and excising the redundant skin. Three conditions in which a blepharoplasty of the lower lid may be indicated and not considered cosmetic are:

1. **Ectropion**—A condition in which the margin of the upper or lower eyelid turns outward. When the lower lid is involved, involuntary tearing often constitutes the most annoying symptom. Surgery consists of removing a portion of the inside of the lid to cause the eyelid to turn inward. This is a functional correction.

2. **Entropion**—A condition in which the margin of the upper or lower eyelid turns in, causing the eyelashes to rub against and irritate the eyeball. If a secondary infection occurs, scarring of the cornea may ensue with subsequent loss of vision. Therefore, correcting the condition in the early stages of development is important. Surgery consists of cutting away a portion of the inside of the eyelid in a way that causes the eyelid to turn outward. This is a functional correction.

3. **Lid Lesions**—Most often a chalazion that is a cyst-like mass resulting in chronic inflammation of the meibomian gland in the eyelid. This may also be called a meibomian or tarsal cyst. Another lesion is a hordeolum or sty, which is an infection of the eyelash and is associated with whitish pus under the skin. When medical treatment fails to alleviate the condition, surgery may be preformed to remove the affected area. Tumors constitute the third type of lesion that might require surgical care.

In a blepharoplasty, the pockets of fat in the upper and lower lids beneath the skin are removed. The ellipse of skin has to be cut off to elevate the drooping eyebrow. The margins are sewn together with the final suture line lying with the eyebrow's upper hairline. The redundant skin of the lower lid is undermined, and the excess fat is removed along with the redundant skin. The wound is then sutured with fine silk.

The structure line in the upper eyelid partially coincides with the old; the one in the lower lid is disguised by the eyelashes. The rest of the two sutures coincide with the natural creases about the eye.

**Breast Augmentation**—Surgical enlargement of the breast by use of implants. Implants come in various types but are most often gel- or fluid-filled sacs.

**Breast Prosthesis**—An artificial sac implanted in the chest muscles to replace or enlarge the breast. Many types of prostheses are available.

**Breast Reconstruction**—A procedure in which an implant is placed under the skin or muscle of the chest wall to restore the contour of a missing breast. This procedure is usually covered when it is used to restore the appearance of patients who have had a mastectomy due to cancer, fibroadenoma, or fibrocystic breast disease. Claims submitted for breast reconstruction should include the diagnosis of the underlying disease and the date of the previously performed mastectomy. In cases of breast cancer, only those charges submitted for reconstruction for the removed breast are considered covered expenses. Charges submitted for reduction mammoplasty on the unaffected side (to make the unaffected breast appear similar in size and shape to the reconstructed breast) are considered cosmetic and are usually not covered.

*Asymmetry* is a condition in which the breasts are grossly dissimilar in size, shape, or arrangement on the chest wall. Since a slight discrepancy in the breasts is normal, the condition must be severe to be considered functional.

**Breast Reduction**—Surgical procedure to reduce the size of the breast. This may be covered in extreme cases (usually when over one pound of fat is removed on each side).

**Chemical Peel or Chemical Abrasion**—This has the same affect as dermabrasion except that caustic chemicals such as phenol or trichloracetic acid (TCA) are used. The technique creates a superficial chemical burn which, when healed, has flattened fine wrinkles and tightened the skin. This is considered purely cosmetic.

**Cheiloplasty**—Surgery for the lips. The lips, like the skin and mucous membranes of other parts of the body, are subject to precancerous and cancerous lesions. These lesions most often occur in fair-skinned persons with a long history of exposure to sunlight.

A common precancerous condition is known as *hyperkeratosis*, a condition in which the mucosa of the lip becomes paler, thinner, and more fragile with numerous cracks and fissures. Gradually, ulcerations appear which continue to break down and heal. Treatment consists of removing all of the involved lip surface and advancing the inner lining of the lip to cover the defect. This procedure is called *lip stripping and resurfacing* and is considered medically necessary.

A cheiloplasty can also be done to make the lips narrower, to enlarge thin lips, and to create a "cupid's bow" (the dip in the edge line of the upper lip). When done for these reasons, cheiloplasty would be considered cosmetic.

**Cleft Lip and Palate**—A birth defect in which the two sides of the face fail to unite properly in the early stage of prenatal development, resulting in a fissure or split in the lip and/or palate (roof) of the mouth. A cleft lip may occur unilaterally or bilaterally. An incomplete cleft lip occurs when a bridge of skin connects the cleft and noncleft sides. If a skin bridge does not exist, the cleft is complete. Deformity of the nose usually accompanies a cleft lip in the form of distortion and displacement of the lower lateral nasal cartilage.

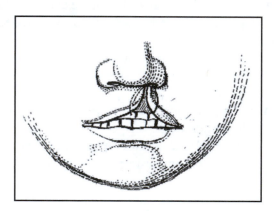

Surgery to correct a cleft lip or palate is scheduled when a child is old enough to tolerate the procedure safely, usually at about 10 weeks of age with a weight of about 10 pounds and a hemoglobin of 10g. By that time, the tissues are large enough to allow accurate repair. Further correction of the nasal deformity, often with simultaneous revision of minor lip irregularities, may be done when the child is older and final surgery may be delayed until adolescence to allow for full maturity of the facial features. Services to correct this congenital defect are considered functional.

However, claims for services related to cleft lip (and possibly palate) repair in persons older than adolescent age should be reviewed for possibly purely cosmetic repair and not functional repair of the defect.

**Collagen or Zyderm Injections**—Zyderm is a medical grade of collagen (taken from cows), which is injected into fine lines or small defects in the skin. It is a temporary measure which plumps up the indented areas, making them appear less pronounced. Usually, supplemental injections must be performed about every six to nine months. Collagen injections are strictly cosmetic.

**Congenital Anomaly**—A birth defect. Depending on the defect, a congenital abnormality may or may not be covered by a plan.

**Dermabrasion**—A procedure using abrasive materials (sandpaper, emery paper, or wire brushes) to remove acne scars, birthmarks, fine wrinkles, or other skin defects. When the skin grows back, the surface irregularities have been smoothed away. Although this is considered a cosmetic procedure, check the plan guidelines because it may be covered to restore the skin to the appearance of a presickness state. Some plans may cover dermabrasion for cases of severe acne.

**Deviated Nasal Septum**—A condition in which the dividing wall between the two nasal cavities is deflected (turned) away from the center of the nose.

**Electrolysis Epilation**—Removal of hair by destruction of the hair follicle (root) with an electric current. For women, the usual diagnosis submitted is hirsutism, which is a condition of adult male hair growth in a female. Electrolysis does not treat the underlying condition, which is a hormonal imbalance, and is therefore considered purely cosmetic.

**Gynecomastia**—A swelling of the breast tissue in the male. If an underlying hormonal disease has been ruled out, the condition is treated by removing a small section of the breast tissue. This may be considered eligible under some plans.

**Hair Transplantation**—Moving healthy hair follicles from one location on the body to another location, usually the head. Alopecia areata is a condition in which patchy areas of baldness occur. Alopecia means the absence of hair from areas where it normally occurs. Male pattern baldness (androgenic alopecia) is loss of hair from the crown of the head. This occurs in about 30% of adult males. A few medications have been shown to assist in regrowing hair in some instances. Transplantation treats the symptoms and not the condition. Therefore, it is usually considered purely cosmetic.

**Hypertrophied/Macromastia Breasts**—An abnormal enlargement of the female breasts caused by hormonal factors or obesity. The condition may require a mastectomy when the weight of the breast tissue causes physical complaints. Among the symptoms present are shoulder, neck, and back pain; numbness of the hand and arm caused by the bra straps compressing the brachial plexus (the group of nerves in the area between the neck and the shoulder that innervate the arm); and chronic inflammation of the skin of the opposed surfaces (intertrigo). Documentation to substantiate the functional nature of this procedure includes pre and postoperative photos, admission history, and physical examination information including the patient's height and weight, discharge summary, operative report, and pathology report.

Each administrator has their own guidelines. Therefore, all claims involving hypertrophied breasts should be researched before payment, after verification of the applicable guidelines.

**Keloid**—A thick scar resulting from excessive growth of fibroid tissue. Any open wound can develop keloid scarring. Therefore, this scarring may occur following surgery. Keloid scar surgery is not usually considered cosmetic.

**Lipectomy**—The surgical removal of fatty tissue. The removal of this fatty tissue may be accomplished by standard surgical techniques (incisional approach) or by liposuction, which consists of "sucking" out the fatty tissue through a vacuum tube inserted through small incisions. Regardless of the method used, the surgical removal of the redundant fatty tissue is considered cosmetic.

**Mammoplasty**—Surgery to reduce (reduction mammoplasty) or enlarge (augmentation mammoplasty) the size of the breast.

*Amastia* or *amazia* is defined as the congenital absence of mammary tissue. These terms refer to masculine breast characteristics in an adult female. Amastia can be unilateral (one-sided) or bilateral (two-sided).

*Hypomastia* or *hypomazia* is defined as abnormal smallness of the mammary gland and, like amastia, it can affect one or both breasts. In cases in which one breast is normal and the other is markedly small or absent, asymmetry results. Augmentation mammoplasty is performed for both of these conditions.

**Mastectomy**—Excision or amputation of the breast, usually required as a result of a malignant disease. This is not the same as a reduction mammoplasty. The three types of mastectomies are:

1. *Radical mastectomy* is the removal of the breast tissue (mammary gland), pectoral muscles, axillary lymph nodes, and associated skin and subcutaneous tissue. This procedure is used for the treatment of cancer but may result in the partial loss of arm movement. Usually, radical mastectomy is followed by reconstructive surgery to restore the appearance of the remaining tissue.

2. *Modified radical mastectomy* is the same as the radical procedure except that the pectoral muscles are left intact. This procedure can usually be performed during the earlier stages of cancer (stage I or II). Modified radical mastectomy is usually also followed by reconstructive procedures.

3. *Subcutaneous mastectomy* is a technique in which most of the breast tissue is removed but the skin and areola are preserved. Unlike the other two methods, immediate reconstruction can usually be done by inserting a Silastic prosthesis into the subcutaneous pocket left by the excision of the breast tissue or under the pectoralis major muscle. Subcutaneous mastectomy and reconstruction for multipathology breasts (i.e., fibrocystic disease, fibroadenoma) consists of removing the mammary tissue and inserting a prosthesis (implant) under the remaining skin to maintain the breast contour. The surgery is used to treat chronic mastitis in patients who experience incapacitating breast pain or those who have repeated breast biopsies of the cystic nodules to rule out cancer.

To determine the medical necessity of a mastectomy, the documentation requested from the physician should include a history of removal of the lumps or repeated aspirations of the cysts as well as the laboratory results of the previous biopsies.

**Mentoplasty/Genioplasty**—Surgery to change the size and shape of the chin with an implant. This procedure is done for a small (microgenic) or moderately receding chin in persons in whom there is no underlying defect with the jaw itself. A small incision is made under the chin and a silicone implant is inserted, giving increased prominence to the chin.

**Otoplasty**—Plastic surgery to change the position or configuration of the ear or ears. The most common deformities that require an otoplasty are:

- **Protruding or Lop Ears**—Ears set at a greater than 25-degree angle from the skull. They may protrude due to cartilage deformities to such an extent that they form a right angle on the side of the head. In lop ears, the ear is bent upon itself. Prominent ears are usually caused by lack of definition of the antihelical fold. This defect is referred to in the diagnosis and operative report.

The best age to perform corrective surgery for these conditions is about 13 to 14 years, when the ear has attained almost maximum growth. However, because of the emotional and psychological problems associated with these conditions, surgery may be done before the child reaches school age. This surgery is usually considered cosmetic.

- **Microtia**—A congenital defect characterized by a small, malformed, malpositioned ear remnant. A hearing deficit is almost always present in affected children. Repair begins at age five or six years and is performed in a series of surgeries. The surgery is considered reconstructive.

**Palatoplasty**—Plastic surgery of the palate, usually to correct a cleft palate.

**Panniculectomy**—Removal of a sheet or layer of fatty tissue. This procedure is most often done to remove excess fatty tissue from the abdomen.

**"-Plasty"**—The surgical suffix that means to mold or shape.

**Ptosis**—Drooping or sagging of an organ part.

**Removal of Tattoos**—This procedure is always considered cosmetic.

**Rhinoplasty**—Cosmetic repair of the external part of the nose to change its size or shape. This procedure does not involve the internal functioning of the nose, although it is performed entirely within the nose to prevent scarring.

A rhinoplasty consists of five major steps:

1. Elevating the skin from the bony and cartilaginous dorsum.
2. Removing the hump or lowering a prominent dorsum.
3. Narrowing the nasal pyramid to compensate for the flatness caused by the hump removal.
4. Shortening the nose if necessary.
5. Modeling the tip or lower cartilaginous complex to proportions consistent with the previous steps.

Key words to look for in determining whether surgery on the nose is cosmetic are "modifications of alar cartilages" and "lowering the dorsum." It is never necessary to modify the alar cartilages or lower the dorsum other than for cosmetic reasons. It is also never necessary to do alar base excisions for functional reasons. In fact, this constricts the airway and is against the principle of improving air flow.

Rhinoplasties are often combined with a septoplasty or submucous resection. Therefore, proper claim investigation is essential to determine whether and what part of the nasal procedure is necessary to correct a functional defect versus what part is for purely cosmetic purposes.

The test used to document airway obstruction is called *rhinomanometry*. It is the measurement of the airflow and pressure within the nose during respiration, and the resistance or obstruction is calculated. Unfortunately, this test is not often performed.

The structures of the nose responsible for airway obstruction are the septum and the nasal turbinates. The septum is made up of the downward projection of the ethmoid bone at the back, the vomer bone at the bottom, and the triangular-shaped septal cartilage. It divides the nasal cavity (internal nose) into two wedge-shaped cavities.

An accident can displace the septal cartilage where it meets the vomer or ethmoid bones, causing one side of the nasal cavity to become narrower and to obstruct the airway.

**Rhytidectomy**—Surgical removal of wrinkles. This procedure is usually cosmetic unless it interferes with the normal function of a body part.

**Rhytidoplasty (facelift)**—Removal of facial wrinkles. Wrinkles are related to the absorption of subcutaneous fat, a decrease in the thickness and elasticity of the skin, and a failure in adherence of the skin to the deeper tissues—all processes that are part of the normal physiology of aging. This is possibly one of the most graphic examples of a purely cosmetic procedure.

**Senile Ptosis of the Eyelids**—A condition in which the skin of the eyelids sags or droops. This may cause vision impairment.

**Septoplasty**—Surgical correction of a deviated nasal septum, the dividing wall between the two nasal cavities. This involves only the internal functioning of the nose and is usually covered. Septoplasty or submucous resection of the septum involves undermining the mucous membrane that covers the septum. This procedure is also referred to as "raising the mucoperichondrial and mucoperiosteal flaps." The cartilage is then cut into at its base so as to allow it to be moved over and straightened.

**Submental Lipectomy**—Removal of fat deposits under the chin. The region under the chin (submental region) and the neck often requires special attention. A submental lipectomy through a separate incision may be required to remove the fat deposits beneath the chin, thus correcting double chins. Suturing and repositioning of the neck muscle (platysma) is done to obliterate jowls. This is usually considered cosmetic.

**Submucous Resection**—Removal of a portion of the nasal septum.

**TMJ Surgery**—Osteoplastic surgery of the jaw for prognathism (projection of the jaw(s) beyond the projection of the forehead), micrognathism (abnormal smallness of jaws), and other variations may be cosmetic or functional, depending on the degree of malocclusion.

**Turbinates**—Bony projections from the sidewalls of the internal nose. The purpose of the turbinates is to warm and moisten air. Each nasal cavity is divided into three passageways by the turbinates. A submucous resection of the turbinates consists of undermining the mucous membrane that covers them and removing a portion of the bone, thereby enlarging the nasal passageway. A submucous resection is a functional correction, and is therefore an eligible expense.

**Wart and Mole Removal**—Moles and warts are discolorations of the skin which protrude above the normal skin elevation. Often warts and moles are associated with other diseases and conditions, especially cancer. Therefore, many plans will cover the removal of warts and moles.

# On the Job Now

**Directions:** Answer the following questions without looking back at the material just covered. Write your answers in the space provided.

1. List the documents that must be reviewed during a claim investigation when the restorative or cosmetic nature of the procedure is not obvious.

    1. _____

    2. _____

    3. _____

    4. _____

    5. _____

2. Why do providers take preoperative and postoperative photographs of a patient? _____

    _____

    _____

3. What is the procedure for requesting and using preoperative and postoperative photographs to process a claim? _____

    _____

    _____

    _____

    _____

    _____

# Obesity Surgery

**Exogenous obesity** is obesity caused by overeating. Treatment for this condition is not considered treatment of a disease and is usually not covered by most plans until the level of obesity reaches a point at which it is life threatening. Most administrators have defined this level as being 100 pounds or 30% over the weight considered optimal for a person of a particular height and bone frame.

**Endogenous obesity**—is obesity caused by an internal malfunction, usually hormonal (i.e., thyroid disorder). Treatment for this type of obesity or for the underlying cause is considered treatment of a disease and is eligible under most plans. This is a comparatively rare condition.

Most administrators require the following documentation to be submitted before the scheduled treatment for review:

- Current weight and height.
- Frame type (small, medium, large).
- History of weight loss in the past (i.e., what diets have been tried, what level of success).
- Concurrent medical complications such as high blood pressure or diabetes.
- Family history of obesity or other health problems.

The following three procedures are the most common procedures used to combat exogenous obesity:

1. **Gastric Balloon/Garren Gastric Bubble**—A procedure in which a balloon is inserted into the stomach, thus giving the impression of being "full." Since many overweight people eat not because they are hungry but because of habit or compulsion, this has not been an effective method. In addition, many complications, including death, have resulted from this procedure. Therefore, it is no longer considered an accepted medical practice.

2. **Gastric Bypass**—A procedure in which the stomach is bypassed, allowing food to empty directly into the large intestine. The theory behind this procedure is that the food, nutrients, and fats are not thoroughly broken down and digested, resulting in fewer calories being accessible to the body for storing. Therefore, weight is lost. This is usually considered to be a permanent procedure, although it can be reversed. See CPT® code 43846.

3. **Gastric Stapling**—A procedure in which a portion of the stomach is stapled off so as to reduce the size of the stomach. This procedure decreases the amount of food that may be eaten at a single meal. See CPT® code 43843.

Most procedures for obesity surgery have side effects. Some of the side effects may be so severe for some people that the procedure will need to be reversed. Therefore, only the severely obese should consider any of these methods of treatment.

The alternatives to surgery include the following services that are usually not covered under benefit plans:

- Special diets and dietary supplements.
- HCG (human chorionic gonadotropin) and vitamin injections.
- Acupuncture.
- Appetite suppressants.
- Biofeedback.
- Hypnosis.
- Hospital confinements for weight reduction.
- Exercise programs.
- Health centers, weight loss centers, or other similar programs.
- Diet books and instructions.

## Practice Pitfalls

Many insurance companies will wait until receipt of the surgeon's billing prior to paying any assistant surgeon or anesthesiologist bill. This is because the primary surgeon usually has a better understanding of the actual surgical procedures performed and to ensure that the assistant surgeon and anesthesiologist have billed properly.

If a surgeon is a PPO provider but the assistant surgeon or anesthesiologist is not, some insurance carriers will not penalize the patient for not using a PPO assistant surgeon or anesthesiologist, because the patient does not normally select the assistant surgeon or anesthesiologist.

# Cosurgeons

Under some circumstances, two surgeons, usually with similar skills, may operate simultaneously as primary surgeons performing distinct, separate parts of a total surgical service. These are referred to as **cosurgeons**. For example, two surgeons may simultaneously apply skin grafts to different parts of the body or two surgeons may repair different fractures of the same patient.

When a claim is received for cosurgeons, plan guidelines or administrative guidelines need to be referred to before processing. Usually cosurgeon procedures are referred to a consultant, supervisor, or Medical Review Department before processing.

# Assistant Surgeons

Complex surgeries may require a primary surgeon and an assistant surgeon. The **assistant surgeon** may do the closing of the operative wound, hemostasis of the wound edges, and suturing of vessels. The job of the assistant surgeon is to assist the primary surgeon as required. Since the assistant surgeon is not the physician primarily responsible for the patient, the UCR allowance is considerably less than that for the surgeon.

The first consideration is that the complexity of the surgical procedure must medically require an assistant (see Appendix C for Assistant Surgeon Procedures). Obviously, an assistant surgeon would not be covered for minor surgery (i.e., acne surgery).

As a rule, the following guidelines may be used in determining whether an assistant is required:

1. The place of service is either a hospital (inpatient or outpatient), or a surgi-center. Seldom are major surgeries performed in an office.

2. Follow-up days are listed in the *RVS* for each procedure. Services without follow-up days are usually not complex enough to require an assistant.

The allowance for an assistant surgeon is 20% of the surgery allowance (UCR). Modifier -80 is used to designate the assistant surgeon's fee.

**Example:** Procedure 15570 has a unit value of 10.0. The conversion factor is $38.50. Therefore,

10 units × $38.50 = $385.  20% of $385 = $77.

Based on the previously stated guidelines, $77 would be considered the UCR fee for an assistant surgeon.

Some procedures do not require the expertise of an M.D. assistant, but do require technical help. For these procedures, physician assistants (PA's) are often used. When these professionals are used in lieu of an M.D. assistant, Modifier -81 is used. The allowed amount is usually calculated at 10%–15% of the surgeon's allowance, depending on the insurance carrier's practice and plan definition. However, the most common percentage used is 10%.

**Example:** Procedure 15570 has a unit value of 10 units. The conversion factor for surgery is $38.50. Therefore,

10 units × $138.50 = $385. $385 × 10% = $38.50;

therefore, the allowable amount for the PA is $38.50.

It should be noted that although an assistant surgeon is considered medically necessary when a C-section is performed, the physician's coding should be reviewed. The assistant is entitled to 20% (or 10% if a PA) of the delivery only and not the global code that includes the antepartum and postpartum care.

If there is more than one procedure performed, the multiple/bilateral guidelines apply. The reasoning is that the assistant surgeon allowable is 20% of the surgeon's allowable. Thus, the first procedure would be calculated at 20% of the allowed amount and the subsequent procedures would be calculated at the allowed amount × 50% × 20%.

# Podiatry

**Podiatry** is an area of medicine that provides services for the feet. The services are usually provided by a podiatrist with the professional designation D.P.M. (Doctor of Podiatric Medicine).

The joints of the feet are very complex. When surgery is performed, the claims that are received by the claims examiner will also be complex. In this chapter we will discuss some of the procedures performed on the foot and some guidelines that have been established regarding payment of podiatry claims.

# On the Job Now

1. What are therapeutic procedures? _____

   _____

2. What is the difference between a cosmetic procedure and a reconstructive procedure? _____

   _____

3. Define lump sum billing in relation to maternity charges. _____

   _____

4. When would charges for amniocentesis or chromosomal analysis usually be covered? _____

   _____

5. Are collagen injections a cosmetic procedure? _____

6. What is the name of the surgical procedure for excision or amputation of the breast? _____

7. What is a deviated nasal septum? _____

   _____

8. Modifier _____ is used to designate the assistant surgeon's fee.

9. The allowance for an assistant surgeon is _____ of the surgery allowance.

10. Would an assistant surgeon be required for acne surgery? _____

## Practice Pitfalls

Because of the complexity of podiatry claims, most administrators have special handling guidelines for podiatric care and for podiatric surgery. Many plans have provisions that place a UCR limitation and a daily maximum on podiatric claims. In addition, most of these claims may also be referred to a consultant for review, prior to payment.

The UCR fee allowance for podiatric surgery is determined the same way as any other surgical procedure. The most common problem in determining the correct UCR allowance is the excessive detail in which the surgery is sometimes described. At times, the podiatrist describes and bills each procedure independently, even though some procedures are incidental to the major operation performed. Refer to the Surgery section in this chapter for further information on multiple, bilateral, and incidental surgeries. The following four handling procedures may be helpful in identifying the correct breakdown of the surgeries performed:

1. Separate the procedures performed on each foot. The foot that has the most or major surgery is identified as the primary foot.

2. List the independent procedures and identify the metatarsal or phalange by digit (i.e., great toe #1, second toe #2).

3. Determine whether more than one procedure has been performed on one joint, one toe, or adjacent parts of the foot. If this has been identified, no additional allowance is made for secondary procedures because all such procedures are to be considered incidental (part of the major procedure).

4. After all the independent procedures for both the primary and secondary foot have been identified, the correct CPT® surgical procedure code can be located.

# Surgical Coding for Podiatry

To select the correct CPT® code, identify the diagnosis and the required procedures necessary to correct the medical problem. For example, a bill with a diagnosis of "hammertoe" may list service for an arthroplasty, a capsulotomy, and a tenotomy with a separate charge for each procedure. The benefit for correction of the diagnosis (hammertoe), repair of hammertoe (CPT® code 28285), should be allowed. No additional allowance is available for each separate procedure because they are included in the hammertoe repair CPT® code. The following eight rules are important to consider when determining the correct surgical codes:

1. Only one bunion surgery is allowable per foot.
2. Only one bone operation is allowable per toe.
3. Only one capsulotomy/tenotomy is allowable per metatarsal.
4. No increase is allowable for K wires (stabilizing wires placed in the foot). These are considered a necessary part of the procedure and do not warrant an extra benefit.
5. Generally, one operation is allowable per incision.
6. Taylor's bunion is not a bunion.
7. Unna's boot (gauze soaked in zinc oxide) is considered part of the surgery itself and does not warrant an additional allowance. When the boot is used for treatment of leg ulcers, additional benefits may be allowed.
8. Flexible casts are nothing more than a tape or bandage and do not warrant a casting benefit.

Remember that these are general guidelines only. The actual administration of podiatry claims varies greatly among companies. Therefore, you should refer to the benefit plan summary prior to claim payment.

# Conditions of the Foot and Treatment Procedures

The following are explanations of common foot conditions and some of the procedures performed to treat or correct problems.

Foot surgeries usually involve some incision of the skin and, in some cases, of the bone. Skin heals in phases. In the first phase, skin grows together, which allows stitches to be removed. The scar may look slightly inflamed. Some redness and swelling are normal. After about six months, the scar blends with the surrounding skin. However, scarring varies according to the individual.

Bone also heals in phases. A bone-like "cement" forms first, bridging the affected bone and enabling it to bear some weight. Later, this extra bone dissolves. The healing process varies from person to person and also depends on the health and age of the person.

**Ligaments** are flexible bands of fiber joining bone to bone. **Joints** are where two bones meet. Thirty-three complex joints in each foot permit flexibility.

## Bunions

A **bunion** is an enlargement of a bone in a joint at the base of the big toe. Bunions are most often inherited. Contrary to what many people believe, bunions are not caused by tight shoes, although tight-fitting shoes can aggravate them. The simplest bunion procedure is the Silver procedure. The Silver procedure does not involve any surgery in the first metatarsal interspace; all other bunion procedures do.

The McBride procedure is performed to remove the bump on the outside of the first metatarsal, remove the sesamoid, and sever the abductor and short tendon. If tenotomies are not performed, the procedure is a Silver.

Reverdin or Reverdin and Green bunionectomy involves the removal of the bunion on the outside of the first metatarsal and a wedge osteotomy of the first metatarsal to bring the toe into proper alignment.

The Austin, Reverdin, Peabody, Mitchell, Wilson, and Rue bunionectomies all involve some kind of osteotomy in the head of the metatarsal and all have the same CPT® of 28296. A metatarsal base osteotomy is a valid second procedure (28306).

The Akin osteotomy involves the removal of a cylindrical wedge of the proximal phalanx of the great toe and is closed with a screw, wire, or pin. This cylindrical wedge can be taken from either the distal or proximal end of the phalanx. If done with the Akin bunionectomy, the CPT® code is 28298. When the Akin osteotomy and bunionectomy are performed at the same time, there should be one surgery per foot.

The Keller bunionectomy with Silastic implant involves the removal of a bunion from the first metatarsal and excision of the head of the proximal phalanx with insertion of the Silastic head into the end of the phalanx so that it forms a new gliding joint.

### Positional Bunions

A **positional bunion** develops when a bony growth on the side of the metatarsal bone enlarges the joint, forcing the joint capsule to stretch over it. As this growth pushes the big toe toward the others, the tendons on the inside tighten. This then forces the big toe further out of alignment. The bunion presses against the shoe, irritating the skin and causing increased pain.

In treatment of a positional bunion (positional bunionectomy), the bump is removed (**see Figure 7–1**). A wedge of the joint capsule may also be removed to reposition it. Tight tendons may also have to be released. A special wooden shoe or splint may be required for about three weeks postoperatively.

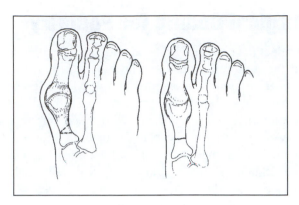

**■ Figure 7–2** Structural Bunionectomy

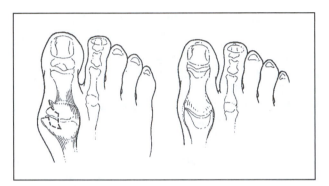

**■ Figure 7–1** Positional Bunionectomy

## Structural Bunions

A mild **structural bunion** occurs when the angle between the first and second metatarsal bones increases to a point at which it is greater than normal. The increased angle of the metatarsal makes the big toe bow toward the other toes. This is usually an inherited tendency. Treatment of a structural bunion (structural bunionectomy) involves repositioning the bone (**see Figure 7–2**). A splint or a special shoe may be required for about six weeks postoperatively.

A structural bunion becomes severe when the angle between the metatarsal bones of the first and second toes grows greater than the angle of a mild structural bunion. The big toe bows toward the others, sometimes causing the second and third toes to buckle.

For a severe structural bunion, a base osteotomy may be performed to remove a wedge of bone so that the metatarsal can be repositioned. Tiny K wires or screws may be used to stabilize the bone.

The foot and ankle may be immobilized with a cast; no weight should be placed on the foot for several weeks.

## Degenerative Disease

Degenerative disease is not a bunion, but it is often associated with bunions. This is because an untreated bunion can increase wear and tear on the joint of the big toe, break down the cartilage, and pave the way for degenerative diseases such as arthritis, osteoarthritis, and rheumatoid arthritis.

Treatment of degenerative conditions involves removal of all bunions; the degenerated joint is then removed and replaced with a silastic (plastic) implant. A splint or a special shoe may be worn for several weeks. However, the ability to walk may return within one or two days after surgery.

## Taylor's Bunionectomy

Taylor's procedure is not a bunion operation but the removal of a small bone portion of the fifth metatarsal. It is often done with an osteotomy. When the portion of the fifth metatarsal is removed, it may accompany an incidental removal of the outside of the first phalanx.

## Hammertoes

**Hammertoes** are inherited muscle imbalances or abnormal bone lengths that can make the toes buckle under, causing their joints to contract. Subsequently, the tendons shorten. A flexible hammertoe is one in which the buckled joint can be straightened manually with the hand. These may progress and become rigid over time. Rigid hammertoes are fixed and cannot be manually straightened. Corns, irritation, pain, and loss of function are common symptoms and may be more severe in rigid than in flexible hammertoes.

## Surgical Repair

There are two different types of hammertoe repair: simple and radical. Regardless of the procedure, only one hammertoe operation is allowable per toe. Some of the more common hammertoe repair procedures are tenotomy, capsulotomy, osteotomy, arthroplasty, and arthrodesis.

A **tenotomy** and **capsulotomy** are performed to release the buckling and the top and bottom tendons. The joint capsules may also have to be cut (**see Figure 7–3**). When a tenotomy and capsulotomy are performed on the same joint, only one operation is allowable per joint.

When an osteotomy is performed in conjunction with a tenotomy and capsulotomy, the additional procedure is incidental.

An **arthroplasty** is a procedure in which a portion of the joint is surgically removed and the toe is straightened. The resulting gap will fill in with fibrous tissue. Removal of the joint and fusion of the bones constitute an alternative treatment.

The fifth (little) toe may curl inward beneath the fourth toe so that the nail faces outward. This inherited problem results in corns and pain. A derotation anthroplasty is performed to remove a wedge of skin and bone to uncurl (derotate) the toe. A bandage, splint, and sometimes a surgical shoe are required for several weeks following surgery.

## Plantar Calluses

A **metatarsal plantar callus** occurs when the metatarsal bone is longer or lower than the others so that it hits the ground first at every step with more force than it is equipped to handle. As a result, the skin under this bone thickens and becomes hardened into a callus. The callus causes irritation and pain. The treatment is a V osteotomy in which the metatarsal bone is cut in a V shape. The end of the bone is then lifted and aligned with the other bones. The V shape holds the bone in its new position, preventing it from rocking to the left or the right.

A fifth metatarsal plantar callus is caused by walking improperly on the outside of the foot. The extra pressure may cause the skin under the bone to thicken, causing irritation and pain.

## Dwyer Osteotomy Surgical Procedure

The **Dwyer procedure** is the treatment for a deformity of the calcaneus or large heel bone. It consists of a wedge resection of a portion of the calcaneus bone and is closed with a staple, pin, or screw fixation.

A **dorsal osteotomy** is performed by removing a small wedge of bone from the top (dorsal) side of the base of the fifth metatarsal bone. This elevates the bone and relieves pressure on the callus. The bone is then fixated with tiny wires or screws.

## Bone Spurs

A **bone spur** is a bony overgrowth on the bone. Bone spurs have a variety of causes and usually result in pain, interfere with the use of the foot, and detract from its appearance.

A **heel spur** is an overgrowth on the heel bone. It may be stimulated by muscles that pull from the heel bone along the bottom of the foot. High-arched feet are especially apt to have excessively tight muscles in this area.

Treatment of bone spurs involves releasing the band of tight muscles to relieve the stress. The bone spur is then surgically removed (**see Figure 7–4**). Crutches may be required for up to two weeks after surgery to avoid weight bearing on the foot.

A bone spur may occur alone or with a hammertoe, usually resulting in pain and interfering with the use of the foot. An overgrowth under the toenail can press up into the tissue underneath the growth plate, deforming the nail above. This is especially painful when shoes are worn.

### Common Surgical Procedures

The most common exostosis (bony growth) on the foot is the heel spur. In most cases, surgery is the most effective way to treat a heel spur. A plantar fasciotomy

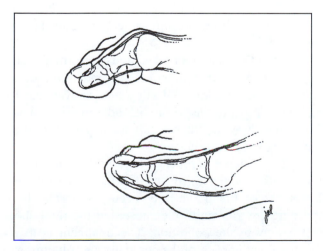

■ **Figure 7–3** Tenotomy and Capsulotomy

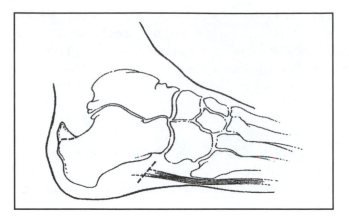

**■ Figure 7–4** Treatment of Bone Spur

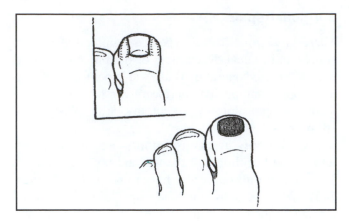

**■ Figure 7–5** Treatment of Ingrown Toenail

performed at the same time as a surgery for heel spurs is an incidental procedure, since a fasciotomy must be done to cut through the area before the heel spur is located. In many cases, the use of **orthosis** (an orthopedic appliance) is as effective as the surgery.

Treatment for subungual exostosis is performed to smooth down the spur with a tiny rasp. The rasp resembles a dental burr and is inserted through a small incision.

### Ingrown Toenails

An **ingrown toenail** is a nail where one or both corners or sides of the nail grow into the skin of the toe. Irritation, redness, an uncomfortable sensation of warmth, swelling, pain, and infection can result.

#### Surgical Procedures

Removal of a nail margin can be done with or without the excision of the root or matrix. To allow surgical benefits for the total excision of the nail and matrix, it must be indicated that the root and matrix are being permanently removed. Excision of subungual exostosis is sometimes used to describe the removal of one or two margins. This is not a separate procedure.

On a partial ingrown toenail, only one or two sides grow into the skin. The treatment is a partial matrixectomy in which a wedge of the nail and the underlying nail bed are removed. The nail portion can be surgically removed with a scalpel or by chemical means. This is a simple and brief procedure.

In severe cases of ingrown toenails, the entire nail grows into the skin on both sides. This is called a completely ingrown toenail. Usually, significant pain is present. Treatment is a total **matrixectomy** in which the nail and growth plate are removed either surgically

or chemically **(see Figure 7–5)**. The body then produces a "**false nail**," that is, tough skin that mimics a real nail. This false nail usually grows in within a few months after the surgery.

### Warts

**Warts** are caused by a virus and are contagious. They often grow in groups and spread to the fingers and other areas of the body. Warts occurring on the soles of the feet are called plantar warts, which are painful and may affect walking. Usually, these warts grow on the soles, but may occur on the toes or on the top of the foot. Treatment entails scooping out the wart with a curette, a spoon-shaped surgical instrument. The base is then cauterized (burned either electrically or chemically) to discourage regrowth.

### Neuromas

A **neuroma** is a tumor arising from the connective tissue of the nerves. Although there are four interspaces, neuromas most often occur in the second interspace. Neuromas are commonly bilateral, but rarely does more than one occur on the same foot or in the first interspace.

If any other surgical procedure is performed on the first toe or on the M-P joint of the second, third, fourth, or fifth toes, no additional allowance is available for removal of neuromas from the adjacent interspace. This procedure should not call for any increased allowance for microsurgery.

When a nerve is pinched between two metatarsal bones (usually the third and fourth metatarsal), enlargement of the nerve may occur. Abnormal bone structure contributes to the cause, but too-tight shoes can aggravate the condition. The treatment is to remove a small portion of the nerve. As a result, this area is permanently numbed.

## Ganglions

**Ganglions** are fluid-filled sacs that may grow on a joint capsule or tendon **(see Figure 7–6)**. The location and size vary. The cause is unknown. Ganglions cause irritation, swelling, and pain when they press against nerves.

Treatment involves excision of the ganglion by separating it from the surrounding tissues. If not removed completely, a ganglion may grow back.

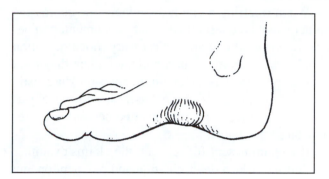

■ **Figure 7–6** Ganglion

## Miscellaneous

**High-arched feet** (pes cavus) are caused by an imbalance of muscles and nerves and are often inherited. High arches can cause various problems such as calluses and foot, heel, ankle, or tendon pain. Treatment depends on specific problems. Usually, surgery or orthosis is prescribed.

**Flat feet** (pes planus) are also hereditary and are caused by a muscle imbalance. Feet with low, relaxed arches may create problems such as hammertoes and bunions; arch, foot, and leg fatigue; calf pain, and an overly tight heel cord (which makes the foot even flatter). Loose joints may move too freely, causing pain and instability. Surgery and orthoses may also be used to treat this condition. **Orthotic devices** are prescribed custom-made arch supports that fit inside most shoes and "bring the floor up to your feet." To make this support, a plaster impression of the feet is made. The orthotic device is made of leather, plastic, or other material, depending on the particular foot problem based on the impression.

# On the Job Now

**Directions:** Fill in the blank spaces with the correct word without looking back at the material just covered.

1. A _____ is an enlargement of a bone in a joint at the base of the big toe. They are most often inherited.

2. _____ are also hereditary and are caused by a muscle imbalance.

3. _____ are inherited muscle imbalances or abnormal bone lengths that can make the toes buckle under, causing their joints to contract. Subsequently, the tendons shorten.

4. _____ are caused by an imbalance of muscles and nerves and are often inherited.

5. An _____ occurs when one or both corners or sides of the nail grow into the skin of the toe.

6. A _____ occurs when the metatarsal bone is longer or lower than the others so that it hits the ground first at every step with more force than it is equipped to handle. As a result, the skin under this bone thickens and becomes hardened into a callus.

7. A _____ is a tumor arising from the connective tissue of the nerves.

8. A _____ is a bony overgrowth on the bone.

9. _____ are caused by a virus and are contagious. They often grow in groups and spread to the fingers and other areas of the body.

## Assistant Surgeon for Podiatry

Because of the complexity of the bones, joints, and tendons in the foot, many podiatric surgeries that are performed on an inpatient basis require an assistant surgeon. However, some of these surgeries may also require an assistant surgeon when performed in a doctor's office.

## Practice
# Pitfalls

Because of the difficulty in determining allowable expense and the correct surgical allowance, questionable claim situations should be referred to a supervisor, review department, or consultant. Following are some guidelines or situations that may warrant a consultant's review:

1. Charges for the insertion or removal of K wire.

2. Microsurgical repair of nerves.

3. Serial surgery. (**Serial surgery** is surgery on several individual toes or joints with one surgical procedure being performed in a single operative visit, i.e., surgery on one toe followed by surgery on another toe one week later, followed by still other surgeries after that. Or, it is surgery on one joint, followed by surgery on a different joint of the same toe at a later date.) It can last days, weeks, or even months.

4. Fragmented fees billed at 100% for each procedure. This situation may also include misrepresented CPT® codes.

5. Vascular studies (i.e., temperature gradient studies, Doppler studies, or plethysmography). These tests can be considered medically necessary in certain situations or for certain conditions (i.e., diabetes, peripheral vascular disease). Test results and the patient's history are needed for review.

6. Possible unnecessary services or procedures.

   These can include:

   • Use of nitrous oxide anesthesia.

   • Operating room charge for office surgery.

   • Preoperative sedatives.

   • Use of steroid injections, arthrocentesis, or power equipment on the day of surgery.

   • Rental of TENS unit.

   • More than two postoperative x-rays. The exception is in the case of major bone surgery and delayed bunion surgery.

It is generally accepted medical practice to allow an assistant surgeon when doing soft tissue work. The exception to this is for ingrown toenails. Multiple or bilateral procedures may also require an assistant surgeon.

Single-toe procedures for excision of dome and simple hammertoe procedures usually do not warrant the use of an assistant surgeon.

When allowed, the assistant surgeon's benefits are paid according to the standard policy provisions for assistant surgeons.

When referring a claim for review, the claims examiner should request all necessary documentation before referring the claim. Necessary documentation includes the operating report and the patient diagnosis and history as well as the claim. In addition, diagnostic tests, before and after photos, x-rays, and the physician's daily office notes may also be necessary for review on some claims.

If a claim is sent for referral, the claims examiner should first make a determination and payment on any and all services that are not being questioned. Written notification should accompany the payment regarding which services are being held pending a consultant's review.

When the consultant's review is received, some services may be allowed and others denied. The claims examiner should verify the plan guidelines and benefits, and make a payment determination on the claim.

The consultant's report and the name, address, and phone number of the consultant are the property of the company and should never be given to the claimant. This information should be retained as part of the claim file.

## Surgery Modifiers

Following are some examples of modifiers frequently used with surgery procedures.

-22 Unusual Procedural Services.

-32 Mandated Services.

-47 Anesthesia by Surgeon.

-50 Bilateral Procedure.

-51 Multiple Procedures.

-52 Reduced Services.

-54 Surgical Care Only.

-55 Postoperative Management Only.

-56 Preoperative Management Only.

-57 Decision for Surgery.

-62 Two Surgeons.

-66   Surgical Team.

-80   Assistant Surgeon.

-81   Minimum Assistant Surgeon.

# Anesthesia

**Anesthesia** is the artificially induced loss of feeling and sensation with or without loss of consciousness. The four kinds of anesthesia administration are:

1. General anesthesia.
2. Regional anesthesia.
3. Intravenous (IV) sedation.
4. Acupuncture.

## General Anesthesia

**General anesthesia** produces a state of unconsciousness. It may be brought about by inhalation of gases such as ether, nitrous oxide, and ethylene or by drugs administered intravenously; such as sodium pentothal. General anesthesia produces preliminary excitement, replaced by a loss of voluntary control. Loss of consciousness occurs when the anesthetic reaches the brain, with hearing being the last sense to be lost. Most major operations, particularly on the upper abdomen, chest, head, and neck, are performed under general anesthesia. A number of side effects may accompany general anesthesia, many of which cannot be controlled or predicted. General anesthesia is considered more dangerous than other forms of anesthesia. Therefore, anesthesiologists have one of the highest malpractice insurance rates.

Prior to surgery requiring general anesthesia, the anesthesiologist usually meets with the patient to assess his or her general health and record age, weight, concurrent medical problems, family history, and other pertinent data. Anesthesiologists are reluctant to administer general anesthesia to patients who are extremely obese or who have blood pressure or respiratory problems because they have the highest risk factors.

General anesthesia can be used in outpatient surgery. However, it requires a prolonged postoperative recovery period (usually two to four hours), and therefore is commonly reserved for use in a facility setting (outpatient hospital, surgi-center). The administration of general anesthesia in a doctor's or dentist's office is considered very dangerous, although some specialists do so routinely.

## Regional Anesthesia

**Regional anesthesia** is the loss of sensation of a part of the body due to the interruption of nerve conduction. While regional anesthesia is in effect, the patient remains conscious. This method is adequate for many operations and is considerably less dangerous than general anesthesia. Regional anesthesia can be safely performed on an outpatient basis. The three types of regional anesthesia are topical, local, and nerve block.

**Topical anesthesia** is applied directly to the surface of the area to be anesthetized. The conjunctiva and mucous membranes of the mouth, throat, urethra, and bladder are examples of areas that are most effectively anesthetized by a topical application.

**Local anesthesia** affects only a localized area. The drug is directly introduced by injection into the skin and subcutaneous tissues. The anesthesia injection wears off very quickly; therefore, only short procedures can be performed painlessly. Superficial biopsies, mole excisions, and suturing of lacerations are the most common procedures performed with local anesthesia.

For a **nerve block anesthesia**, a drug is injected close to the nerve so that the nerve impulses are interrupted, thereby producing a loss of sensation.

Spinal anesthesia is a specialized type of nerve block. The spinal nerves are blocked in either the subarachnoid or the epidural space. The term **spinal anesthesia** generally refers to nerves blocked in the subarachnoid space. **Epidural anesthesia** refers to the nerves blocked in the epidural space. Epidural anesthesia is frequently used for maternity claims.

According to the American Society of Anesthesiologists (ASA) guidelines, the anesthesia value for maternity claims is base units + time units. Since the epidural is administered throughout labor and the physician is not in constant attendance, many insurance carriers and PPO organizations have developed special guidelines for maternity anesthesia. To process these claims accurately, be sure to develop a full understanding of the office procedures.

Another type of spinal anesthetic is a **saddle block**. This is so named because the injection produces a loss of feeling in the region of the body that corresponds to the area that makes contact with a riding saddle (buttocks, perineum, and thighs). Spinal anesthesia was formerly used frequently for normal deliveries. Now, it is mainly used on operations within the peritoneal cavity and on the lower extremities.

## Intravenous Sedation

**Intravenous (IV) sedation** is a medication composed of a sedative and a painkiller administered intravenously. A semiconscious state is produced. A common mixture is meperidine (Demerol) and diazepam (Valium). This type of anesthesia is often used in dental surgical procedures and in many diagnostic procedures such as bronchoscopy and esophagogastro-duodenoscopy in which the surgical invasion is obtained through an existing orifice. This type of anesthesia is commonly referred to as "twilight sleep."

## Acupuncture

Acupuncture can be used as another form of anesthesia. There are more than 1000 acupuncture locations on the body. A different physiological effect is produced in each location or combination of locations. Sometimes, only one needle is necessary to achieve the desired result; other times many needles are required. The patient remains awake and can talk during the procedure. Acupuncture works similarly to the way nerve block anesthesia works. Although this type of anesthesia is popular in China, it is also used in the United States.

## Hypnosis

**Hypnosis** is a state where the subconscious mind is allowed to take over and the conscious mind is more or less inactive. Some patients will choose hypnosis rather than conventional forms of anesthesia.

Most plans do not cover hypnosis services, though a few may allow coverage for hypnosis used in lieu of covered anesthesia.

| ANESTHESIA CODES | |
|---|---|
| Head | 00100 – 00222 |
| Neck | 00300 – 00352 |
| Thorax | 00400 – 00474 |
| Intrathoracic | 00500 – 00580 |
| Spine and Spinal Cord | 00600 – 00670 |
| Upper Abdomen | 00700 – 00797 |
| Lower Abdomen | 00800 – 00882 |
| Perineum | 00902 – 00952 |
| Pelvis (Except Hip) | 01112 – 01190 |
| Upper Leg (Except Knee) | 01200 – 01274 |
| Knee and Popliteal Area | 01320 – 01444 |
| Lower Leg | 01462 – 01522 |
| Shoulder and Axilla | 01610 – 01682 |
| Upper Arm and Elbow | 01710 – 01782 |
| Forearm, Wrist, and Hand | 01810 – 01860 |
| Radiological Procedures | 01905 – 01933 |
| Burn, Excisions or Debridement | 01951 – 01953 |
| Obstetric | 01958 – 01969 |
| Other Procedures | 01990 – 01999 |

**Table 7–2** **Anesthesia Codes**

# Anesthesia CPT® Coding

The coding for anesthesia services depends on the area of the body being operated on. Anesthesia CPT® codes range from 00100–01999 **(see Table 7–2)**. Since specific surgeries are usually not included in these codes, there are no special circumstances for any given body area. For that reason we will list the subsections without further comment.

# Anesthesia Handling Procedures

An anesthesiologist may be classified as either a **hospital staff anesthesiologist** (employed by the hospital) or an **independent anesthesiologist** (self-employed or not employed by the hospital). Charges made by a hospital for the services of a staff anesthesiologist are usually covered as a hospital ancillary expense.

Charges by an outside anesthesiologist vary according to plan provision, but are usually covered under either a separate Basic anesthesia benefit or under a Major Medical benefit. When processing claims, do not confuse the professional anesthesia expense with the charges that may appear on a hospital

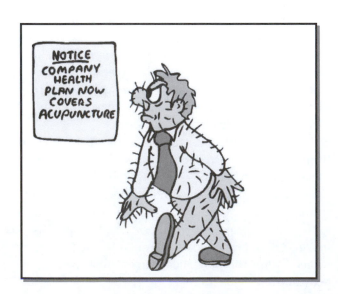

bill. The anesthesia charges on a hospital bill are for the actual anesthesia drug, the anesthesia machine, and other associated supplies.

Anesthesia may be administered by any of the following individuals:

Medical doctor (M.D.)

Anesthesiologist (Anes.)

Certified registered nurse anesthetist (CRNA)

Anesthetic assistant (AA)

## RVS Ground Rules

The American Society of Anesthesiologists developed a coding system which has been adopted by the *CPT*®. The CPT® code range for anesthesia is 00100–01999. The RVS uses 00100–01999 or 10000–69999 (same as surgery) for coding anesthetic services. Anesthesia unit values are listed in the *RVS* for procedures that require that anesthesia be administered by an anesthesiologist. Remember that local anesthesia is never allowable separately. Therefore, anesthesia benefits are those that are allowed on procedures that require more than a local anesthesia.

These units (for all schedules) are used when:

• The anesthesia is personally administered by a licensed physician, and

• The physician remains in constant attendance during the procedure for the sole purpose of administering and monitoring the anesthesia service.

## Basic/Base Units

The basic or base anesthesia units are designed to allow for the usual pre and postoperative care, the administration of anesthesia, and the administration of fluids or blood incident to the anesthesia or surgery. Usually monitoring services such as ECG, blood pressure oximetry, capnography, mass spectrometry, and monitoring of blood gases are also included in the basic value and should not be billed separately.

Remember that the surgical unit values include surgery, local infiltration, and digital block or topical anesthesia.

## Time Units

The length of time that a person is under anesthesia determines the amount of money that will be considered allowable for the procedure. Anesthesia time begins when the anesthesiologist starts to physically prepare the patient for the induction of anesthesia in the operat-

ing room area (or its equivalent). The time ends when the anesthesiologist is no longer in constant attendance, usually when the patient is ready for postoperative supervision.

There are two ways of calculating the anesthesia time, depending on individual payer guidelines:

**1.** Actual time.
**2.** Block time.

### Actual Time

Some carriers allow one time unit for each fifteen minutes, regardless of the amount of time a patient is under anesthesia. Any fractional portions of a fifteen minute block (i.e., five minutes) are calculated to the nearest tenth of a unit. Thus, each 1.5 minutes is worth 0.1 units.

### Block Time

For the first four hours, time units are computed by allowing 1.0 time unit for each 15 minutes. Or, if less than 15 minutes, 1.0 unit is allowed for spans between five and 15 minutes. After four hours, 1.0 unit is allowed for each 10 minutes. If less than 10 minutes, 1.0 unit is allowed for spans between five and 10 minutes. The reason for this is that the risks of injury or adverse effects significantly increase with time. Therefore, extra compensation is provided for extended anesthesia time.

For example, if the anesthesia time were 50 minutes, a total of 4.0 time units would be allowed (1.0 unit for every 15 minutes = 3.0 units, plus 1.0 unit for the additional five minutes). Therefore, the same number of units would be allowed for a 50-minute procedure, a 55-minute procedure, or a one-hour procedure. **Table 7–3** is an example of anesthesia Block Time units.

Many anesthesiologists bill time according to a military clock, that is, by a 24-hour standard. When using military time, do not worry about converting the time to a regular clock. The regular time is unimportant. Instead, concentrate only on determining the time units involved. For example:

**1.** Total time: 13:15 to 14:25
    13:15 to 14:15 = 1 hour = 4.0 units
    14:15 to 14:25 = <u>10 min = 1.0 unit</u>
                1 hr 10 min = 5.0 units
**2.** Total time: 15:20 to 18:25
    15:20 to 18:20 = 3 hours = 12.0 units
    18:20 to 18:25 = <u>5 min = 1.0 unit</u>
                3 hr 5 min = 13.0 units

| Anesthesia Time | Units of Occurrence |
|---|---|
| 5 min – 19 min | 1 unit |
| 20 – 34 min | 2 units |
| 35 min – 49 min | 3 units |
| 50 min – 1 hr 04 min | 4 units |
| 1 hr 5 min – 1 hr 19 min | 5 units |
| 1 hr 20 min – 1 hr 34 min | 6 units |
| 1 hr 35 min – 1 hr 49 min | 7 units |
| 1 hr 50 min – 2 hr 4 min | 8 units |
| 2 hr 5 min – 2 hr 19 min | 9 units |
| 2 hr 20 min – 2 hr 34 min | 10 units |
| 2 hr 35 min – 2 hr 49 min | 11 units |
| 2 hr 50 min – 3 hr 4 min | 12 units |
| 3 hr 5 min – 3 hr 19 min | 13 units |
| 3 hr 20 min – 3 hr 34 min | 14 units |
| 3 hr 35 min – 3 hr 49 min | 15 units |
| 3 hr 50 min – 4 hr 4 min | 16 units |
| 4 hr 5 min – 4 hr 14 min | 17 units |
| 4 hr 15 min – 4 hr 24 min | 18 units |
| 4 hr 25 min – 4 hr 34 min | 19 units |
| 4 hr 35 min – 4 hr 44 min | 20 units |
| 4 hr 45 min – 4 hr 54 min | 21 units |
| 4 hr 55 min – 5 hr 4 min | 22 units |

**Table 7–3 Example of Anesthesia Block Time Units**

**Exceptions:**

Time units are usually not allowed for the following procedures/situations:

- Regional anesthesia upper or lower extremity (01995).
- Daily management of epidural of subarachnoid drug administration (01996).
- Administration of epidural anesthesia for maternal delivery (62282).
- Anesthesia for patient of extreme age, under one year or over 70 years (99100).
- Anesthesia complicated by use of total body hypothermia (99116).
- Anesthesia complicated by use of controlled hypotension (99135).
- Anesthesia complicated by emergency conditions (99140).

These codes are normally paid at the base units multiplied by the conversion factor. No allowance is made for time units.

# On the Job Now

**Directions:** Answer the following questions without looking back at the material just covered. Write your answers in the space provided.

1. What are the anesthesia charges on a hospital bill for? _____
_____
_____

2. What four individuals are qualified to administer anesthesia?
   1. _____
   2. _____
   3. _____
   4. _____

3. When does anesthesia time begin and end? _____
_____
_____
_____
_____

# Calculating Anesthesia

The anesthesia allowance is calculated by adding the basic units to the time units and multiplying that amount by the conversion factor. This procedure applies to all schedules.

> Basic Unit Value for the procedure
> + Time Unit Value
> + Modifier Unit Value (if applicable)
> Total Anesthesia Value

Total Anesthesia Value × plan/Basic Conversion Factor = Anesthesia basic allowance or plan UCR.

## Multiple Procedures

For anesthesia claims with multiple procedures, the basic units for the major procedure (the procedure with the greatest number of basic units) are the only basic units allowed. The basic units for the secondary procedure are not taken into account. The additional expense is accommodated by allowing the extra time units necessitated for completion of the multiple procedures.

## Network Anesthesia

Carriers which pay different percentages for network and nonnetwork providers will often pay the anesthesiologist at the network rate if the chosen surgeon is a network provider, regardless of whether the anesthesiologist is a part of their network or not. This is because the surgeon usually chooses the anesthesiologist. Thus, the patient is not penalized for a choice they were not allowed to make.

# Modifiers

In addition to the modifiers listed above which denote who performed the services, some carriers use additional modifiers for anesthesia services.

**Physical status modifiers** are represented by the initial P, followed by a single digit from 1 to 6.

P1: A normal healthy patient

P2: A patient with mild systemic disease

P3: A patient with severe systemic disease

P4: A patient with severe systemic disease that is a constant threat to life

P5: A moribund patient who is not expected to survive without the operation

P6: A declared brain-dead patient whose organs are being removed for donor reasons

**Optional modifiers** denote special conditions. The following are the valid anesthesia two-digit modifier codes (for additional information, consult your $CPT^{®}$):

-22: Unusual services

-23: Unusual anesthesia

-32: Mandated services

-51: Multiple procedures, but not bilateral

Some carriers require that a modifier be used to identify who performed the anesthesia service, and the type of service. These modifiers are HCPCS Level II modifiers. The following modifier codes are used for this purpose:

AA: Anesthesia services performed by an anesthesiologist.

AD: Anesthesia was medically supervised by a physician for more than four concurrent procedures.

QK: Medically directed by a physician; two through four concurrent procedures.

QX: Anesthesia administered by a CRNA with medical direction by a physician.

QY: Medical direction on one CRNA by an anesthesiologist.

QZ: Anesthesia administered by a CRNA without medical direction by a physician.

## Unusual Circumstances

Occasionally the use of modifier -22 or -23 will indicate that unusual procedures were performed. This modifier is often used to explain why the amount of time shown on an anesthesia claim is greater than usual. **Unusual services** are services that are rarely provided, unusual, or variable and may warrant an additional anesthesia fee. These situations can include:

- Severe or multiple injuries.
- Procedures in the head, neck, or shoulder region which can disrupt the administration of anesthesia.
- Unusual or lengthy monitoring.
- Procedures where care must be taken to avoid certain areas of the body.
- Procedures or situations where the patient must be placed in an unusual position (i.e., sitting).

When processing these claims, the examiner should request a copy of the operative report, the hospital medical records, detailed records from the anesthesiologist regarding the services performed, and the length of time under anesthesia. These reports will provide information to determine if the correct code was billed by the anesthesiologist, or if additional complications were involved which could increase the amount of time the anesthesiologist was in attendance with the patient.

Some insurance carriers will allow an additional percentage for unusual services claims (i.e., an additional 25% benefit), and some will allow a specific amount of units (i.e., an additional three units is not uncommon). Additionally, there are a number of other carriers who do not allow any additional benefit. The rationale for not allowing more is that the additional time involved in the procedure is enough to compensate the anesthesiologist for the unusual services. Be sure to consult plan guidelines prior to processing claims with unusual services modifiers. Many of these claims may need to be referred for medical review.

## Qualifying Circumstances

Many anesthesia services are provided under particularly difficult circumstances, depending on factors such as extraordinary conditions of the patient, notable operative conditions, and unusual risk factors. This section includes a list of important qualifying circumstances that make a significant impact on the character of the anesthesia service provided. These procedures would not be reported alone, but as additional procedures qualifying an anesthesia procedure or service. More than one may be selected.

99100    Anesthesia for patient of extreme age, under one year or over 70 years.

99116    Anesthesia complicated by use of total body hypothermia.

99135    Anesthesia complicated by use of controlled hypotension.

99140    Anesthesia complicated by emergency conditions. Most plans require emergency conditions to be specified. Treatment is considered emergency treatment when its delay would lead to a significant increase in the threat to life or body part.

Many providers will allow additional units for qualifying circumstances.

### Example:

99100 – 1 additional unit
99116 – 5 additional units

99135 – 5 additional units
99140 – 2 additional units

## Examining Tips

Many insurance carriers will allow additional units for some modifiers.

### Example:

P1 – No additional value
P2 – No additional value
P3 – 1 additional unit
P4 – 2 additional units
P5 – 3 additional units
P6 – No additional units

# Monitored Anesthesia Care

**Monitored anesthesia care (MAC)** is the monitoring of a patient's vital signs during an operation in anticipation of the need for general anesthesia. This can be due to:

- The anticipation of an adverse physiological reaction by the patient to the procedure.
- Patients with low pain thresholds or who may experience intense pain.
- Expected expansion of the operative field (i.e., a mass is biopsied under a local anesthetic; however, if the surgeon locates additional tumors, more radical surgery would be done during the same operative session).
- Combative patients.
- Neonatal or pediatric patients who may become frightened or combative.
- Mentally impaired patients who may become uncooperative due to their impairment.
- The administration of drugs which are required to be administered by an anesthesiologist, even though they may not produce unconsciousness in a patient.

In order for an anesthesiologist to be reimbursed for MAC, the following services are required:

- Preoperative visit and evaluation, including medical history, anesthesia history, taking of medication information, and physical exam.

- Preoperative evaluation of all available pertinent reports (lab, x-ray, etc.).
- Patient discussion and informed consent.
- Monitoring of vital signs during the operative procedure, including oxygenation, ventilation, circulation, temperature, and maintenance of the patient's airway.
- Diagnosis and treatment of any clinical problems which occur during the procedure.
- Administration of medications or other agents to ensure patient safety and comfort during the procedure.
- Postoperative patient management, including evaluation of the patient, time based record of vital signs and level of consciousness, reporting of any complications, adverse reactions, or unusual events.
- Post anesthesia visits (as needed).
- A complete record of all drugs used and amounts.

In order for MAC to be reimbursed, the anesthesiologist must be present during the entire operative procedure. If all above requirements are met, a MAC anesthesiologist is reimbursed at the same amount as routine anesthesiology since the same level of attention and care is required.

The modifier -QS on the claim will denote that the claim is for MAC services.

# Medical Direction of Anesthesiology

At times, the actual monitoring of the patient will be performed by an anesthesia assistant or a Certified Registered Nurse Anesthetist (CRNA) under the direction of a physician. In such cases, the physician is responsible for:

- The preoperative evaluation of the patient.
- Ordering the drugs.
- Determining the anesthesia treatment plan.
- Handling or participating in the most demanding anesthesia procedures, including induction and emergence.
- Monitoring the course of anesthesia and the patient's situation at frequent intervals.
- Handling any emergency situations.
- Providing all postanesthesia care.

The assistant anesthesiologist or CRNA is responsible for:

- Understanding the anesthesia plan.
- The continuous administration of the anesthesia.
- Monitoring the patient's vitals.
- Remaining in contact with the physician and summoning her if needed.

This allows a directing physician to handle anesthesia for several patients at the same time. However, most payers limit the number of patients a physician may direct at one time to four or less.

In such cases, most carriers will split the anesthesiologist allowance to 50% for the directing physician and 50% for the assistant anesthesiologist or CRNA, provided the directing physician is not directing the care of more than four patients concurrently. If the physician is directing the care of more than four patients at a time, some payers will reduce reimbursement to 25% for the directing physician and 75% for the assistant anesthesiologist or CRNA. Others will consider the anesthesiologist's services to be supervisory. In other words, they are simply overseeing the work of the assistant anesthesiologist or CRNA, not directing their work. Reimbursement for supervisory anesthesiologists is often calculated at three base units per procedure. No time units are allowed, unless an anesthesiologist can document that they were present and attending during the induction of the anesthesia. If this can be documented, one time unit is allowed.

Anesthesiologists are required to certify the number of patients for whom concurrent care was handled at any given time during the operative session.

# Pain Control

Occasionally an anesthesiologist may be called upon to perform services to ease intractable or chronic pain. **Intractable pain** is pain which is hard to manage and is often severe enough to limit a patient's movement or abilities.

In such cases, relief may be obtained through an injection or intravenous infusion of pain medication.

Many insurance carriers will allow payment for these services if certain conditions are met, as follows:

- The pain cannot be managed through other means (i.e., oral or traditional pain medications).
- The pain is severe enough that it interferes with daily living.

- A complete medical evaluation has been performed to asses the source of the pain.
- All other reasonable medical treatments (including psychological approaches) were considered or tried and found to be unsuccessful or potentially harmful.
- Electrical stimulation (TENS) was found to be unsuccessful.
- Pharmacological or physical therapy programs were found to be unsuccessful or potentially harmful.

Often block treatments for intractable pain are limited to three per year. Medical records should be requested to evaluate the success of the treatment. These cases will often need to be referred for review.

## Patient Controlled Anesthesia

Some conditions allow the patient to administer their own pain medication (or anesthetic). This is often done through an **infusion pump**. This is a machine which contains medication and administers a small dose when a button is depressed. The machine is attached to the outside of the body, with a line running into a vein (for intravenous medications) or under the skin (for subcutaneous medications). Safeguards on the machine prevent an overdose and prevent a second dose from being administered before a first dose has had a chance to take effect.

Infusion pumps have been shown to provide equal or better pain relief with a lower overall dosage level.

Many carriers will allow benefits for the placement and use of an infusion pump if all of the following criteria are met:

- The unit and pain medication are prescribed by a licensed physician.
- The medical condition being treated is a covered expense.
- The medical condition being treated requires long-term pain control.

- The pain is manageable by pharmacological means and no other pain control (or very limited additional pain control) is necessary.
- The unit is used in a hospital setting, or, if used in a home setting, the use is monitored by an RN on a regular basis.

As with many other new forms of anesthesia, plan guidelines vary widely. Be sure to check contract provisions before processing infusion pump claims. If the plan does allow for payment, there will often be separate charges for the infusion pump, professional charges for the placement of the infusion pump, and charges for the medications to be placed in the infusion pump.

## Miscellaneous

Epidural anesthesia is often provided during labor for normal deliveries. Time of administration tends to run four or more hours. Some administrators provide their own rules, and some plans do not cover anesthesia during labor at all. Therefore, verify the guidelines that apply to the plan you are processing.

General anesthesia is usually administered when shock therapy is provided. Many plans do not cover it for this purpose or may have special handling guidelines. Verify before processing.

A standby anesthetist may be asked to be available while diagnostic procedures are performed on a patient who may require emergency surgery. If the anesthesiologist is not rendering treatment, administering anesthesia, monitoring vital signs, etc., but is merely making a charge for being available, the charge is usually not a covered expense. However, verify first before processing.

If surgery is cancelled for medical reasons prior to the surgery, the anesthesiologist may be allowed reimbursement for evaluation and management. In such cases, an E&M code should be used. Full documentation of the reason for the cancellation of surgery should be included with the claim.

# CHAPTER REVIEW

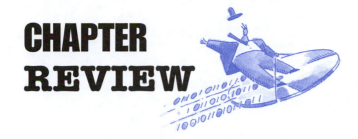

## Summary

- Surgery charges may be the most complicated charges you will encounter. That is why there are so many guidelines covering surgery, multiple surgery, assistant surgery, and cosmetic surgery. If for any reason you are unsure, request the medical opinion of a senior examiner or technical person.

- The use of an assistant surgeon always depends on the medical necessity of the procedure performed.

- The charges for podiatry services vary from simple to complex.

- Because podiatry surgery guidelines vary from company to company, check with the administrator before processing these types of claims.

- Anesthesia plays an important role in patient care. Anesthesia in certain situations has been shown to help the patient recover more rapidly than if anesthesia were not used.

- The guidelines we have just covered will enable you to process anesthesia charges no matter what method or type of anesthesia is administered.

- There is almost always an anesthesia charge when major surgery is performed, and you as the claims examiner are responsible for processing these charges.

- Use the preceding guidelines to calculate anesthesia time and to identify the provider of services (anesthesiologist, nurse anesthetist, or surgeon).

## Assignments

Complete the Questions for Review.
Complete Exercises 7–1 through 7–12.

## Questions for Review

**Directions:** Answer the following questions without looking back at the material just covered. Write your answers in the space provided.

1. Define surgery. _____

_____

2. Are cosmetic surgical procedures usually covered by benefit plans? _____

3. What are the four types of surgical procedures? (List and define.)

1. _____

_____

2. _____

_____

3. _____

_____

4. _____

_____

4. What does the physician's charge for surgery performed in the office generally include? _____

_____

5. Identify two situations that would warrant separate payment for preoperative care.

_____

_____

6. What does the surgical unit value include? _____

_____

7. When is the follow-up care allowed separately? _____

_____

8. What are cosurgeons? _____

_____

9. What are By Report procedures and what other term may be used to indicate these procedures? _____

_____

10. What services are normally provided in maternity cases? _____

_____

11. What is podiatric surgery? _____

_____

12. Define ligaments. _____

_____

13. How many complex joints are in the foot? _____

14. How many bunion surgeries are normally allowed per foot? _____

15. What is an orthotic device? _____

_____

**16.** What are the four methods of anesthesia administration?

1. _____

2. _____

3. _____

4. _____

**17.** What is the ASA code range for anesthesia? _____

**18.** What is the RVS code range for anesthesia? _____

**19.** The total anesthesia unit values consist of _____ and _____ units.

**20.** (True or False?) Most plans cover anesthesia for shock therapy. _____

If you were unable to answer any of these questions, refer back to that section and then fill in the answers.

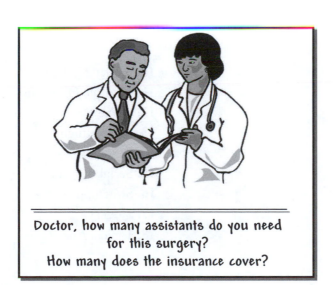

Doctor, how many assistants do you need
for this surgery?
How many does the insurance cover?

# Exercise 7-1

**Directions:** Find and circle the words listed below. Words can appear horizontally, vertically, diagonally, forward, or backward.

```
Y V M N R O P V V J P E R K N S I S Q T O H
P M K U I E C M C I J Q C I T C E X S O T Y
L G O W L H C R U J D O W R F C P E Q P P P
A N L T W T U O O P L S U I I X R U T I N N
N I U T O A I K N B N C G V P I Z W X C I O
T Q D F Z E Q P E S T O R X A U R B C A A S
A C M Z L Q T L L U T E I L C R M W X L P I
R Y L P X K D S R E S R S S V H L I W A E S
C D L D H D U A O L P U U P U Z A O I N L E
A U Y Z A R L Y A L R R M C N F N M L E B R
L T X S G B P U K G A P O S T W N Y L S A U
L C E E U T S X E F T S N C B I O I O T T T
U V R N G U X R X A L F R B E K O K U H C C
S Y I Y N I Y Q J N W J K O Y D E N Z E A N
A O M U H A M M E R T O E S D R U W H S R U
N S E R U D E C O R P K C O L B E R E I T P
S Y A D P U W O L L O F F Q H P A P E A N U
B S H E C L C F Y F X L M B C V S P O S I C
E Z M T N P P U V Z Y K D W F H T M L R U A
Y W E V I Q R D X M N S B N F O F M I A T K
N E R V E B L O C K A N E S T H E S I A R M
G L O B A L A P P R O A C H X G Z E K H L J
```

1. Unusual Services
2. Block Procedures
3. By Report
4. Dorsal Osteotomy
5. Follow Up Days
6. Global Approach
7. Hammertoes
8. Hypnosis
9. Infusion Pump

10. Intractable Pain
11. Mulitple Procedures
12. Nerve Block Anesthesia
13. Reconstruction
14. Saddle Block
15. Serial Surgery
16. Structural Bunion
17. Surgery
18. Topical Anesthesia

# Exercise 7-2

**Directions:** Complete the crossword puzzle by filling in a word from the keywords that fits each clue.

**Across**

7. Surgeries that involve a pair of similar body parts.
11. An overgrowth on the heel bone.
18. A surgical procedure performed solely to improve appearance.
19. An imbalance of muscles and nerves and is often inherited.
20. Flexible bands of fiber joining bone to bone.
21. A contagious growth caused by a virus.

**Down**

1. Anesthesia that affects only a localized area.
2. Denote special conditions. For additional information consult your *CPT*®.
3. A procedure in which a portion of the joint is surgically removed and the toe is straightened.

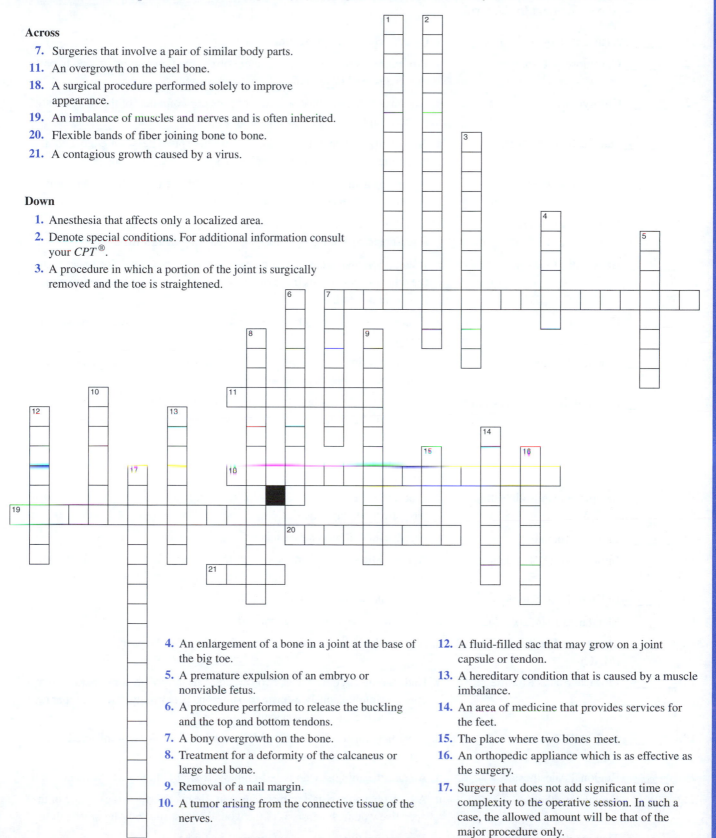

4. An enlargement of a bone in a joint at the base of the big toe.
5. A premature expulsion of an embryo or nonviable fetus.
6. A procedure performed to release the buckling and the top and bottom tendons.
7. A bony overgrowth on the bone.
8. Treatment for a deformity of the calcaneus or large heel bone.
9. Removal of a nail margin.
10. A tumor arising from the connective tissue of the nerves.

12. A fluid-filled sac that may grow on a joint capsule or tendon.
13. A hereditary condition that is caused by a muscle imbalance.
14. An area of medicine that provides services for the feet.
15. The place where two bones meet.
16. An orthopedic appliance which is as effective as the surgery.
17. Surgery that does not add significant time or complexity to the operative session. In such a case, the allowed amount will be that of the major procedure only.

# Exercise 7-3

**Directions:** Match the following terms with the proper definition by writing the letter of the correct definition in the space next to the term.

1. _____ Assistant Surgeon

2. _____ Chromosomal Analysis

3. _____ Cosurgeons

4. _____ Diagnostic Procedures

5. _____ Endogenous Obesity

6. _____ Epidural Anesthesia

7. _____ Exogenous Obesity

8. _____ False Nail

9. _____ General Anesthesia

10. _____ Hospital Staff Anesthesiologist

11. _____ In Vitro Fertilization

12. _____ Independent Anesthesiologist

13. _____ Ingrown Toenail

14. _____ Intravenous (IV) Sedation

15. _____ In Utero Fetal Surgery

16. _____ Metatarsal Plantar Callus

17. _____ Monitored Anesthesia Care (MAC)

18. _____ Physical Status Modifiers

19. _____ Positional Bunion

20. _____ Regional Anesthesia

21. _____ Spinal Anesthesia

22. _____ Therapeutic Procedures

a. Obesity caused by overeating.

b. Procedures performed to remove or correct the functioning of a body part that is diseased or injured.

c. Anesthesia that produces the loss of sensation of a part of the body due to the interruption of nerve conduction.

d. A specialized type of nerve block where the spinal nerves are blocked in either the subarachnoid or the epidural space.

e. A bony growth on the side of the metatarsal bone that enlarges the joint, forcing the joint capsule to stretch over it.

f. Modifiers that are used to indicate various physical conditions and are represented by the initial P, followed by a single digit from 1 to 6.

g. A condition that occurs when the metatarsal bone is longer or lower than the others so that it hits the ground first at every step with more force than it is equipped to handle.

h. A nail where one or both corners or sides of the nail grow into the skin of the toe.

i. The monitoring of a patient's vital signs during an operation in anticipation of the need for a general anesthesia.

j. Surgery on a fetus while it is in the mother's womb; and also to remove the fetus from the womb, perform surgery, and return it back to the womb, with the pregnancy continuing to term.

k. Obesity caused by an internal malfunction, usually hormonal (i.e., thyroid disorder).

l. Procedures performed to determine the presence of disease or the cause of the patient's symptoms.

m. Anesthesia that produces a state of unconsciousness.

n. A diagnostic study performed on the fluid to study the number and structure of the chromosomes to determine whether any abnormalities are present.

o. An anesthesiologist employed by the hospital.

p. A tough skin that mimics a real nail.

q. Anesthesia which blocks the nerves in the epidural space.

r. Under some circumstances, two surgeons, usually with similar skills, may operate simultaneously as primary surgeons performing distinct, separate parts of a total surgical service.

s. A medication composed of a sedative and a painkiller administered intravenously. A semiconscious state is produced.

t. An anesthesiologist who is self-employed or not employed by the hospital.

u. A surgeon who assists a primary surgeon. He may perform the closing of the operative wound, hemostasis of the wound edges, and suturing of vessels.

v. The fertilization of the ovum within a test tube.

# Exercises **7-4** through **7-12**

**Directions:** Process on a Payment Worksheet each of the surgery, assistant surgery, and anesthesia service claims found on the following pages. Refer to Appendices A, B, and C for contracts and additional information.

   When processing the multiple surgery claims exercises use the global UCR processing guidelines when computing UCR. All insureds are eligible for coverage under their respective plans. Amounts paid for each claim throughout this book should be accumulated and carried forward to subsequent claims.

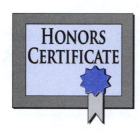

## Honors Certification[TM]

The Honors Certification[TM] challenge for this chapter consists of a written test of the information in this chapter. Additionally you will be given nine claims to process, using the contracts contained in this book. Each incorrect answer will result in a deduction of up to 5% from your grade. You must achieve a score of 80% or higher to pass this test. If you fail the test on your first attempt, you may retake the test one additional time. The items included in the second test may be different from those in the first test.

PLEASE
DO NOT
STAPLE
IN THIS
AREA

□□□ PICA

ROVER INSURERS INC
5931 ROLLING ROAD
RONSON CO 81369

APPROVED MOB-0938-0008

# HEALTH INSURANCE CLAIM FORM

PICA □□□

| 1. | MEDICARE | MEDICAID | CHAMPUS | CHAMPVA | GROUP HEALTH PLAN | FECA BLK LUNG | OTHER | 1a. INSURED'S I.D NUMBER (FOR PROGRAM IN ITEM 1) |
|---|---|---|---|---|---|---|---|---|
| | ☐ (Medicare #) | ☐ (Medicaid #) | ☐ (Sponsor's SSN) | ☐ (VA File #) | ☒ (SSN or ID) | ☐ (SSN) | ☐ (ID) | 999 99 NIN |

| 2. PATIENT'S NAME (Last, First, Middle Initial). | 3. PATIENT'S BIRTH DATE | 4. INSURED'S NAME (Last, First, Middle Initial) |
|---|---|---|
| BOSSY BETTY B | MM 09 DD 19 YY CCYY-47  SEX M ☐ F ☒ | SAME |

| 5. PATIENT'S ADDRESS (No., Street) | 6. PATIENT'S RELATIONSHIP TO INSURED | 7. INSURED'S ADDRESS (No., Street) |
|---|---|---|
| 7991 BAGEL BLVD | Self ☒  Spouse ☐  Child ☐  Other ☐ | |

| CITY | STATE | 8. PATIENT STATUS | CITY | STATE |
|---|---|---|---|---|
| BARSTOW | NY | Single ☐  Married ☒  Other ☐ | | |

| ZIP CODE | TELEPHONE (Include Area Code) | | ZIP CODE | TELEPHONE (INCLUDE AREA CODE) |
|---|---|---|---|---|
| 10012 | (914) 555 3399 | Employed ☒  Full-Time Student ☐  Part-Time Student ☐ | | |

| 9. OTHER INSURED'S NAME (Last, First, Middle Initial) | 10. IS PATIENT'S CONDITION RELATED TO: | 11. INSURED'S POLICY GROUP OR FECA NUMBER |
|---|---|---|
| | | 21088NIN |

| a. OTHER INSURED'S POLICY OR GROUP NUMBER | a. EMPLOYMENT? (CURRENT OR PREVIOUS) ☐ YES ☒ NO | a. INSURED'S DATE OF BIRTH  MM DD YY  SEX M ☐ F ☐ |
|---|---|---|

| b. OTHER INSURED'S DATE OF BIRTH  MM DD YY  SEX M ☐ F ☐ | b. AUTO ACCIDENT?  PLACE (State) ☐ YES ☒ NO | b. EMPLOYER'S NAME OR SCHOOL NAME  NINJA CORPORATION |
|---|---|---|

| c. EMPLOYER'S NAME OR SCHOOL NAME | c. OTHER ACCIDENT? ☐ YES ☒ NO | c. INSURANCE PLAN NAME OR PROGRAM NAME  ROVER INSURERS INC |
|---|---|---|

| d. INSURANCE PLAN NAME OR PROGRAM NAME | 10d. RESERVED FOR LOCAL USE | d. IS THERE ANOTHER HEALTH BENEFIT PLAN? ☐ YES ☒ NO  if yes, return to and complete item 9 a-d |
|---|---|---|

READ BACK OF FORM BEFORE COMPLETING & SIGNING THIS FORM

12. PATIENT'S OR AUTHORIZED PERSON'S SIGNATURE I authorize the release of any medical or other information necessary to process this claim. I also request payment of government benefits either to myself or to the party who accepts assignment below.

SIGNED **SIGNATURE ON FILE** DATE

13. INSURED'S OR AUTHORIZED PERSON'S SIGNATURE I authorize payment of medical benefits to the undersigned physician or supplier for services described below.

SIGNED **SIGNATURE ON FILE**

| 14. DATE OF CURRENT: ◄ ILLNESS (1st symptom) ◄ INJURY (Accident) PREGNANCY (LMP)  MM 02 DD 06 YY YY | 15. IF PATIENT HAS HAD SAME OR SIMILAR ILLNESS, GIVE FIRST DATE  MM DD YY | 16. DATES PATIENT UNABLE TO WORK IN CURRENT OCCUPATION  MM DD YY  MM DD YY  FROM   TO |
|---|---|---|

| 17. NAME OF REFERRING PHYSICIAN OR OTHER SOURCE | 17a. I.D. NUMBER OF REFERRING PHYSICIAN | 18. HOSPITALIZATION DATES RELATED TO CURRENT SERVICES  MM DD YY  MM DD YY  FROM 02 06 YY  TO 02 14 YY |
|---|---|---|

| 19. RESERVED FOR LOCAL USE | 20. OUTSIDE LAB? ☐ YES ☐ NO  $ CHARGES |
|---|---|

| 21. DIAGNOSIS OR NATURE OF ILLNESS OR INJURY, (RELATE ITEMS 1,2,3, OR 4 TO ITEM 24E BY LINE) | 22. MEDICAID RESUBMISSION CODE  ORIGINAL REF. NO. |
|---|---|
| 1. 410 .91    3. ___ . ___ | |
| 2. ___ . ___    4. ___ . ___ | 23. PRIOR AUTHORIZATION NUMBER |

| 24. A. DATE(S) OF SERVICE | | | | | | B. Place of Service | C. Type of Service | D. PROCEDURES, SERVICES, OR SUPPLIES (Explain Unusual Circumstances) | | E. DIAGNOSIS CODE | F. $ CHARGES | | G. DAYS OR UNITS | H. EPSDT Family Plan | I. EMG | J. COB | K. RESERVED FOR LOCAL USE |
|---|---|---|---|---|---|---|---|---|---|---|---|---|---|---|---|---|---|
| From | | | To | | | | | CPT/HCPS | MODIFIER | | | | | | | | |
| MM | DD | YY | MM | DD | YY | | | | | | | | | | | | |
| 02 | 06 | YY | 02 | 06 | YY | 21 | 1 | 33217 | -51 | 1 | 245 | 00 | 1 | | | | |
| 02 | 06 | YY | 02 | 06 | YY | 21 | 1 | 33225 | | 1 | 500 | 00 | 1 | | | | |
| 02 | 06 | YY | 02 | 06 | YY | 21 | 1 | 33240 | -51 | 1 | 295 | 00 | 1 | | | | |

| 25. FEDERAL TAX I.D. NUMBER  SSN EIN | 26. PATIENT'S ACCOUNT NO. | 27. ACCEPT ASSIGNMENT? (For govt. claims, see back) | 28. TOTAL CHARGE | 29. AMOUNT PAID | 30. BALANCE DUE |
|---|---|---|---|---|---|
| 70-0089773  ☐ ☒ | 001   939 | ☒ YES ☐ NO | $ 1040 00 | $ 0 00 | $ 1040 00 |

| 31. SIGNATURE OF PHYSICIAN OR SUPPLIER INCLUDING DEGREES OR CREDENTIALS (I certify that the statements on the reverse apply to this bill and are made a part thereof.)  SIGNED *Abe Domin MD* DATE 02/11/YY | 32. NAME AND ADDRESS OF FACILITY WHERE SERVICES WERE RENDERED (If other than home or office)  HEADACHE HOSPITAL  2000 HAZARD STREET  HELP NY 12899 | 33. PHYSICIAN'S, SUPPLIERS BILLING NAME, ADDRESS, ZIP CODE & PHONE #  ABE DOMIN MD   NETWORK PROVIDER  9909 DATEWAY DRIVE STE 9A  DOVE NY 12899  (914) 555 5199  PIN# A21212   GRP# |
|---|---|---|

(APPROVED BY AMA COUNCIL ON MEDICAL SERVICE 8/88)   **PLEASE PRINT OR TYPE**

FORM CMS-1500  (12-90)
FORM OWCP-1500   FORM RRB-1500
FORM AMA-OP050591

**Exercise 7–4**

PLEASE DO NOT STAPLE IN THIS AREA

WINTER INSURANCE CO
9763 WESTERN WAY
WHITTIER CO  82963

APPROVED MOB-0938-0008

□□□ PICA

# HEALTH INSURANCE CLAIM FORM

PICA □□□

| 1. | MEDICARE | MEDICAID | CHAMPUS | CHAMPVA | GROUP HEALTH PLAN | FECA BLK LUNG | OTHER | 1a. INSURED'S I.D NUMBER (FOR PROGRAM IN ITEM 1) |
|---|---|---|---|---|---|---|---|---|
| | ☐ (Medicare #) | ☐ (Medicaid #) | ☐ (Sponsor's SSN) | ☐ (VA File #) | ☒ (SSN or ID) | ☐ (SSN) | ☐ (ID) | 444 44 ABC |

| 2. PATIENT'S NAME (Last, First, Middle Initial). | 3. PATIENT'S BIRTH DATE | 4. INSURED'S NAME (Last, First, Middle Initial) |
|---|---|---|
| DINGBAT DANNY D | MM 04  DD 24  YY CCYY-10   M ☒  F ☐ | DINGBAT DANA D |

| 5. PATIENT'S ADDRESS (No., Street) | 6. PATIENT'S RELATIONSHIP TO INSURED | 7. INSURED'S ADDRESS (No., Street) |
|---|---|---|
| 404 DOORWAY DRIVE | Self ☐  Spouse ☐  Child ☒  Other ☐ | SAME |

| CITY | STATE | 8. PATIENT STATUS | CITY | STATE |
|---|---|---|---|---|
| DENVER | ND | Single ☒  Married ☐  Other ☐ | | |

| ZIP CODE | TELEPHONE (Include Area Code) | | ZIP CODE | TELEPHONE (INCLUDE AREA CODE) |
|---|---|---|---|---|
| 58444 | (701) 555 3344 | Employed ☐  Full-Time Student ☒  Part-Time Student ☐ | | |

| 9. OTHER INSURED'S NAME (Last, First, Middle Initial) | 10. IS PATIENT'S CONDITION RELATED TO: | 11. INSURED'S POLICY GROUP OR FECA NUMBER: |
|---|---|---|
| | | 36928ABC |

| a. OTHER INSURED'S POLICY OR GROUP NUMBER | a. EMPLOYMENT? (CURRENT OR PREVIOUS) ☐ YES  ☒ NO | a. INSURED'S DATE OF BIRTH  MM 04  DD 04  YY CCYY -37   M ☐  F ☒ |
|---|---|---|

| b. OTHER INSURED'S DATE OF BIRTH  MM  DD  YY   SEX  M ☐  F ☐ | b. AUTO ACCIDENT?  PLACE (State)  ☐ YES  ☒ NO | b. EMPLOYER'S NAME OR SCHOOL NAME  ABC CORPORATION |
|---|---|---|

| c. EMPLOYER'S NAME OR SCHOOL NAME | c. OTHER ACCIDENT?  ☒ YES  ☐ NO | c. INSURANCE PLAN NAME OR PROGRAM NAME  WINTER INSURANCE COMPANY |
|---|---|---|

| d. INSURANCE PLAN NAME OR PROGRAM NAME | 10d. RESERVED FOR LOCAL USE | d. IS THERE ANOTHER HEALTH BENEFIT PLAN?  ☐ YES  ☒ NO  *if yes*, return to and complete item 9 a-d |
|---|---|---|

READ BACK OF FORM BEFORE COMPLETING & SIGNING THIS FORM

12. PATIENT'S OR AUTHORIZED PERSON'S SIGNATURE I authorize the release of any medical or other information necessary to process this claim. I also request payment of government benefits either to myself or to the party who accepts assignment below.

SIGNED  SIGNATURE ON FILE            DATE _____

13. INSURED'S OR AUTHORIZED PERSON'S SIGNATURE I authorize payment of medical benefits to the undersigned physician or supplier for services described below.

SIGNED  SIGNATURE ON FILE

| 14. DATE OF CURRENT:  ILLNESS (1st symptom)  INJURY (Accident)  PREGNANCY (LMP)  MM 01  DD 26  YY | 15. IF PATIENT HAS HAD SAME OR SIMILAR ILLNESS, GIVE FIRST DATE  MM  DD  YY | 16. DATES PATIENT UNABLE TO WORK IN CURRENT OCCUPATION  MM  DD  YY  MM  DD  YY  FROM  TO |
|---|---|---|

| 17. NAME OF REFERRING PHYSICIAN OR OTHER SOURCE | 17a. I.D. NUMBER OF REFERRING PHYSICIAN | 18. HOSPITALIZATION DATES RELATED TO CURRENT SERVICES  MM 01  DD 26  YY  MM 02  DD 08  YY  FROM  TO |
|---|---|---|

| 19. RESERVED FOR LOCAL USE | 20. OUTSIDE LAB?  ☐ YES  ☐ NO  $ CHARGES |
|---|---|

21. DIAGNOSIS OR NATURE OF ILLNESS OR INJURY, (RELATE ITEMS 1,2,3, OR 4 TO ITEM 24E BY LINE)

1. | 807 . 01
2. | 823 . 32
3. | 800 . 40
4. | E884 . 9

| 22. MEDICAID RESUBMISSION  CODE  ORIGINAL REF. NO. |
|---|
| 23. PRIOR AUTHORIZATION NUMBER |

| 24. A. DATE(S) OF SERVICE |  |  |  |  |  | B. Place of Service | C. Type of Service | D. PROCEDURES, SERVICES, OR SUPPLIES (Explain Unusual Circumstances)  CPT/HCPS  MODIFIER | | E. DIAGNOSIS CODE | F. $ CHARGES | G. DAYS OR UNITS | H. EPSDT Family Plan | I. EMG | J. COB | K. RESERVED FOR LOCAL USE |
|---|---|---|---|---|---|---|---|---|---|---|---|---|---|---|---|---|
| From MM | DD | YY | To MM | DD | YY | | | | | | | | | | | |
| 01 | 26 | YY | 01 | 26 | YY | 21 | 1 | 21800 | | 1 4 | 560 00 | 1 | | Y | | |
| 01 | 26 | YY | 01 | 26 | YY | 21 | 1 | 27758 | -51 | 2 4 | 215 00 | 1 | | Y | | |
| 01 | 26 | YY | 01 | 26 | YY | 21 | 1 | 27784 | -51 | 2 4 | 200 00 | 1 | | Y | | |
| 01 | 26 | YY | 01 | 26 | YY | 21 | 1 | 62000 | -51 | 3 4 | 150 00 | 1 | | Y | | |

| 25. FEDERAL TAX I.D. NUMBER  SSN EIN | 26. PATIENT'S ACCOUNT NO. | 27. ACCEPT ASSIGNMENT? (For govt. claims, see back) | 28. TOTAL CHARGE | 29. AMOUNT PAID | 30. BALANCE DUE |
|---|---|---|---|---|---|
| 70-2883888  ☐ ☒ | 001  434 | ☒ YES  ☐ NO | $ 1125 00 | $  0 00 | $ 1125 00 |

| 31. SIGNATURE OF PHYSICIAN OR SUPPLIER INCLUDING DEGREES OR CREDENTIALS (I certify that the statements on the reverse apply to this bill and are made a part thereof.)  SIGNED *Ray Machine MD*  DATE 02/08/YY | 32. NAME AND ADDRESS OF FACILITY WHERE SERVICES WERE RENDERED (If other than home or office)  HACKIM HOSPITAL  1000 HIDE STREET  HUSHTOWN ND 58444 | 33. PHYSICIAN'S, SUPPLIERS BILLING NAME, ADDRESS, ZIP CODE & PHONE #  RAY MACHINE MD  4044 ROOMER ROAD STE 4R  ROLLER ND 58444  (701) 555 1144  PIN# I78904   GRP# |
|---|---|---|

(APPROVED BY AMA COUNCIL ON MEDICAL SERVICE 8/88)   **PLEASE PRINT OR TYPE**

FORM CMS-1500  (12-90)
FORM OWCP-1500    FORM RRB-1500
FORM AMA-OP050591

**Exercise 7–5**

PLEASE DO NOT STAPLE IN THIS AREA

□□□ PICA

BALL INSURANCE CARRIERS
3895 BUBBLE BLVD STE 283
BOXWOOD CO 85926

APPROVED MOB-0938-0008

# HEALTH INSURANCE CLAIM FORM

PICA □□□

| 1. | MEDICARE | MEDICAID | CHAMPUS | CHAMPVA | GROUP HEALTH PLAN | FECA BLK LUNG | OTHER | 1a. INSURED'S I.D NUMBER | (FOR PROGRAM IN ITEM 1) |
|---|---|---|---|---|---|---|---|---|---|
| | ☐ (Medicare #) | ☐ (Medicaid #) | ☐ (Sponsor's SSN) | ☐ (VA File #) | ☒ (SSN or ID) | ☐ (SSN) | ☐ (ID) | 555 55 XYZ | |

**2. PATIENT'S NAME (Last, First, Middle Initial).**
PATIENT PATTY P

**3. PATIENT'S BIRTH DATE**
MM 05 DD 15 YY CCYY -35 SEX M ☐ F ☒

**4. INSURED'S NAME (Last, First, Middle Initial)**
SAME

**5. PATIENT'S ADDRESS (No., Street)**
655 PAIN LANE

**6. PATIENT'S RELATIONSHIP TO INSURED**
Self ☒ Spouse ☐ Child ☐ Other ☐

**7. INSURED'S ADDRESS (No., Street)**

CITY PEN   STATE PA

**8. PATIENT STATUS**
Single ☒ Married ☐ Other ☐
Employed ☒ Full-Time Student ☐ Part-Time Student ☐

CITY   STATE

ZIP CODE 15522   TELEPHONE (Include Area Code) (878) 555 3355

ZIP CODE   TELEPHONE (INCLUDE AREA CODE)

**9. OTHER INSURED'S NAME (Last, First, Middle Initial)**

**10. IS PATIENT'S CONDITION RELATED TO:**

**11. INSURED'S POLICY GROUP OR FECA NUMBER:**
62958XYZ

**a. OTHER INSURED'S POLICY OR GROUP NUMBER**

**a. EMPLOYMENT? (CURRENT OR PREVIOUS)**
☐ YES ☒ NO

**a. INSURED'S DATE OF BIRTH**
MM DD YY SEX M ☐ F ☐

**b. OTHER INSURED'S DATE OF BIRTH**
MM DD YY SEX M ☐ F ☐

**b. AUTO ACCIDENT?** PLACE (State)
☐ YES ☒ NO |_____|

**b. EMPLOYER'S NAME OR SCHOOL NAME**
XYZ CORPORATION

**c. EMPLOYER'S NAME OR SCHOOL NAME**

**c. OTHER ACCIDENT?**
☐ YES ☒ NO

**c. INSURANCE PLAN NAME OR PROGRAM NAME**
BALL INSURANCE CARRIERS

**d. INSURANCE PLAN NAME OR PROGRAM NAME**

**10d. RESERVED FOR LOCAL USE**

**d. IS THERE ANOTHER HEALTH BENEFIT PLAN?**
☐ YES ☒ NO   *if yes*, return to and complete item 9 a-d

READ BACK OF FORM BEFORE COMPLETING & SIGNING THIS FORM

**12. PATIENT'S OR AUTHORIZED PERSON'S SIGNATURE** I authorize the release of any medical or other information necessary to process this claim. I also request payment of government benefits either to myself or to the party who accepts assignment below.

SIGNED **SIGNATURE ON FILE**   DATE

**13. INSURED'S OR AUTHORIZED PERSON'S SIGNATURE** I authorize payment of medical benefits to the undersigned physician or supplier for services described below.

SIGNED **SIGNATURE ON FILE**

**14. DATE OF CURRENT:** ◄ ILLNESS (1st symptom) ◄ INJURY (Accident) PREGNANCY (LMP)
MM 02 DD 02 YY YY

**15. IF PATIENT HAS HAD SAME OR SIMILAR ILLNESS, GIVE FIRST DATE** MM DD YY

**16. DATES PATIENT UNABLE TO WORK IN CURRENT OCCUPATION**
MM DD YY   MM DD YY
FROM   TO

**17. NAME OF REFERRING PHYSICIAN OR OTHER SOURCE**

**17a. I.D. NUMBER OF REFERRING PHYSICIAN**

**18. HOSPITALIZATION DATES RELATED TO CURRENT SERVICES**
MM DD YY   MM DD YY
FROM 02 16 YY TO 02 16 YY

**19. RESERVED FOR LOCAL USE**

**20. OUTSIDE LAB?**   $ CHARGES
☐ YES ☐ NO

**21. DIAGNOSIS OR NATURE OF ILLNESS OR INJURY, (RELATE ITEMS 1,2,3, OR 4 TO ITEM 24E BY LINE)**

1. |___233__.0___  3. |_____.____
2. |_____.____  4. |_____.____

**22. MEDICAID RESUBMISSION CODE**   ORIGINAL REF. NO.

**23. PRIOR AUTHORIZATION NUMBER**

| 24. A DATE(S) OF SERVICE From | | | To | | | B Place of Service | C Type of Service | D PROCEDURES, SERVICES, OR SUPPLIES (Explain Unusual Circumstances) CPT/HCPS | MODIFIER | E DIAGNOSIS CODE | F $ CHARGES | G DAYS OR UNITS | H EPSDT Family Plan | I EMG | J COB | K RESERVED FOR LOCAL USE |
|---|---|---|---|---|---|---|---|---|---|---|---|---|---|---|---|---|
| MM | DD | YY | MM | DD | YY | | | | | | | | | | | |
| 02 | 16 | YY | 02 | 16 | YY | 22 | 1 | 19125 | -51 | 1 | 360 00 | 1 | | | | |
| 02 | 16 | YY | 02 | 16 | YY | 22 | 1 | 19126 | | 1 | 740 00 | 4 | | | | |
| | | | | | | | | | | | | | | | | |
| | | | | | | | | | | | | | | | | |
| | | | | | | | | | | | | | | | | |
| | | | | | | | | | | | | | | | | |

**25. FEDERAL TAX I.D. NUMBER** SSN ☐ EIN ☒
70-1312131

**26. PATIENT'S ACCOUNT NO**
001   535

**27. ACCEPT ASSIGNMENT?** (For govt. claims, see back)
☐ YES ☒ NO

**28. TOTAL CHARGE**
$ 1100 00

**29. AMOUNT PAID**
$ 0 00

**30. BALANCE DUE**
$ 1100 00

**31. SIGNATURE OF PHYSICIAN OR SUPPLIER INCLUDING DEGREES OR CREDENTIALS** (I certify that the statements on the reverse apply to this bill and are made a part thereof.)

SIGNED *Sam A Piller MD* DATE 03/01/YY

**32. NAME AND ADDRESS OF FACILITY WHERE SERVICES WERE RENDERED** (If other than home or office)
HELPER HOSPITAL
25450 HAMMER AVE
HUMMER TOWN PA 15522

**33. PHYSICIAN'S, SUPPLIERS BILLING NAME, ADDRESS, ZIP CODE & PHONE #**
SAM A PILLER MD
155 SOFT AVENUE STE 505P
SUMMER VILLE PA 15522
(878) 555 0055
PIN# J48748   GRP#

(APPROVED BY AMA COUNCIL ON MEDICAL SERVICE 8/88)   **PLEASE PRINT OR TYPE**

FORM CMS-1500   (12-90)
FORM OWCP-1500   FORM RRB-1500
FORM AMA-OP050591

**Exercise 7–6**

PLEASE
DO NOT
STAPLE
IN THIS
AREA

□□□ PICA

ROVER INSURERS INC
5931 ROLLING ROAD
RONSON CO 81369

APPROVED MOB-0938-0008

## HEALTH INSURANCE CLAIM FORM

PICA □□□

| 1. MEDICARE   MEDICAID   CHAMPUS   CHAMPVA   GROUP HEALTH PLAN   FECA BLK LUNG   OTHER | 1a. INSURED'S I.D NUMBER   (FOR PROGRAM IN ITEM 1) |
|---|---|
| □ (Medicare #)  □ (Medicaid #)  □ (Sponsor's SSN)  □ (VA File #)  ☒ (SSN or ID)  □ (SSN)  □ (ID) | 999 99 NIN |

| 2. PATIENT'S NAME (Last, First, Middle Initial). | 3. PATIENT'S BIRTH DATE   MM DD YY   SEX | 4. INSURED'S NAME (Last, First, Middle Initial) |
|---|---|---|
| BOSSY BETTY B | 09  19  CCYY -47   M □   F ☒ | SAME |

| 5. PATIENT'S ADDRESS (No., Street) | 6. PATIENT'S RELATIONSHIP TO INSURED | 7. INSURED'S ADDRESS (No., Street) |
|---|---|---|
| 7991 BAGEL BLVD | Self ☒  Spouse □  Child □  Other □ | |

| CITY | STATE | 8. PATIENT STATUS | CITY | STATE |
|---|---|---|---|---|
| BARSTOW | NY | Single □  Married ☒  Other □ | | |

| ZIP CODE | TELEPHONE (Include Area Code) | | ZIP CODE | TELEPHONE (INCLUDE AREA CODE) |
|---|---|---|---|---|
| 12899 | (914) 555 3399 | Employed ☒  Full-Time Student □  Part-Time Student □ | | |

| 9. OTHER INSURED'S NAME (Last, First, Middle Initial) | 10. IS PATIENT'S CONDITION RELATED TO: | 11. INSURED'S POLICY GROUP OR FECA NUMBER: |
|---|---|---|
| | | 21088NIN |

| a. OTHER INSURED'S POLICY OR GROUP NUMBER | a. EMPLOYMENT? (CURRENT OR PREVIOUS)   □ YES  ☒ NO | a. INSURED'S DATE OF BIRTH   MM DD YY   SEX   M □   F □ |
|---|---|---|

| b. OTHER INSURED'S DATE OF BIRTH   MM DD YY   SEX   M □   F □ | b. AUTO ACCIDENT?   PLACE (State)   □ YES  ☒ NO | b. EMPLOYER'S NAME OR SCHOOL NAME   NINJA CORPORATION |
|---|---|---|

| c. EMPLOYER'S NAME OR SCHOOL NAME | c. OTHER ACCIDENT?   □ YES  ☒ NO | c. INSURANCE PLAN NAME OR PROGRAM NAME   ROVER INSURERS INC |
|---|---|---|

| d. INSURANCE PLAN NAME OR PROGRAM NAME | 10d. RESERVED FOR LOCAL USE | d. IS THERE ANOTHER HEALTH BENEFIT PLAN?   □ YES  ☒ NO   *if yes*, return to and complete item 9 a-d |
|---|---|---|

READ BACK OF FORM BEFORE COMPLETING & SIGNING THIS FORM

12. PATIENT'S OR AUTHORIZED PERSON'S SIGNATURE I authorize the release of any medical or other information necessary to process this claim. I also request payment of government benefits either to myself or to the party who accepts assignment below.

SIGNED **SIGNATURE ON FILE**   DATE _____

13. INSURED'S OR AUTHORIZED PERSON'S SIGNATURE I authorize payment of medical benefits to the undersigned physician or supplier for services described below.

SIGNED **SIGNATURE ON FILE**

| 14. DATE OF CURRENT:  ◄ ILLNESS (1st symptom)  INJURY (Accident)  PREGNANCY (LMP)   MM DD YY   02  06  YY | 15. IF PATIENT HAS HAD SAME OR SIMILAR ILLNESS, GIVE FIRST DATE   MM DD YY | 16. DATES PATIENT UNABLE TO WORK IN CURRENT OCCUPATION   MM DD YY   MM DD YY   FROM   TO |
|---|---|---|

| 17. NAME OF REFERRING PHYSICIAN OR OTHER SOURCE | 17a. I.D. NUMBER OF REFERRING PHYSICIAN | 18. HOSPITALIZATION DATES RELATED TO CURRENT SERVICES   MM DD YY   MM DD YY   FROM 02 06 YY  TO 02 14 YY |
|---|---|---|

| 19. RESERVED FOR LOCAL USE | 20. OUTSIDE LAB?   □ YES  □ NO   $ CHARGES |
|---|---|

21. DIAGNOSIS OR NATURE OF ILLNESS OR INJURY, (RELATE ITEMS 1,2,3, OR 4 TO ITEM 24E BY LINE)

1. 410 .91           3. ____ . ____
2. ____ . ____        4. ____ . ____

| 22. MEDICAID RESUBMISSION CODE   ORIGINAL REF. NO. |
|---|
| 23. PRIOR AUTHORIZATION NUMBER |

| 24. A. DATE(S) OF SERVICE From MM DD YY | To MM DD YY | B. Place of Service | C. Type of Service | D. PROCEDURES, SERVICES, OR SUPPLIES (Explain Unusual Circumstances) CPT/HCPS   MODIFIER | E. DIAGNOSIS CODE | F. $ CHARGES | G. DAYS OR UNITS | H. EPSDT Family Plan | I. EMG | J. COB | K. RESERVED FOR LOCAL USE |
|---|---|---|---|---|---|---|---|---|---|---|---|
| 02 06 YY | 02 06 YY | 21 | 1 | 33217  -80  -51 | 1 | 49 00 | 1 | | Y | | |
| 02 06 YY | 02 06 YY | 21 | 1 | 33225  -80 | 1 | 100 00 | 1 | | Y | | |
| 02 06 YY | 02 06 YY | 21 | 1 | 33240  -80  -51 | 1 | 59 00 | 1 | | Y | | |
| | | | | | | | | | | | |
| | | | | | | | | | | | |
| | | | | | | | | | | | |

| 25. FEDERAL TAX I.D. NUMBER   SSN EIN | 26. PATIENT'S ACCOUNT NO | 27. ACCEPT ASSIGNMENT? (For govt. claims, see back) | 28. TOTAL CHARGE | 29. AMOUNT PAID | 30. BALANCE DUE |
|---|---|---|---|---|---|
| 70-0089779   □ ☒ | 001   939 | ☒ YES  □ NO | $ 208 00 | $ 0 00 | $ 208 00 |

| 31. SIGNATURE OF PHYSICIAN OR SUPPLIER INCLUDING DEGREES OR CREDENTIALS (I certify that the statements on the reverse apply to this bill and are made a part thereof.)   SIGNED *Tim Percher MD*  DATE 02/19/YY | 32. NAME AND ADDRESS OF FACILITY WHERE SERVICES WERE RENDERED (If other than home or office)   HEADACHE HOSPITAL  2000 HAZARD STREET  HELP NY 12899 | 33. PHYSICIAN'S, SUPPLIERS BILLING NAME, ADDRESS, ZIP CODE & PHONE #   TIM PERCHER MD   NETWORK PROVIDER  99 TANK STREET STE 9T  TREE NY 12899  (914) 555 2599   PIN# B00369   GRP# |
|---|---|---|

(APPROVED BY AMA COUNCIL ON MEDICAL SERVICE 8/88)     **PLEASE PRINT OR TYPE**

FORM CMS-1500   (12-90)
FORM OWCP-1500   FORM RRB-1500
FORM AMA-OP050591

**Exercise 7–7**

PLEASE
DO NOT
STAPLE
IN THIS
AREA
□□□ PICA

WINTER INSURANCE CO
9763 WESTERN WAY
WHITTIER CO 82963

APPROVED MOB-0938-0008

# HEALTH INSURANCE CLAIM FORM

PICA □□□

| | | | | | | | | |
|---|---|---|---|---|---|---|---|---|
| 1. MEDICARE | MEDICAID | CHAMPUS | CHAMPVA | GROUP HEALTH PLAN | FECA BLK LUNG | OTHER | 1a. INSURED'S I.D NUMBER | (FOR PROGRAM IN ITEM 1) |
| □ (Medicare #) | □ (Medicaid #) | □ (Sponsor's SSN) | □ (VA File #) | ☒ (SSN or ID) | □ (SSN) | □ (ID) | 444 44 ABC | |

2. PATIENT'S NAME (Last, First, Middle Initial).
**DINGBAT DANNY D**

3. PATIENT'S BIRTH DATE
MM 04 DD 24 YY CCYY -10   SEX M ☒  F □

4. INSURED'S NAME (Last, First, Middle Initial)
**DINGBAT DANA D**

5. PATIENT'S ADDRESS (No., Street)
**404 DOORWAY DRIVE**

6. PATIENT'S RELATIONSHIP TO INSURED
Self □  Spouse □  Child ☒  Other □

7. INSURED'S ADDRESS (No., Street)
**SAME**

CITY **DENVER**   STATE **ND**

8. PATIENT STATUS
Single ☒  Married □  Other □
Employed □  Full-Time Student ☒  Part-Time Student □

CITY   STATE

ZIP CODE **58444**   TELEPHONE (Include Area Code) **(701) 555 3344**

CITY   STATE
ZIP CODE   TELEPHONE (INCLUDE AREA CODE)

9. OTHER INSURED'S NAME (Last, First, Middle Initial)

10. IS PATIENT'S CONDITION RELATED TO:

11. INSURED'S POLICY GROUP OR FECA NUMBER:
**36928ABC**

a. OTHER INSURED'S POLICY OR GROUP NUMBER

a. EMPLOYMENT? (CURRENT OR PREVIOUS)
□ YES  ☒ NO

a. INSURED'S DATE OF BIRTH
MM 04 DD 04 YY CCYY -37   SEX M □  F ☒

b. OTHER INSURED'S DATE OF BIRTH
MM DD YY   SEX M □  F □

b. AUTO ACCIDENT?   PLACE (State)
□ YES  ☒ NO

b. EMPLOYER'S NAME OR SCHOOL NAME
**ABC CORPORATION**

c. EMPLOYER'S NAME OR SCHOOL NAME

c. OTHER ACCIDENT?
☒ YES  □ NO

c. INSURANCE PLAN NAME OR PROGRAM NAME
**WINTER INSURANCE COMPANY**

d. INSURANCE PLAN NAME OR PROGRAM NAME

10d. RESERVED FOR LOCAL USE

d. IS THERE ANOTHER HEALTH BENEFIT PLAN?
□ YES  ☒ NO   *if yes*, return to and complete item 9 a-d

READ BACK OF FORM BEFORE COMPLETING & SIGNING THIS FORM
12. PATIENT'S OR AUTHORIZED PERSON'S SIGNATURE I authorize the release of any medical or other information necessary to process this claim. I also request payment of government benefits either to myself or to the party who accepts assignment below.

SIGNED **SIGNATURE ON FILE**   DATE

13. INSURED'S OR AUTHORIZED PERSON'S SIGNATURE I authorize payment of medical benefits to the undersigned physician or supplier for services described below.

SIGNED **SIGNATURE ON FILE**

14. DATE OF CURRENT: ◄ ILLNESS (1st symptom) INJURY (Accident) PREGNANCY (LMP)
MM 01 DD 26 YY YY

15. IF PATIENT HAS HAD SAME OR SIMILAR ILLNESS, GIVE FIRST DATE   MM DD YY

16. DATES PATIENT UNABLE TO WORK IN CURRENT OCCUPATION
FROM MM DD YY   TO MM DD YY

17. NAME OF REFERRING PHYSICIAN OR OTHER SOURCE

17a. I.D. NUMBER OF REFERRING PHYSICIAN

18. HOSPITALIZATION DATES RELATED TO CURRENT SERVICES
FROM MM 01 DD 26 YY YY   TO MM 02 DD 07 YY YY

19. RESERVED FOR LOCAL USE

20. OUTSIDE LAB?
□ YES  □ NO   $ CHARGES

21. DIAGNOSIS OR NATURE OF ILLNESS OR INJURY, (RELATE ITEMS 1,2,3, OR 4 TO ITEM 24E BY LINE)

1. |_____807_.01_____    3. |_____800_.40_____
2. |_____823_.32_____    4. |_____E884_.9_____

22. MEDICAID RESUBMISSION CODE   ORIGINAL REF. NO.

23. PRIOR AUTHORIZATION NUMBER

| 24. A DATE(S) OF SERVICE | | | | | | B Place of Service | C Type of Service | D PROCEDURES, SERVICES, OR SUPPLIES (Explain Unusual Circumstances) CPT/HCPS   MODIFIER | | E DIAGNOSIS CODE | F $ CHARGES | G DAYS OR UNITS | H EPSDT Family Plan | I EMG | J COB | K RESERVED FOR LOCAL USE |
|---|---|---|---|---|---|---|---|---|---|---|---|---|---|---|---|---|
| From MM | DD | YY | To MM | DD | YY | | | | | | | | | | | |
| 01 | 26 | YY | 01 | 26 | YY | 21 | 1 | 21800 | -80 | 1 | 132 00 | 1 | | Y | | |
| 01 | 26 | YY | 01 | 26 | YY | 21 | 1 | 27758 | -80 -51 | 2 | 35 00 | 1 | | Y | | |
| 01 | 26 | YY | 01 | 26 | YY | 21 | 1 | 27784 | -80 -51 | 2 | 50 00 | 1 | | Y | | |
| 01 | 26 | YY | 01 | 26 | YY | 21 | 1 | 62000 | -80 -51 | 3 | 40 00 | 1 | | Y | | |

25. FEDERAL TAX I.D. NUMBER   SSN EIN
**70-0089775**   □ ☒

26. PATIENT'S ACCOUNT NO
**001 434**

27. ACCEPT ASSIGNMENT? (For govt. claims, see back)
□ YES  ☒ NO

28. TOTAL CHARGE
$ 257 00

29. AMOUNT PAID
$ 0 00

30. BALANCE DUE
$ 257 00

31. SIGNATURE OF PHYSICIAN OR SUPPLIER INCLUDING DEGREES OR CREDENTIALS (I certify that the statements on the reverse apply to this bill and are made a part thereof.)

SIGNED *Rod Didogy MD*   DATE 02/07/YY

32. NAME AND ADDRESS OF FACILITY WHERE SERVICES WERE RENDERED (If other than home or office)
**HACKIM HOSPITAL**
**1000 HIDE STREET**
**HUSHTOWN ND 58444**

33. PHYSICIAN'S, SUPPLIERS BILLING NAME, ADDRESS, ZIP CODE & PHONE #
**ROD DIOLOGY MD**
**4557 DREAMER DRIVE STE 41D**
**DAYS ND 58444**
**(710) 555 6044**
PIN# **C32109**   GRP#

(APPROVED BY AMA COUNCIL ON MEDICAL SERVICE 8/88)   **PLEASE PRINT OR TYPE**

FORM CMS-1500 (12-90)
FORM OWCP-1500   FORM RRB-1500
FORM AMA-OP050591

**Exercise 7–8**

BALL INSURANCE CARRIERS
3895 BUBBLE BLVD STE 283
BOXWOOD CO 85926

APPROVED MOB-0938-0008

□□□ PICA

# HEALTH INSURANCE CLAIM FORM

PICA □□□

| 1. MEDICARE | MEDICAID | CHAMPUS | CHAMPVA | GROUP HEALTH PLAN | FECA BLK LUNG | OTHER | 1a. INSURED'S I.D NUMBER (FOR PROGRAM IN ITEM 1) |
|---|---|---|---|---|---|---|---|
| ☐ (Medicare #) | ☐ (Medicaid #) | ☐ (Sponsor's SSN) | ☐ (VA File #) | ☒ (SSN or ID) | ☐ (SSN) | ☐ (ID) | 555 55 XYZ |

2. PATIENT'S NAME (Last, First, Middle Initial).
PATIENT PATTY P

3. PATIENT'S BIRTH DATE  MM 05 DD 15 YY CCYY -35  SEX M ☐ F ☒

4. INSURED'S NAME (Last, First, Middle Initial).
SAME

5. PATIENT'S ADDRESS (No., Street)
655 PAIN LANE

6. PATIENT'S RELATIONSHIP TO INSURED
Self ☒ Spouse ☐ Child ☐ Other ☐

7. INSURED'S ADDRESS (No., Street)

CITY PEN  STATE PA

8. PATIENT STATUS
Single ☒ Married ☐ Other ☐
Employed ☒ Full-Time Student ☐ Part-Time Student ☐

CITY  STATE

ZIP CODE 15522  TELEPHONE (Include Area Code) (878) 555 3355

ZIP CODE  TELEPHONE (INCLUDE AREA CODE)

9. OTHER INSURED'S NAME (Last, First, Middle Initial)

10. IS PATIENT'S CONDITION RELATED TO:

11. INSURED'S POLICY GROUP OR FECA NUMBER:
62958XYZ

a. OTHER INSURED'S POLICY OR GROUP NUMBER

a. EMPLOYMENT? (CURRENT OR PREVIOUS) ☐ YES ☒ NO

a. INSURED'S DATE OF BIRTH  MM DD YY  SEX M ☐ F ☐

b. OTHER INSURED'S DATE OF BIRTH  MM DD YY SEX M ☐ F ☐

b. AUTO ACCIDENT? PLACE (State) ☐ YES ☒ NO

b. EMPLOYER'S NAME OR SCHOOL NAME
XYZ CORPORATION

c. EMPLOYER'S NAME OR SCHOOL NAME

c. OTHER ACCIDENT? ☐ YES ☒ NO

c. INSURANCE PLAN NAME OR PROGRAM NAME
BALL INSURANCE CARRIERS

d. INSURANCE PLAN NAME OR PROGRAM NAME

10d. RESERVED FOR LOCAL USE

d. IS THERE ANOTHER HEALTH BENEFIT PLAN? ☐ YES ☒ NO *if yes*, return to and complete item 9 a-d

12. PATIENT'S OR AUTHORIZED PERSON'S SIGNATURE
SIGNED SIGNATURE ON FILE  DATE

13. INSURED'S OR AUTHORIZED PERSON'S SIGNATURE
SIGNED SIGNATURE ON FILE

14. DATE OF CURRENT: MM 02 DD 02 YY YY
15. IF PATIENT HAS HAD SAME OR SIMILAR ILLNESS.
16. DATES PATIENT UNABLE TO WORK IN CURRENT OCCUPATION FROM TO

17. NAME OF REFERRING PHYSICIAN OR OTHER SOURCE
17a. I.D. NUMBER OF REFERRING PHYSICIAN
18. HOSPITALIZATION DATES RELATED TO CURRENT SERVICES FROM 02 16 YY TO 02 16 YY

19. RESERVED FOR LOCAL USE
20. OUTSIDE LAB? ☐ YES ☐ NO  $ CHARGES

21. DIAGNOSIS OR NATURE OF ILLNESS OR INJURY
1. 233 .0
2.
3.
4.

22. MEDICAID RESUBMISSION CODE  ORIGINAL REF. NO.
23. PRIOR AUTHORIZATION NUMBER

| 24. A DATE(S) OF SERVICE From MM DD YY  To MM DD YY | B Place of Service | C Type of Service | D PROCEDURES, SERVICES, OR SUPPLIES CPT/HCPS MODIFIER | E DIAGNOSIS CODE | F $ CHARGES | G DAYS OR UNITS | H EPSDT Family Plan | I EMG | J COB | K RESERVED FOR LOCAL USE |
|---|---|---|---|---|---|---|---|---|---|---|
| 02 16 YY 02 16 YY | 22 | 1 | 19125 -80 -51 | 1 | 72 00 | 1 | | | | |
| 02 16 YY 02 16 YY | 22 | 1 | 19126 -80 | 1 | 160 00 | 4 | | | | |

25. FEDERAL TAX I.D. NUMBER 70-0089774  SSN ☐ EIN ☒
26. PATIENT'S ACCOUNT NO 001 535
27. ACCEPT ASSIGNMENT? ☒ YES ☐ NO
28. TOTAL CHARGE $ 232 00
29. AMOUNT PAID $ 0 00
30. BALANCE DUE $ 232 00

31. SIGNATURE OF PHYSICIAN OR SUPPLIER
SIGNED Ann Tiseptic MD DATE 03/02/YY

32. NAME AND ADDRESS OF FACILITY WHERE SERVICES WERE RENDERED
HELPER HOSPITAL
25450 HAMMER AVE
HUMMER TOWN PA 15522

33. PHYSICIAN'S, SUPPLIERS BILLING NAME, ADDRESS, ZIP CODE & PHONE #
ANN TISEPTIC MD
232 AMSTER AVE STE 228A
AFTERALL PA 15522
(878) 555 1055
PIN# D98761  GRP#

(APPROVED BY AMA COUNCIL ON MEDICAL SERVICE 8/88)  **PLEASE PRINT OR TYPE**
FORM CMS-1500 (12-90) FORM OWCP-1500 FORM RRB-1500 FORM AMA-OP050591

**Exercise 7–9**

PLEASE
DO NOT
STAPLE
IN THIS
AREA

ROVER INSURERS INC
5931 ROLLING ROAD
RONSON CO 81369

APPROVED MOB-0938-0008

□□□ PICA

# HEALTH INSURANCE CLAIM FORM

PICA □□□

| 1. | MEDICARE | MEDICAID | CHAMPUS | CHAMPVA | GROUP HEALTH PLAN | FECA BLK LUNG | OTHER | 1a. INSURED'S I.D NUMBER (FOR PROGRAM IN ITEM 1) |
|---|---|---|---|---|---|---|---|---|
| | ☐ (Medicare #) | ☐ (Medicaid #) | ☐ (Sponsor's SSN) | ☐ (VA File #) | ☒ (SSN or ID) | ☐ (SSN) | ☐ (ID) | 999 99 NIN |

2. PATIENT'S NAME (Last, First, Middle Initial).
BOSSY BETTY B

3. PATIENT'S BIRTH DATE
MM 09 DD 19 YY CCYY -47
SEX M ☐ F ☒

4. INSURED'S NAME (Last, First, Middle Initial)
SAME

5. PATIENT'S ADDRESS (No., Street)
7991 BAGEL BLVD

6. PATIENT'S RELATIONSHIP TO INSURED
Self ☒ Spouse ☐ Child ☐ Other ☐

7. INSURED'S ADDRESS (No., Street)

CITY
BARSTOW
STATE NY

8. PATIENT STATUS
Single ☐ Married ☒ Other ☐
Employed ☒ Full-Time Student ☐ Part-Time Student ☐

CITY
STATE

ZIP CODE
12899
TELEPHONE (Include Area Code)
(914) 555 3399

ZIP CODE
TELEPHONE (INCLUDE AREA CODE)

9. OTHER INSURED'S NAME (Last, First, Middle Initial)

10. IS PATIENT'S CONDITION RELATED TO:

11. INSURED'S POLICY GROUP OR FECA NUMBER:
21088NIN

a. OTHER INSURED'S POLICY OR GROUP NUMBER

a. EMPLOYMENT? (CURRENT OR PREVIOUS)
☐ YES ☒ NO

a. INSURED'S DATE OF BIRTH
MM DD YY
SEX M ☐ F ☐

b. OTHER INSURED'S DATE OF BIRTH
MM DD YY
SEX M ☐ F ☐

b. AUTO ACCIDENT? PLACE (State)
☐ YES ☒ NO

b. EMPLOYER'S NAME OR SCHOOL NAME
NINJA ENTERPRISES

c. EMPLOYER'S NAME OR SCHOOL NAME

c. OTHER ACCIDENT?
☐ YES ☒ NO

c. INSURANCE PLAN NAME OR PROGRAM NAME
ROVER INSURER INC

d. INSURANCE PLAN NAME OR PROGRAM NAME

10d. RESERVED FOR LOCAL USE

d. IS THERE ANOTHER HEALTH BENEFIT PLAN?
☐ YES ☒ NO *if yes*, return to and complete item 9 a-d

READ BACK OF FORM BEFORE COMPLETING & SIGNING THIS FORM

12. PATIENT'S OR AUTHORIZED PERSON'S SIGNATURE I authorize the release of any medical or other information necessary to process this claim. I also request payment of government benefits either to myself or to the party who accepts assignment below.

SIGNED SIGNATURE ON FILE
DATE

13. INSURED'S OR AUTHORIZED PERSON'S SIGNATURE I authorize payment of medical benefits to the undersigned physician or supplier for services described below.

SIGNED SIGNATURE ON FILE

14. DATE OF CURRENT: ◄ ILLNESS (1st symptom) INJURY (Accident) PREGNANCY (LMP)
MM 02 DD 06 YY YY

15. IF PATIENT HAS HAD SAME OR SIMILAR ILLNESS. GIVE FIRST DATE MM DD YY

16. DATES PATIENT UNABLE TO WORK IN CURRENT OCCUPATION
FROM MM DD YY TO MM DD YY

17. NAME OF REFERRING PHYSICIAN OR OTHER SOURCE

17a. I.D. NUMBER OF REFERRING PHYSICIAN

18. HOSPITALIZATION DATES RELATED TO CURRENT SERVICES
FROM MM 02 DD 06 YY YY TO MM 02 DD 14 YY YY

19. RESERVED FOR LOCAL USE

20. OUTSIDE LAB? ☐ YES ☐ NO $ CHARGES

21. DIAGNOSIS OR NATURE OF ILLNESS OR INJURY, (RELATE ITEMS 1,2,3, OR 4 TO ITEM 24E BY LINE)

1. 410 . 91        3. __ . __
2. __ . __          4. __ . __

22. MEDICAID RESUBMISSION CODE ORIGINAL REF. NO.

23. PRIOR AUTHORIZATION NUMBER

| 24. A DATE(S) OF SERVICE From MM DD YY | To MM DD YY | B Place of Service | C Type of Service | D PROCEDURES, SERVICES, OR SUPPLIES (Explain Unusual Circumstances) CPT/HCPS \| MODIFIER | E DIAGNOSIS CODE | F $ CHARGES | G DAYS OR UNITS | H EPSDT Family Plan | I EMG | J COB | K RESERVED FOR LOCAL USE |
|---|---|---|---|---|---|---|---|---|---|---|---|
| 02 06 YY | 02 06 YY | 21 | 1 | 00534 | 1 | 430 00 | 1 | | Y | | |
| | | | | 1708-1848 (Actual Time) | | | | | | | |

25. FEDERAL TAX I.D. NUMBER SSN ☐ EIN ☒
70-3539779

26. PATIENT'S ACCOUNT NO.
001 939

27. ACCEPT ASSIGNMENT? (For govt. claims, see back)
☒ YES ☐ NO

28. TOTAL CHARGE
$ 430 00

29. AMOUNT PAID
$ 0 00

30. BALANCE DUE
$ 430 00

31. SIGNATURE OF PHYSICIAN OR SUPPLIER INCLUDING DEGREES OR CREDENTIALS (I certify that the statements on the reverse apply to this bill and are made a part thereof.)

SIGNED Tom Sillitis MD DATE 02/20/YY

32. NAME AND ADDRESS OF FACILITY WHERE SERVICES WERE RENDERED (If other than home or office)
HEADACHE HOSPITAL
2000 HAZARD STREET
HELP NY 12899

33. PHYSICIAN'S, SUPPLIERS BILLING NAME, ADDRESS, ZIP CODE & PHONE #
TOM SILLITIS MD        NETWORK PROVIDER
9909 TRIMMER STREET STE 1T
TRAVEL NY 12899
(914) 555 6789
PIN# E34567        GRP#

(APPROVED BY AMA COUNCIL ON MEDICAL SERVICE 8/88)

**PLEASE PRINT OR TYPE**

FORM CMS-1500 (12-90)
FORM OWCP-1500    FORM RRB-1500
FORM AMA-OP050591

**Exercise 7–10**

PLEASE
DO NOT
STAPLE
IN THIS
AREA
□□□ PICA

WINTER INSURANCE CO
9763 WESTERN WAY
WHITTIER CO 82963

APPROVED MOB-0938-0008

# HEALTH INSURANCE CLAIM FORM

PICA □□□

| 1. MEDICARE  MEDICAID  CHAMPUS  CHAMPVA  GROUP HEALTH PLAN  FECA BLK LUNG  OTHER | 1a. INSURED'S I.D NUMBER (FOR PROGRAM IN ITEM 1) |
|---|---|
| ☐ (Medicare #)  ☐ (Medicaid #)  ☐ (Sponsor's SSN)  ☐ (VA File #)  ☒ (SSN or ID)  ☐ (SSN)  ☐ (ID) | 444 44 ABC |

| 2. PATIENT'S NAME (Last, First, Middle Initial). | 3. PATIENT'S BIRTH DATE | 4. INSURED'S NAME (Last, First, Middle Initial) |
|---|---|---|
| DINGBAT DANNY D | MM 04  DD 24  YY CCYY -10   SEX M ☒  F ☐ | DINGBAT DANA D |

| 5. PATIENT'S ADDRESS (No., Street) | 6. PATIENT'S RELATIONSHIP TO INSURED | 7. INSURED'S ADDRESS (No., Street) |
|---|---|---|
| 404 DOORWAY DRIVE | Self ☐  Spouse ☐  Child ☒  Other ☐ | SAME |

| CITY | STATE | 8. PATIENT STATUS | CITY | STATE |
|---|---|---|---|---|
| DENVER | ND | Single ☒  Married ☐  Other ☐ | | |
| ZIP CODE | TELEPHONE (Include Area Code) | Employed ☐  Full-Time Student ☒  Part-Time Student ☐ | ZIP CODE | TELEPHONE (INCLUDE AREA CODE) |
| 58444 | (701) 555 3344 | | | |

| 9. OTHER INSURED'S NAME (Last, First, Middle Initial) | 10. IS PATIENT'S CONDITION RELATED TO: | 11. INSURED'S POLICY GROUP OR FECA NUMBER: |
|---|---|---|
| | | 36928ABC |
| a. OTHER INSURED'S POLICY OR GROUP NUMBER | a. EMPLOYMENT? (CURRENT OR PREVIOUS) ☐ YES ☒ NO | a. INSURED'S DATE OF BIRTH  MM 04  DD 04  YY CCYY -37   SEX M ☐  F ☒ |
| b. OTHER INSURED'S DATE OF BIRTH  MM  DD  YY    SEX M ☐  F ☐ | b. AUTO ACCIDENT?  PLACE (State) ☐ YES ☒ NO | b. EMPLOYER'S NAME OR SCHOOL NAME  ABC CORPORATION |
| c. EMPLOYER'S NAME OR SCHOOL NAME | c. OTHER ACCIDENT? ☒ YES ☐ NO | c. INSURANCE PLAN NAME OR PROGRAM NAME  WINTER INSURANCE COMPANY |
| d. INSURANCE PLAN NAME OR PROGRAM NAME | 10d. RESERVED FOR LOCAL USE | d. IS THERE ANOTHER HEALTH BENEFIT PLAN? ☐ YES ☒ NO   *if yes*, return to and complete item 9 a-d |

READ BACK OF FORM BEFORE COMPLETING & SIGNING THIS FORM

12. PATIENT'S OR AUTHORIZED PERSON'S SIGNATURE I authorize the release of any medical or other information necessary to process this claim. I also request payment of government benefits either to myself or to the party who accepts assignment below.

SIGNED **SIGNATURE ON FILE**   DATE _____

13. INSURED'S OR AUTHORIZED PERSON'S SIGNATURE I authorize payment of medical benefits to the undersigned physician or supplier for services described below.

SIGNED **SIGNATURE ON FILE**

| 14. DATE OF CURRENT: ◄ ILLNESS (1st symptom) ◄ INJURY (Accident) PREGNANCY (LMP)  MM 01  DD 26  YY YY | 15. IF PATIENT HAS HAD SAME OR SIMILAR ILLNESS, GIVE FIRST DATE  MM  DD  YY | 16. DATES PATIENT UNABLE TO WORK IN CURRENT OCCUPATION  FROM  MM  DD  YY   TO  MM  DD  YY |
|---|---|---|
| 17. NAME OF REFERRING PHYSICIAN OR OTHER SOURCE | 17a. I.D. NUMBER OF REFERRING PHYSICIAN | 18. HOSPITALIZATION DATES RELATED TO CURRENT SERVICES  FROM 01 26 YY  TO 02 08 YY |
| 19. RESERVED FOR LOCAL USE | | 20. OUTSIDE LAB?  ☐ YES ☐ NO   $ CHARGES |

21. DIAGNOSIS OR NATURE OF ILLNESS OR INJURY, (RELATE ITEMS 1,2,3, OR 4 TO ITEM 24E BY LINE)

1. | 807 . 01        3. | 800 . 40
2. | 823 . 32        4. | E884 . 9

| 22. MEDICAID RESUBMISSION CODE | ORIGINAL REF. NO. |
|---|---|
| 23. PRIOR AUTHORIZATION NUMBER | |

| 24. A. DATE(S) OF SERVICE From — To  MM DD YY  MM DD YY | B. Place of Service | C. Type of Service | D. PROCEDURES, SERVICES, OR SUPPLIES (Explain Unusual Circumstances) CPT/HCPCS  MODIFIER | E. DIAGNOSIS CODE | F. $ CHARGES | G. DAYS OR UNITS | H. EPSDT Family Plan | I. EMG | J. COB | K. RESERVED FOR LOCAL USE |
|---|---|---|---|---|---|---|---|---|---|---|
| 01 26 YY 01 26 YY | 21 | 1 | 01480 | 1 4 | 170 00 | | | Y | | |
| 01 26 YY 01 26 YY | 21 | 1 | 00520 | 2 4 | 240 00 | | | Y | | |
| 01 26 YY 01 26 YY | 21 | 1 | 00215 | 3 4 | 300 00 | | | Y | | |
| | | | 1820-2140 (Block Time) | | | | | | | |

| 25. FEDERAL TAX I.D. NUMBER   SSN EIN | 26. PATIENT'S ACCOUNT NO. | 27. ACCEPT ASSIGNMENT? (For govt. claims, see back) | 28. TOTAL CHARGE | 29. AMOUNT PAID | 30. BALANCE DUE |
|---|---|---|---|---|---|
| 60-3539774   ☐ ☒ | 001        434 | ☐ YES ☒ NO | $ 710 00 | $ 0 00 | $ 710 00 |

| 31. SIGNATURE OF PHYSICIAN OR SUPPLIER INCLUDING DEGREES OR CREDENTIALS (I certify that the statements on the reverse apply to this bill and are made a part thereof.)  SIGNED *Perry Cardiectomy MD*  DATE 02/07/YY | 32. NAME AND ADDRESS OF FACILITY WHERE SERVICES WERE RENDERED (If other than home or office)  HACKIM HOSPITAL 1000 HIDE STREET HUSHTOWN ND 58444 | 33. PHYSICIAN'S, SUPPLIERS BILLING NAME, ADDRESS, ZIP CODE & PHONE #  PERRY CARDIECTOMY MD 4404 CLOVER COURT STE 4C COOL ND 58442 (701) 555 1234  PIN# PEC004    GRP# |
|---|---|---|

(APPROVED BY AMA COUNCIL ON MEDICAL SERVICE 8/88)   **PLEASE PRINT OR TYPE**   FORM CMS-1500 (12-90) FORM OWCP-1500   FORM RRB-1500 FORM AMA-OP050591

**Exercise 7–11**

PLEASE DO NOT STAPLE IN THIS AREA
□□□ PICA

BALL INSURANCE CARRIERS
3895 BUBBLE BLVD STE 283
BOXWOOD CO 85926

APPROVED MOB-0938-0008

# HEALTH INSURANCE CLAIM FORM

PICA □□□

| 1. | MEDICARE | MEDICAID | CHAMPUS | CHAMPVA | GROUP HEALTH PLAN | FECA BLK LUNG | OTHER | 1a. INSURED'S I.D NUMBER | (FOR PROGRAM IN ITEM 1) |
|---|---|---|---|---|---|---|---|---|
| | ☐ (Medicare #) | ☐ (Medicaid #) | ☐ (Sponsor's SSN) | ☐ (VA File #) | ☒ (SSN or ID) | ☐ (SSN) | ☐ (ID) | 555 55 XYZ | |

2. PATIENT'S NAME (Last, First, Middle Initial).
PATIENT PATTY P

3. PATIENT'S BIRTH DATE
MM 05 DD 15 YY CCYY-35  SEX M ☐ F ☒

4. INSURED'S NAME (Last, First, Middle Initial).
SAME

5. PATIENT'S ADDRESS (No., Street)
655 PAIN LANE

6. PATIENT'S RELATIONSHIP TO INSURED
Self ☒ Spouse ☐ Child ☐ Other ☐

7. INSURED'S ADDRESS (No., Street)

CITY PEN    STATE PA

8. PATIENT STATUS
Single ☒ Married ☐ Other ☐
Employed ☒ Full-Time Student ☐ Part-Time Student ☐

CITY    STATE

ZIP CODE 15522    TELEPHONE (Include Area Code) (878) 555 3355

ZIP CODE    TELEPHONE (INCLUDE AREA CODE)

9. OTHER INSURED'S NAME (Last, First, Middle Initial)

10. IS PATIENT'S CONDITION RELATED TO:

11. INSURED'S POLICY GROUP OR FECA NUMBER:
62958XYZ

a. OTHER INSURED'S POLICY OR GROUP NUMBER

a. EMPLOYMENT? (CURRENT OR PREVIOUS)
☐ YES ☒ NO

a. INSURED'S DATE OF BIRTH
MM DD YY    SEX M ☐ F ☐

b. OTHER INSURED'S DATE OF BIRTH
MM DD YY    SEX M ☐ F ☐

b. AUTO ACCIDENT?    PLACE (State)
☐ YES ☒ NO

b. EMPLOYER'S NAME OR SCHOOL NAME
XYZ CORPORATION

c. EMPLOYER'S NAME OR SCHOOL NAME

c. OTHER ACCIDENT?
☐ YES ☒ NO

c. INSURANCE PLAN NAME OR PROGRAM NAME
BALL INSURANCE CARRIERS

d. INSURANCE PLAN NAME OR PROGRAM NAME

10d. RESERVED FOR LOCAL USE

d. IS THERE ANOTHER HEALTH BENEFIT PLAN?
☐ YES ☒ NO    if yes, return to and complete item 9 a-d

READ BACK OF FORM BEFORE COMPLETING & SIGNING THIS FORM
12. PATIENT'S OR AUTHORIZED PERSON'S SIGNATURE I authorize the release of any medical or other information necessary to process this claim. I also request payment of government benefits either to myself or to the party who accepts assignment below.

SIGNED SIGNATURE ON FILE    DATE

13. INSURED'S OR AUTHORIZED PERSON'S SIGNATURE I authorize payment of medical benefits to the undersigned physician or supplier for services described below.

SIGNED SIGNATURE ON FILE

14. DATE OF CURRENT: ◄ ILLNESS (1st symptom) ◄ INJURY (Accident) PREGNANCY (LMP)
MM 02 DD 16 YY YY

15. IF PATIENT HAS HAD SAME OR SIMILAR ILLNESS. GIVE FIRST DATE MM DD YY

16. DATES PATIENT UNABLE TO WORK IN CURRENT OCCUPATION
MM DD YY    MM DD YY
FROM    TO

17. NAME OF REFERRING PHYSICIAN OR OTHER SOURCE

17a. I.D. NUMBER OF REFERRING PHYSICIAN

18. HOSPITALIZATION DATES RELATED TO CURRENT SERVICES
MM DD YY    MM DD YY
FROM 02 16 YY    TO 02 16 YY

19. RESERVED FOR LOCAL USE

20. OUTSIDE LAB?    $ CHARGES
☐ YES ☐ NO

21. DIAGNOSIS OR NATURE OF ILLNESS OR INJURY, (RELATE ITEMS 1,2,3, OR 4 TO ITEM 24E BY LINE)
1. |__233__.0__    3. |_____.___
2. |_____.___    4. |_____.___

22. MEDICAID RESUBMISSION CODE    ORIGINAL REF. NO.

23. PRIOR AUTHORIZATION NUMBER

| 24. A DATE(S) OF SERVICE | | B Place of Service | C Type of Service | D PROCEDURES, SERVICES, OR SUPPLIES (Explain Unusual Circumstances) | | E DIAGNOSIS CODE | F $ CHARGES | G DAYS OR UNITS | H EPSDT Family Plan | I EMG | J COB | K RESERVED FOR LOCAL USE |
|---|---|---|---|---|---|---|---|---|---|---|---|---|
| From MM DD YY | To MM DD YY | | | CPT/HCPS | MODIFIER | | | | | | | |
| 02 16 YY | 02 16 YY | 22 | 1 | 00400 | | 1 | 175 00 | 1 | | | | |
| | | | | 0145-0235 | | | | | | | | |
| | | | | (Actual Time) | | | | | | | | |

25. FEDERAL TAX I.D. NUMBER    SSN ☐ EIN ☒
70-3539775

26. PATIENT'S ACCOUNT NO.
001 535

27. ACCEPT ASSIGNMENT? (For govt. claims, see back)
☒ YES ☐ NO

28. TOTAL CHARGE
$ 175 00

29. AMOUNT PAID
$ 0 00

30. BALANCE DUE
$ 175 00

31. SIGNATURE OF PHYSICIAN OR SUPPLIER INCLUDING DEGREES OR CREDENTIALS (I certify that the statements on the reverse apply to this bill and are made a part thereof.)

SIGNED Diane Ignosis MD DATE 02/18/YY

32. NAME AND ADDRESS OF FACILITY WHERE SERVICES WERE RENDERED (If other than home or office)
HELPER HOSPITAL
25450 HAMMER AVE
HUMMER TOWN PA 15522

33. PHYSICIAN'S, SUPPLIERS BILLING NAME, ADDRESS, ZIP CODE & PHONE #
DIANE IGNOSIS MD
656 DAIRY DRIVE STE 101D
DEER PA 15522
(878) 555 2455
PIN# G40039    GRP#

(APPROVED BY AMA COUNCIL ON MEDICAL SERVICE 8/88)    PLEASE PRINT OR TYPE

FORM CMS-1500 (12-90)
FORM OWCP-1500    FORM RRB-1500
FORM AMA-OP050591

**Exercise 7–12**

# 8

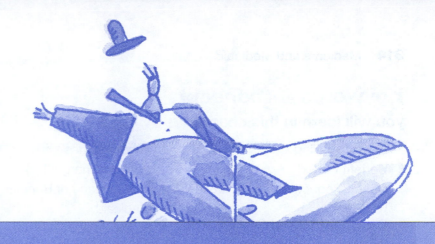

# Medicare
## and Medicaid

## After completion of this chapter
**you will be able to:**

- Explain the impact of TEFRA and DEFRA on health insurance plans.
- State the eligibility requirements for Medicare.
- Describe the two types of Medicare coverage and the benefits for each.
- List the types of nonparticipating facilities that Medicare will not cover.
- List the differences on a CMS-1500 between billing for Medicare and billing other insurance carriers.
- State the exceptions when a patient may submit a bill themselves.
- Describe what Acceptance of Assignment is and how it affects billing.
- List the claims that require acceptance of assignment.

- Describe "assignment of benefits" and how it can affect the amount collected on a Medicare claim.
- State the most common reasons for a "not medically necessary" denial and describe how this affects the amount collected from the patient.
- Show how a DRG benefit is calculated with a given scenario.
- Properly coordinate benefits with Medicare.
- Define and explain Medicare supplement programs.
- Properly estimate Medicare benefits in a given scenario.
- Explain and describe DRG billing.
- Describe the purpose of the Medicaid program.
- List Medicaid eligibility requirements.
- Explain what the HIPD form is and how to use it.

## Keywords and concepts

**you will learn in this chapter:**

- Balance Billing
- Benefit Period
- Deficit Reduction Act of 1984 (DEFRA)
- Diagnosis-Related Group (DRG)
- End-Stage Renal Disease (ESRD)
- Health Insurance Payment Demand (HIPD)

- Intermediaries
- Limiting Charge (LC)
- Maintenance of Benefits
- Medicaid
- Medicare
- Medicare Allowance
- Medicare Remittance Notice
- Medicare Summary Notice
- Medicare Supplements

- Nonparticipating Physicians
- Outliers
- Part A
- Part B
- Participating Physicians
- Reasonable Charges
- Tax Equity and Fiscal Responsibility Act of 1982 (TEFRA)

**Medicare** is the Federal Health Insurance Benefit Plan for the Aged and Disabled, Title XVII of Public Law 89-97 of the Social Security Act. This program is for people 65 years of age or older and certain persons who are totally disabled.

Social Security Administration (SSA) offices throughout the United States take applications for Medicare, determine eligibility, and provide general information about the program. The actual processing of the claims is administered by many different insurance companies, usually one or two within each state. Consequently, as an examiner you will see diversity in the application or denial of benefits and in the Medicare Remittance Notice (MRN) forms. The **Medicare Remittance Notice** is used to convey payments to providers who accept assignment for Medicare claims. The **Medicare Summary Notice** (MSN) is an explanation of benefits sent to the Medicare beneficiary, detailing the processing of claims submitted for payment.

## TEFRA/DEFRA

The **Tax Equity and Fiscal Responsibility Act of 1982 (TEFRA)**—and amendments to it—has redirected the financial responsibility for medical coverage of active employees age 65 years and older and their spouses aged 65 years and older. When this federal program was introduced, it was determined that Medicare would be the primary payer for persons who have reached their 65th birthday, regardless of employment status.

Initially, TEFRA regulations did not apply to spouses over age 65 of active employees who were under 65 years of age. The **Deficit Reduction Act of 1984 (DEFRA)**, effective January 1, 1985, amended TEFRA so that now spouses age 65 years and older of active employees who are under age 65 can elect their primary coverage as either Medicare or the private group plan.

The employers affected by these Acts are those who regularly employ 20 or more workers for each working day in at least 20 weeks of the current or preceding calendar year. Employees of such employers must be offered coverage under the group plan on the same basis as other employees. An election form choosing the primary plan must be completed and signed by each employee who is, or becomes, affected.

If coverage is chosen under the employer's group plan, the group plan will be the primary payer on all medical services and Medicare will be the secondary payer. If coverage under the group plan is rejected and Medicare is chosen, the employee/spouse by law can be covered only by Medicare. The group plan will not provide secondary coverage.

Employers with fewer than 20 employees are exempt from the TEFRA/DEFRA regulations, and Medicare is the primary carrier for their active employees and spouses age 65 years or older. Medicare is also primary for all retired employees and for active employees and their spouses under age 65 who are totally disabled with conditions other than end-stage renal disease (ESRD).

After it has been determined that the group plan is subject to TEFRA/DEFRA, it becomes necessary to determine the individual's eligibility for Medicare.

## Medicare Eligibility

Medicare eligibility is based on three principles:

1. Age.
2. Disability.
3. ESRD.

An individual is eligible for Medicare coverage on the first day of the month in which he or she reaches age 65. Persons born on the first day of the month are eligible on the first day of the month preceding their birth date.

**Example:**

Birthday: June 15, eligible for Medicare on June 1

Birthday: June 1, eligible for Medicare on May 1

Medicare coverage for totally disabled persons begins on the first of the 25th month from the date approved for Social Security Disability or Railroad Retirement benefits. Those covered include disabled workers of any age, disabled widows between the ages of 50 and 65, disabled beneficiaries age 18 and over who receive Social Security benefits because of disability before age 22, the blind, and railroad retirement annuitants.

**End-stage renal disease (ESRD)** is the condition in which a person's kidneys fail to function. As a result, the patient needs dialysis treatments (refer to the Physician's, Clinical, and Hospital Services Claims chapter for a review of this type of service). Because of the many problems associated with ESRD, patients are considered to be totally disabled, even though some persons with this disease continue to work. As a result, the following special rules apply to ESRD patients.

The employer's group health plan is the primary payer for the first 30 months after a patient (under age 65) with ESRD becomes eligible for Medicare. This 30-month period begins based on the earlier of:

- The month in which a regular course of renal dialysis is initiated.
- The month in which the patient is hospitalized for a kidney transplant.

Medicare is the secondary payer during this 30-month period but will revert to the primary status

beginning with the 31st month. As a general rule, all services under a dialysis program are Medicare-assigned.

## Providers of Service

Providers of services and medical equipment suppliers under Medicare must meet all licensing requirements of the state in which they are located. To be a participating provider under the Medicare program, they must meet additional Medicare requirements before payments can be made for their services. Medicare does not pay for the following care received in nonparticipating facilities:

- Hospital care.
- Skilled nursing facility.
- Home health agency.
- Hospice.
- Outpatient rehabilitation.
- Dialysis facilities.
- Ambulatory surgical centers.
- Independent physical therapists.
- Independent occupational therapists.
- Clinical laboratories.
- Portable x-ray suppliers.
- Rural health clinics.

## The Parts of Medicare

There are four parts to the Medicare program: Part A, Part B, Part C, and Part D. The services covered under the four parts of Medicare are as follows:

1. **Part A** is considered the basic plan or hospital insurance. This part covers facility charges for acute inpatient hospital care, skilled nursing, home health care, and hospice care.
2. **Part B** is the medical (supplementary, voluntary) insurance that covers physician services, outpatient hospital services, home health care, outpatient speech and physical therapy, and durable medical equipment.
3. **Part C** is the Medicare advantage portion and includes coverage in an HMO, PPO, and so on.
4. **Part D** is the prescription drug component (effective 2006).

## Part A

Part A, the hospital coverage portion of Medicare, is automatic on enrollment for the following individuals:

- All people age 65 and over, if entitled to (a) monthly Social Security benefits, or (b) pensions under the Railroad Retirement Act.
- All people who reached the age of 65 before 1968, whether or not under the Social Security or Railroad Retirement Programs.
- Workers who reached 65 in 1975 or after need 20 quarters of Social Security work credits if female, or 24 quarters of Social Security work credits if male, to be fully insured.
- Some spouses may receive Medicare benefits derived strictly from their eligible spouse's work credits. Using the eligible spouse's social security number with the appropriate letter behind it designates benefits are based on the eligible spouse.

Effective July 1, 1973, all people age 65 years and over who are not otherwise eligible for Part A may enroll by paying the full cost of such coverage, provided they also enroll in Part B.

Undocumented immigrants may be eligible for coverage in the Medicare program if they have been U.S. residents for five years.

Part A claims are processed by private insurance companies called **intermediaries**.

### Benefits

There is a Part A deductible amount that is taken from the first inpatient hospital admission. The use of Medicare benefits for an inpatient is measured by benefit periods. A **benefit period** begins with the first day of admission to the hospital. A benefit period ends after the patient has been discharged from the hospital or skilled nursing facility for a period of 60 consecutive days (including the day of discharge). A new benefit period begins and another inpatient deductible would be taken if the patient were readmitted.

For 2006, the Part A deductible is $952 per benefit period. If a member remains in the hospital for an extended period of time, additional copayments are required. Medicare deducts the copay amount from the billed amount and then pays the amount in excess of the copay.

The 2006 inpatient hospital copayments are as follows:

- 1st day–60th day = Deductible only, no additional copayment.
- 61st day–90th day = $238 copayment per day.

- 91st day–150th day = $476 copayment per day.

These days are known as the 60-day Lifetime Reserve. These copayments are not renewable.

For skilled nursing facilities (SNF), there is a separate copayment schedule and requirement. To be eligible for this benefit, a doctor must certify the necessity of skilled nursing and rehabilitative care on a daily basis. Custodial care is not covered nor is it available for occasional rehabilitative care. In addition, the Medicare intermediary approves the stay.

The 2006 SNF copayments are as follows:

- 1st day–20th day = No copayment. Because admission is usually from an acute care facility, during which time the deductible was met, 100% of the allowable is generally paid by Medicare.
- 21st day–100th day = $119 copayment per day.

Multiple admissions can occur during a calendar year. However, the maximum number of allowable days is 100 per benefit period.

## Part B

Part B is the supplementary medical insurance, which covers physician and outpatient hospital services. It is considered a supplemental plan because each participant must pay a stipulated amount each month for the benefits. Private insurance companies, called carriers, process Part B claims.

The rules, limits, and maximums under this coverage are subject to change annually.

### Benefits

The 2006 deductible is $124 per calendar year. After the deductible has been satisfied, generally 80% of the approved charge will be paid.

Beginning January 1, 2006, the Medicare Part B deductible will be indexed to the increase in the average cost of Part B services for Medicare beneficiaries. In other words, the amount charged for the Part B deductible will depend on the amount spent by Medicare for payments for services.

## Services That Are Not Covered Under Medicare Part A or Part B

Medicare does not cover everything. Items and services that are not covered include, but are not limited to the following:

- Acupuncture.
- Deductibles, coinsurance, or copayments when you get healthcare services.

- Dental care and dentures (with only a few exceptions).
- Cosmetic surgery.
- Custodial care (help with bathing, dressing, using the bathroom, and eating) at home or in a nursing home.
- Eye refractions.
- Healthcare you get while traveling outside of the United States.
- Hearing aids and hearing exams for the purpose of fitting a hearing aid.
- Hearing tests (other than for fitting a hearing aid) that have not been ordered by your doctor.
- Long-term care, such as custodial care in a nursing home.
- Orthopedic shoes (with only a few exceptions).
- Prescription drugs—most prescription drugs are not covered.
- Routine foot care such as cutting of corns or calluses (with only a few exceptions).
- Routine eye care and most eyeglasses.

- Routine or yearly physical exams (unless within the first six month of coverage for Part B).
- Screening tests and screening laboratory tests (some exceptions apply).
- Shots (vaccinations) (some exceptions apply).
- Some diabetic supplies (like syringes or insulin unless the insulin is used with an insulin pump or you join a Medicare Prescription Drug Plan).

## Part C

Medicare beneficiaries may choose to have covered items and services furnished to them through a Medicare Health Maintenance Organization. If a Medicare beneficiary selects this coverage, they are required to receive services according to the selected carrier's arrangements. When patients are enrolled in a Medicare HMO, claims for these patients must be submitted to the HMO.

## Part D

In an effort to provide better health coverage for Medicare beneficiaries, starting in the year 2006 Medicare beneficiaries will receive limited coverage for prescription drug benefits.

# On the Job Now

**Directions:** Answer the following questions without looking back at the material just covered. Write your answers in the space provided.

1. What is the difference between Medicare Part A and Part B? _____

_____

_____

_____

2. List five services that are not covered under Medicare Part A or Part B.

1. _____

2. _____

3. _____

4. _____

5. _____

3. Medicare Part A claims are processed by private companies called _____

4. How much is the 2006 Medicare Part A deductible? _____

5. How much is the 2006 Medicare Part B deductible? _____

# Approved or Reasonable Charges

Medicare payments are based on "**reasonable charges**," which are the amounts approved by the Medicare carrier based on what is considered reasonable for the geographic area in which the doctor practices. Because of the way that the approved amounts are determined and because of high rates of inflation in medical care prices, the approved amounts are often significantly less than the actual charges billed by providers. The charge approved by the carrier is the lowest of either of the following: the charge billed by the provider, or the prevailing charge (based on all the customary charges in the locality for each type of service) as determined by Medicare.

Since the participating provider must write off the amounts that are more than the Medicare approved amount, many providers have refused to participate in Medicare. Unfortunately, the member, who is often on a fixed income, is then held responsible for a large portion of the billed amount from the nonparticipating provider.

# Medicare Assignment of Benefits

A participating provider must agree to accept assignment on all Medicare claims. By doing this, the payment goes directly to the provider for all claims, rather than to the member. In addition, the provider has agreed to accept the amount approved by the Medicare carrier as payment in full for the covered services. The patient is not responsible for any amount over the Medicare-approved amount. In such a case, the secondary carrier is also not responsible for the amount in excess of the Medicare-approved amount.

## Physicians Who Accept Medicare Assignment

When a physician agrees to accept Medicare assignment for a bill, Medicare pays the physician directly for that bill. The physician may bill the patient only for any deductibles or coinsurance that Medicare has deducted from the assigned bill. As a result, the total fee that a physician may receive from Medicare and from beneficiaries for an assigned bill is limited by what Medicare deems an appropriate fee for the particular service or procedure (the "**Medicare allowance**").

To encourage physicians to accept assignment, the Medicare allowance is higher for physicians who agree to accept assignment for all bills for Medicare-eligible persons. These physicians are called "**participating physicians**." Thus, participating physicians agree not to practice "**balance billing**," or charging patients for more than the Medicare allowance.

The phrase "participating physician" can be confusing because physicians who sign these agreements are not the only ones who treat Medicare patients. Physicians who treat Medicare-eligible patients but who decide whether to accept assignment on a case-by-case basis are called "**nonparticipating physicians**." In exchange for the freedom to make this choice for each patient, nonparticipating physicians receive only 95% of the allowed amount that Medicare participating physicians receive.

## Mandatory Assignment

Providers may usually accept or not accept Medicare assignment. However, there are some services that require acceptance of assignment. These include:

- Clinical diagnostic laboratory services.
- Medicare patients who also are eligible for Medicaid.
- Ambulatory surgery centers.
- Method II home dialysis supplies and equipment.
- Physician's assistant, nurse midwives, nurse specialists, nonphysician anesthetists, clinical psychologists, and clinical social workers services.
- All physicians, nonphysician practitioners, and suppliers must take assignment on all claims for drugs and biologicals furnished to any patient enrolled in Medicare Part B.

## Limiting Charges

A **limiting charge** (**LC**) is the maximum amount that the federal government allows nonparticipating physicians to charge Medicare patients for a given service. The limiting charge applies to services billed on a nonassigned basis. The limiting charge for these services is 115% of the nonparticipating fee schedule amount.

Balance billing by nonparticipating physicians is strictly limited to this amount. Participating physicians are not affected because they are not allowed to balance bill Medicare patients for any services. The limiting charge applies only to physicians' services. Ambulance companies and other nonphysician providers are not subject to limiting charge regulations.

Following are two examples of how this rule affects the payment of claims.

**Example 1.** Participating provider; accepts assignment.

| Billed Charge | Medicare Approved Amount | Medicare Pays | Member Pays |
|---|---|---|---|
| $42 | $35 | $35 to ded = 0 pd (2006 Part B deductible $124) | $35 (ded) |
| $90 | $75 | $75 to ded = 0 pd | $75 (ded) |
| $480 | $400 | $400 − $14 to ded = $386 × 80% = $308.80 pd | $14 (ded) + $77.20 (20%) = $91.20 |

**Example 2.** Nonparticipating provider; does not accept; assignment.

| Billed Charge | Medicare Approved Amount | Medicare Pays | Member Pays |
|---|---|---|---|
| $42 | $33.25 ($35 × 95%) | $33.25 to ded = 0 pd | $33.25 (ded) + 4.99 (LC 15%) = $38.24 |
| $90 | $71.25 ($75 × 95%) | $71.25 to ded = 0 pd | $71.25 (ded) + 10.69 (LC 15%) = $81.94 |
| $480 | $380.00 ($400 × 95%) | $380.00 − $19.50 = $360.50 × 80% = $288.40 | $19.50 (ded) + $72.10 (20%) + $57.00 (LC 15%) = $148.60 |

Some providers routinely write off any amounts not covered by Medicare. This practice is prohibited by law, as it means that Medicare covers 100% of the bill. Thus, there is no monetary incentive to the patient not to overuse services.

# Coordination of Benefits with Medicare

There are a variety of ways in which group health plans coordinate their payments with Medicare when Medicare is primary and the group plan is secondary. The most common methods in use include the following:

- Nonduplication of Medicare.
- Maintenance of benefits.
- Coordination of benefits.
- Medicare supplemental coverage.

# Nonduplication of Medicare

Calculation of benefits under the nonduplication approach is the same as with COB except that allowable expenses are those that are listed as covered expenses under the group plan. To compute benefits under this approach, use the following guidelines:

1. Regular group benefits are computed. Apply all eligibility requirements, deductibles, limitations, and maximums. This is the plan's normal liability (NL).
2. If the claim is Medicare-assigned, the Medicare-approved amount is used as the base. This will give you the balance amount.

# Practice Pitfalls

The following are additional examples of limiting charges for balance billing by nonparticipating providers.

**Example 1.** Participating provider; accepts assignment.

| Billed Charge | Medicare Approved Amount | Medicare Pays | Member Pays |
|---|---|---|---|
| $182 | $135 | $135 − $124 to ded = $11 × 80% = $8.80 pd (2006 Part B deductible $124) | $124 (ded) + 2.20 (20%) = $126.20 |

**Example 2.** Nonparticipating provider; does not accept assignment.

| Billed Charge | Medicare Approved Amount | Medicare Pays | Member Pays |
|---|---|---|---|
| $182 | $128.25 ($135 × 95%) | $128.25 − $124 to ded = $4.25 × 80% = $3.40 pd (2006 Part B deductible $124) | $124 (ded) + .85 (20%) + $19.24 (LC 15%) = $144.09 |

## Practice
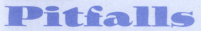

Following are two examples of calculation of benefits using the nonduplication of Medicare benefits approach:

**Example 1.** Plan benefits: $150 deductible; no charges have been applied toward the deductible amount. 80% payable for all expenses, participating provider; Medicare-assigned.

| Billed Charges | Plan Allowed Charges | Plan Normal Liability (NL) | Medicare Allowed Amount | Medicare Payment | Payment |
|---|---|---|---|---|---|
| $175.00 Office Visit | $125.00 | $0.00 ($125 applied to ded) | $125.00 | $.80 ($125 − $124 ded = $1 × 80%) | $260.00 Lesser of Plan or Medicare allowed −$108.80 Medicare/Primary Payer Payment $151.20 Balance Due **$124.80 Payment Made by Plan** |
| $165.00 Lab | $150.00 | $100.00 ($150 − $25 ded = $125 × 80%) | $135.00 | $108 ($135 × 80%) | The plan pays the lesser of the NL ($124.80) or the Balance Due ($151.20). |
| $31.00 Meds | $31.00 | 24.80 ($31 × 80%) | $0.00 | $0.00 (Not Covered) | The patient's out-of-pocket amount is $26.40 ($151.20 − $124.80). |
| **Totals** $371.00 | $306.00 | $124.80 | $260.00 | $108.80 | |

**Example 2.** Same plan benefits as in #1, nonparticipating provider; not Medicare-assigned.

| Billed Charges | Plan Allowed Charges | Plan Normal Liability (NL) | Medicare Allowed Amount | Medicare Payment | Payment |
|---|---|---|---|---|---|
| $175.00 Office Visit | $125.00 | $0.00 ($125 applied to ded) | $118.75 | $0.00 ($118.75 applied to ded) | $284.05 Lesser of Plan Allowed or MBBA ($247 × 115% = $284.05) −$98.40 Medicare/Primary Payer Payment $185.65 Balance Due **$124.80 Payment Made by Plan** |
| $165.00 Lab | $150.00 | $100.00 ($150 − $25 ded = $125 × 80%) | $128.25 | $98.40 ($128.25 − $5.25 ded = $123.00 × 80%) | The plan pays the lesser of the NL ($124.80) or the Balance Due ($185.65). |
| $31.00 Meds | $31.00 | 24.80 ($31 × 80%) | $0.00 | $0.00 (Not Covered) | The patient's out-of-pocket amount is $60.85 ($185.65 − $124.80). |
| **Totals** $371.00 | $306.00 | $124.80 | $247.00 | $98.40 | |

**a.** Subtract the amount paid by Medicare from the Medicare-approved amount.

**b.** Compare the balance with the plan's normal liability (the amount determined in 1).

    **1.** If the normal liability amount is equal to or greater than the balance amount, the balance amount is paid by the plan.

    **2.** If the normal liability amount is less than the balance amount, the normal liability amount is paid.

**3.** If the claim is not Medicare-assigned, the base is the lesser of the plan's eligible expense or the Medicare balance billable amount (MBBA).

**a.** Subtract the amount paid by Medicare from the plan's approval amount (calculated in 1).

**b.** Compare the balance with the plan's normal liability (the amount determined in number 1).

    **1.** If the normal liability amount is equal to or greater than the balance amount, the balance is paid by the plan.

    **2.** If the normal liability (NL) amount is less than the balance, the normal liability amount is paid.

**4.** The credit reserve is calculated based on the difference between the plan's liability (calculated in number 1) and the amount actually paid by the plan.

## Maintenance of Benefits

**Maintenance of benefits** refers to a provision in many group health plans that allows the person who has Medicare to "maintain" the same group benefits as members who do not have Medicare. Benefit credits are not established. To determine the benefits payable under this provision, use the following guidelines:

**1.** Compute the normal liability (NL), both Basic or Major Medical benefits, that would be payable in the absence of Medicare (perform a line-for-line calculation). Apply all eligibility requirements, deductibles, limitations, and contractual maximums.

**2.** Determine the amount the provider is allowed to collect (the Medicare-allowed amount if the claim is assigned, or the Medicare balance billable amount [MBBA] if the claim is not assigned).

**3.** Use the lesser of number 1 or number 2 as the base.

**4.** Compare the amount paid by Medicare to the base.

**5.** If the amount paid by Medicare is greater than the base, no payment will be issued by the plan. The insured has received at least the same in benefits as he would have received under the plan.

**6.** If the base is greater than the amount paid by Medicare, pay the difference. The insured will now have received the amount they would have received if there was no Medicare coverage, up to the amount of the Medicare-allowed amount or the balance billing limit.

Under maintenance of benefits, when a group plan and Medicare are both providing benefits on the same expenses, the total benefits provided should equal what the benefit would have been under the group plan alone as if the member did not have Medicare. However, since most plans exclude any amount for which there would be no charge in the absence of the insurance, the Medicare allowed amount (on assigned claims) or Medicare balance billable amount (on nonassigned claims) must be taken into consideration.

Regular group benefits are provided for charges covered by the group plan but not covered at all by Medicare.

## Standard Coordination of Benefits

Standard COB with Medicare is calculated as with any other COB claim. Allowable expenses are based on the amount approved by Medicare on an assigned claim; or the amount approved by the plan or Medicare, whichever is greater, on a nonassigned claim. However, payment is only made up to the Medicare-allowable amount on assigned claims, and up to the MBBA amount on nonassigned claims. If the plan's normal liability is greater than the payment made, the difference between the plan's normal liability and the payment is reserved for future claims payments. Also, as with other COB claims, allowable expenses are considered those payable in whole or part by one or both plans. Benefit credit reserve is established and used to cover allowable expenses. See **Figure 8–1** for Medicare Secondary Payer rules.

## Medicare Secondary Payer

| If the patient... | And this condition exists... | Then the program pays first... | And this program pays second... |
|---|---|---|---|
| Is age 65 or older, and is covered by a group health plan through a current employer or spouse's current employer... | The employer has fewer than 20 employees... | **Medicare** | group health plan |
| | The employer has 20 or more employees, or at least one employer is a multi-employer group that employs 20 or more individuals... | group health plan | **Medicare** |
| Has an employer retirement plan and is age 65 or older or is disabled and age 65 or older... | The patient is entitled to Medicare... | **Medicare** | Retiree coverage |
| Is disabled and covered by a large group health plan from work, or is covered by a family member who is working... | The employer has fewer than 100 employees... | **Medicare** | large group health plan |
| | The employer has 100 or more employees, or at least one employer is a multi-employer group that employs 100 or more individuals... | large group health plan | **Medicare** |
| Has end-stage renal disease and group health plan coverage... | Is in the first 30 months of eligibility or entitlement to Medicare... | group health plan | **Medicare** |
| | After 30 months... | **Medicare** | group health plan |
| Has end-stage renal disease and COBRA coverage... | Is in the first 30 months of eligibility or entitlement to Medicare... | COBRA | Medicare |
| | After 30 months... | **Medicare** | COBRA |
| Is covered under Workers' Compensation because of job-related illness or injury... | The patient is entitled to Medicare... | Workers' Compensation (for health care items or services related to job-related illness or injury) | **Medicare** |
| Has black lung disease and is covered under the Federal Black Lung Program... | The patient is eligible for the Federal Black Lung Program... | Federal Black Lung Program (for health care services related to black lung disease) | **Medicare** |
| Has been in an auto accident where no-fault or liability insurance is involved... | The patient is entitled to Medicare... | No-fault or liability insurance (for accident-related health care services) | **Medicare** |
| Is age 65 or older OR is disabled and covered by Medicare and COBRA... | The patient is entitled to Medicare... | **Medicare** | COBRA |
| Has Veterans Health Administration (VHA) benefits... | Receives VHA authorized health care services at a non-VHA facility... | VHA | Medicare may pay when the services provided are Medicare-covered services and are not covered by the VHA |

■ **Figure 8–1** Medicare Secondary Payer Rules

# Practice
# Pitfalls

The following are two examples of calculation of benefits using the maintenance of benefits approach.

**Example 1.** Plan benefits: $150 deductible; no charges have been applied toward the deductible amount. 80% payable for all expenses. Participating provider; Medicare-assigned.

| Billed Charges | Plan Allowed Charges | Plan Normal Liability (NL) | Medicare Allowed Amount | Medicare Payment | Payment |
|---|---|---|---|---|---|
| $175.00 Office Visit | $125.00 | $0.00 ($125 applied to ded) | $125.00 | $.80 ($125 − $124 ded = $1 × 80%) | $124.80 Base <br> −$108.80 Medicare/Primary Payer Payment <br> **$16.00 Payment Made by Plan** |
| $165.00 Lab | $150.00 | $100.00 ($150 − $25 ded = $125 × 80%) | $135.00 | $108 ($135 × 80%) | $260.00 Lesser of the Plan or Medicare Allowed |
| $31.00 Meds | $31.00 | 24.80 ($31 × 80%) | $0.00 | $0.00 (Not Covered) | The patient's out-of-pocket amount is $135.20 ($260.00 − $108.80 − $16.00). |
| **Totals** $371.00 | $306.00 | $124.80 | $260.00 | $108.80 | |

**Example 2.** Same plan benefits as in #1, nonparticipating provider; not Medicare-assigned.

| Billed Charges | Plan Allowed Charges | Plan Normal Liability (NL) | Medicare Allowed Amount | Medicare Payment | Payment |
|---|---|---|---|---|---|
| $175.00 Office Visit | $125.00 | $0.00 ($125 applied to ded) | $118.75 | $0.00 ($118.75 applied to ded) | $124.80 Base <br> −$98.40 Medicare/Primary Payer Payment <br> **$26.40 Payment Made by Plan** |
| $165.00 Lab | $150.00 | $100.00 ($150 − $25 ded = $125 × 80%) | $128.25 | $98.40 ($128.25 − $5.25 ded = $123.00 × 80%) | $284.05 Lesser of Plan Allowed or MBBA ($247 × 115%). |
| $31.00 Meds | $31.00 | 24.80 ($31 × 80%) | $0.00 | $0.00 (Not Covered) | The patient's out-of-pocket amount is $159.25 ($284.05 − $98.40 − $26.40) |
| **Totals** $371.00 | $306.00 | $124.80 | $247.00 | $98.40 | |

# Practice
# Pitfalls

The following are examples or calculation of benefits using standard coordination of benefits.

**Example 1.** Plan benefits: $150 deductible; no charges have been applied toward the deductible amount. Participating provider; Medicare-assigned.

| Billed Charges | Plan Allowed Charges | Plan Normal Liability (NL) | Medicare Allowed Amount | Medicare Payment | Payment |
|---|---|---|---|---|---|
| $175.00 Office Visit | $125.00 | $0.00 ($125 applied to ded) | $125.00 | $.80 ($125 − $124 ded = $1 × 80%) | $260.00 Medicare Allowed Amount −$108.80 Medicare/Primary Payer Payment $151.20 Balance Due **$124.80 Payment Made by Plan** |
| $165.00 Lab | $150.00 | $100.00 ($150 − $25 ded = $125 × 80%) | $135.00 | $108 ($135 × 80%) | The plan pays the lesser of the NL ($124.80) or the difference; up to the Medicare allowed amount. |
| $31.00 Meds | $31.00 | 24.80 ($31 × 80%) | $0.00 | $0.00 (Not Covered) | The patient's out-of-pocket amount is $26.40 ($151.20 − $124.80). |
| **Totals** $371.00 | $306.00 | $124.80 | $260.00 | $108.80 | |

**Example 2.** Same plan benefits as in #1, nonparticipating provider; not Medicare-assigned.

| Billed Charges | Plan Allowed Charges | Plan Normal Liability (NL) | Medicare Allowed Amount | Medicare Payment | Payment |
|---|---|---|---|---|---|
| $175.00 Office Visit | $125.00 | $0.00 ($125 applied to ded) | $118.75 | $0.00 ($118.75 applied to ded) | $284.05 (MBBA Amount) ($247 × 115%) −$98.40 Medicare/Primary Payer Payment $185.65 Balance Due **$124.80 Payment Made by Plan** |
| $165.00 Lab | $150.00 | $100.00 ($150 − $25 ded = $125 × 80%) | $128.25 | $98.40 ($128.25 − $5.25 ded = $123.00 × 80%) | Plan pays the lesser of the NL ($124.80) or the Balance Due ($185.65); up to the balance billing limit. |
| $31.00 Meds | $31.00 | 24.80 ($31 × 80%) | $0.00 | $0.00 (Not Covered) | The patient's out-of-pocket amount is $60.85 ($185.65 − $124.80). |
| **Totals** $371.00 | $306.00 | $124.80 | $247.00 | $98.40 | |

**Example 3.** Benefits payable at 85% of PPO schedule. Deductible $150, deductible satisfied. Participating provider; Medicare-assigned.

| Billed Charges | Plan Allowed Charges | Plan Normal Liability (NL) | Medicare Allowed Amount | Medicare Payment | Payment |
|---|---|---|---|---|---|
| $5,000.00 Inpatient Hospital Charges | $2,200.00 PPO Contract Rate | $1,870.00 (PPO allowance $2,200 × 85%) | $4,000.00 | $2,438.40 ($4,000.00 − $952 (2006 inpatient ded) = $3048.00 × 80%) | **$1,561.60 Payment Made by Plan** The payment includes the inpatient deductible amount ($952.00) + $609.60 (20% copayment). |

In example 3 the PPO provider has a contractual obligation to provide care on this claim for $2,200. This is due to a contract between the provider and the PPO. Amounts over $2,200 are not usually collectible.

Until early 1999, the insurance carrier had no liability in this example because Medicare paid more than the normal liability and because the provider is part of the plan network and contractually has to write off charges over $2,200. This would leave no patient responsibility and no insurance liability.

However, providers claimed that insurance carriers and PPO's were in violation of the Social Security Act antikickback clause. This section of the Act basically states that an insurance company or PPO cannot make a provider write off the Medicare patient responsibility amount. Therefore, the patient responsibility amount is payable by the insurance carrier up to the plan's normal liability in the absence of Medicare. Thus, the plan must pay the $1,561.60 patient responsibility amount on this claim since their normal liability is higher than this amount.

## Medicare Supplement

**Medicare supplements** are separate plans written exclusively for Medicare participants. A supplement plan may be written with optional benefits the policyholder wants. Common options are as follows:

- Physicians' services—Covers Part B deductible and 20% coinsurance for reasonable charges. "Reasonable charges" means that amounts reduced by Medicare because of prevailing fees are not covered under the plan even though the plan's prevailing fee may be higher than that of Medicare when the bill is assigned. If the bill is not assigned, the plan's UCR or Medicare's UCR is the amount allowable, whichever is greater.
- Hospital services—Covers Part A deductible and may or may not cover the various copays not covered by Medicare.

With the changes in Medicare, supplemental plans have become more flexible. Therefore, the benefits can be complex and comprehensive, or very basic. Read plan provisions carefully to determine which items are covered and which are not. Since the purpose of a Medicare supplement plan is to cover the patient's responsibility, many charges that are covered are paid at 100%.

# On the Job Now

**Directions:** Answer the following questions without looking back at the material just covered. Write your answers in the space provided.

1. Explain how you would compute benefits under each method for payment.

    a. Nonduplication of Medicare _____

    _____

    b. Maintenance of benefits _____

    _____

    c. Coordination of benefits _____

    _____

    d. Medicare supplemental coverage _____

    _____

2. Why can the benefits for Medicare supplemental plans fall into a wide range of being complex and comprehensive, or very basic? _____

# Estimating Medicare Coverage

Sometimes a member is entitled to Medicare but has not enrolled. In this circumstance, many policies specify that the group plan will estimate what Medicare would have paid if the person had been enrolled properly, or the policy may specify instead that benefits may be reduced only when the member is actually enrolled in Medicare. In this situation, the regular plan benefits will be provided and the Medicare payment will not be estimated.

To estimate the Medicare payment, use the following as a guideline:

**Hospital: Part A**
1. Provide full benefits toward the Medicare deductible and coinsurance amounts.
2. Provide regular group benefits for services or items covered by the group plan but not covered by Medicare.

**Professional: Part B**
1. Determine the plan's UCR for the billed charges.
2. The UCR amount is considered the estimated Medicare-approved amount.
3. Multiply 80% of the estimated approved amount (#2). This is your estimated Medicare payment.
4. Once you have estimated Medicare's payment, you can proceed with calculating the coordination of benefits (as shown above).

# Diagnosis-Related Group Billing

In the early 1980s, Medicare instituted **diagnosis-related group (DRG)** payments for inpatient hospital claims. Under DRG, a flat rate payment is made based on the patient's diagnosis rather than the hospital's itemized billing. If the hospital can treat the patient for less, it keeps the savings. If treatment costs more, the hospital must absorb the loss. Neither Medicare nor the patient is responsible for the excess amount.

## Exceptions

Provisions have been made for cases atypically expensive (based on the diagnosis) because of complications or an abnormally long confinement. Known as **outliers**, these cases will be reimbursed on an itemized or cost percentage basis rather than DRG. The bill from the hospital must indicate that it is an outlier.

## Exclusions

Excluded from DRG are long-term care, children's care, and psychiatric and rehabilitative hospitals. Some states have obtained waivers from DRG, so you should consult your state Department of Insurance to determine which states are excluded.

## DRG Benefit Payment Calculations

As shown in the following examples, the maximum liability under a plan consists of only the following expenses:

- Those covered by the plan.
- Those that the insured is legally obligated to pay.

## Practice Pitfalls

**Example 1.** Itemized hospital bill exceeds Medicare DRG allowance.

| | |
|---|---|
| Hospital Bill | $8,700 |
| DRG Allowance | $7,000 |
| Medicare Payment | $6,048 (DRG Allowance – $952 [2006 Medicare inpatient deductible]) |
| Member's Responsibility | $ 952 |
| Hospital Write-off | $1,700 |

Although the Medicare DRG allowance is less than the itemized hospital bill, the insured is legally obligated to pay only the $952 Part A deductible. Therefore, the difference between the itemized hospital bill amount and the DRG allowance is excluded as not covered. The plan's benefits would be based on the DRG allowance of $7,000, with the $1,700 reflected as not covered because it may exceed the DRG allowance.

**Example 2.** Medicare DRG allowance exceeds itemized billed amount.

| | |
|---|---|
| Hospital Bill | $ 8,700 |
| DRG Allowance | $10,000 |
| Medicare Payment | $ 9,048 (DRG Allowance – $952 [2006 Medicare inpatient deductible]) |
| Member's Responsibility | $ 952 |

Although the Medicare payment exceeds the itemized hospital bill, the insured is legally obligated to pay the $952 Part A deductible. Handling of this type of billing also varies. Check the payer guidelines before processing the claim.

## Medicaid

The Medicaid program was established under Title XIX of the Social Security Act of 1965. **Medicaid** is a jointly funded federal-state entitlement program, designed to provide healthcare services to certain low-income and needy people. It covers children, the aged, blind or disabled, and people who are eligible to receive federally assisted income maintenance payments. The purpose of this program is to provide the needy with access to medical care.

Medicaid is the largest program providing medical and health-related services to America's neediest people. Within broad national guidelines which the federal government provides, each state:

1. Establishes its own eligibility standards.
2. Determines the type, amount, duration, and scope of services.
3. Sets the rate of payment for services.
4. Administers its own program.

Thus, the Medicaid program varies considerably from state to state.

By law, Medicaid is always secondary to private group healthcare plans. If Medicaid inadvertently pays primary, it will exercise its right of recovery and seek reimbursement from the private plan. Again, the private plan by law is required to process Medicaid's request for reimbursement and pay back to Medicaid the monies it paid the Medicaid provider.

The regulations governing eligibility under the Medicaid program are complex. Individuals may be entitled to coverage due to medical, family, or financial situations. The fact that the individual has private insurance does not preclude him from being eligible for Medicaid benefits.

The Medicaid program does not process its own claims. Medicaid contracts with other organizations who act as the fiscal intermediary, similar to Medicare. The intermediary processes the claims according to specifications set forth by the Medicaid program.

The rates under Medicaid are based on the results of reimbursement studies conducted by the Department of Health Services. Reimbursement for hospital inpatient services is based on each facility's "reasonable cost" of services as determined from audit cost reports and annual limitations on reimbursable increases in cost.

If the patient is covered by private insurance in addition to Medicaid, the provider may bill the patient's private insurance. There is a three-year statute of limitations from the date of service for recovering payment. In addition, there is a three-year subrogation right.

For a claimant's services to be covered under Medicaid, the claimant must be a Medicaid beneficiary and the provider must be an approved Medicaid provider. To be an approved provider, the provider of services must agree to accept Medicaid's determination of approved amounts as binding. This is similar to Medicare's approved amount on assigned claims, where the provider is not allowed to bill the patient for any amount not approved by Medicaid. In recent years, many providers have dropped out of the Medicaid program because Medicaid's allowances and payments were extremely low. Some were even lower than those provided by Medicare.

## Health Insurance Payment Demand

The **Health Insurance Payment Demand (HIPD)**, commonly referred to as "hippid," is a bill that lists the healthcare services paid by the Medicaid program on behalf of a person who has indicated she has other healthcare coverage benefits available. Insurers/plans are to reimburse the Medicaid program for those services to the extent of the plan's available benefits, or the amount paid by Medicaid, whichever is less. If the private plan is not liable for a particular service, the reason for this must be explained on the HIPD, along with indications of what was paid.

The HIPD is a computer-generated list that includes the following:

- The patient's name.
- The policyholder name.
- The policy number.
- The provider.
- The diagnosis.
- The treatment provided.
- The dates of services.
- The charges.
- Payments previously made by Medicaid on each service.

Return Address

Attention: Claims Manager

Warning! Enclosed is confidential information. This information is provided to you so that you may determine the liability of your company or your health insurance carrier to repay the Medicaid program on behalf of the individual listed. This is pursuant to State Code Sections 100XX et sq., 140XX.XX, or 141XX. Any person may be subject to civil or criminal penalties for disclosure, publication, or other use, or for permitting or causing this confidential information to be disclosed, published, or used except as necessary to accomplish the above-mentioned purpose or with specific written permission from the Medicaid beneficiary, personal representative, or guardian (if a minor).

Enclosed are Health Insurance Payment Demands (HIPDs) for claims for healthcare services paid by the Medicaid program for individuals who indicate that they have healthcare coverage with your organization.

Payment to the extent of your contractual obligation is now due. Medicaid should be reimbursed for all amounts that it has paid as shown on the following form. When making payment on this claim, please indicate the HIPD number and the patient's Medicaid number on your check. Mark the amount of payment for each service on the state copy and the HIPD. If a service or services are not covered, a complete explanation of the reason for nonpayment should be indicated on the enclosed HIPD Processing Form. The HIPD Processing Form may be reproduced for use within your office.

If you are unable to identify the claimant as an insured policyholder under your plan, mark the HIPD box 4a and return. If you need additional information to locate the claimant or confirm eligibility, list the precise information needed. Additional information that would facilitate future HIPD processing (i.e., Group name, policy #), which is not listed on the HIPD, may be noted under response #4d (Other) on the HIPD Processing Form.

If this HIPD should be sent to another department or location, indicate the appropriate department and the complete address and return the HIPD to us. We will update our files with the proper information.

All policyholders that provide coverage for the claimant listed are indicated under the claimant's name. This information is for use in coordinating benefits with other health insurance carriers.

Thank you for your cooperation. If you have any questions, please write us at the address indicated above.

Sincerely

Jane Doe, Chief
Health Insurance Unit
Recovery Branch

■ **Figure 8–2** HIPD Cover Letter

The HIPD is usually accompanied by a cover letter (**see Figure 8–2**). The state's Recovery Unit will also supply the HIPD Processing Form, which is used by the payer when responding to a HIPD. It is completed by the carrier and then sent to Medicaid with the state's copy of the HIPD. A sample of the front of this form is shown in **Figure 8–3**. The forms may differ from state to state, but they usually contain similar information.

# Health Insurance Payment Demand
# (HIPD) Processing Form

Please Return State Copy of HIPD to:

Please feel free to write on the HIPD. In addition, complete the appropriate information below and return with the HIPD.

Patient Name (Medicaid Beneficiary): _____    Medicaid #: _____

HIPD Number(s) (From the upper-right-hand corner of the HIPD): _____

HIPD Billing Date(s) (From the upper right corner of the HIPD): _____

☐ 1. The enclosed check(s) for $ _____ represents payment of our liability under this policy. For any charges considered ineligible, see Number 3 below.

☐ 2. Charges previously considered (if additional space is needed, please use reverse side).

      Payee _____    Amount $ _____    Date _____

      Address _____    Date(s) of Service _____

      Payee _____    Amount $ _____    Date _____

      Address _____    Date(s) of Service _____

3.   Claimant is ineligible due to:

    ☐ a. Claimant's policy is no longer in effect. Termination date: _____

    ☐ b. Claimant was not covered on date of service. Coverage date(s) _____ to _____

    ☐ c. Claimant's group was not insured on date of service. Coverage date(s) _____ to _____

      If liable carrier is known, provide complete name and address: _____

    ☐ d. Claimant was not a covered dependent on date of service. Explain: _____

    ☐ e. Services are not covered expenses under the policy. Why?

      ☐ Policy does not cover convalescent care.  ☐ Policy covers in-hospital services only.

      ☐ Policy does not cover drugs, vision, etc.  ☐ Other _____

    ☐ f. Maximum benefit of $ _____ per _____ (time period) has been exhausted.

    ☐ g. Charges do not exceed policy deductible. Deductible is $ _____ per _____

    ☐ h. Other reasons (specify) _____

4.   This HIPD is being returned or processing is being delayed due to:

    ☐ a. We are unable to identify individual/group as our insured. We need: _____

    ☐ b. Dual coverage is indicated. We need: _____

    ☐ c. Additional information is needed on the following service(s): _____

    ☐ d. Other (specify): _____

■ **Figure 8–3** HIPD Processing Form

# HIPD Handling Procedures

When a HIPD is received, the following eight procedures will assist in its handling and in filling out the HIPD processing form.

1. Determine whether or not the patient is eligible under the plan shown. If not, complete item #3. If the information provided on the HIPD is incomplete and you are unable to identify the member or patient, complete item #4.

2. Determine whether the charges shown were previously paid under the plan. If so, no payment is due Medicaid. Complete item #2.

3. If no payment has been made for the charges in question and payments were due, calculate the normal plan benefits. Do not request an attending physician's statement because the HIPD constitutes sufficient proof of loss.

4. Usually, a line-by-line comparison is made between the amount paid by Medicaid and the amount payable under the private plan. However, it is also possible to do a total-by-total comparison. To do this, subtract the amounts paid by Medicaid for expenses not covered by the private plan from the total Medicaid payment.

5. Pay the lesser of:
   a. The normal private plan benefit, or
   b. The total Medicaid payment, as adjusted in #4. The payment by the private plan to Medicaid should never exceed the total adjusted Medicaid payment. The draft should be made payable to Health Care Deposit Fund (or the source included on the form).

6. If payment has previously been made, complete item #2. If some or all of the charges are not covered under the terms of the plan, complete item #3 or #4.

7. Send the completed HIPD Processing Form, the state copy of the HIPD, and the benefit draft (if benefits are payable) to the Health Recovery Bureau for your state (or the source included on the form).

8. Retain one copy of the HIPD in the claim file.

After payment has been made to Medicaid, the plan's full liability has been discharged. This is true even if the payment made is less than the payment that would have been made in the absence of Medicaid.

These instructions apply only if the HIPD has been received. If the claims file indicates that the claimant is eligible for Medicaid but the state has not submitted a HIPD, any charges received should be handled in the usual manner. When processing a HIPD billing, all plan provisions except the timely filing limitations apply. Check with your supervisor for company procedures on handling HIPDs.

# CHAPTER REVIEW

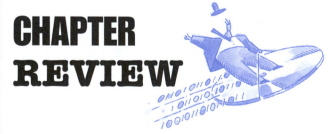

## Summary

- Medicare is administered through the Health Care Financing Administration.
- Each year, rules and guidelines for payment and covered charges are established.
- Claims examiners must stay informed of the changes in the Medicare system. This can be accomplished by subscribing to the Medicare bulletin that is usually published by the fiscal intermediary for Medicare in the local area.
- By using the Medicare bulletins and applying the guidelines we have covered in this chapter, claims examiners will establish a consistent approach to processing Medicare claims, which will result in competent and accurate claim decisions.
- Medicaid guidelines vary from state to state.
- Medicaid bulletins are produced to assist you in interpreting the rules for coverage and to determine which charges Medicaid covers.
- These bulletins are available to Medicaid providers and are primarily used by billers; however, they may be helpful to the claims examiner. Contact your Medicaid intermediary for copies of the bulletins.

## Assignments

Complete the Questions for Review.
Complete Exercise 8–1 through 8–4.

**Note:** All Medicare benefits and exclusions are correct as of the date of printing. For updated benefits, contact your local Social Security Administration.

## Questions for Review

**Directions:**  Answer the following questions without looking back at the material just covered. Write your answers in the space provided.

1. What is Medicare? _____

   _____

2. On what three criteria is Medicare eligibility based?

   1. _____

   2. _____

   3. _____

3. Medicare _____ is considered the basic plan or hospital insurance.

4. Medicare _____ is the medical insurance that covers doctors' services, outpatient services, and so on.

5. What does it mean when a provider accepts assignment of benefits in relation to Medicare? _____

   _____

   _____

6. What is the purpose of the Medicaid program? _____

   _____

7. (True or False?) By law, Medicaid is always primary to private group health insurance plans. _____

8. In what situation are providers allowed to bill or submit a claim to the Medicaid beneficiary? _____

   _____

9. The _____ is a bill that lists the healthcare services paid by the Medicaid program on behalf of a person who has indicated that he or she has other healthcare coverage benefits available.

10. For a claimant's services to be covered under Medicaid, the claimant must be a _____ and the provider must be an _____.

   If you were unable to answer any of these questions, refer back to that section and then fill in the answers.

# Exercise 8-1

**Directions:** Using the attached Medicare Remittance Notice, compute the COB payment amount for the claims that are listed on the notice. Be sure to check plan provisions for the type of COB that should be performed.

## MEDICARE REMITTANCE NOTICE

DATE: FEBRUARY 27, CCYY
CHECK SEQUENCE NO.: 2AF-01241351-2
PAGE 1 OF 1

| BENEFICIARY NAME | SVC FR MO-DY | TO DY-YR | PLACE TYPE | PROCEDURE DESCRIPTION | AMOUNT BILLED | AMOUNT APPROVED | SEE NOTE | DEDUCTIBLE | COINSURANCE | PAYMENT | SECONDARY CARRIER UCR | SECONDARY CARRIER LIABILITY | PAYMENT AMOUNT |
|---|---|---|---|---|---|---|---|---|---|---|---|---|---|
| **HELGA HEARTACHE** | 02-06 | 02-06 | 23 | 93000 | 340.00 | 297.18 | 56 | | | | | | |
| | 02-06 | 02-06 | 23 | 93545 | 770.00 | 699.23 | 56 | | | | | | |
| | 02-06 | 02-06 | 23 | 85025 | 40.00 | 21.21 | 56 | | | | | | |
| | 02-06 | 02-06 | 23 | 86901 | 45.00 | 27.34 | 56 | | | | | | |
| | 02-06 | 02-06 | 23 | 85610 | 30.00 | 19.57 | 56 | | | | | | |
| Accepts assignment | CLAIM NOTE | | | TOTALS | 1,225.00 | 1,064.53 | 442 | 124.00 | 188.11 | 752.42 | 846.32 | 507.79 | |
| **BARRY BROKEN** | 01-26 | 01-26 | 23 | 992885 | 882.00 | 699.00 | 56 | | | | | | |
| Accepts assignment | CLAIM NOTE | | | TOTALS | 882.00 | 699.00 | 442 | 124.00 | 115.00 | 460.00 | 882.00 | 433.80 | |
| **HELGA HEARTACHE** | 02-09 | 02-09 | 21 | 33217 | 245.00 | 189.46 | 56 | | | | | | |
| | 02-09 | 02-09 | 21 | 33225 | 500.00 | 167.38 | 56 | | | | | | |
| | 02-09 | 02-09 | 21 | 33240 | 295.00 | 295.00 | | | | | | | |
| Accepts assignment | CLAIM NOTE | | | TOTALS | 1,040.00 | 651.84 | 442 | 0.00 | 130.37 | 521.47 | 895.63 | 716.51 | |
| **ALMA ALVAREZ** | 02-02 | 02-02 | 11 | 99213 | 330.00 | 227.56 | 56 | | | | | | |
| Does not accept assignment | CLAIM NOTE | | | TOTALS | 330.00 | 227.56 | 442 | 124.00 | 20.71 | 82.85 | 289.44 | 145.06 | |
| **ALMA ALVAREZ** | 02-02 | 02-02 | 11 | 76092 | 165.00 | 127.57 | 56 | | | | | | |
| Accepts assignment | CLAIM NOTE | | | TOTALS | 165.00 | 127.57 | 442 | 0.00 | 25.51 | 102.06 | 124.07 | 105.56 | |
| **BARRY BROKEN** | 01-26 | 01-26 | 21 | 70260-27 | 70.00 | 61.12 | 56 | | | | | | |
| | 01-26 | 01-26 | 21 | 71020-27 | 55.00 | 43.21 | 56 | | | | | | |
| | 01-26 | 01-26 | 21 | 735502-7 | 80.00 | 70.88 | 56 | | | | | | |
| | 01-26 | 01-26 | 21 | 73590-27 | 100.00 | 83.83 | 56 | | | | | | |
| | 01-26 | 01-26 | 21 | 70450-27 | 325.00 | 180.67 | 56 | | | | | | |
| | 01-26 | 01-26 | 21 | 73718-27 | 770.00 | 622.39 | 56 | | | | | | |
| Accepts assignment | CLAIM NOTE | | | TOTALS | 1,400.00 | 1,062.10 | 442 | 0.00 | 212.42 | 849.68 | 1,203.30 | 1,082.97 | |
| **HELGA HEARTACHE** | 02-06 | 02-06 | 23 | 99285 | 1,600.00 | 1,306.70 | 56 | | | | | | |
| | 02-06 | 02-06 | 23 | 99285 | 420.00 | 383.13 | 56 | | | | | | |
| Does not accept assignment | CLAIM NOTE | | | TOTALS | 2,020.00 | 1,689.83 | 442 | 0.00 | 337.97 | 1,351.86 | 1,595.78 | 1,156.62 | |
| **BARRY BROKEN** | 01-26 | 01-26 | 21 | 21800 | 560.00 | 499.99 | 56 | | | | | | |
| | 01-26 | 01-26 | 21 | 27758 | 215.00 | 116.32 | 56 | | | | | | |
| | 01-26 | 01-26 | 21 | 27784 | 200.00 | 159.56 | 56 | | | | | | |
| | 01-26 | 01-26 | 21 | 62000 | 150.00 | 130.99 | | | | | | | |
| Accepts assignment | CLAIM NOTE | | | TOTALS | 1,125.00 | 906.86 | 442 | 0.00 | 181.37 | 725.49 | 975.80 | 878.22 | |

HELGA HEARTACHE - Ninja
BARRY BROKEN - ABC
ALMA ALVAREZ - XYZ

56 - Medicare limits payment to this amount.
63 - Medicare considers follow-up care to be an integral part of the surgery with no additional allowance.
92 - An assistant surgeon is not considered medically necessary for this surgery.
442 - Total for these charges.

# Exercise **8-2**

**Directions:** Find and circle the words listed below. Words can appear horizontally, vertically, diagonally, forward, or backward.

```
C B L U E C G E A S M R R P T M T M B K G K N C M
L E D Q X N U N P P H F U W D A E U U V Y F E D E
U O W W H F D O I U G G X K W D F V F T V L E Y D
O R J U V P T S I L F S Y Q I Z O E S R U T M E I
C O A W S A A A T A L Z S C P N C T E U P P C C C
U V Z W M D K R Y A F I A W J W B A I W K B J U A
Q J K Y T R R Q O D G R B D B E T B J A B A B F R
Y K O C M K Z U S V E E H E G D N V I N Z S V O E
H S F K B V B P T A I C R C C J A M X H S F K E S
F S M L Y Y P W L Q N E G E M N H F Q E U E Q U U
L E Y Z P K E L S E Q A W C N G A L F L G K U R P
U N M W S H O O R N K V D L G A A L W U T Z P T P
N V V E E W P U R T U Q D T T W L G A E M D M S L
S E G R A H C E L B A N O S A E R D O B B D K P E
Q V Q N O J A V P I B F E V F B D V I A R J E B M
L M C N U E Z F O R H J G M L L S D T S A S H Y E
N E C M I R F W H S L G D I F N D K A C E Q K X N
Y P A R T I C I P A T I N G P H Y S I C I A N S T
R R C N U G W A Y T R F X O N B P J S T Y W S O S
I A P T X C G O S H A N E G M J C G K E K L X E V
H C B D L Q P H S R B F H F Y L I I E H R C Y D V
J X E K C N W L W N E Z D C F O G T S T X T V O K
Z O N J V T Q C R K P V W A G I B Q H Y J P E O B
X H F I U P L K M D L V B A C C X T I L D N U X K
A T S V J I W J E P U H I P S Y I Z M D P L Z V G
```

1. Balance Billing
2. End Stage Renal Disease
3. Medicare Allowance
4. Medicare Supplements
5. Participating Physicians
6. Reasonable Charges

# Exercise 8-3

**Directions:** Complete the crossword puzzle by filling in a word from the keywords that fits each clue.

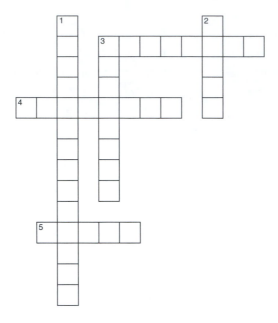

## Across

**3.** A jointly funded federal-state entitlement program, designed to provide healthcare services to certain low-income and needy people.

**4.** DRG cases which are atypically expensive (based on the diagnosis) because of complications or an abnormally long confinement.

**5.** The Medicare medical insurance which covers doctor's services, outpatient hospital services, home healthcare, outpatient speech and physical therapy, and durable medical equipment.

## Down

**1.** The maximum amount that the Federal Government allows nonparticipating physicians to charge Medicare patients for a given service.

**2.** The Medicare basic plan or hospital insurance which covers facility charges for acute inpatient hospital care, skilled nursing, home healthcare, and hospice care.

**3.** The Federal Health Insurance Benefit Plan for the Aged and Disabled.

# Exercise 8-4

**Directions:** Match the following terms with the proper definition by writing the letter of the correct definition in the space next to the term.

1. _____ Deficit Reduction Act of 1984

    a. A federal act that redirected the financial responsibility for medical coverage of active employees age 65 years and older and their spouses aged 65 years and older to Medicare.

2. _____ Diagnosis Related Group Billing

    b. Physicians who treat Medicare-eligible patients but who decide whether to accept assignment on a case-by-case basis.

3. _____ Health Insurance Payment Demand

    c. A bill that lists the healthcare services paid by the Medicaid program on behalf of a person who has other healthcare coverage benefits available.

4. _____ Maintenance of Benefits

    d. A flat rate payment is made based on the patient's diagnosis rather than the hospital's itemized billing.

5. _____ Nonparticipating Physicians

    e. The Act that amended TEFRA so that spouses aged 65 years and older of active employees who are under age 65 can elect their primary coverage as either Medicare or the private group plan.

6. _____ Tax Equity and Fiscal Responsibility Act of 1982

    f. A COB provision in many group health plans that allows the person who has Medicare to "maintain" the same group benefits as members who do not have Medicare.

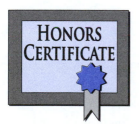

## Honors Certification™

The Honors Certification™ challenge for this chapter consists of a written test of the information contained within this chapter. Each incorrect answer will result in a deduction of up to 5% from your grade. You must achieve a score of 85% or higher to pass this test. If you fail the test on your first attempt, you may retake the test one additional time. The items included in the second test may be different from those in the first test.

# 9
# Workers'
## Compensation

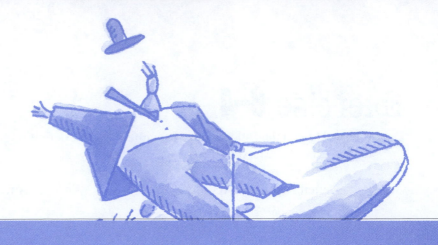

## After completion of this chapter
**you will be able to:**

- Describe the eligibility requirements and basic benefits of Workers' Compensation.
- List situations or places that would be covered by workers' compensation if an accident were to occur.
- List the types of claims workers' compensation provides coverage for.
- Describe the three disability levels for workers' compensation claims.
- Describe the benefits provided by workers' compensation coverage.
- List the types of issues that most of the new workers' compensation laws deal with.

- Describe the Doctor's First Report and how it is used.
- State the information that should be included in a Doctor's First Report and Subsequent Progress Reports.
- List the factors that may delay the close of a workers' compensation case.
- List signs to look for that may indicate fraud or abuse of a workers' compensation case.
- Describe how third party liability on a workers' compensation case can affect the claim.
- Properly complete lien documents.

## Keywords and concepts
**you will learn in this chapter:**

- Company Activities
- Death Benefits
- Doctor's First Report of Occupational Injury or Illness (First Report)
- Job-Related Injuries

- Lien
- Nondisability Claims
- Occupational Illnesses
- Permanent and Stationary
- Permanent Disability
- Physician's Final Report

- Rehabilitation Benefit
- Subjective Findings
- Temporary Disability
- Vocational Rehabilitation
- Work Hardening
- Workers' Compensation (WC)

**Workers' Compensation (WC)** is a separate medical and disability reimbursement program which provides 100% coverage for job related injuries, illnesses, or conditions arising out of and in the course of employment. The employer, by law, is responsible for the benefits due to an injured worker for work related injuries and illnesses. WC insurance includes benefits for medical care expenses, disability income, and death benefits.

When a claim is received for treatment of an accident, it is important to obtain a statement of exactly what happened so that you can determine if a claim is covered by WC or by the patient's regular insurance. **Job-related injuries** include any injuries which happen during the performance of work-related duties, whether they are in or out of the office. **Occupational illnesses** are considered to be any disorders, illnesses, or conditions which arise at work or from exposure to factors at work. Occupational illnesses may be caused by inhaling, directly contacting, absorbing, or ingesting a hazardous agent. Some occupational illnesses may take years to develop, or remain latent for a number of years before flaring up. For this reason, some states have WC laws which cover workers for years after they cease active employment in a field. For example, construction workers who dealt repeatedly with asbestos may develop asbestosis years after exposure.

Federal WC programs cover federal workers, coal miners (black lung program), longshoremen, and harbor workers. State WC laws cover everyone else. States set up their own guidelines, with the federal government mandating a minimum level of benefits.

Each state's WC Appeals Board has the sole authority to oversee the rights and benefits of an injured or ill worker. It is through this Appeals Board that an applicant (employee) will file their WC application.

As a general limitation, most health insurance plans specify that the claimant will not be entitled to payment for "bodily injury or disease resulting from and arising out of any employment or occupation for compensation or profit."

Most health insurance plans will investigate and then provide benefits for medical care if they suspect that a claim is work-related. Because the resolution of a WC case usually takes one to two years, private plans are obligated to pay the benefits for which the member is entitled, and then file a lien with the member and the WC Board to recover plan losses when the case is settled.

Once the WC carrier has accepted liability for the claim, the plan will discontinue providing benefits for medical care. At that point, the claim would be denied on the basis that it is work-related.

# Employee Activities

The following section contains some general guidelines as to what constitutes an injury or illness as recognized by a WC Board in most states based on the type of activity, not the type of injury.

## Company Activities

**Company activities** can be defined as the following:

1. An injury sustained while attending an activity sponsored by an employer for the purpose of obtaining some business gain. (i.e., company party for morale purposes; sporting activity for which the employee is provided transportation, and/or the company gains advertisement by virtue of having the employee wear a company "athletic shirt").

2. An injury sustained during an activity for which the company provides remuneration.

3. An injury sustained while in the course of a person's occupation.

## Use of Company Vehicles

Most WC laws provide coverage for an injury sustained while driving or as an authorized passenger in a company vehicle. This is true whether the injury is incurred in the course of the person's occupation, or if the vehicle is provided as a part of the employee's benefits to use to and from work.

The law's interpretation of "in the course of employment" is very different from most laymen's interpretation. For instance, someone injured while eating lunch at a company-sponsored event may be considered covered by WC. Therefore, always do an investigation and let the claims specialist handle the final determination.

## Business Trips

Most WC laws provide coverage for a person who is on a business trip. This coverage is applicable as long as the person is engaged in employment duties. Of course, there are always exceptions to this rule.

## Company Parking Lot

Most WC laws provide that if an employee is injured in a parking lot which is owned by or maintained by this employer and furnished to the employee free of charge, he/she may be covered under WC. In addition, coverage would extend, in some instances, to an injury sustained by the employee while on neutral ground between the parking lot and the place of employment. An exception would be if such incidents were specifically excluded in the WC law, or if the injuries were sustained from willful or negligent actions on the part of the employee.

Usually, WC is not liable for injuries sustained in a parking lot which is owned by the employer and for which a rental fee is charged for the parking space. In such instances, the employee has a free choice to park elsewhere, which would relieve the employer of any and all responsibility.

## Occupational Disease

Most of the time, coverage will extend to employees who contract a disease that develops by working within a certain industry. For instance, most states provide compensation for individuals working with asbestos material over a period of years who then develop as-

bestosis or silicosis. Likewise, individuals can develop dermatitis from working with certain chemicals, such as those found in the exterminating industry.

Sometimes a claimant may have an occupational illness which is submitted to the WC Board and a concurrent nonoccupational illness for which he/she may be reimbursed under the plan. In such instances, a separate billing should be completed by the provider indicating those charges that were solely for the treatment of the nonoccupational disability.

## Types of Claims

Workers' Compensation provides benefits for:

1. Medical expenses, including medical services, hospital treatment, surgery, medications, prosthetics or appliances, and durable medical equipment.
2. Temporary disability, allowing payments to continue to the employee even though they are not currently working. Payments are based on the employee's salary and the length of the disability. Payments are usually not taxable as income.
3. Permanent disability, either in the form of weekly or monthly payments, or as a lump sum distribution.
4. Death, to compensate spouses and dependents for the loss of an employee. Some states also provide for a burial benefit to help cover the cost of funeral services.
5. Rehabilitation, to cover rehabilitation services or vocational retraining for permanently disabled workers who are unable to continue in their present position.

There are three types of WC claims. They are nondisability claims, temporary disability claims, and permanent disability claims.

## Nondisability Claims

**Nondisability claims** are for minor injuries that will not require the patient to be kept from his job. The patient is able to continue working throughout the extent of the injury. On the first visit to the physician, the physician should complete a **"Doctor's First Report of Occupational Injury or Illness (First Report)."** This form and a copy of the bill should be submitted to the WC carrier. If you receive a claim with an attached First Report, consult company guidelines regarding whether the claim should be pended for a WC determination or paid with a lien attached.

## Temporary Disability Claims

**Temporary disability** claims are when the patient is not able to perform his or her job requirements until he or she recovers from the injury involved. When a physician sees a patient in this situation, a First Report will be submitted and ongoing reports will be issued every two to three weeks until the patient is discharged to return to work.

Each state has a waiting period before temporary disability becomes effective, usually three to seven days (except in the Virgin Islands where the waiting period is one day). During temporary disability, the employee is paid a portion of their salary as a tax-free benefit. Temporary disability ends when the patient is able to return to work, even with limitations or to a different department, or when the patient's condition ceases to improve and the patient is left with a permanent disability. Most health care plans do not have a disability benefit (for either temporary or permanent disability) or death benefits. Therefore, the health claims examiner should not receive a disability claim. If one is received, it should be denied as not a covered benefit.

## Permanent Disability Claims

**Permanent disability** usually commences after temporary disability when it is determined that the patient will not be able to return to work. The physician will prepare a discharge report stating that the patient is "**permanent and stationary**." This means that nothing more can be done and the patient will have the disability for the rest of his or her life. The WC Board will review the case and, if determined to be permanent, a compromise and release will be issued. This is a settlement from the insurance carrier for a payment to the injured party.

The amount of the settlement is based upon the age of the disabled worker, the amount of money they were making at the time of the injury, and the severity of the injury. The older an employee is, the higher the disability rating. This is due to the idea that a younger patient has a better chance of finding other employ-ment or of being retrained for another job than an older worker would. Additionally, death benefits and rehabilitation benefits may be provided.

## Death Benefits

**Death Benefits** compensate the family of a deceased employee for the loss of income which the employee would have provided to the family. Some states also provide a burial benefit to assist with the funeral and burial expenses for the employee.

## Rehabilitation Benefits

If an employee is found to have a permanent disability, some states allow for a **rehabilitation benefit**. This benefit can be provided to retrain the employee in a physical ability which will help them to seek future employment (i.e., proper use of a wheelchair, use of the left hand when a person loses their right hand).

Some states participate in a "**work hardening**" program, wherein an employee is assigned therapy similar to their work in an attempt to strengthen them and build up their endurance toward a full day's work. Often employees in such a program will be returned to work on a limited or restricted basis. Physicians, therapists, employers, insurance carriers, and all others concerned with the employee's case must keep in constant communication to ensure that the patient is not returned to work either sooner or later than possible.

Many states also allow for **vocational rehabilitation** or retraining in a different job field when the employee is unable to return to their former position. This can include courses in colleges and vocational schools, or on-the-job training programs. Often employees are paid a weekly allowance (as in the case of temporary disability) while they are attending school and for a limited time after graduation. The time after graduation is to allow them time to locate a job. The employee is then considered to be off temporary disability and have returned to work. Vocational rehabilitation can also include job guidance, resume preparation, and placement services.

## Doctor's Reports Needed to Process a Claim

If a member is being treated for a work related injury, all records relating to the injury and treatment should be kept separate from the patient's regular medical records. Since employers are covering the costs of

# On the Job Now

1. What kind of claim would be filed if the patient is not able to perform his or her job requirements? _____

_____

2. What kind of claim would be filed if the patient is able to continue working throughout the injury? _____

_____

3. What is the "work hardening" program? _____

_____

_____

treatment, privacy guidelines are somewhat different than the normal privacy agreement between the member and provider. In WC cases, the agreement is actually between the provider and the employer, not the employee. The employer may request to see records regarding the injury, and these records may be subpoenaed. No information pertaining to the employee's non-work related treatment should be made a part of this file, so that confidentiality between the provider and the member is not breached for non-work related treatments and conditions.

A claims examiner may need a copy of the following reports to process a claim properly:

- Doctor's First Report
- Subsequent Progress Reports
- Physician's Final Report

Adjudication is when the claim or benefit case has been closed. Delay of adjudication can occur due to unresolved factors of the case.

## Doctor's First Report

Regardless of the type of claim or benefits, the doctor must file a First Report of Injury (**see Figure 9–1**). This form may have a different name, depending on the state; however, nearly all states require the completion of a similar form. This form requests basic information regarding the date, time, and location of the injury/illness and the treatment, the patient's subjective

complaints and objective findings, the diagnosis, and the treatment needed. **Subjective findings** are those that cannot be discerned by anyone other than the patient (i.e., pain, discomfort). The physician should give an opinion as to the extent of pain, description of activities that produce pain, and any other findings. A treatment plan should also be indicated.

Physicians must make a report of injury, disability, or death within a specified time period. This varies from immediately upon knowledge of the incident to within 30 days. Different states set different time limits and different requirements for reporting. There may also be different levels of injury (i.e., injury, disability, death).

This report is considered a legal document and it should be signed in ink by the physician. All information should be typed or printed clearly. The original copy of the form should be sent to the insurance carrier. One copy is retained in the patient's records, and many providers also send a copy to the employer.

If the physician chooses to send a narrative report along with the standard report, the following information should be included:

- A history of the accident, injury or illness.
- Diagnosis.
- Any connection between the primary injury and any subsequent injuries, especially if the interrelating factors between the primary and secondary injuries are not immediately discernable.
- Subjective and objective findings.

STATE OF CONFUSION

# DOCTOR'S FIRST REPORT OF OCCUPATIONAL INJURY OR ILLNESS

Within five days of your initial examination, for every occupational injury or illness, send two copies of this report to the employer's workers' compensation insurance carrier or the insured employer. Failure to file a timely doctor's report may result in assessment of a civil penalty. In the case of diagnosed or suspected pesticide poisoning, send a copy of the report to Division of Labor Statistics and Research, P.O. Box 555555, Anytown, USA 12345-6789, and notify your local health officer by telephone within 24 hours.

| | PLEASE DO NOT USE THIS COLUMN |
|---|---|
| **1. INSURER NAME AND ADDRESS** | |
| **2. EMPLOYER NAME** | Case No. |
| 3. Address:        No. and Street        City        Zip | Industry |
| 4. Nature of business (e.g., food manufacturing, building construction, retailer of women's clothes.) | County |

| | | | |
|---|---|---|---|
| 5. **PATIENT NAME** (first name, middle initial, last name) | 6. Sex ☐Male ☐Female | 7. Date of  Mo.  Day  Yr. Birth: | Age |
| 8. Address:   No. and Street   City   Zip | | 9. Telephone number ( ) | Hazard |
| 10. Occupation (Specific job title) | | 11. Social Security Number - - | Disease |
| 12. Injured at:   No. and Street   City   County | | | Hospitalization |
| 13. Date and hour of injury   Mo. Day Yr.  Hour or onset of illness  ____ a.m. ____ p.m. | | 14. Date last worked   Mo.  Day  Yr. | Occupation |
| 15. Date and hour of first   Mo. Day Yr.  Hour examination or treatment  ____ a.m. ____ p.m. | | 16. Have you (or your office) previously treated patient?  ☐Yes ☐No | Return Date/Code |

Patient please complete this portion, if able to do so. Otherwise, doctor please complete immediately, inability or failure of a patient to complete this portion shall not affect his/her rights to workers' compensation under the California Labor Code.

17. **DESCRIBE HOW THE ACCIDENT OR EXPOSURE HAPPENED.** (Give specific object, machinery or chemical. Use reverse side if more space is required.)

18. **SUBJECTIVE COMPLAINTS** (Describe fully. Use reverse side if more space is required.)

19. **OBJECTIVE FINDINGS** (Use reverse side if more space is required.)
A. Physical examination

B. X-ray and laboratory results (State if none or pending.)

20. **DIAGNOSIS** (if occupational illness specify etiologic agent and duration of exposure.) Chemical or toxic compounds involved? ☐Yes ☐No
ICD-9cm Code ___ ___ ___ - ___ ___

21. Are your findings and diagnosis consistent with patient's account of injury or onset of illness?   ☐Yes ☐No   If "no", please explain.

22. Is there any other current condition that will impede or delay patient's recovery?   ☐Yes ☐No   If "yes", please explain.

23. **TREATMENT RENDERED** (Use reverse side if more space is required.)

24. If further treatment required, specify treatment plan/estimated duration.

25. If hospitalized as inpatient, give hospital name and location    Date  Mo.  Day  Yr.  Estimated stay
admitted

26. WORK STATUS -- Is patient able to perform usual work?   ☐Yes ☐No
If "no", date when patient can return to:   Regular work ___/___/___
Modified work ___/___/___   Specify restrictions _____

Doctor's Signature _____    License Number _____
Doctor Name and Degree (please type) _____    IRS Number _____
Address _____    Telephone Number _____

FORM 5021 (Rev. 4)

■ **Figure 9–1**  Copy of a Doctor's First Report

## Progress Reports

Following the First Report, the physician should follow up with progress reports (sometimes called supplemental reports) every two or three weeks. Although many states have forms for progress reports, they may also allow a narrative report to be filed rather than requiring completion of the specified form. Progress reports should also be sent at the end of a hospitalization even if the patient is expected to be readmitted later. This report often serves as both a report on the patient's condition and as a bill.

If the patient's condition changes significantly, a Reexamination Report, or a detailed progress report, should be filed with the insurance carrier.

## Physician's Final Report

By obtaining a copy of these reports, a health claims examiner can monitor a patient's progress. Then, if claims are received at a later time, it is easier to determine if subsequent treatment is related to the original WC injury or not. If it is determined to be related to the WC injury, the claim should be denied and the patient should submit the claim to the WC insurance carrier.

The WC carrier will often wait until the physician indicates that the patient's condition is permanent and stationary before finalizing a claim. The physician should then notify the WC carrier that no further treatment is needed (or that no further treatment will significantly alter the patient's condition) and that the patient has been discharged. This is called the **Physician's Final Report**. Some states require the final report be submitted on a specified form, and some states use the same form for both subsequent and final reports. The Physician's Final Report should indicate that the patient has been discharged, the level of the patient's permanent disability, if any, and the balance due on the patient's account (usually provided as a patient's statement showing services, dates of service, charges, and any payments rendered). Once this information is received, the WC carrier will establish the level of permanent disability (if any), medical and other expenses will be paid, and the case will be closed.

## Delay of Adjudication

When a patient is released to work, all benefits have been paid, and the case is closed, the claim is said to have been adjudicated. Often adjudication occurs within two to eight weeks after the physician submits the report stating that the patient has been discharged and is able to return to work.

If the patient suffers a permanent disability, adjudication can take much longer, especially if the level of permanent disability is protested and a lawsuit ensues. Additional factors which may delay the close of a case include:

1. Confusion or questions on any of the reports submitted by the employer, employee, or physician. This can include conflicting information from one or more parties, vague or ambiguous terminology (especially by the physician), or illegible items.
2. Omitted information on a report, including incomplete forms, boxes not filled in, or signatures not included.
3. Incorrect billing or questions on the billing provided by the physician.
4. Insufficient progress reports to update the insurance carrier on the status of the patient.

# On the Job Now

**Directions:** Answer the following questions without looking back at the material just covered. Write your answers in the space provided.

1. Why should a member's records relating to the work related injury and treatment be kept separate from the patient's regular medical records? _____

_____

2. When is a patient's claim considered adjudicated? _____

_____

3. Answer the following three part question.

   **1.** Which report is considered a legal document? _____

   **2.** Should it be typed/printed or handwritten? _____

   **3.** How should it be signed? _____

## Fraud and Abuse

Unfortunately, fraud and abuse occur frequently in the WC system. Many employees, employers, providers, and insurance carriers find it easy to defraud the system and reap significant financial awards.

In the past there have been few deterrents to abusing the system. It was frequently possible to find a doctor who was willing to testify that injuries were more serious than was first thought. Likewise, numerous lawyers stepped in and set up relationships with doctors to produce claims where no actual injury or illness existed. This is especially true when work-related stress became a popular diagnosis for any one of a number of ailments.

## Practice
## Pitfalls

While most claims are legitimate, the health claims examiner should recognize what constitutes fraud. Following are some signs of fraud or abuse to look out for.

An injured employee who:

- Cannot clearly describe the pain or injury, or whose description changes each time details of the incident are related.

- Is overly dramatic regarding their injury.

- Complains of an injury which cannot be substantiated by medical evidence. This may include soft tissue injuries which cannot be seen on an x-ray, or a patient who insists there is a serious injury, even when there is medical evidence to the contrary.

- Delays the reporting of an injury, especially an injury that is reported on a Monday when the employee claims it happened on Friday.

- Reports the injury to an attorney or regulatory agency prior to reporting the injury to their employer.

- Changes physicians frequently, or shows up for a first treatment, but seems unhappy with the diagnosis and changes physicians. Patient may be seeking a physician who will grant additional time off or will testify to a greater degree of injury.

- An employee who is a short-term worker, or who was scheduled to terminate employment just after the injury occurred.

- Has a history of curious or an excessive amount of WC claims.

A medical provider who:

- Orders or performs unnecessary procedures or tests.

- Inflates the severity of the injury to qualify for higher reimbursement (i.e., lists a fracture as open rather than closed, bills for a high complexity exam rather than a moderate complexity exam).

- Charges for services that were never performed, or adds additional procedures onto existing claims.

- Makes multiple referrals to a lab, clinic, or hospital and receives a referral fee from these organizations.

- States that an injury exists and needs treatment when no injury is actually present.

- Sends in duplicate billings with information changed (i.e., dates) to make it appear services were performed more than once.

- Files many claims with subjective injuries (i.e., pain, strain, emotional disturbance, inability to perform certain functions).

- Files claims for several employees of the same company which show similar injuries (i.e., injuries for which reports or x-rays may be duplicated).

An attorney who:

- Pressures an insurer to process and pay immediately.

These instances suggest signs a health claims examiner should look for. If an examiner suspects fraud, it should be reported to the appropriate authority immediately. If an examiner becomes aware of fraud by any means, the claim file should be noted and the information referred to a supervisor. An examiner can be guilty of fraud if they knew of the fraud and did nothing to prevent it. This is true even if the examiner receives no money from the fraud.

## Liens

Since it can take months or even years for a WC claim to be paid by the WC insurance carrier, many health insurance carriers will pay these claims, then place a lien to recoup the money when the claim is settled. A **lien** is a legal document that expresses claim on the property of another for payment of a debt (**see Figure 9–2**). A lien is completed and submitted to the attorney representing the injured party to be paid upon monetary settlement of the WC claim.

A lien should be sent along with copies of the EOBs. Whenever additional payments are made, a copy of the EOB should be submitted to the attorney so that all payments will be included in the lien. All services must be for the care of the injury covered under the WC claim.

Many states have a special lien form for WC purposes. These forms can be obtained through the local Division of Industrial Accidents. (A sample copy of a state lien form is shown in **Figure 9–3**.) The claims examiner should complete the lien form and send copies to the WC appeals board, the patient's attorney, the patient, and the WC insurance carrier. A copy should also be kept for the claims files.

If a lien is not filed, all monies recovered at the close of the case technically belong to the member. It is then the member's responsibility to cover the medical expenses. If any liens are filed, the member must first pay the liens, and then pay any other resultant expenses. Therefore, if the lawyer files a lien and his fees exhaust most of the money, there will be little or none left for other expenses. If at all possible, members should be persuaded to pay for medical services prior to settlement of the claim.

If a lien is filed, the examiner should have their copy of the lien letter signed by the patient and their attorney. This makes the attorney responsible for payment of the physician's bills. If the attorney does not remit the necessary funds from the member's settlement, the attorney must cover the payments for medical services.

A lien should have a specified time limit on it, often a period of one year. If settlement has not been reached by that time, or there are ongoing charges on the member's account relating to the WC injury, an amended lien should be filed. The subsequent lien should state the balance of the patient's account and should have the word AMENDED stamped across the top or below the Appeals Board Case Number.

The examiner should place all files with liens in a special section and hold them until the cases have been settled. It is illegal to continually bill or harass the member when a lien agreement has been signed. In effect, the lien acknowledges the insurance carrier's agreement to wait for reimbursement until the case has been settled. The examiner should contact the member's attorney at least once every three months for an update on the case and to determine when settlement is expected to occur. The attorney should also be contacted within two weeks after the date settlement is expected, to find out the results of the case and ask when reimbursement will be provided to pay the claim.

In some states, the law provides that the insurance carrier will be paid prior to the attorney or member collecting any monies from the settlement. Statutes in your state should be checked to protect you. If your state has such a provision, attorneys may not collect their fee and then state that insufficient funds were recovered to cover the outstanding medical expenses. Some states also allow the insurance carrier to bill the member for any funds which were not received from the settlement. Once again, check with the laws of your state to determine if members can be billed or if any amounts not collected should be written off.

Liens are an inexpensive way of ensuring that the insurance carrier will be reimbursed for payments made. The cost is much less than suing the member and assures that payment will be received when the dispute between the member and the WC insurance carrier is settled. A lien is a legal document that will be recognized by the court and will provide protection in the event of litigation.

TO: Attorney _____

_____

_____, Confusion

RE: Medical Reports and Insurance Carrier Lien

FOR_____


I do hereby authorize the above insurance carrier to furnish you, my attorney, with a full report of any records and resultant payments of myself in regard to the accident in which I was involved.

I hereby authorize and direct you, my attorney, to pay directly to said insurance carrier such sums as may be due and owed for payment of medical services rendered me or the provider of services both by reason of this accident and by reason of any other bills that are due, and to withhold such sums from any settlement, judgment or verdict as may be necessary to adequately protect said insurance carrier. And I hereby further give a lien on my case to said insurance carrier against any and all proceeds of any settlement, judgment or verdict which may be paid to you, my attorney, or myself as the result of the injuries for which I have been treated or injuries in connection therewith.

I fully understand that I am directly and fully responsible for reimbursement of any payments for all medical bills submitted for services rendered and that this agreement is made solely for said insurance carrier's additional protection and in consideration of its awaiting payment. And I further understand that such payment is not contingent on any settlement, judgment or verdict by which I may eventually recover said fee.


Dated: _____    Patient's Signature: _____



The undersigned being attorney of record for the above patient does hereby agree to observe all the terms of the above and agrees to withhold such sums from any settlement, judgment or verdict as may be necessary to adequately protect said insurance carrier named above.


Dated: _____    Attorney's Signature: _____
Mr./Ms. Attorney:  Please sign, date, and return one copy to our office at once.

Keep one copy for your records.

■ **Figure 9–2** Copy of a Lien Letter

# WORKERS' COMPENSATION APPEALS BOARD

## STATE OF CONFUSION

# CASE NO. _____

### NOTICE AND REQUEST FOR ALLOWANCE OF LIEN

_____

LIEN CLAIMANT                                                                 ADDRESS

VS.

_____

INJURED WORKER                                                               ADDRESS

_____

EMPLOYER                                                                       ADDRESS

_____

INSurance CARRIER                                                            ADDRESS

The undersigned hereby requests the Workers' Compensation Appeals Board to determine and allow as a lien the sum of

_____ dollars ($_____) against

any amount now due or which may hereafter become payable as compensation to _____

                                                                                  INJURED WORKER

on account of injury sustained by him/ her on _____.

                                                                  DATE

This request and claim for lien is for: (Mark appropriate box)
- ❑ The reasonable expense incurred by or on behalf of said injured worker for medical treatment to cure or relieve from the effects of said injury; or
- ❑ The reasonable medical expense incurred to prove a contested claim; or
- ❑ The reasonable value of living expenses of said injured worker or of his dependents, subsequent to the injury, or
- ❑ The reasonable living expenses of the wife or minor children, or both, of said injured worker, subsequent to the date of injury, where such injured worker has deserted or is neglecting his family; or
- ❑ The reasonable fee for interpreter's services performed on _____.
                                                                           DATE

NOTE: ITEMIZED STATEMENTS MUST BE ATTACHED

The undersigned declares that he delivered or mailed a copy of this lien claim to each of the above-named parties on

_____

ATTORNEY FOR LIEN CLAIMANT                                              DATE

_____

ADDRESS OF ATTORNEY FOR LIEN CLAIMANT                                   LIEN CLAIMANT

### INJURED WORKER'S CONSENT TO ALLOWANCE OF LIEN

*I consent to the requested allowance of a lien against my compensation.*

_____

ATTORNEY FOR INJURED WORKER                                             INJURED WORKER

DEPARTMENT OF INDUSTRIAL RELATIONS
DIVISION OF INDUSTRIAL ACCIDENTS

■ **Figure 9–3** Copy of a State Lien Form

## Reversals

Occasionally an accident which was thought to be WC will turn out not to be. This can happen when a patient hides or omits facts regarding when and how the accident occurred. It can also be found that there is a nonindustrial, underlying condition which caused the accident. For example, a patient may have epilepsy and suffer a seizure at work. Any injuries directly received on the job site could be considered WC; however, the treatment of the underlying epileptic condition would not be WC.

In some cases the employee may be found to be negligent in their actions, or willfully not abiding by established workplace rules. In such cases, injuries sustained as the result of negligence of the employee may not be considered industrial accidents. For example, if the employee is told they must refrain from wearing hoop earrings, but they chose to anyway, they may be considered liable if the earrings are caught on machinery and ripped from the ear, resulting in an injury.

In such cases, the WC board would deny payment on the claim. All claims for treatment should then be paid by the member's regular insurance carrier. Thus, the claims and subsequent payments would become part of the patient's regular file.

# CHAPTER REVIEW

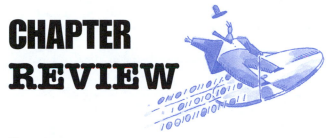

## Summary

- WC insurance is a separate medical insurance program that covers work-related injuries, disabilities, and death. A wide range of activities may be covered under WC laws.

- WC provides nondisability claims, temporary disability claims, permanent disability claims, death benefits, and rehabilitation benefits to injured workers.

- Vocational rehabilitation or training in a different job field is allowed by many states.

- The Doctor's First Report of Injury/Illness is a major factor in the employer's or insurance company's decision to accept or contest the workers' compensation claim. The basic information requested on the form is the date, time, and location of the injury/illness and treatment rendered.

- The Physician's Final Report is usually the last report, stating that the patient has been discharged.

- The physician must notify the WC carrier that no further treatment is needed.

- The claim is said to be adjudicated when all the benefits have been paid and the patient is released to work.

- Some factors that may delay the close of a case are confusion or questions on any of the reports, omitted information on a report, incorrect billing or questions on the billing, and insufficient progress reports.

## Assignments

Complete the Questions for Review.
Complete Exercise 9–1 through 9–3.

## Questions for Review

**Directions:**  Answer the following questions without looking back at the material just covered. Write your answers in the space provided.

1. What is Workers' Compensation? _____

_____

2. What items are likely to cause a delay in adjudication of a case? _____

_____

_____

_____

3. What do you do if a patient says he has a WC injury but he has nothing from the employer to prove it? _____

_____

_____

4. What is a lien? _____

_____

5. Why should you file a lien? _____

_____

6. What signatures should you get on a lien? _____

_____

7. Define Temporary Disability. _____

_____

8. Define Permanent Disability. _____

_____

9. What is a nondisability claim? _____

_____

10. If an employee is injured while at a company sponsored game, is it considered a WC case? _____

_____

If you were unable to answer any of these questions, refer back to that section and then fill in the answers.

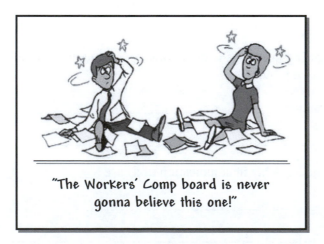

"The Workers' Comp board is never gonna believe this one!"

# Exercise 9-1

**Directions:** Find and circle the words listed below. Words can appear horizontally, vertically, diagonally, forward, or backward.

```
Z S E S C N U E V H T U Q Z F A L G N T M W V
T C H Z M O L B X C M X N D D W Y U J X E Q M
S I N B P I M G F V Z F G F N U E T J E T A P
N W R D R T A P D S R G F F X Q G A C N I V W
S L Q E X A T L A F N C T W Q T D T A U P Y E
K V E R G S F Q C N Y Y D Z Q U D U A P Y Y C
B V R D H N N B R Y Y Z Q K O T M R Q D O D M
T I F E N E B N O I T A T I L I B A H E R Y K
V V E F E P R D C P M I C U C V N P D T T B N
L O G I I M F V K U Z A L T H Y G H R P C M W
O T L U B O W H T S K Q E I I H K O V F I B V
X K R S P C M G T K U J K N B V I M K U C R O
K B M I A S Y B D W K R N M Q A I D X F X W N
Q A V Z N R U P Z B B R J C I O S T P B Z M V
W J D O O E S A K Y Y K B O T I N I I W B A S
R R H E Z K A P C S O Y P D Y I F D D E R D S
Z F J A L R V B Q Q D J A W V N H B I N S C N
U E S S P O F T K F J N O M M O L E N D O X J
U G X O V W N T A R Y F A X S Q X A F S Z N G
J O B R E L A T E D I N J U R I E S P T N Q J
S C U U T U T K P X N T M W Z J W K T C R W W
R O V M H H D I U Y W C W B X I O Z J P C Q R
S V Q Q I M D V W U Q F L F L C G U T D G Q W
```

1. Company Activities
2. Job-Related Injuries
3. Nondisability Claims
4. Rehabilitation Benefit
5. Workers' Compensation

# Exercise 9-2

**Directions:** Complete the crossword puzzle by filling in a word from the keywords that fits each clue.

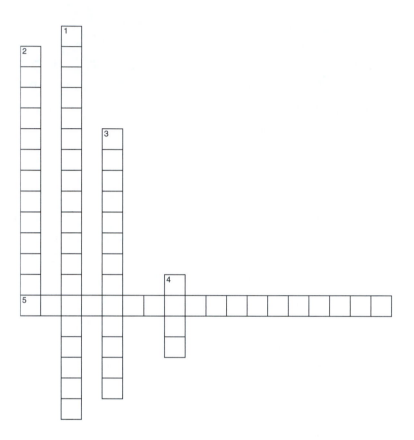

## Across

**5.** Findings that cannot be discerned by anyone other than the patient.

## Down

**1.** When it is determined that the patient will not be able to return to work.

**2.** Benefits which compensate the family of a deceased employee for the loss of income which the employee would have provided to the family.

**3.** A program wherein an employee is assigned therapy similar to their work in an attempt to strengthen them and build up their endurance toward a full day's work.

**4.** A legal document that expresses claim on the property of another for payment of a debt.

# Exercise 9-3

**Directions:** Match the following terms with the proper definition by writing the letter of the correct definition in the space next to the term.

1. _____ Doctor's First Report of Occupational Injury or Illness

2. _____ Occupational Illnesses

3. _____ Permanent and Stationary

4. _____ Temporary Disability

5. _____ Vocational Rehabilitation

a. Retraining in a different job field when the employee is unable to return to their former position.

b. Claims for when the patient is not able to perform his or her job requirements until he or she recovers from the injury involved.

c. Any disorders, illnesses, or conditions which arise at work or from exposure to factors at work.

d. A term meaning that nothing more can be done and the patient will have the disability for the rest of his or her life.

e. The report completed by a doctor at a Workers' Compensation patient's first visit.

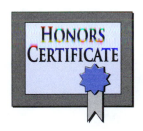

## Honors Certification™

The Honors Certification™ challenge for this chapter constitutes a written test of the information contained within this chapter. Each incorrect answer will result in a deduction of up to 5% from your grade. You must achieve a score of 80% or higher to pass this test. If you fail the test on your first attempt, you may retake the test one additional time. The items included in the second test may be different from those in the first test.

# 10

# Managed
## Care Claims

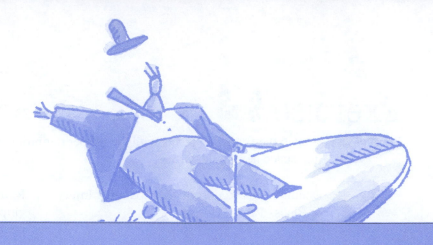

## After completion of this chapter
**you will be able to:**

- Describe the main types of managed care organizations and how they work.
- List the common HMO benefits.
- Describe the various types of Preferred Provider Organizations and how they work.
- Describe how risk for expenses is shared between groups/IPAs and the HMO.
- Explain how providers are reimbursed in a capitation agreement.

- List the information that must be included on member appeals of denied HMO claims.
- Properly generate a payment to an outside provider using a given scenario.
- Properly complete a denial notice.
- Describe stoploss and the procedures for obtaining stoploss reimbursement from the HMO.

## Key words and concepts
**you will learn in this chapter:**

- Capitation
- Eligibility Roster
- Group Model
- Independent Physician Associations (IPAs)

- Individual Practice Organizations (IPOs)
- Medical Groups
- Network Model
- Preventive Coverage

- Primary Care Provider (PCP)
- Staff Model
- Stoploss
- Treatment Authorization Request (TAR)
- Withhold

The health insurance industry has been transformed in recent years with the rise of managed care networks and health maintenance organizations. Managed care is a system for organizing the delivery of health services so that the cost of care is reduced and the quality of care is maintained or improved. Managed care plans (MCPs) were created in an attempt to bring healthcare under control by having providers share some of the financial risks of healthcare with the patient and the insurance carrier. Managed care techniques are most often practiced by organizations and professionals which assume part or all of the risk associated with providing the medical care for a defined population of patients. It is best described as a multifaceted system for providing healthcare while maintaining costs.

There are many different types of managed care organizations, including Health Maintenance Organizations, Preferred Provider Organizations, Gatekeeper PPOs, Exclusive Provider Organizations, Physician Hospital Organizations, and Management Service Organizations, just to mention a few. Several of these types of care were previously discussed in the Introduction chapter under "Types of Insurance." In this chapter we will focus on processing claims in a Health Maintenance Organization setting.

## Health Maintenance Organizations

Under an HMO setup, members pay a set amount every month, and the HMO agrees to provide all their care or to pay for the covered care they cannot provide. The HMO hires physicians and sets up hospitals (or contracts with existing physicians and hospitals). The member chooses a specific provider for their care (called a **primary care provider or primary care physician [PCP]**). Members can sign up for HMO coverage through their employer or with an individual policy.

Many HMOs require a copayment amount from the member for each visit, usually a nominal fee of $10 to $50. This is the entire amount the patient must pay.

Additionally, members often receive benefits that are not usually covered under regular indemnity plans; such as annual physicals, mammograms, and pap smears. Another benefit is the lack of paperwork for the patient since the provider completes any paperwork for reimbursement.

The member is locked into visiting one physician or provider. If the member wishes to see a provider other than their PCP, they must usually seek preapproval from the HMO or must cover the costs themselves.

There are several different types of HMO organizations. The most common include:

- **Staff model.** This is the original concept of HMO services. A physician or provider is hired to work at the HMO's own facility. They are usually paid a salary and may receive additional bonuses. The provider works only for the HMO and sees no outside patients.
- **Group model.** The HMO contracts with providers or provider groups to provide services. These practitioners agree to see only HMO members, but they do so at their own facilities.

### Staff Model HMOs

In a staff HMO, the HMO owns the facility and hires the staff. When a patient comes for a visit, the copayment amount is collected from the patient by the HMO. This money is kept by the HMO and added to premiums to cover their costs of doing business.

The practitioners on staff, whether physicians, nurses, or specialists (i.e., x-ray technicians, cardiac specialists, etc.) are paid a standard salary based on the work they do and the hours they are at work. The amount stays the same regardless of the number of patients they see or the number of procedures they perform.

The HMO covers all costs, including the costs of the facilities, equipment and supplies, and personnel (including doctors, nurses, specialists, accountants, and any other personnel needed to keep the company running).

In this arrangement, appointments are often made through the HMO, rather than through the provider. This allows the HMO to monitor the number of patients the provider sees and the services performed. If the patient needs additional services (i.e., a referral to a specialist, lab tests, x-rays, etc.), the staff provider will input information into a system, letting the HMO know that these services are needed.

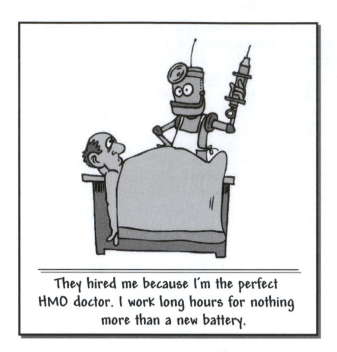

They hired me because I'm the perfect HMO doctor. I work long hours for nothing more than a new battery.

Since providers are not reimbursed per procedure, there is little benefit to performing or ordering services the patient does not need.

Additionally, if an HMO feels a provider is referring too many patients for additional services, they will limit the number of referrals he may make or may insist on additional documentation to justify the services.

In this model, there are no claims to process since all costs and services are handled by the HMO.

## Group Model HMOs

In a Group model HMO, a facility or Group bands together to provide services for HMO patients at their own facilities. This is much like the staff model HMO in that the providers receive a salary based on their qualifications and working hours. However, rather than receiving payment directly from the HMO, they receive their salary from the Group. The Group itself receives a capitation amount from the HMO to cover a wide range of services.

**Example:** The HMO signs up 10,000 members who each pay an average premium of $150 per month. The HMO contracts with a Group to provide all provider visits, outpatient x-ray and DXL charges, and outpatient/minor surgery charges for 1,000 of these patients (other Groups will handle the remaining patients). In exchange for these services, the HMO will pay a capitated payment of $50 per member for these 1,000 members. Thus, the Group receives

$50,000 per month to cover these services. The Group then hires or contracts with providers to work for them for a salary. Thus, the providers are paid from this pool of money a set amount each month.

If there are any services which the Group is contracted to provide, but cannot supply themselves, they must cover the cost of these services.

**Example:** The Group contract requires the Group to provide chiropractic services for those patients who need it. However, there is not enough need for the Group to keep a chiropractor on staff on a regular basis. Thus, the Group will make an arrangement with a chiropractor to provide these services at a reduced fee (say $50 per visit). Then, when patients need chiropractic services, they are referred to this contracted chiropractor. The chiropractor collects the copayment amount from the patient (i.e., $20), and the remaining $30 for the visit is paid to the chiropractor by the Group.

If the patient needs services which are not covered by the provider Group (i.e., hospital services), they are referred back to the HMO. The HMO will then provide these services at one of their facilities. These facilities may be either wholly owned by the HMO and thus paid as a staff model, or they may be another Group who has contracted with the HMO to provide all inpatient hospital treatment. If the hospital is a staff arrangement, the HMO covers all costs. If it is a Group arrangement, they receive a capitated amount (i.e., $75 per person per month). Any amount remaining from the premiums after all Groups have been paid their capitated amounts are used to cover the costs of services which they are contractually obligated to cover, but for which there is no provider under contract (i.e., prescriptions).

In a Group setup, patients may see different doctors in the Group each time they visit the Group offices. The copayment amount for each visit is collected by the Group and is used to cover their costs (including staff, facilities and supplies).

Some HMOs are contracting with hospitals to take over a specified number of beds or a wing of an existing hospital rather than building their own facilities. This has come about due to the increased costs associated with building a new hospital facility and the lowered utilization of hospitals. With HMOs, doctors are encouraged to shorten the length of stay at hospitals. Thus, some hospitals have only 40% to 50% of their beds filled at any given time. Sharing a facility can be a good way to provide an HMO the resources and treatment options needed while at the same time increasing the revenues of the hospital. HMO personnel are usually used to care for patients at these facilities.

## Individual Practice Organizations (IPOs)

**Individual Practice Organizations** or IPOs (sometimes called Independent Practice Associations) are legal entities, comprised of a network of private physicians, who have organized to negotiate contracts with insurance companies and HMOs.

There are two arms to this type of organization. The HMO arm acts as an insurer, oversees the program, enrolls members, collects premiums, and handles the claims. The medical Group arm organizes physicians and contracts with the HMO for discounted rates on services. The medical Group as a whole is paid a capitation amount for each member, and the Group oversees the care of the members and attempts to control costs.

The individual physicians (who are members of the medical Groups) agree to see patients in their own offices along with their regular fee-for-service clients. These providers are able to easily gather a large number of patients by joining the IPO, and at the same time retain their autonomy and freedom, unlike the traditional HMO doctors who were hired by the HMO and placed on salary.

This type of arrangement allows the HMO to add numerous doctors, giving patients a wider freedom of choice. Since doctors are paid a capitation amount according to the number of members they see, there is no additional cost to the HMO for adding more doctors.

**Network model.** In this type of arrangement the HMO contracts with several providers in a locale, allowing some overlap of geographic area. This allows more of a choice for subscribers and allows an HMO to increase its subscriber base without worrying about unduly overloading a single provider. In the network model, providers see not only the HMO members, but continue to see their regular fee-paying patients as well.

There are two payment types within HMOs; those that utilize capitation, and those that pay according to services provided. Capitation pays a provider a set amount per month for the treatment of a patient. The provider is paid each month, regardless of whether or not the patient visits the provider. The savings of being paid for those that do not visit is usually offset by those people who require more treatment than the average member.

Most HMOs require the Group or IPO to have a certain number of physicians in varying specialties. For example, they must often have a general practitioner or internist, a pediatrician, an OB-GYN, a cardiologist, etc. This allows the Group to treat all aspects of the patient's care and to provide appropriate services to all members who choose that Group/IPO as their PCP.

## HMO Coverage

Most HMOs offer a higher level of coverage than traditional indemnity plans. For example, not only do HMOs cover physician visits and necessary testing but also treatment by a specialist (when the patient is referred by their PCP) is often covered. HMOs also tend to cover prenatal care, emergency care, home health care, skilled nursing care, drug and alcohol abuse treatment, physical therapy, allergy treatment, and inhalation therapy, often to a higher degree than coverage provided by indemnity plans. Most physician visits require a small copayment from the member.

Hospitalization is usually covered in full by most HMO plans. However, many plans require a per-day inpatient copayment, and if a patient is seen in the emergency room there often is a copayment.

Additionally, HMOs often cover preventive services. **Preventive coverage** provides for services such as an annual physical, cancer screening (pap smears, mammograms, etc.), flu shots, immunizations, and well-baby care. Many HMO plans also cover health education, cessation of smoking classes, nutrition counseling (especially for diabetics and those needing weight control), or exercise classes. Traditional indemnity plans either limit or restrict coverage of such services.

Eye exams for both children and adults are covered by most HMOs; however, additional vision services (glasses, contacts, etc.) may not be covered.

For those plans that cover prescription drugs, there often is a small copayment required from the member for each prescription. Prescriptions are often limited to a 30-day supply, but many HMOs have no limit to the number of prescriptions that may be filled in a month.

Mental health treatments often require a higher copayment than physician visits and are often limited to short-term care. There also are usually limits on the number of visits.

Physical therapy is often covered only for a brief period of time and only if significant improvement is expected for the patient.

Controversial or experimental procedures (i.e., temporomandibular joint (TMJ) surgery, laser surgery, and gastric stapling) often are not covered. Cosmetic procedures are almost never covered.

Those HMOs that are federally qualified must provide the following minimum benefits:

1. Preventive care.
2. All hospital inpatient services with no limits on costs or days.
3. Hospital outpatient diagnosis and treatment services, including rehabilitative services, with some limitations.
4. Skilled nursing home and home healthcare services.
5. Short-term detoxification treatment for drug and alcohol abuse.
6. Medical treatment and referral for substance abuse.

# Groups/Independent Physician Associations

**Medical groups** are groups of physicians who are signed under or work for the same company. **Independent Physician Associations (IPAs)** are groups of providers who have banded together for the sole purpose of signing a contract with an MCP.

Most MCPs require the group or IPA to have a certain number of physicians in varying specialties. For example, they must often have a general practitioner or internist, a pediatrician, an obstetrician, a gynecologist, or a cardiologist. This allows the group to treat all aspects of the patient's care and to provide appropriate services to all members who choose that Group/IPA as their PCP.

## MCP to Group/IPA Risk

MCPs often use existing providers to deliver care to their patients by signing the providers to contracts. They introduce a mechanism for financial risk-sharing by providing cost incentives to providers in order to contain their expenditures (i.e., the provider is paid a set amount, regardless of the services they provide to the patient).

In many MCP situations, the risk for patient services is shared between the Group/IPA and the MCP. The contract between the MCP and the Group/IPA will outline who is responsible for what services and any conditions or limitations that apply to those services.

Risk determinations are usually considered to be:

- **No risk**—the MCP collects and keeps the monthly capitation amount, and merely pays providers on a fee-for-service basis for the treatment rendered to members. This is similar to a regular insurance carrier setup, except that the member pays only the copay amount, not deductibles or copayment percentage. This arrangement is almost never seen.
- **Partial risk**—the MCP is responsible for most services; however, the capitation covers basic services.
- **Shared risk**—the MCP and the Group/IPA share the responsibility for services. A contract will designate which services or treatments are covered by the MCP and which are covered by the provider.
- **Full risk**—the Group/IPA is responsible for most, if not all of the services. The MCP is just in the business of selling policies and writing contracts with groups/IPAs.

Most MCP contracts with providers are on a shared-risk basis. The MCP will provide a list to the Group/IPA of all possible services (often indicated by CPT® codes and descriptions), and an indication of who is responsible for those services (**see Figure 10–1**). A letter code will often designate who is responsible for payment for that service (i.e., G = Group/IPA responsibility, H = MCP/HMO responsibility, etc.).

This document also will list any services that are denied and the appropriate copayment amount for many of these services.

## Group/IPA to Physician Risk

In addition to the MCP transferring all or part of the risk to the Group/IPA, the Group/IPA may transfer some or all of their risk to an individual capitated provider as well. The levels of risk transferred to the capitated provider include:

- **No risk**—the Group/IPA keeps the entire capitation payment and providers are paid on a fee-for-service basis. There are usually no withholds or bonuses as part of the provider's contract. However, there will often be a fee schedule incorporated as part of the contract agreement, so the amount that the provider receives for services will be determined by the fee schedule.

| Covered Services | MEDICARE | | COMMERCIAL | | | | | | |
|---|---|---|---|---|---|---|---|---|---|
| | Standard[1] | Medi-Medi | AMG | Rocky | CAT | MIPC | CAIT | SBA | RICE |
| Abortion - Elective (CPT 59840 - 59841)<br>Note: Refer to Super Panel contracts for financial responsibility for specific procedures | G/P[1] | G/P[2] | G/P[2] | G/P[1] | G/P[2] | G/P[2,3] | G/P[4] | G/P[4] | G/P[4] |
| Abortion - Therapeutic (CPT 59812 - 59857)<br>If the life of the mother could be endangered if the fetus is carried to term, or in cases of fetal genetic defect. | - | G | G | G | G | G | G | G | G |
| Acupuncture | - | - | - | - | - | - | - | - | G |
| Acute Care | | | | | | | | | |
| • Facility Component | P | P | P | P | P | P | P | P | P |
| • Hospital Based Physicians, including clinical and anatomical pathologist (CPT 80002 - 83999), radiologist (CPT 70010 - 76499), anesthesiologist (CPT 00100 - 01999, 99100 - 99140) | P | P | P | P | P | P | P | P | P |
| • Professional Component, including consultations and follow up care visits (CPT 99217 - 99239, 99251 - 99275) | G | G | G | G | G | G | G | G | G |
| • Closed panel physicians under contract with a hospital for test reading (e.g. EKG)[5] | P | P | P | P | P | P | P | P | P |
| • Special services and reports, miscellaneous (CPT 99000 - 99090, 99175 - 99199) | G | G | G | G | G | G | G | G | G |

[1]Not covered except in cases of rape or incest, or when the life of the mother would be endangered if the fetus were brought to term.
[2]Covered for the first thirteen (13) weeks of pregnancy only.
[3]Copay for HIPC is the same as for in-patient hospitalization.
[4]Covered through the second trimester (24 weeks) of pregnancy only.
[5]Plan to confirm closed panel status.

**Legend: G = Medical Group Responsibility; P = Plan/HMO Responsibility; G/P = Shared Responsibility; -- = Not Covered**

This chart shows a sampling of CPT codes and the party that bears responsibility for covering costs for each procedure under numerous different plans. It is important to check the correct column for the plan being processed to determine if services are covered or not.

■ **Figure 10–1** Distribution of Responsibility

- **No referral risk transferred**—all or part of the payment to the provider involves risk, but the risk is not tied to referrals. Only the capitation amount, bonuses, and withholds are at risk (i.e., the provider may perform more services than the capitation, withholds, and bonuses cover). Under this arrangement, referral means any service not provided for by the provider. Essentially, it is expected that the capitation, withholds, and bonuses are the only payments for any and all care that the provider renders to the member. The provider is not responsible for paying for referrals, and the amount of money paid to the provider is not affected by the decision of the provider to make referrals to other providers.

- **Referral risk is transferred, but is not substantial**—part of the payment to the provider is dependent on the decisions the provider makes to refer patients to other providers. However,

that part of the payment is not substantial (i.e., is under 25%). Therefore, if this type of provider makes too many patient referrals to other providers, up to 25% of his or her capitation amount may be withheld.

- **Substantial risk for referrals is transferred, but stoploss protection is in place**—if more than 25% of total payments to the provider are at risk for referrals, the medical Group/IPA must have aggregate or per-patient stoploss protection in place. **Stoploss** protection means that if the costs to the provider exceed a specified amount, the provider will be reimbursed by the group/ IPA for at least 90% of expenditures over that amount.

In general, the higher the risk that is transferred to the provider, the higher the capitation amount. If less risk is transferred to the provider, the Group/IPA keeps a higher percentage of the capitation amount to cover its expenses.

# On the Job Now

**Directions:** Fill in the blank spaces with the correct word without looking back at the material just covered.

1. Most HMO contracts with providers are on a _____ basis.

2. In addition to the _____ transferring all or part of the risk to the Group/IPA, the Group/IPA may turn around and transfer some or all of their risk to an individual _____.

3. In general, the _____ the risk that is transferred to the provider, the _____ the capitation amount.

# Capitation Payments

**Capitation** is the practice of paying a provider a set amount per month to provide treatment to MCP members and for providing other administrative duties. When a contract is signed between an MCP and a provider, an agreement is made regarding a capitated fee. This fee often is dependent on the type of plan under which the patient is covered. Varying factors such as the gender and age of the patient and their overall health also may be considered. The provider and MCP will also agree which services are covered by the capitation amount.

Often, capitation amounts pay for all the basic treatment the patient needs during the month. If the patient does not see the physician that month, the physician keeps the fee. If the patient becomes ill and requires treatment, the physician is expected to provide the necessary services without additional compensation by the MCP. Usually, the amount saved and the extra amount spent balance out.

The capitation amount for each provider is determined by those who are included on either the active or new member roster. The PCP usually receives capitation payments for the previous month. The amount of the capitation payment will vary according to the coverages or plans that have been selected. Additional amounts may be provided for patients who have entered a hospice or skilled nursing care facility, as well as those who have been diagnosed with specific diseases (i.e., HIV or ESRD).

The MCP may retain a portion of the monthly capitation amount to protect the HMO from inadequate patient care or financial management by the PCP. This amount is called a **withhold**. They also may withhold a portion to ensure the quality of care given to patients and promptness of payments to outside providers. This amount is outlined in the contract signed by the group and the MCP.

## Practice Pitfalls

The 123 MCP withholds 3% of the capitation amount to cover financial insolvency and unpaid claims by the Group/IPA. If all obligations have been met, this amount will be returned when the group terminates its contract with the MCP. Additionally, the 123 MCP will withhold 5% of the capitation for its Medical Management Incentive Program. This program stipulates that the 5% will be reimbursed to the Group/IPA if the following guidelines are met:

- 25% of the withheld amount will be reimbursed if the provider/Group/IPA has submitted less than their budgeted amount of hospital expenses which are covered by the HMO.

- 10% of the amount will be reimbursed for customer satisfaction. The MCP will randomly survey patients to determine their satisfaction with the provider and the services rendered. If the provider is above the average in customer satisfaction, he or she will receive this amount.

- 10% of the withheld amount will be reimbursed for low disenrollment. If the provider/group maintains less than 2% disenrollment (those terminating MCP coverage or transferring to another provider), then they will receive this amount.

- 40% of the withheld amount will be reimbursed for quality of care. This will be determined by a review of medical records by the MCP. If the Medical Review Panel agrees with the treatment given at least 80% of the time, the provider will receive this amount.

- 15% of the withheld amount will be reimbursed for protocol compliance. This is calculated as follows:

  - 5% for compliance with all facility requirements as determined by an audit of the facility.
  - 5% for timeliness of claim payments.
  - 5% for timeliness in submission of all contractually required statements to the MCP.

If the provider meets all the stipulations outlined, they will keep the 5% quality care amount.

## Billing for Services

Although the monthly capitation amount covers most services, some services will be reimbursed on a fee-for-service basis. This means that the provider will bill the MCP for these services when they are performed. Most agreements between a provider and an MCP will have a list of those services that are covered by the capitation amount, or those that are considered to be on a fee-for-service basis. Fee-for-service procedures are usually billed on a CMS-1500 form the same as non-MCP services, or they may be electronically billed if required.

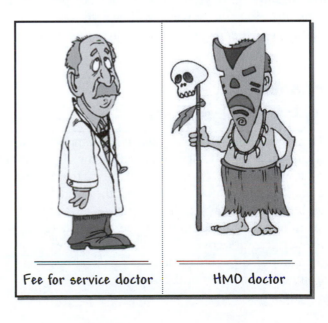

| Fee for service doctor | HMO doctor |

# Authorizations, Referrals, and Second Opinions

In an effort to contain their costs, MCPs will often require preauthorizations for treatment that is their financial responsibility. They may also require a Second Surgical Opinion regarding the proposed treatment.

## Preauthorization

Most MCPs require that the provider or member obtain preauthorization for services which are the financial responsibility of the MCP. This is often done on a **Treatment Authorization Request (TAR)** form. The provider lists the diagnosis and proposed treatment plan along with any needed follow-up care.

The TAR is submitted to the MCP for approval, and the MCP evaluates the proposed treatment and informs the provider and member whether or not they will cover the services. If the MCP decides that the services are not necessary, they will deny payment. The provider and member must then decide whether they will abandon the treatment, seek authorization for an alternate treatment, or if they will go ahead with the treatment with the understanding that the patient is completely responsible for the charges.

The MCP may decide that a Second Surgical Opinion (SSO) is needed before they make a determination. In such a case, the member must have the SSO performed prior to the services and with enough time for the MCP to evaluate the second surgeon's response to determine whether or not they will cover the services.

Often a TAR approval will be valid for a limited time, usually 30 days. If services are not performed within that time, the provider will need to complete an additional TAR and obtain another preauthorization. In the case of ongoing treatments (i.e., chemotherapy, dialysis), the provider may need to obtain monthly authorization of services covered by the MCP.

All routine follow-up care and/or hospital stays should be included in the one authorization.

If a specific date of surgery is listed on the TAR and the surgery is approved, the surgery should have been performed on the date indicated on the TAR. If there is no date listed, TARs are often good for 30 days from the date of approval. Services must have been performed within that time period for the TAR approval to be valid. If a TAR was approved but services were not performed within the required time period, and no additional TAR was submitted, the Group/IPA may be responsible for payment of services, not the MCP.

The TAR approval will also indicate the number of days allowed for the patient to remain in the hospital (if it is an inpatient admit). Any days beyond this are not covered by the MCP unless an additional TAR was submitted and approved, verifying the need for additional services.

Different rules may apply for inpatient admission for psychiatric care or chemical dependency.

## Emergency TARs

Many MCPs have an emergency request procedure which allows faxing of the TAR and overnight approval.

If the member is unable to wait the 24 hours for treatment, they should seek assistance in the emergency room of the nearest hospital. The hospital will then contact the MCP for an emergency treatment request. Many MCPs have a clause that the member must seek emergency treatment at an MCP facility if possible. Only if the emergency is threatening to life or limb, should the member go to a non-MCP facility.

In such cases, the hospital is required to provide life-saving measures. Any measures not required to sustain life must be approved by the MCP before they are rendered. Many hospitals are aware of this situation and will immediately call the MCP before treating an MCP member who has sought treatment at their facility.

The MCP will do an immediate review of the patient's situation and authorize individual services. However, each service will need to be authorized prior to being rendered, unless it is necessary to sustain the life of the patient.

If the patient is stable, the MCP will often have the patient transferred to their own facility for treatment.

## Practice Pitfalls

**Example:** John Johnson received approval for treatment in the MCP hospital facility for surgery to remove gallstones. During the surgery, there were complications which necessitated the need for an additional three days in the hospital. A TAR was not submitted for the additional three days. Therefore, the services are covered for the main surgery, but the additional three days are the financial responsibility of the member or the Group.

## Practice

# Pitfalls

**Example:** June Jenkins was involved in a diving accident. When she was pulled from the water, she was not breathing and it appeared her neck was broken. At the emergency room, the doctors were able to perform life-saving measures (i.e., CPR, insertion of a respirator tube). However, before being able to do a spinal x-ray or MRI, authorization was needed from the MCP. Only when the MCP authorized these procedures would the hospital be assured of payment on the services done to determine the extent of her injury. If the hospital had performed these services prior to receiving authorization, June would have been responsible for full payment on the unauthorized procedures.

If the Group/IPA is considered financially responsible for emergency room services, then they are responsible for managing the member's utilization of ER services and for paying the cost of these services. The group must provide written information to its members on how to access these services. The Group/IPA must have procedures for the authorization of these services. Payment may not be denied based on lack of notification or lack of authorization for these services.

If the member seeks ER services from a noncontracted provider, the Group/IPA usually has 30 minutes to respond from the time of the noncontracted provider's first call. Lack of response means that the ER may provide whatever services it deems necessary to treat the emergency situation and the Group/IPA is often obligated to pay for all charges.

## Utilization Review

Many insurance carriers began creating utilization review departments in an effort to control costs and avoid unnecessary procedures. While this process was started with traditional insurance carriers, managed care carriers have taken the concept a step further, creating complete UR departments and reviewing every outside procedure which may require additional costs.

Additionally, UR committees are becoming more selective in the items and providers they choose to review. Those procedures which are nearly always allowed; such as a cystourethroscopy, are being automatically allowed, while more questionable procedures; such as MRIs on the knees, are being reviewed. Additionally, some insurers are tracking the records of providers. Those that are known for ordering tests or procedures that are nearly always necessary are less closely watched than those who have a history of ordering questionable procedures.

## Specialist Referrals

If a member requests to see a specialist, the PCP must discuss the request with the member. If the request is denied, the procedures for denial of services must be followed, including the sending of a denial letter to the member.

If the PCP agrees with the member's request or recommends the member to see a specialist, an appropriate referral form should be completed and approved by the Group/IPA. The decision to refer or not to refer a member is a medical judgment which should be made by the PCP and the Group/IPA, especially since the financial responsibility for these visits often falls with the PCP or Group/IPA. Of course if the member wishes a referral to a specialist for a service that is the financial responsibility of the MCP, preauthorization must be obtained.

If the referral authorization is approved, a written notice must advise the member of the name, address, and phone number of the specialist and must either state an appointment time or inform the member of how to schedule an appointment.

The Group/IPA is required to have contracts with its specialists. They must maintain contracts with a sufficient number of specialists so that members are not inconvenienced by excessive appointment waiting times.

## Second Opinions

If a member requests a specific treatment and the MCP determines that this treatment or service is not medically necessary, would be detrimental to the patient, or would provide no medical benefit to the member, they may deny the service (i.e., refuse to cover the treatment). The denial letter should contain a statement regarding why services are denied.

Many MCPs have a second opinion policy designed to resolve differences of opinion regarding proposed treatment among PCP, members, specialists, and the MSP. Second opinions are often provided in the following instances:

- At the request of the member before a surgical or other invasive procedure.

- If the PCP's opinion is contrary to the member's expressed expectations, even after the physician has counseled the member.

- If the opinion of the PCP differs substantially from the recommended treatment plan of the specialist on the case.
- At the request of the MCP.

There are several steps to the second opinion process:

1. A request is made by the PCP, member, consultant, or MCP for a second opinion. This request may be either verbal or in writing.

2. The patient's chart is documented with the request.

3. An internal review is done. This is a second opinion performed by another physician affiliated with the same Group/IPA as the PCP.

4. If the member is still dissatisfied or if the two opinions differ substantially, an external review may be performed. This is an opinion provided by a physician who is not a member of the Group/IPA to which the member belongs. If the member is still dissatisfied, they may contact the MCP to request the external review. The MCP reviews the records and, if they deem it necessary to have an external review, they will inform the PCP and the member. The MCP may send the member to a physician of their choosing.

5. All records are forwarded to the MCP's Chief Medical Officer who makes a determination of the proper course of treatment. The PCP will then be informed of the decision, and it is their responsibility to carry out the proposed treatment plan. This may mean treating the patient themselves or referring the member to a specialist for treatment.

Financial responsibility for second opinions is usually split among the Group/IPA and the MCP as follows:

1. The Group/IPA is responsible for the internal review.

2. The MCP is responsible for the external review unless the Group/IPA failed to document the internal review, did not properly complete a TAR and obtain authorization before sending the member for an external review, or if the opinion of the external review physician differs substantially from the Group/IPA decision.

All activities regarding the second opinion process must be thoroughly documented in the patient's record. Any time the MCP must bear financial responsibility for

any services, including the external review, a TAR must be completed and the treatment preauthorized.

Because of substantial delays in receiving authorizations and/or referrals, and member complaints, some MCPs are now allowing members to refer themselves for a second opinion. However, they are limited to obtaining a second opinion from another provider who is affiliated with the same MCP, and the number of times they may refer themselves for a second opinion is limited (i.e., once every six months).

## Denials of Service after a Second Opinion

Once the member has exhausted the second opinion process or chooses not to proceed with the process (i.e., accepts the decision of the internal review), the Group/IPA must send a denial letter to the member. A copy of this letter must also be sent to the MCP with any supporting documentation.

This letter must state the patient's name, the date services were requested, the services that were requested, and the reason for the denial of services.

The MCP will often keep a log of these denials. If they feel a Group/IPA is denying too many treatments, they may ask for a review of the record to monitor the quality of care given to the patients.

# Miscellaneous Services

Certain rules may apply to select types of service under an MCP agreement. These services can include outpatient surgery, emergency room services, durable medical equipment, and prescriptions.

## Outpatient Surgery

Some MCPs will provide a list of surgeries that must be performed in an outpatient setting. This is most often done in a shared risk contract when the Group/IPA is financially responsible for outpatient services and the MCP is responsible for inpatient services.

It is important to know which surgeries must be performed on an outpatient basis. If these guidelines are not followed, the Group/IPA may be financially responsible for all inpatient costs in relation to the surgery.

The examiner should be aware of this list and keep it handy. If a claim is received for inpatient surgery that should have been performed on an outpatient basis, the claim should be denied and returned to the provider/PCP.

If the provider feels the surgery should have been performed inpatient due to complications or other circumstances, a TAR should have been submitted and approval received prior to surgery.

# On the Job Now

**Directions:** Answer the following questions without looking back at the material just covered. Write your answers in the space provided.

1. What form is usually submitted for a member to obtain preauthorization for services which are the financial responsibility of the MCP? _____

2. Who is financially responsible for second opinions? _____

_____

3. What is the utilization review? _____

_____

_____

## Prescription Coverage

When an MCP offers prescription coverage to a member, there are often limitations as follows:

1. The member must purchase the drugs from an MCP contracted facility. If they obtain prescriptions from a noncontracted pharmacy, the member will bear the cost of the pharmacy services. There may be exceptions to this rule for emergency situations, situations where the patient is outside the service area, or if the prescription is not available from a contracted pharmacy.

2. They may limit drugs and medications to a 30 day supply.

3. They will usually only cover prescription drugs. Over-the-counter medications are usually not covered.

4. They may only include oral and topical drugs. Injectable drugs are often not covered under the pharmacy benefit. They may, however, be covered under the medical benefit. This is especially true for injectable medications which the patient needs for survival (i.e., insulin for a diabetic).

5. They may also insist that the generic equivalent of a drug be prescribed if it is available. If there is no generic equivalent, the MCP will often cover the brand name at the standard copayment amount. However, if there is a generic equivalent, the MCP may only cover the cost of the generic equivalent. Thus, the member will be charged the standard

copay, plus the difference between the generic and the brand name medication.

Some generic drugs are not the same as their brand name counterparts. They may have a similar but different active ingredient, or they may be in a different dosage amount from the brand name drug. In such a case, they are not considered to be therapeutically equivalent. For these drugs, the MCP may require the physician to prescribe the generic drug, or they may allow the full benefit for the brand name drug.

## Claim Payments

Now that you understand some of the basic rules regarding eligibility, preauthorizations, referrals and second opinions, we will discuss processing an MCP claim. Below is a brief overview of the process. Each item will then be discussed in more detail.

1. Check the member's eligibility, which contract they are covered under, and who their PCP is.

2. Check the member's contract to determine if the services are covered and any copayment or other amounts.

3. Determine who is financially responsible for payment on the claim by using the Distribution of Responsibility chart.

4. Check if the proper referrals, preauthorizations, or second opinions were done.

5. If the referrals, preauthorizations, or second opinions were done, process the claim.

6. If the referrals were not done, deny or reduce benefits accordingly and process the claim.

To process the claim:

1. Determine the allowed amount for the procedure.

2. Determine if there should be a reduction of benefits due to improper referrals, incomplete authorizations, or other limitations.

3. Subtract the amount of any copayment given by the member.

4. Pay the remaining amount.

## Check Member Eligibility

When processing MCP claims, as with other types of claims, eligibility is the first item to consider. Check the **eligibility roster** to determine the effective dates of the patient's coverage, what contract they are covered under, and their PCP (the Group/IPA responsible for their primary care).

The MCP's providers will often have three eligibility rosters to consider:

1. The **active member roster** lists those whose coverage has continued into the next month. This usually means the insured or their employer has paid the monthly premium to continue coverage for another month.

2. The **new member roster** shows those patients who have signed up for MCP coverage and have chosen the provider as their PCP. The new member roster also shows those patients who have recently chosen this provider as their PCP.

3. The **terminated member roster** shows those members whose coverage has been terminated.

The claims examiner will often have a computerized eligibility roster which shows not only the dates the member was eligible, but also what plan they are covered under and who their primary care physician is. The plan the patient is covered under will not only determine the covered services, but will also determine who is responsible for payment of each individual service.

## Check the Member's Contract

Once you have determined the plan, go through the member's contract. As with other contracts, this will list the items covered, the amount of copayments, and any excluded items. Any amounts that are excluded would be automatically denied.

## Determine Financial Responsibility

For items that are covered, you will need to determine who is responsible for payment of the item. When a Group or a provider signs up with an MCP, they agree to cover certain services in exchange for a capitation amount. When each provider signs up, they will sign up for certain plans. They may be providers on some plans, but not on others.

Refer to the Distribution of Responsibility chart (**see Figure 10–1**). This is a chart (often many pages long) that will show who is responsible for the payment on each plan. This will be either the provider (regardless of whether it is a group of individual provider), or the MCP. On some items, the responsibility may be shared. In these cases you will need to refer to the specific contract. This will explain in greater detail who has financial responsibility for the services.

Items are often listed on the Distribution of Responsibility chart by CPT® number. If a chart lists items alphabetically, it may be necessary to look up the procedure code in the *CPT*® to determine what the service is. Additionally, many Distribution of Responsibility charts that are listed alphabetically may have an indexed listing by CPT® code in the back.

Once you have located the proper procedure code, follow the line across until you are under the plan name for the plan the member is covered under. Determine whether the responsibility is with the provider or the MCP. Be sure to check if there are any provisions regarding coverage. These will often be referenced by a small number with a more detailed explanation at the bottom of the page (i.e., see abortion on **Figure 10–1**).

If the provider is responsible for payment of the services, these items are considered covered by the capitation amount and no further payment is due on those services. Check who the provider was on the claim. If the provider submitting the claim was the member's PCP, then charges should be denied as being covered by the capitation amount. If the provider on the claim is not the PCP, the claim should be forwarded to the PCP for payment.

If there are services that the PCP is responsible for and services that the MCP is responsible for on the same claim, process the claim and pay those items the MCP is responsible for. Items the PCP is responsible for should be denied and the claim should be forwarded to the PCP for further processing, if needed.

## Check Referrals, Preauthorizations, or Second Opinions

Those items that are the financial responsibility of the MCP should have had referrals or preauthorizations performed. In some cases a second opinion may also have been required. Check to be sure that all the proper paperwork was done.

If the paperwork was not done, check the contract to determine what the impact will be on the coverage of those services.

The preauthorization will often be accessible by computer, so the claims examiner should be able to check it quickly and easily. Often a preauthorization number will be included on the claim (see block 23 on the CMS-1500). If a preauthorization number is not included, you must check the system for the preauthorization. Not having a preauthorization number on the claim is often not considered a valid reason for denying payment on a service since the claims examiner has access to that information.

If the referrals, preauthorizations, or second opinions were done, process the claim.

If the referrals were not done, deny or reduce benefits accordingly and process the claim.

## Patient Encounter Forms

The Group/IPA must report all patient encounters (i.e., visits) to the MCP. This is true regardless of whether the visit occurs at the Group/IPA or at one of its contracted providers. This reporting is often done using an encounter form. If the Group/IPA does not have data regarding an encounter (which may happen if they are not contractually obligated to cover the services), but they receive information regarding the encounter, they should report what they know of the encounter to the MCP.

The MCP may specify the use of a designated form for reporting encounters, or they may use the CMS-1500.

Encounters for consultation, second opinions, and other outside visits should be reported prior to adjudication and/or payment of the claim.

Some MCPs have their providers or Group/IPAs report patient encounters on a CMS-1500. When this is done, the only difference between this and a normal CMS-1500 is in block 24F, the charges. If the charges are covered by a capitation amount, then there is no charge for these services. Therefore, the indicated charges will be $0. The total charges and the balance due will likewise be $0.

If there are services which a provider renders which are not covered by the normal capitation amount, the amount for these charges should be placed in block 24F. Some MCPs may have providers or Group/IPAs submit charges that are the MCP's responsibility on a separate claim form from those that are covered under capitation. Thus, two claim forms for the same provider, patient, and dates of service may be necessary.

# On the Job Now

**Directions:** Answer the following questions without looking back at the material just covered. Write your answers in the space provided.

1. List the four things a claims examiner needs to check before a claim can be processed, denied, or reduced.

   1. _____

   2. _____

   3. _____

   4. _____

2. Under what circumstances would a payment be covered by the capitation amount? _____

   _____

3. Under what circumstances would a payment be denied as being covered by the capitation amount?

   _____

   _____

# Processing the Claim

You are now ready to begin the actual calculations to process the claim. When claims are submitted, they will often be accompanied by a Claim Transmittal Form (see Figure 10–2). This form will indicate the type of claim being submitted and the authorization number for these claims.

## Determine the Allowed Amount

Start by determining the allowed amount for the procedure. Most MCPs will have a fee schedule which will list each CPT® code and the allowed amount for that code. Some MCPs that cover a wide area may have an RVS and Conversion Factor Report. In these cases, calculate the allowed amount using these factors in the same way you would calculate indemnity.

If there is a contracted amount for services, the terms in the contract should be adhered to. Usually a fee schedule will accompany contracted terms. This fee schedule may be different for each provider with which the Group/IPA contracts. The proper contract should be pulled and the correct allowed amount determined.

## Calculate Any Reduced Benefits

If the member or PCP did not obtain the proper referrals, preauthorizations, or second opinions, determine the impact on the payment. This will often be stated in either the contract with the member (if it was the member's responsibility to obtain the proper paperwork) or the MCP's contract with the Group/IPA.

If the benefits are reduced, calculate the impact of the reduction (i.e., if benefits are reduced to 50% if preauthorization is not obtained, multiply the allowed amount by 50%).

Be sure that you look at all paperwork carefully. If the preauthorization allowed three days of inpatient care and the member spent four days in the hospital, services for the last day may not be covered or may be reduced. In such a case, you may need to request an itemized billing to determine the dates that services were provided so you can determine which services should be denied.

## Subtract the Copayment

Check the member's contract. Each item should list a copayment amount if a copayment is required from the member. Be sure you are checking the proper category. Often there will be different copayment amounts for different types of services.

The amount of the member's copayment is always subtracted from the allowed amount. If the provider neglected to collect this amount at the time services were rendered, they are responsible for contacting the patient and collecting it. Thus, even if the claim states that no money was collected from the member, the copayment amount should always be subtracted.

## Pay the Remaining Amount

Calculate any reduced benefits and subtract the copayment amount, then pay the remaining amount. Since the member is always responsible for the copayment, and usually only the copayment, any resulting benefits are generally due to the provider. The member should not have paid more than the copayment amount. If the member did pay more than the copayment amount, the provider is responsible for reimbursing the member for any amounts they overpaid.

An EOB should accompany all claim payments, showing the calculation of the benefits and providing an explanation for why any services were denied or reduced. A notice should also accompany the EOB, stating that this is the contracted amount for this service and no amounts other than the copayment may be collected from the member.

Of course if you are working for a staff model HMO, there is no payment due for those services rendered by the HMO owned facility. This is because the providers in this type of facility are paid a salary, regardless of the members they see or the services they perform.

# Denial of a Claim or Service

If a claim or service is denied, a denial letter must be included with the EOB, indicating the reason for the denial. The denial notice must also include a statement that the provider has the right to appeal the denial within 60 days, and the address of where to file an appeal. If it is believed that services were not medically necessary or were not true emergency services, then the claim must be sent through a medical review process. The medical review should use the presenting diagnosis, rather than the discharge diagnosis, as the basis for their decision making, and must consider the member's understanding of the medical circumstances which led to the emergency service.

All denial notices must contain an explicit reason, in layman's terms, of why the service(s) are being denied. If the MCP provides a list of denial reasons, then the appropriate denial reason should be written on the denial letter. You may not use a code unless you indicate the meaning of that code on the denial letter.

Additionally, all denial letters must meet the following criteria:

1. The decision to deny must be correct and based upon approved medical practices.

2. The denial reason must be clear to the member and CMS-approved denial reasons must be used.

3. The denial letter must include mandated appeals language and the correct health plan address.

4. The denial letter must be sent to the appropriate parties (the provider, the member, or both).

5. The denial notice must be issued within required time frames.

## Appeals

Any member or provider has the right to appeal a denied claim. All denial letters, by law, must include a statement indicating that the receiver has the right to appeal the decision and whom to contact to begin the appeal process.

If a member or provider appeals a denied claim, the MCP will review the claim and make a determination of whether to uphold or reverse the denial. If the MCP determines that the services should have been covered and the services were the financial responsibility of the Group/IPA, it will inform the Group/IPA of its decision and will instruct the Group/IPA to pay the claim.

## Reinsurance/Stoploss

**Stoploss** is an attempt to limit payments by an insured person or a Group/IPA in the case of a catastrophic illness or injury to a member.

Many MCP have a stoploss or reinsurance clause included in them. This clause may state that the Group/IPA will be financially responsible for the first set amount (i.e., $7,000) in expenses for each member in a contract year. After those expenses have been paid, the MCP will reimburse the Group/IPA for verified expenses which exceed the set amount.

If the provider's contract has a stoploss clause, it is important that the claims examiner be aware of the amount. Any services which exceed that set amount should be covered by the MCP.

Often the MCP will require that a claim for reimbursement be submitted on specific forms. An example of this form is shown in **Figure 10–3**.

Provider Network Services
CLAIMS TRANSMITTAL FORM

Date:

To:    Claims Services

From: _____, Administrator for _____

The attached claims are the responsibility of [the MCP].

Authorization Number

_____ Inpatient Hospital (IP) Charges

_____ Outpatient Surgery (OPS) Facility Charges

_____ Anesthesia for approved IP or OPS

_____ Radiology for approved IP, OPS or SNF

_____ Pathology for approved IP, OPS or SNF

_____ Emergency services which resulted in admission to Inpatient status

_____ Ambulance

_____ Durable Medical Equipment

_____ Dialysis Facility Charges

_____ Radiation Therapy

_____ Member not on roster for date of service. Include relevant roster page(s).

NOTE: Use a separate form for each type of Plan expense. Multiple providers may be grouped if the authorization number is the same.

[The MCP] will not send denial notices for services which are the responsibility of the Group/IPA.

Refer to the Medical Services Agreement for questions of coverage and financial responsibility.

■ **Figure 10–2**  Transmittal Form

**Excess Risk Limit Cost Summary**

I.  Group Name: _____          Enrollee Name: _____          II.

    Address: _____             Enrollee PF#: _____

    _____                      Date of Elegibility: _____

    Contact Person: _____      Contract Year: _____

    Phone Number: _____        For HIV/AIDS cases, list qualifying hospital stays:

    Date Submitted: _____

| | | |
|---|---|---|
| | **Type of submission** | |
| __ Original | | __ Medicare |
| __ Supplemental | | __ Commercial |
| __ Resubmittal | | __ OO Care |
| __ AIDS/HIV | | __ CCC |

_____    _____    _____

_____    _____    _____

III.

| Provider of Service / Provider # | Date of Service | CPT, RVS, or SMA code | Units | Billed Amount | Amount Paid | For HMO use only |
|---|---|---|---|---|---|---|
| | | | | | | |
| | | | | | | |
| | | | | | | |
| | | | | | | |
| | | | | | | |
| | | | | | | |
| | | | | | **TOTAL THIS PAGE:** | | |

■ **Figure 10–3** Excess Risk (Stoploss) Form

# CHAPTER REVIEW

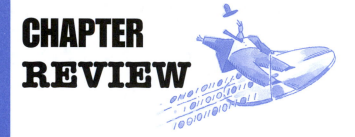

## Summary

- Managed care contracts were created in an attempt to bring healthcare costs under control by having doctors share some of the financial risks of healthcare with the patient and the insurance carrier.
- HMOs are one of the most common managed care trends.

- A written contract will dictate those services which the provider will cover and those which the MCP will cover.
- For those services that are the financial responsibility of the MCP, the provider will submit a claim. The claim must be processed and paid or denied in a timely manner.
- The rules governing payment of MCP claims will vary from those of indemnity claims.
- In an MCP, the financial responsibility must be considered along with whether or not preauthorizations, referrals, or second opinions were handled properly.

## Assignments

Complete the Questions for Review.
Complete Exercises 10–1 through 10–8.

## Questions for Review

**Directions:** Answer the following questions without looking back into the material just covered. Write your answers in the space provided.

1. What is an HMO? _____

_____

2. In a _____, a facility or Group bands together to provide services for HMO patients at their own facilities.

3. What is a capitation payment? _____

_____

4. What is a TAR and what is its purpose? _____

_____

5. What is stoploss? _____

_____

If you were unable to answer any of the questions, refer back to that section and then fill in the answers.

# Exercise **10–1**

**Directions:** Find and circle the words listed below. Words can appear horizontally, vertically, diagonally, forward, or backward.

```
A C K H Z Q Q G M D I E V C Q Z N W V F
W H S K W S O X R L Y F I Q M K I B A N
X T B M L D U S P O I N T V Q Z V S F Z
Q A I O O Q J X E C U O C R S O P W W C
P I L L R U B Q D P H P D J D I E J W M
F H L O E I W B H H L E M J T T F P C S
N E T W O R K M O D E L C O V C N G L C
K W W O N N B P M L I C G E D T Y V S T
X G S D A P A M C V W J R P K E L S C F
Q Z F Z W Q E P S C Y N X I F G L T N E
R V B D L Z G L Y P O P J S X Y U O L C
Q E X S U X O Q S I M B Y T K B N P I E
R J C H M P M X T M N P K S U B L L Q E
J A K K L D N A Z F H R W X P Z T O C U
I B H Y Z B Z S X O Y H N C T Y N S K Y
B G X O J I H G N U H Q H V J F Q S B J
O R U T L U G I I N P Z U J Y S T M U U
U O D I B G Y E V K X Y U C M N K G E J
H V T G V B F A Z I M O V Z E L K R G E
O U Q I F R N B Z U C W M Y C X O Q S G
```

1. Group Model
2. Network Model
3. Stoploss

# Exercise 10-2

**Directions:** Complete the crossword puzzle by filling in a word from the keywords that fits each clue.

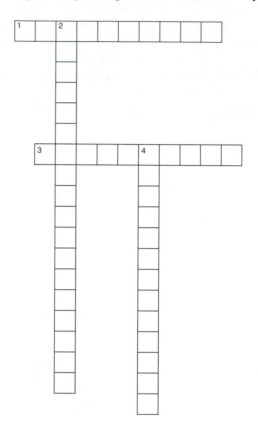

**Across**

1. A monthly fee paid to a provider in exchange for handling the healthcare needs of a patient.
3. An HMO that hires physicians or providers to work at the HMO's own facility.

**Down**

2. Items such as an annual physical, cancer screening (pap smears, mammograms, etc.), flu shots, immunizations, and well-baby care.
4. Groups of physicians who are signed under or work for the same company.

# Exercise **10-3**

**Directions:** Match the following terms with the proper definition by writing the letter of the correct definition in the space next to the term.

1. _____ Eligibility Roster

2. _____ Individual Practice Organizations

3. _____ Primary Care Provider

4. _____ Treatment Authorization Request

a. A legal entity, comprised of a network of private physicians who have organized to negotiate contracts with insurance companies and HMOs.

b. The provider a member has chosen who is responsible for all their healthcare needs.

c. A form used to request authorization for services which are the financial responsibility of the HMO.

d. A listing which shows the effective dates of the patient's coverage, what contract they are covered under, and their primary care provider.

# Exercises **10-4** through **10-8**

**Directions:** Process on a Payment Worksheet the following Managed Care claims found on the following pages. Use the Small Group HMO contract, the Distribution of Responsibility, and the Fee Schedule found in Appendix A to process the claims. Refer to Appendices B and C for additional information.

All insureds are eligible for coverage under their respective plans. There are no beginning financials for members. This is their first claim. Amounts paid for each claim should be accumulated and carried forward to subsequent claims.

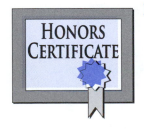

### Honors Certification™

The Honors Certification™ challenge for this chapter consists of a written test of the information contained within this chapter. Additionally you will be given three claims to process, using the contracts contained in this book. Each incorrect answer will result in a deduction of up to 5% from your grade. You must achieve a score of 80% or higher to pass this test. If you fail the test on your first attempt, you may retake the test one additional time. The items included in the second test may be different from those in the first test.

PLEASE
DO NOT
STAPLE
IN THIS
AREA
□□□ PICA

SUMMER INSURANCE CO
70065 SUNNY STREET
SANDY CITY CO 82936

APPROVED MOB-0938-0008

# HEALTH INSURANCE CLAIM FORM

PICA □□□

| 1. MEDICARE | MEDICAID | CHAMPUS | CHAMPVA | GROUP HEALTH PLAN | FECA BLK LUNG | OTHER | 1a. INSURED'S I.D NUMBER (FOR PROGRAM IN ITEM 1) |
|---|---|---|---|---|---|---|---|
| ☐ (Medicare #) | ☐ (Medicaid #) | ☐ (Sponsor's SSN) | ☐ (VA File #) | ☒ (SSN or ID) | ☐ (SSN) | ☐ (ID) | 222 22 ROC |

| 2. PATIENT'S NAME (Last, First, Middle Initial). | 3. PATIENT'S BIRTH DATE | 4. INSURED'S NAME (Last, First, Middle Initial) |
|---|---|---|
| MORPHINE MIKE M | MM 02 DD 12 YY CCYY-45 SEX M ☒ F ☐ | MORPHINE MINDY M |

| 5. PATIENT'S ADDRESS (No., Street) | 6. PATIENT'S RELATIONSHIP TO INSURED | 7. INSURED'S ADDRESS (No., Street) |
|---|---|---|
| 522 MUSHROOM STREET | Self ☐ Spouse ☒ Child ☐ Other ☐ | SAME |

| CITY | STATE | 8. PATIENT STATUS | CITY | STATE |
|---|---|---|---|---|
| MIGRAINE | ME | Single ☐ Married ☒ Other ☐ | | |

| ZIP CODE | TELEPHONE (Include Area Code) | | ZIP CODE | TELEPHONE (INCLUDE AREA CODE) |
|---|---|---|---|---|
| 04022 | (207) 555 3322 | Employed ☒ Full-Time Student ☐ Part-Time Student ☐ | | |

| 9. OTHER INSURED'S NAME (Last, First, Middle Initial) | 10. IS PATIENT'S CONDITION RELATED TO: | 11. INSURED'S POLICY GROUP OR FECA NUMBER: |
|---|---|---|
| | | 67980ROC |

| a. OTHER INSURED'S POLICY OR GROUP NUMBER | a. EMPLOYMENT? (CURRENT OR PREVIOUS) | a. INSURED'S DATE OF BIRTH |
|---|---|---|
| | ☐ YES ☒ NO | MM 12 DD 22 YY CCYY -45 SEX M ☐ F ☒ |

| b. OTHER INSURED'S DATE OF BIRTH | b. AUTO ACCIDENT? PLACE (State) | b. EMPLOYER'S NAME OR SCHOOL NAME |
|---|---|---|
| MM DD YY SEX M ☐ F ☐ | ☐ YES ☒ NO | ROCKY CORPORATION |

| c. EMPLOYER'S NAME OR SCHOOL NAME | c. OTHER ACCIDENT? | c. INSURANCE PLAN NAME OR PROGRAM NAME |
|---|---|---|
| | ☒ YES ☐ NO | SUMMER INSURANCE COMPANY |

| d. INSURANCE PLAN NAME OR PROGRAM NAME | 10d. RESERVED FOR LOCAL USE | d. IS THERE ANOTHER HEALTH BENEFIT PLAN? |
|---|---|---|
| | | ☐ YES ☒ NO **if yes**, return to and complete item 9 a-d |

READ BACK OF FORM BEFORE COMPLETING & SIGNING THIS FORM

12. PATIENT'S OR AUTHORIZED PERSON'S SIGNATURE I authorize the release of any medical or other information necessary to process this claim. I also request payment of government benefits either to myself or to the party who accepts assignment below.

SIGNED **SIGNATURE ON FILE**    DATE _____

13. INSURED'S OR AUTHORIZED PERSON'S SIGNATURE I authorize payment of medical benefits to the undersigned physician or supplier for services described below.

SIGNED **SIGNATURE ON FILE**

| 14. DATE OF CURRENT: ◄ ILLNESS (1st symptom) ◄ INJURY (Accident) PREGNANCY (LMP) | 15. IF PATIENT HAS HAD SAME OR SIMILAR ILLNESS, GIVE FIRST DATE | 16. DATES PATIENT UNABLE TO WORK IN CURRENT OCCUPATION |
|---|---|---|
| MM 01 DD 30 YY YY | MM DD YY | FROM MM DD YY TO MM DD YY |

| 17. NAME OF REFERRING PHYSICIAN OR OTHER SOURCE | 17a. I.D. NUMBER OF REFERRING PHYSICIAN | 18. HOSPITALIZATION DATES RELATED TO CURRENT SERVICES |
|---|---|---|
| | | FROM MM DD YY TO MM DD YY |

| 19. RESERVED FOR LOCAL USE | 20. OUTSIDE LAB? $ CHARGES |
|---|---|
| HURRY HOSPITAL 8000 HALLS WAY HUNTERSVILLE ME 04022 | ☐ YES ☐ NO |

| 21. DIAGNOSIS OR NATURE OF ILLNESS OR INJURY, (RELATE ITEMS 1,2,3, OR 4 TO ITEM 24E BY LINE) | 22. MEDICAID RESUBMISSION CODE / ORIGINAL REF. NO. |
|---|---|
| 1. 729 . 5 ⎯⎯⎯ 3. ___ . ___ | |
| 2. ___ . ___ 4. ___ . ___ | 23. PRIOR AUTHORIZATION NUMBER |

| 24. A. DATE(S) OF SERVICE From MM DD YY | To MM DD YY | B. Place of Service | C. Type of Service | D. PROCEDURES, SERVICES, OR SUPPLIES (Explain Unusual Circumstances) CPT/HCPS \| MODIFIER | E. DIAGNOSIS CODE | F. $ CHARGES | G. DAYS OR UNITS | H. EPSDT Family Plan | I. EMG | J. COB | K. RESERVED FOR LOCAL USE |
|---|---|---|---|---|---|---|---|---|---|---|---|
| 01 30 YY | 01 30 YY | 41 | 1 | A0429 | 1 | 355 \| 00 | 1 | | | | |
| | | | | | | | | | | | |
| | | | | | | | | | | | |
| | | | | | | | | | | | |
| | | | | | | | | | | | |
| | | | | | | | | | | | |

| 25. FEDERAL TAX I.D. NUMBER | SSN EIN | 26. PATIENT'S ACCOUNT NO. | 27. ACCEPT ASSIGNMENT? (For govt. claims, see back) | 28. TOTAL CHARGE | 29. AMOUNT PAID | 30. BALANCE DUE |
|---|---|---|---|---|---|---|
| 70 6659776 | ☐ ☒ | A001125 232 | ☒ YES ☐ NO | $ 355 \| 00 | $ | $ 355 \| 00 |

| 31. SIGNATURE OF PHYSICIAN OR SUPPLIER INCLUDING DEGREES OR CREDENTIALS (I certify that the statements on the reverse apply to this bill and are made a part thereof.) | 32. NAME AND ADDRESS OF FACILITY WHERE SERVICES WERE RENDERED (If other than home or office) | 33. PHYSICIAN'S, SUPPLIERS BILLING NAME, ADDRESS, ZIP CODE & PHONE # |
|---|---|---|
| SIGNED *Anna Bell* DATE *02/14/YY* | | AMAZING AMBULANCE SERVICE 21 ARCH WAY APPLEVILLE ME 04022 (207) 555 8882 |
| | | PIN# A21342    GRP# |

(APPROVED BY AMA COUNCIL ON MEDICAL SERVICE 8/88)    **PLEASE PRINT OR TYPE**

FORM CMS-1500 (12-90)
FORM OWCP-1500    FORM RRB-1500
FORM AMA-OP050591

# Exercise 10–4

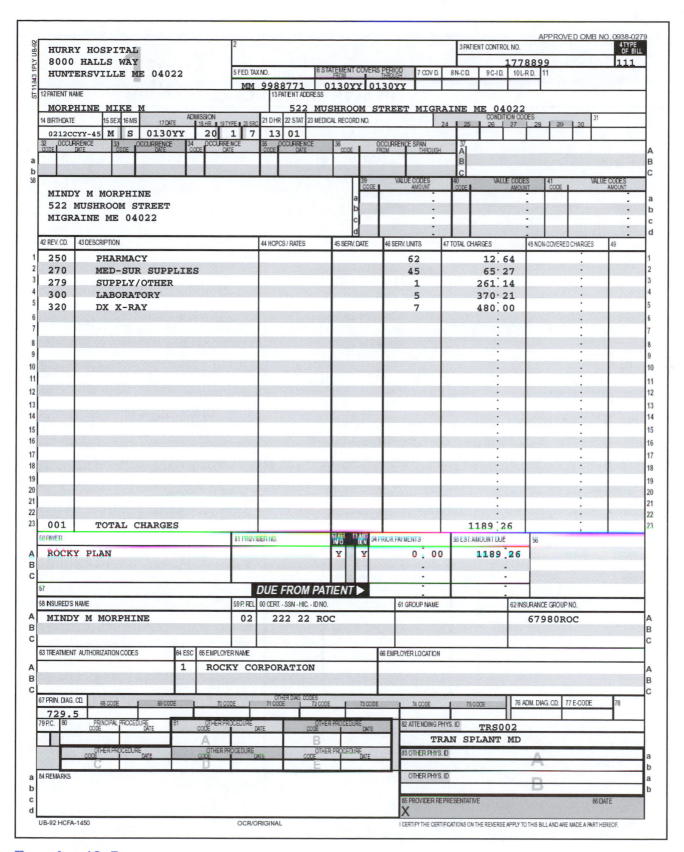

APPROVED OMB NO. 0938-0279

| | | | |
|---|---|---|---|
| HURRY HOSPITAL<br>8000 HALLS WAY<br>HUNTERSVILLE ME 04022 | 2 | 3 PATIENT CONTROL NO.<br>1778899 | 4 TYPE OF BILL<br>111 |

| 5 FED. TAX NO. | 6 STATEMENT COVERS PERIOD FROM THROUGH | 7 COV D. | 8 N-C D. | 9 C-I D. | 10 L-R D. | 11 |
|---|---|---|---|---|---|---|
| MM 9988771 | 0130YY 0130YY | | | | | |

| 12 PATIENT NAME | 13 PATIENT ADDRESS |
|---|---|
| MORPHINE MIKE M | 522 MUSHROOM STREET MIGRAINE ME 04022 |

| 14 BIRTHDATE | 15 SEX | 16 MS | 17 DATE | ADMISSION<br>18 HR. | 19 TYPE | 20 SRC | 21 D HR | 22 STAT | 23 MEDICAL RECORD NO. | CONDITION CODES<br>24 25 26 27 28 29 30 | 31 |
|---|---|---|---|---|---|---|---|---|---|---|---|
| 0212CCYY-45 | M | S | 0130YY | 20 | 1 | 7 | 13 | 01 | | | |

| 32 OCCURRENCE CODE DATE | 33 CODE OCCURRENCE DATE | 34 CODE OCCURRENCE DATE | 35 CODE OCCURRENCE DATE | 36 CODE | OCCURRENCE SPAN FROM THROUGH | 37 A B C |
|---|---|---|---|---|---|---|
| a | | | | | | |
| b | | | | | | |

38

MINDY M MORPHINE
522 MUSHROOM STREET
MIGRAINE ME 04022

| 39 CODE | VALUE CODES AMOUNT | 40 CODE | VALUE CODES AMOUNT | 41 CODE | VALUE CODES AMOUNT |
|---|---|---|---|---|---|
| a | | | | | |
| b | | | | | |
| c | | | | | |
| d | | | | | |

| 42 REV. CD. | 43 DESCRIPTION | 44 HCPCS / RATES | 45 SERV. DATE | 46 SERV. UNITS | 47 TOTAL CHARGES | 48 NON-COVERED CHARGES | 49 |
|---|---|---|---|---|---|---|---|
| 1 | 250 | PHARMACY | | | 62 | 12.64 | | 1 |
| 2 | 270 | MED-SUR SUPPLIES | | | 45 | 65.27 | | 2 |
| 3 | 279 | SUPPLY/OTHER | | | 1 | 261.14 | | 3 |
| 4 | 300 | LABORATORY | | | 5 | 370.21 | | 4 |
| 5 | 320 | DX X-RAY | | | 7 | 480.00 | | 5 |
| 6 | | | | | | | | 6 |
| 7 | | | | | | | | 7 |
| 8 | | | | | | | | 8 |
| 9 | | | | | | | | 9 |
| 10 | | | | | | | | 10 |
| 11 | | | | | | | | 11 |
| 12 | | | | | | | | 12 |
| 13 | | | | | | | | 13 |
| 14 | | | | | | | | 14 |
| 15 | | | | | | | | 15 |
| 16 | | | | | | | | 16 |
| 17 | | | | | | | | 17 |
| 18 | | | | | | | | 18 |
| 19 | | | | | | | | 19 |
| 20 | | | | | | | | 20 |
| 21 | | | | | | | | 21 |
| 22 | | | | | | | | 22 |
| 23 | 001 | TOTAL CHARGES | | | | 1189.26 | | 23 |

| 50 PAYER | 51 PROVIDER NO. | 52 REL INFO | 53 ASG BEN | 54 PRIOR PAYMENTS | 55 EST. AMOUNT DUE | 56 |
|---|---|---|---|---|---|---|
| A | ROCKY PLAN | | Y | Y | 0.00 | 1189.26 | |
| B | | | | | | | |
| C | | | | | | | |

| 57 | DUE FROM PATIENT ▶ |
|---|---|

| 58 INSURED'S NAME | 59 P. REL | 60 CERT. - SSN - HIC. - ID NO. | 61 GROUP NAME | 62 INSURANCE GROUP NO. |
|---|---|---|---|---|
| A | MINDY M MORPHINE | 02 | 222 22 ROC | | 67980ROC |
| B | | | | | |
| C | | | | | |

| 63 TREATMENT AUTHORIZATION CODES | 64 ESC | 65 EMPLOYER NAME | 66 EMPLOYER LOCATION |
|---|---|---|---|
| A | | 1 | ROCKY CORPORATION | |
| B | | | | |
| C | | | | |

| 67 PRIN. DIAG. CD. | 68 CODE | 69 CODE | 70 CODE | OTHER DIAG. CODES<br>71 CODE 72 CODE 73 CODE | 74 CODE | 75 CODE | 76 ADM. DIAG. CD. | 77 E-CODE | 78 |
|---|---|---|---|---|---|---|---|---|---|
| 729.5 | | | | | | | | | |

| 79 P.C. | 80 | PRINCIPAL PROCEDURE CODE DATE | 81 | OTHER PROCEDURE CODE DATE | OTHER PROCEDURE CODE DATE | 82 ATTENDING PHYS. ID | TRS002 |
|---|---|---|---|---|---|---|---|
| | | | | A | B | | TRAN SPLANT MD |

| | OTHER PROCEDURE CODE DATE | OTHER PROCEDURE CODE DATE | OTHER PROCEDURE CODE DATE | 83 OTHER PHYS. ID | A |
|---|---|---|---|---|---|
| | C | D | E | OTHER PHYS. ID | B |

| a | 84 REMARKS | 85 PROVIDER REPRESENTATIVE<br>X | 86 DATE |
|---|---|---|---|
| b | | | |
| c | | | |
| d | | | |

UB-92 HCFA-1450          OCR/ORIGINAL          I CERTIFY THE CERTIFICATIONS ON THE REVERSE APPLY TO THIS BILL AND ARE MADE A PART HEREOF.

**Exercise 10–5**

PLEASE DO NOT STAPLE IN THIS AREA

SUMMER INSURANCE CO
70065 SUNNY STREET
SANDY CITY CO 82936

APPROVED MOB-0938-0008

☐☐☐ PICA

# HEALTH INSURANCE CLAIM FORM

PICA ☐☐☐

**1.** MEDICARE ☐ (Medicare #)  MEDICAID ☐ (Medicaid #)  CHAMPUS ☐ (Sponsor's SSN)  CHAMPVA ☐ (VA File #)  GROUP HEALTH PLAN ☒ (SSN or ID)  FECA BLK LUNG ☐ (SSN)  OTHER ☐ (ID)

**1a.** INSURED'S I.D NUMBER (FOR PROGRAM IN ITEM 1): 222 22 ROC

**2.** PATIENT'S NAME (Last, First, Middle Initial): MORPHINE MIKE M

**3.** PATIENT'S BIRTH DATE: MM 02 DD 12 YY CCYY-45  SEX M ☒ F ☐

**4.** INSURED'S NAME (Last, First, Middle Initial): MORPHINE MINDY M

**5.** PATIENT'S ADDRESS (No., Street): 522 MUSHROOM STREET

**6.** PATIENT'S RELATIONSHIP TO INSURED: Self ☐ Spouse ☒ Child ☐ Other ☐

**7.** INSURED'S ADDRESS (No., Street): SAME

CITY: MIGRAINE  STATE: ME

**8.** PATIENT STATUS: Single ☐ Married ☒ Other ☐  Employed ☒ Full-Time Student ☐ Part-Time Student ☐

CITY:  STATE:

ZIP CODE: 04022  TELEPHONE (Include Area Code): (207) 555 3322

ZIP CODE:  TELEPHONE (INCLUDE AREA CODE):

**9.** OTHER INSURED'S NAME (Last, First, Middle Initial):

**10.** IS PATIENT'S CONDITION RELATED TO:

**11.** INSURED'S POLICY GROUP OR FECA NUMBER: 67980ROC

**a.** OTHER INSURED'S POLICY OR GROUP NUMBER:

**a.** EMPLOYMENT? (CURRENT OR PREVIOUS) YES ☐ NO ☒

**a.** INSURED'S DATE OF BIRTH: MM 12 DD 22 YY CCYY-45  SEX M ☐ F ☒

**b.** OTHER INSURED'S DATE OF BIRTH: MM DD YY  SEX M ☐ F ☐

**b.** AUTO ACCIDENT? YES ☐ NO ☒  PLACE (State)

**b.** EMPLOYER'S NAME OR SCHOOL NAME: ROCKY CORPORATION

**c.** EMPLOYER'S NAME OR SCHOOL NAME:

**c.** OTHER ACCIDENT? YES ☒ NO ☐

**c.** INSURANCE PLAN NAME OR PROGRAM NAME: SUMMER INSURANCE COMPANY

**d.** INSURANCE PLAN NAME OR PROGRAM NAME:

**10d.** RESERVED FOR LOCAL USE

**d.** IS THERE ANOTHER HEALTH BENEFIT PLAN? YES ☐ NO ☒  if yes, return to and complete item 9 a-d

READ BACK OF FORM BEFORE COMPLETING & SIGNING THIS FORM

**12.** PATIENT'S OR AUTHORIZED PERSON'S SIGNATURE ... SIGNED SIGNATURE ON FILE  DATE

**13.** INSURED'S OR AUTHORIZED PERSON'S SIGNATURE ... SIGNED SIGNATURE ON FILE

**14.** DATE OF CURRENT: ILLNESS (1st symptom)/INJURY (Accident)/PREGNANCY (LMP): MM 01 DD 30 YY

**15.** IF PATIENT HAS HAD SAME OR SIMILAR ILLNESS, GIVE FIRST DATE MM DD YY

**16.** DATES PATIENT UNABLE TO WORK IN CURRENT OCCUPATION: FROM   TO

**17.** NAME OF REFERRING PHYSICIAN OR OTHER SOURCE:

**17a.** I.D. NUMBER OF REFERRING PHYSICIAN:

**18.** HOSPITALIZATION DATES RELATED TO CURRENT SERVICES: FROM   TO

**19.** RESERVED FOR LOCAL USE: PRIMARY CARE PHYSICIAN

**20.** OUTSIDE LAB? YES ☐ NO ☐  $ CHARGES

**21.** DIAGNOSIS OR NATURE OF ILLNESS OR INJURY:
1. 729 . 5
2.
3.
4.

**22.** MEDICAID RESUBMISSION CODE  ORIGINAL REF. NO.

**23.** PRIOR AUTHORIZATION NUMBER

| 24. A DATE(S) OF SERVICE From MM DD YY | To MM DD YY | B Place of Service | C Type of Service | D PROCEDURES, SERVICES, OR SUPPLIES CPT/HCPS | MODIFIER | E DIAGNOSIS CODE | F $ CHARGES | G DAYS OR UNITS | H EPSDT Family Plan | I EMG | J COB | K RESERVED FOR LOCAL USE |
|---|---|---|---|---|---|---|---|---|---|---|---|---|
| 02 04 YY | 02 04 YY | 11 | 1 | 99203 | | 1 | 175 00 | 1 | | Y | | |

**25.** FEDERAL TAX I.D. NUMBER: 70 2259772  SSN ☐ EIN ☒

**26.** PATIENT'S ACCOUNT NO.: MIKMD001  232

**27.** ACCEPT ASSIGNMENT? YES ☒ NO ☐

**28.** TOTAL CHARGE: $ 175 00

**29.** AMOUNT PAID: $

**30.** BALANCE DUE: $ 175 00

**31.** SIGNATURE OF PHYSICIAN OR SUPPLIER: SIGNED Sal Pull MD  DATE 02/14/YY

**32.** NAME AND ADDRESS OF FACILITY WHERE SERVICES WERE RENDERED:

**33.** PHYSICIAN'S, SUPPLIERS BILLING NAME, ADDRESS, ZIP CODE & PHONE #:
SAL PULL MD
3500 MARKET BLVD STE 233M
MOUNT ME 04022
(207) 555 0022
PIN# B12730  GRP#

(APPROVED BY AMA COUNCIL ON MEDICAL SERVICE 8/88)   PLEASE PRINT OR TYPE   FORM CMS-1500 (12-90) FORM OWCP-1500  FORM RRB-1500  FORM AMA-OP050591

**Exercise 10–6**

PLEASE
DO NOT
STAPLE
IN THIS
AREA

SUMMER INSURANCE CO
70065 SUNNY STREET
SANDY CITY CO 82936

APPROVED MOB-0938-0008

▫▫▫ PICA

# HEALTH INSURANCE CLAIM FORM

PICA ▫▫▫

| 1. | MEDICARE | MEDICAID | CHAMPUS | CHAMPVA | GROUP HEALTH PLAN | FECA BLK LUNG | OTHER | 1a. INSURED'S I.D NUMBER | (FOR PROGRAM IN ITEM 1) |
|---|---|---|---|---|---|---|---|---|---|

☐ (Medicare #)   ☐ (Medicaid #)   ☐ (Sponsor's SSN)   ☐ (VA File #)   ☒ (SSN or ID)   ☐ (SSN)   ☐ (ID)

222 22 ROC

| 2. PATIENT'S NAME (Last, First, Middle Initial). | 3. PATIENT'S BIRTH DATE | SEX | 4. INSURED'S NAME (Last, First, Middle Initial) |
|---|---|---|---|

MORPHINE MIKE M

MM 02  DD 12  YY CCYY-45   M ☒   F ☐

MORPHINE MINDY M

| 5. PATIENT'S ADDRESS (No., Street) | 6. PATIENT'S RELATIONSHIP TO INSURED | 7. INSURED'S ADDRESS (No., Street) |
|---|---|---|

522 MUSHROOM STREET

Self ☐   Spouse ☒   Child ☐   Other ☐

SAME

| CITY | STATE | 8. PATIENT STATUS | CITY | STATE |
|---|---|---|---|---|

MIGRAINE   ME

Single ☐   Married ☒   Other ☐

| ZIP CODE | TELEPHONE (Include Area Code) | | ZIP CODE | TELEPHONE (INCLUDE AREA CODE) |
|---|---|---|---|---|

04022   (207) 555 3322

Employed ☒   Full-Time Student ☐   Part-Time Student ☐

| 9. OTHER INSURED'S NAME (Last, First, Middle Initial) | 10. IS PATIENT'S CONDITION RELATED TO: | 11. INSURED'S POLICY GROUP OR FECA NUMBER: |
|---|---|---|

67980ROC

| a. OTHER INSURED'S POLICY OR GROUP NUMBER | a. EMPLOYMENT? (CURRENT OR PREVIOUS) | a. INSURED'S DATE OF BIRTH | SEX |
|---|---|---|---|

☐ YES   ☒ NO

MM 12   DD 22   YY CCYY-45   M ☐   F ☒

| b. OTHER INSURED'S DATE OF BIRTH | SEX | b. AUTO ACCIDENT?   PLACE (State) | b. EMPLOYER'S NAME OR SCHOOL NAME |
|---|---|---|---|

MM  DD  YY   M ☐   F ☐

☐ YES   ☒ NO |___

ROCKY CORPORATION

| c. EMPLOYER'S NAME OR SCHOOL NAME | c. OTHER ACCIDENT? | c. INSURANCE PLAN NAME OR PROGRAM NAME |
|---|---|---|

☒ YES   ☐ NO

SUMMER INSURANCE COMPANY

| d. INSURANCE PLAN NAME OR PROGRAM NAME | 10d. RESERVED FOR LOCAL USE | d. IS THERE ANOTHER HEALTH BENEFIT PLAN? |
|---|---|---|

☐ YES   ☒ NO   *if yes*, return to and complete item 9 a-d

READ BACK OF FORM BEFORE COMPLETING & SIGNING THIS FORM

12. PATIENT'S OR AUTHORIZED PERSON'S SIGNATURE I authorize the release of any medical or other information necessary to process this claim. I also request payment of government benefits either to myself or to the party who accepts assignment below.

13. INSURED'S OR AUTHORIZED PERSON'S SIGNATURE I authorize payment of medical benefits to the undersigned physician or supplier for services described below.

SIGNED SIGNATURE ON FILE          DATE _____

SIGNED SIGNATURE ON FILE

| 14. DATE OF CURRENT: | 15. IF PATIENT HAS HAD SAME OR SIMILAR ILLNESS, GIVE FIRST DATE | 16. DATES PATIENT UNABLE TO WORK IN CURRENT OCCUPATION |
|---|---|---|

◄ ILLNESS (1st symptom) ◄ INJURY (Accident) PREGNANCY (LMP)

MM 01  DD 30  YY YY

MM  DD  YY

FROM   MM DD YY   TO   MM DD YY

| 17. NAME OF REFERRING PHYSICIAN OR OTHER SOURCE | 17a. I.D. NUMBER OF REFERRING PHYSICIAN | 18. HOSPITALIZATION DATES RELATED TO CURRENT SERVICES |
|---|---|---|

SAL PULL MD

20 2259772

FROM   MM DD YY   TO   MM DD YY

| 19. RESERVED FOR LOCAL USE | 20. OUTSIDE LAB?   $ CHARGES |
|---|---|

REFERAL ON FILE

☐ YES   ☐ NO

21. DIAGNOSIS OR NATURE OF ILLNESS OR INJURY, (RELATE ITEMS 1,2,3, OR 4 TO ITEM 24E BY LINE)

22. MEDICAID RESUBMISSION CODE   ORIGINAL REF. NO.

1. |   729  .  5   

3. |       .    

23. PRIOR AUTHORIZATION NUMBER

2. |       .    

4. |       .    

| 24. A DATE(S) OF SERVICE | | | | | | B Place of Service | C Type of Service | D PROCEDURES, SERVICES, OR SUPPLIES (Explain Unusual Circumstances) CPT/HCPS   MODIFIER | E DIAGNOSIS CODE | F $ CHARGES | G DAYS OR UNITS | H EPSDT Family Plan | I EMG | J COB | K RESERVED FOR LOCAL USE |
|---|---|---|---|---|---|---|---|---|---|---|---|---|---|---|---|
| From MM | DD | YY | To MM | DD | YY | | | | | | | | | | |
| 02 | 04 | YY | 02 | 04 | YY | 11 | 1 | 73550 | 1 | 75 00 | 1 | | | | |
| 02 | 04 | YY | 02 | 04 | YY | 11 | 1 | 73718 | 1 | 1380 00 | 1 | | | | |
| | | | | | | | | | | | | | | | |
| | | | | | | | | | | | | | | | |
| | | | | | | | | | | | | | | | |
| | | | | | | | | | | | | | | | |

| 25. FEDERAL TAX I.D. NUMBER   SSN EIN | 26. PATIENT'S ACCOUNT NO. | 27. ACCEPT ASSIGNMENT? (For govt. claims, see back) | 28. TOTAL CHARGE | 29. AMOUNT PAID | 30. BALANCE DUE |
|---|---|---|---|---|---|

70 0059770   ☐ ☒

001 232

☒ YES   ☐ NO

$ 1455 00

$

$ 1455 00

31. SIGNATURE OF PHYSICIAN OR SUPPLIER INCLUDING DEGREES OR CREDENTIALS (I certify that the statements on the reverse apply to this bill and are made a part thereof.)

32. NAME AND ADDRESS OF FACILITY WHERE SERVICES WERE RENDERED (If other than home or office)

33. PHYSICIAN'S, SUPPLIERS BILLING NAME, ADDRESS, ZIP CODE & PHONE #

SALLY SAMPLE MD
8000 HALLS WAY
HUNTERSVILLE ME 04022
(207) 555 0242

SIGNED *Sally Sample MD* DATE 02/10/YY

PIN# C74185          GRP#

(APPROVED BY AMA COUNCIL ON MEDICAL SERVICE 8/88)          **PLEASE PRINT OR TYPE**

FORM CMS-1500   (12-90)
FORM OWCP-1500     FORM RRB-1500
FORM AMA-OP050591

# Exercise 10–7

PLEASE
DO NOT
STAPLE
IN THIS
AREA
□□□ PICA

SUMMER INSURANCE CO
70065 SUNNY STREET
SANDY CITY CO 82936

APPROVED MOB-0938-0008

# HEALTH INSURANCE CLAIM FORM

PICA □□□

| 1. MEDICARE | MEDICAID | CHAMPUS | CHAMPVA | GROUP HEALTH PLAN | FECA BLK LUNG | OTHER | 1a. INSURED'S I.D NUMBER (FOR PROGRAM IN ITEM 1) |
|---|---|---|---|---|---|---|---|
| ☐ (Medicare #) | ☐ (Medicaid #) | ☐ (Sponsor's SSN) | ☐ (VA File #) | ☒ (SSN or ID) | ☐ (SSN) | ☐ (ID) | 222 22 ROC |

| 2. PATIENT'S NAME (Last, First, Middle Initial). | 3. PATIENT'S BIRTH DATE | 4. INSURED'S NAME (Last, First, Middle Initial) |
|---|---|---|
| MORPHINE MIKE M | MM 02 DD 12 YY CCYY-45 SEX M ☒ F ☐ | MORPHINE MINDY M |

| 5. PATIENT'S ADDRESS (No., Street) | 6. PATIENT'S RELATIONSHIP TO INSURED | 7. INSURED'S ADDRESS (No., Street) |
|---|---|---|
| 522 MUSHROOM STREET | Self ☐ Spouse ☒ Child ☐ Other ☐ | SAME |

| CITY | STATE | 8. PATIENT STATUS | CITY | STATE |
|---|---|---|---|---|
| MIGRAINE | ME | Single ☐ Married ☒ Other ☐ | | |

| ZIP CODE | TELEPHONE (Include Area Code) | Employed ☒ Full-Time Student ☐ Part-Time Student ☐ | ZIP CODE | TELEPHONE (INCLUDE AREA CODE) |
|---|---|---|---|---|
| 04022 | (207) 555 3322 | | | |

| 9. OTHER INSURED'S NAME (Last, First, Middle Initial) | 10. IS PATIENT'S CONDITION RELATED TO: | 11. INSURED'S POLICY GROUP OR FECA NUMBER: |
|---|---|---|
| | | 67980 ROC |

| a. OTHER INSURED'S POLICY OR GROUP NUMBER | a. EMPLOYMENT? (CURRENT OR PREVIOUS) ☐ YES ☒ NO | a. INSURED'S DATE OF BIRTH MM 12 DD 22 YY CCYY-45 SEX M ☐ F ☒ |
|---|---|---|

| b. OTHER INSURED'S DATE OF BIRTH MM DD YY SEX M ☐ F ☐ | b. AUTO ACCIDENT? PLACE (State) ☐ YES ☒ NO | b. EMPLOYER'S NAME OR SCHOOL NAME ROCKY CORPORATION |
|---|---|---|

| c. EMPLOYER'S NAME OR SCHOOL NAME | c. OTHER ACCIDENT? ☒ YES ☐ NO | c. INSURANCE PLAN NAME OR PROGRAM NAME SUMMER INSURANCE COMPANY |
|---|---|---|

| d. INSURANCE PLAN NAME OR PROGRAM NAME | 10d. RESERVED FOR LOCAL USE | d. IS THERE ANOTHER HEALTH BENEFIT PLAN? ☐ YES ☒ NO if yes, return to and complete item 9 a-d |
|---|---|---|

READ BACK OF FORM BEFORE COMPLETING & SIGNING THIS FORM

12. PATIENT'S OR AUTHORIZED PERSON'S SIGNATURE I authorize the release of any medical or other information necessary to process this claim. I also request payment of government benefits either to myself or to the party who accepts assignment below.

SIGNED SIGNATURE ON FILE        DATE _____

13. INSURED'S OR AUTHORIZED PERSON'S SIGNATURE I authorize payment of medical benefits to the undersigned physician or supplier for services described below.

SIGNED SIGNATURE ON FILE

| 14. DATE OF CURRENT: ◄ ILLNESS (1st symptom) INJURY (Accident) PREGNANCY (LMP) MM 01 DD 30 YY | 15. IF PATIENT HAS HAD SAME OR SIMILAR ILLNESS, GIVE FIRST DATE MM DD YY | 16. DATES PATIENT UNABLE TO WORK IN CURRENT OCCUPATION MM DD YY MM DD YY FROM TO |
|---|---|---|

| 17. NAME OF REFERRING PHYSICIAN OR OTHER SOURCE SAL PULL MD | 17a. I.D. NUMBER OF REFERRING PHYSICIAN 20 2259772 | 18. HOSPITALIZATION DATES RELATED TO CURRENT SERVICES MM DD YY MM DD YY FROM TO |
|---|---|---|

| 19. RESERVED FOR LOCAL USE DME PRESCRIPTION ON FILE | 20. OUTSIDE LAB? ☐ YES ☐ NO $ CHARGES |
|---|---|

21. DIAGNOSIS OR NATURE OF ILLNESS OR INJURY, (RELATE ITEMS 1,2,3, OR 4 TO ITEM 24E BY LINE)

1. |_____ 729 . 5 _____|        3. |_____ . _____|

2. |_____ . _____|        4. |_____ . _____|

| 22. MEDICAID RESUBMISSION CODE | ORIGINAL REF. NO. |
|---|---|
| | |

23. PRIOR AUTHORIZATION NUMBER

| 24. A DATE(S) OF SERVICE | | | | | | B Place of Service | C Type of Service | D PROCEDURES, SERVICES, OR SUPPLIES (Explain Unusual Circumstances) | | E DIAGNOSIS CODE | F $ CHARGES | G DAYS OR UNITS | H EPSDT Family Plan | I EMG | J COB | K RESERVED FOR LOCAL USE |
|---|---|---|---|---|---|---|---|---|---|---|---|---|---|---|---|---|
| From MM | DD | YY | To MM | DD | YY | | | CPT/HCPS | MODIFIER | | | | | | | |
| 02 | 04 | YY | 02 | 04 | YY | 99 | 1 | E0114 | | 1 | 121 00 | 1 | | | | |
| | | | | | | | | | | | | | | | | |
| | | | | | | | | | | | | | | | | |
| | | | | | | | | | | | | | | | | |
| | | | | | | | | | | | | | | | | |
| | | | | | | | | | | | | | | | | |

| 25. FEDERAL TAX I.D. NUMBER SSN EIN 70-8859778 ☐ ☒ | 26. PATIENT'S ACCOUNT NO. 555551  232 | 27. ACCEPT ASSIGNMENT? (For govt. claims, see back) ☒ YES ☐ NO | 28. TOTAL CHARGE $ 121 00 | 29. AMOUNT PAID $ 0 00 | 30. BALANCE DUE $ 121 00 |
|---|---|---|---|---|---|

31. SIGNATURE OF PHYSICIAN OR SUPPLIER INCLUDING DEGREES OR CREDENTIALS (I certify that the statements on the reverse apply to this bill and are made a part thereof.)

SIGNED *Penny Pane*  DATE 02/18/YY

32. NAME AND ADDRESS OF FACILITY WHERE SERVICES WERE RENDERED (If other than home or office)

33. PHYSICIAN'S, SUPPLIERS BILLING NAME, ADDRESS, ZIP CODE & PHONE #

MARVELOUS MEDICAL EQUIPMENT
9 MONEY LANE
MOVE ME 04022
(207) 555 0409

PIN# D36912        GRP#

(APPROVED BY AMA COUNCIL ON MEDICAL SERVICE 8/88)        **PLEASE PRINT OR TYPE**        FORM CMS-1500 (12-90)
FORM OWCP-1500    FORM RRB-1500
FORM AMA-OP050591

**Exercise 10–8**

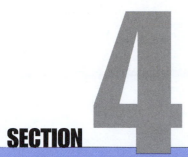

SECTION **4**

## DENTAL CLAIMS EXAMINING GUIDELINES AND PROCEDURES

# 11

# Dental Terminology,
## Anatomy, and Physiology of the Mouth

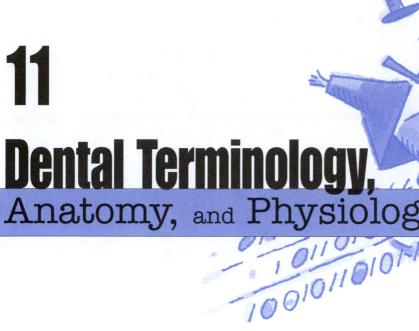

## After completion of this chapter
**you will be able to:**

- Interpret the meaning of common dental terms, including prefixes, suffixes, root words, and combined words.
- Define and explain the use of prefixes, suffixes, and root words.
- Identify and explain the structures of the oral cavity.
- Identify and explain the structures of the jaw.
- List and explain the common diseases of the mouth.
- Name the parts of the tooth and its supporting structures.

- Identify the teeth by types, numbers, and locations.
- Explain the difference between primary and permanent teeth.
- Divide and properly label the teeth into quadrants and sextants.
- Identify the surfaces of the teeth.
- Explain the growth and development of the teeth.
- List and explain the common diseases of the teeth.
- Properly classify dental caries.

## Keywords and concepts
**you will learn in this chapter:**

- Alveolar Process
- Ankyloglossia
- Apex
- Bruxism
- Buccal (B)
- Calculus
- Capillaries
- Cementum
- Cheilitis

- Cheiloschisis
- Cleft Palate
- Complex Cavities
- Compound Cavities
- Crown
- Cuspids (Canines)
- Deciduous Teeth (Primary Teeth)
- Dental Caries or Cavities
- Dental Plaque

- Dentalgia
- Dentin
- Distal (D)
- Edentulous
- Gingivitis
- Gum (Gingiva)
- Hard Palate
- Incisal (I)
- Incisors

- Labial (La, L)
- Lingual (Li)
- Mandible
- Maxilla
- Mesial (M)
- Molars (Tricuspids)
- Mouth
- Mucus
- Neck
- Occlusal (O)
- Occlusion

- Oral Cavity (Cavum Oris)
- Papillae
- Periodontitis
- Periodontosis
- Prefix
- Premolars (Bicuspids)
- Pulp
- Pulp Cavity
- Root
- Root Canal
- Root Word

- Saliva
- Salivary Amylase
- Sialodentitis
- Simple Cavities
- Soft Palate
- Stomatitis
- Suffix
- Taste Buds
- Temporomandibular Joint
- Tongue
- Vestibule

About 75% of all medical terms are derived from Latin and Greek prefixes, suffixes, and roots. A **prefix** is the portion of the word found at the beginning of a term that modifies the meaning of the root word (i.e., *endo*, meaning within, + dontics, meaning teeth = *endo*dontics, meaning within the teeth). Prefixes alter the root word by adding a number (bi- two), a direction, (ab- away from), a location (endo- within), or a description (dis- bad).

A **suffix** is the portion of a word found at the end of a term (i.e., gingi, meaning gum, + *itis*, meaning inflammation = gingiv*itis*, meaning inflammation of the gums). Suffixes also alter the root word, usually by indicating a state of being (-itis).

A **root word** is usually found in the center of a term and identifies the organ or body part involved.

In dental terminology, and less often in medical terminology, it is possible to combine a prefix and suffix to form a word, even though no root word is involved (as in gingivitis). **Table 11–1** presents a list of prefixes and suffixes used in dental terminology. Health claims examiners should become familiar with the prefixes and suffixes to help accurately process dental claims.

The following is a list of common dental terms and procedures. Health claims examiners should become familiar with these terms to help them accurately bill and process dental claims.

## Common Dental Terms and Procedures

**Abrasion**—Wearing away of the surfaces of the teeth as a result of their use in chewing.

**Abscess**—A collection of pus in a cavity formed within the tissue of the body.

**Absorption**—The process of sucking up, taking in, and assimilating certain substances, such as fluids and other matter, by the skin, mucus membranes, blood vessels, or lymphatics.

**Abutment**—A tooth used to support or stabilize one end of a prosthetic appliance, such as a dental bridge.

**Accretion**—An accumulation of foreign matter, such as tartar on the surface of a tooth or decayed matter within the cavity.

**Acid-etch**—In restorative dentistry, a method of etching the tooth enamel with an acid to provide an adhesion of composite filling material to the tooth's surface.

**Acrylic**—A synthetic thermoplastic substance resembling clear glass, but lighter in weight, which permits passage of ultraviolet rays and is used in making dental prostheses and temporary artificial eyes.

| Prefix/Suffix | Meaning | Prefix/Suffix | Meaning |
|---|---|---|---|
| ab- | away from, not | lith- | stone |
| -al | pertaining to | -lysis | loosening, set free, destruction |
| -algia | pain | macr-, macro- | large |
| alveol- | tooth socket | mal- | bad |
| an-, a | without, not | malign- | bad |
| ante- | in front of, before | mandibul- | lower jaw |
| antr- | cavity | maxillo- | upper jaw |
| apic, apex | tip of the root, top | menisci- | pad, disc |
| arthr- | joint | -ment | a way of |
| auto- | self | micr- | small |
| bi- | two | myel- | marrow, spinal cord |
| benign | mild, not cancerous | neo- | new |
| bucc- | cheek | occlud, occlus- | close |
| calc- | stone | odont- | tooth |
| -centesis | punctured | -odyn- | pain |
| cephal- | head | -ologist | a specialist in the study of |
| cervic- | neck | -ology | study of |
| cid- | falling | or- | mouth |
| condyle | knob on the end of a bone | os-, oss- | bone |
| cut- | skin | ost-, oste- | bone |
| de- | down from | -osis | any condition |
| dent- | teeth | -ostomy | create a new opening/passageway |
| -desis | binding, fixation | -otomy | cut into, incision |
| doch- | duct, tube | palat- | roof of mouth |
| dys- | bad | pan- | all |
| -ectomy | surgical removal | parotid | near the ear |
| en- | in | path- | disease |
| end- | inside, within | peri- | about, around |
| esthesia | sensation | -pexy | suspension, fixation |
| ex- | out, from | physio- | nature |
| fistul- | pipe, tube | -plasia | developing, development |
| fistule | pipe, tube | plast- | plastic repair |
| fren- | fold of skin | post- | behind, in back of |
| frenul- | fold of skin | pre- | in front of, before |
| gemin- | twin, double | pro- | in front of, before |
| gen- | originate, produce | pulp | juicy tissue |
| gingiv- | gum | quadr- | four |
| gloss- | tongue | radi- | ray |
| gnath- | jaw | radic- | root |
| grad- | step, stage | retro- | backward |
| gram- | record | sial- | saliva |
| hemi- | half | sinus | hollow space |
| hyper- | above, more than normal, excessive | stom-, stomat- | mouth, opening |
| hypo- | under, beneath, deficient | sub- | under, beneath, below |
| infra- | beneath, below | temporal | on side of skull |
| inter- | between | top- | place |
| intra- | within | trans- | through, across, beyond |
| -ist | one who practices | traum- | wound, injury |
| -itis | inflammation | tri- | three |
| labi- | lip | -trophy | development |
| later- | side | uni- | one |
| lig- | tie | vestibul- | entrance |
| lingu- | tongue | -vulse | twitch, pull |
| | | zygomatic/malar | cheekbone |

**Table 11–1** Dental Prefixes and Suffixes

**Acrylic Resins**—Plastic restorative materials used in making dentures and crowns and as filling material.

**ADA**—American Dental Association.

**Adaptic**—Type of filling (composite); recommended for class I, III, and V restorations.

**Adduct**—To move toward the center or midline.

**Adhesives**—In restorative dentistry, a compound used after the acid-etch to provide an adhesion between the composite and the tooth surface.

**Adjunctive Treatment**—Supplementary and additional therapeutic procedures.

**Adjustment**—An alteration or modification that may be required on a tooth or a denture (after it has been placed in the mouth). Occlusal adjustment is a form of modification.

**Align**—To position properly in relation to another object(s).

**Alloy**—The product of fusing two or more metals; a silver alloy combined with mercury to produce an amalgam for restoration of a destroyed tooth surface.

**Alveolalgia**—Pain in the alveolus or tooth socket following tooth extraction. It may involve osteitis or dry socket.

**Alveolar**—Pertaining to an alveolus.

**Alveolar Osteitis**—A painful condition caused by loss of the blood clot or from an infected socket. Also commonly referred to as "dry socket."

**Alveolectomy**—Shaping of the dental ridges by removal of prominences of bone and excess soft tissue, usually in preparation for construction of a prosthetic appliance.

**Alveolotomy**—Incision into a tooth socket.

**Alveolus**—Bone cavity or a socket in which the root of a tooth is held by the periodontal ligament.

**Alveoplasty**—Surgical excision or revision of the alveolar process to restore a normal contour. It may range from simple alveolectomy in conjunction with extractions to necessary reconstruction of the ridge in preparation for dentures.

**Amalgam**—An alloy of mercury with any other metal. The compound of a basal alloy of silver and tin with mercury, used for restoring teeth. Copper and zinc are usually added as modifying metals to the basal alloy.

**Amputation (Root)**—Excision of the root portion of a tooth. It is usually performed on a multirooted tooth to eliminate a root that cannot be treated.

**Analgesia**—Reduction or loss of sensitivity to pain without loss of consciousness.

**Anesthesia**—Loss of sensation.

**Block**—Anesthesia produced by injecting an anesthetic solution into the nerve trunks supplying the operative field, called *regional block*, or by infiltrating close to the nerves, called *infiltration block*, or by a wall of anesthetic solution injected about the field, called *field block*. In all these methods, the nerve conduction is blocked, and painful impulses fail to reach the brain.

**General**—Loss of sensation with loss of consciousness.

**Infiltration**—Anesthesia induced by the injection of the anesthetic solution directly into the tissues that are to be anesthetized.

**Local**—Anesthesia limited to the local area.

**Regional**—Local anesthesia.

**Anesthetics**—Drugs that produce loss of feeling or sensation either as local or general anesthesia.

**Angle's Classification**—A classification of the forms of malocclusion as established by Edward Hartley Angle, an American orthodontist.

**Class I**—The normal anteroposterior relationship of the lower jaw to the upper jaw. The mesiobuccal cusp of the maxillary first permanent molar occludes in the buccal groove of the mandibular first permanent molar.

**Class II**—The posterior relationship of the lower jaw to the upper jaw. The mesiobuccal cusp of the maxillary first permanent molar occludes mesial to the buccal of the mandibular first permanent molar.

**Class III**—The anterial relationship of the lower jaw to the upper jaw with possible subdivision. The mesiobuccal cusp of the maxillary first permanent molar occludes distal to the buccal groove of the mandibular first permanent molar.

**Ankyloglossia**—Partial or complete fusion of the tongue to the floor of the mouth.

**Ankylosis**—Fixation or true bony union between bones or a tooth to the jaw; abnormal immobility of a joint.

**Anodontia**—Failure of tooth formation; congenital absence of teeth.

**Antagonist**—A tooth in the upper jaw that articulates with a tooth of the lower jaw or vice versa.

**Anterior**—Situated in front; dentally, referring to the teeth at the front of the mouth (i.e., central incisors, lateral incisors, and first bicuspids).

**Anterior Posterior Dysplasia**—An abnormal fit of the maxilla and mandible to each other or to the cranial base.

**Anteversion**—The forward tipping or tilting of the teeth or other surfaces of the oral cavity.

**Antibiotic**—A drug that inhibits or destroys bacterial growth.

**Antiseptic**—A pharmaceutical substance that stops or inhibits the growth of microorganisms.

**Aperture**—An opening.

**Apex**—The terminal end of a cone; a conical end; the terminal end of a root or tooth.

**Apexification**—Removal of dental pulp and treatment of the apex with calcium hydroxide resulting in stimulation of growth of the cementum, which promotes apical closure. It is normally performed in a young patient whose apex is incompletely formed. Root canal therapy is usually performed for an older person.

**Apical**—Pertaining to the apex or conical endings of the roots of the teeth.

**Apical Foramen**—The opening at the end of a root of a tooth through which the tooth receives its nerve and blood supply.

**Apices**—Plural form of apex.

**Apicoectomy**—The excision or resection of the apex of a tooth root, usually following root canal therapy.

**Apicostomy**—A surgical opening through the mucoperiosteum and alveolar bone for access to the apex of a tooth root.

**Aplasis**—Lack of origin or development.

**Appliance**—In dentistry, a device used to replace missing parts, provide function, or perform a therapeutic purpose. Dental prostheses, splints, orthodontic appliances, and obturators are examples of appliances.

> **Craniofacial**—Used to replace and immobilize mandibular or midfacial fractures. Attachments may be external or internal, by means of wires, pins, bars, or headcaps. Holes may be drilled through the craniofacial bones to facilitate placing wires or other attachments.

> **Crozat**—A removable orthodontic appliance.

> **Fixed**—An appliance attached to the teeth by cement or adhesive materials.

> **Fracture**—Device for reduction or fixation of fractures. Pins, screws, and other types of fixation are used in replacing or realigning fractured parts.

> **Hawley**—A removable appliance usually made to fit in the palate against the lingual surfaces of the teeth and used as a retainer after the teeth have been aligned. There are numerous forms and uses.

**Arch, Dental**—The curving structure formed by the crowns of the teeth in their normal position, or by the residual ridge after loss of teeth. The inferior dental arch, or arch of the mandible, is formed by the lower teeth, and the superior dental arch, arch of the maxilla, is formed by the upper teeth.

**Arch Retainer**—An appliance to prevent collapse of the dental arch.

**Arch Wire**—In orthodontics, the main wire framework, which is attached to bands and passes around the entire dental arch, on the lingual surface or facial surface or both, and which serves as the frame of attachment for finger springs.

**Artificial Teeth**—A denture or bridgework composed of two materials – porcelain or plastic. The former is hard, baked vitreous material with specific properties. The latter is less hard, more resilient material with different characteristics and indicated uses.

**Attrition**—The normal or abnormal loss of tooth structure.

**Autogenous Bone Graft**—A bone graft obtained from another part of the same person's body to induce new bone formation in a defect.

**Axis**—A real or imaginary line passing through a body or part, such as the vertical axis of a tooth.

**Backing**—A piece of metal, usually gold, that backs up an artificial bridge or tooth and to which the tooth is soldered or otherwise attached.

**Band**—In orthodontics, a metallic attachment that surrounds and is cemented to the tooth, used to anchor archwires to the teeth.

**Bar**—A connector of two or more parts. It may be used for removable partial dentures, fixed prostheses to provide additional strength, and splinting in treatment of fractures of the teeth and jaws.

**Basal Bone**—The bone-like tissue of the mandible and maxilla other than the alveolar process.

**Base**—A protective material, such as cement, placed over the pulpal area of the tooth (pulp not exposed) to reduce irritation and thermal shock of the pulp. In dentures, the part of a denture that replaces the normal contours of the soft tissues and supports the artificial teeth.

**Baseplate**—A temporary form to represent the base of a denture that is used for making maxillomandibular relation records and for arranging the teeth.

**Bell-crowned**—Pertaining or referring to a tooth crown that is largest at the occlusal surface and tapers to the gum, usually used on incisors and bicuspids.

**Bicuspid**—Having two cusps, as in bicuspid teeth, a premolar.

**Bifurcate**—Fork; divided into two branches; having two roots.

**Bifurcation**—Anatomic area where roots divide into a two-rooted tooth.

**Bilateral**—Having two sides. Any partial denture having a major connector is said to be bilateral, i.e., one on each side.

**Bite, Closed**—A condition in which the upper teeth close too far over the lower, which usually bite into the roof of the mouth.

**Bite Guard**—An appliance that covers the occlusal and incisal surfaces of the teeth. It is used to stabilize the teeth or to provide a flat surface for unobstructive movement of the mandible.

**Bite, Open**—A condition in which the upper and lower incisors do not occlude.

**Bite Plane**—An appliance that covers the palate and is designed to provide resistance to the mandibular incisors where there is contact.

**Bite Raising**—The process of increasing the distance between the occlusal surfaces of the teeth. It may be accomplished by placing appliances or gold inlays or crowns.

**Bitewing Radiograph**—An x-ray showing the crowns of the upper and lower teeth and a portion of the roots and supporting bone.

**Bleaching**—A technique that restores a discolored tooth to its natural color.

**Bone, Alveolar**—A portion of the alveolar process that surrounds the roots of the teeth; a thin plate of bone to which the periodontal ligament is attached. It is pierced by many small openings that transmit blood, lymph vessels, and nerves to the periodontal ligament.

**Bracing**—Resistance to displacement in a lateral direction.

**Bracket**—In orthodontics, an attachment that is either welded or soldered to a band (except a molar band), which secures arch wires to bands.

**Bridge**—A partial denture; bridgework.

   **Fixed**—A bridge that is permanently attached to its abutments.

   **Removable**—A denture that may be removed by the wearer.

   **Removable Fixed**—A bridge that may be removed by the dentist (not by the patient) without mutilation of any of its parts.

**Bridgework**—An appliance made of artificial crowns of teeth to replace missing natural teeth.

**Broken Stress Bridge**—A fixed bridge that includes a rigid connector at one end and a non-rigid connector, or stress breaker, at the other end.

**Bruxism**—The unconscious habit of grinding the teeth, often limited to during sleeping or mental or physical concentration or strain.

**Buccal**—Pertaining to the cheek. The buccal surface of a tooth is a surface next to the cheek.

**Buccal Frenum**—The string-like tissue that attaches the cheeks to the alveolar ridge in the bicuspid region.

**Buccolingual**—Pertaining to the cheek and the tongue.

**Butterfly**—A removable acrylic partial denture for the temporary replacement of front teeth; sometimes referred to as a flipper, provisional partial, or temporary bridge.

**Calcification**—The act of depositing calcific matter or calcium salts during growth. Bones and teeth become calcified.

**Calculus**—A hard calcareous concentration deposited on the surface of the crown or root of a tooth; tartar.

   **Salivary**—Calcareous deposits in the duct of a salivary gland or on the surface of the teeth, which originate from the salivary secretion.

   **Serumal**—Calcareous deposits formed about the teeth by exudation from diseased gums.

**Canine**—The teeth corresponding to the long teeth of a dog, usually referred to as cuspids.

**Cantilever**—A dental prostheses that has one or more abutments at one end while the other end is unsupported.

**Cap**—A substance or structure designed to cover the exposed pulp of the tooth.

**Capping**—The operation of placing a covering over the exposed pulp of a tooth.

> **Direct Pulp**—A capping that provides a direct contact between the material used and the pulp.
>
> **Indirect Pulp**—A capping that applies material to vital or diseased dentin.

**Care**—The total of diagnostic and preventive treatment and restorative services rendered by a licensed dentist.

> **Adequate**—May denote repair of oral damage and the placing of the mouth in a condition to prevent deterioration. It frequently refers to the substitution of a less costly but satisfactory type of service.
>
> **Comprehensive**—All dental services indicated for the restoration and maintenance of oral health.
>
> **Emergency**—Any dental services for unexpected and urgent conditions, such as toothache, acute infection, hemorrhage, accidental injury to teeth and supporting structures, and broken dentures.
>
> **Initial**—Services required for dental needs existing at the time of enrollment in a planned dental program; frequently called mouth rehabilitation.
>
> **Maintenance**—Service required to maintain oral health.
>
> **Minimum**—Generally, oral treatment of acute conditions of teeth and gums.

**Caries**—A molecular depth of bone or teeth, corresponding to ulceration in the soft tissue.

> **Of the Teeth**—A localized, progressive molecular disintegration of the teeth.
>
> **Inter-proximal**—Caries of the surfaces of the teeth in contact with each other.

**Cariogenic**—Conducive to caries.

**Cast**—The positive reproduction of the mouth or teeth in plaster or similar material, upon which a prosthetic appliance is constructed.

**Cavity Classifications**

> **Class I**—Cavities beginning in structural defects such as pits and fissures.
>
> **Class II**—Cavities in proximal surfaces of bicuspids and molars.
>
> **Class III**—Cavities in proximal surfaces of cuspids and incisors that do not involve the incisal edge.
>
> **Class IV**—Cavities in proximal surfaces of cuspids and incisors involving the incisal angle.
>
> **Class V**—Cavities of the gingival third of the labial, buccal, or lingual surfaces of the teeth.
>
> **Class VI**—Cavities on the incisal edges and cusp tips of the teeth.

**Cavity Liner**—A substance that is placed on the walls of the cavity before insertion of a restoration.

**Cement**—In dentistry, an adhesive filling material used for cementing bridges, crowns, and inlays. It may be used as a temporary filling material.

> **Copper Phosphate**—Zinc phosphate cement to which copper oxide has been added; thought to impart germicidal qualities to the cement created.
>
> **Zinc Oxide Eugenol**—A sedative cement used as a temporary filling or a base under restorations, where sedative treatment of the tooth is indicated.

**Cementoenamel Junction**—The portion of the tooth at which the cementum and the enamel join.

**Cementosis**—See hypercementosis.

**Cementum**—The hard calcified tissue that covers the anatomic root of a tooth. It is formed by cementoblast and arranged in layers that cover the root dentin.

**Central Ray**—The x-ray located in the center of the bundle of x-rays that make up the useful beam.

**Cephalometrics**—A scientific study of the measurements of the head.

**Ceramco**—Trade name for a combination of porcelain with metal used in restorations of fixed prosthetics.

**Cervical**—Pertaining to the neck or cervix of the tooth.

**Cervical Anchorage**—In orthodontics, a strap of elastic tape with wire hooks that fits around the back of the patient's neck and is used as a force from outside of the mouth to move teeth distally.

**Cervical Line**—The neck of the tooth; the cementoenamel junction.

**Cervicogingival**—The space between the gingiva and the enamel of the tooth crowns; the space between the gingiva and the cementum in cases in which the gingiva has receded.

**Chamber**—An enclosed area.

    **Pulp**—Pulp cavity or space in the coronal position of the tooth containing the pulp.

**Cleft Lip**—A congenital cleft or defect in the upper lip, usually due to failure of the median nasal and maxillary process to unite.

**Cleft Palate**—A congenital defect due to failure of fusion of embryonic facial process, resulting in a fissure through the palate. It may be complete, extending through both hard and soft palates into the nose, or it may be any degree of incomplete or partial cleft.

**Cohesive**—Uniting together or characterized by cohesion. In dentistry, a property of annealed gold (foil or crystal) that causes separate particles to stick to one another as they are welded when placed in contact with each other by a heavy hand or mallet pressure.

**Coil Spring**—A small wire spring wrapped around the main arch wire in an orthodontic appliance which is used as a force to pull teeth together or to push them apart.

**Cold Cure**—Usually relates to denture relining not requiring laboratory service.

**Collar**—A small part of the root of a denture tooth.

**Complete Denture**—One that replaces all teeth in an arch.

**Composite**—A plastic restorative material that blends resin and quartz crystal with a catalyst.

**Compressive Strength**—The greatest compressive force that can be applied to material before it ruptures.

**Concrescence**—The union of two teeth, after eruption, by fusion of the cementum surfaces.

**Concretion**—In dentistry, a deposit on the surface of a tooth. Also a calculus.

**Condensation**—In dentistry, the packing of a restorative material into the prepared cavity of a tooth.

**Condyle**—The rounded, knuckle-shaped process of the mandible which forms a joint at the temporal bone.

**Condylectomy**—Surgical removal of the condyle.

**Contact Point**—The surface of a tooth that touches the surface of an adjacent tooth.

**Coping**—A thin metal covering over a prepared tooth which is used as a base for the construction of a crown.

**Coronal**—Pertaining to the crown of a tooth.

**Coronoid**—Shaped like the beak of a crown, as the coronoid process of the mandible.

**Coronoid Process**—The more anterior process on the superior border of the ramus.

**Correction of Occlusion**—The correction of malocclusion by elimination of disharmony of occlusal contacts. It may be performed by means of many different methods, depending on the degree or severity, from selective spot grinding to gnathologic evaluation with subsequent treatment to correct any disharmonies.

**Crest Ridge**—The projecting ridge of the alveolar process that surrounds the teeth.

**Cross-Bite**—Bite in which the jaws may be in normal relationship when closed, but the buccal cusp of the upper molars bite into the buccal cusp of the lower molars.

**Crown**—Top part of anything; any structure like a crown.

    **Anatomic**—Portion of a tooth covered by enamel.

    **Artificial**—A cap of metal, plastic, or porcelain process to cover the portion of the tooth that projects beyond the gum line.

    **Clinical**—The portion of the tooth exposed beyond the crest of the gingiva.

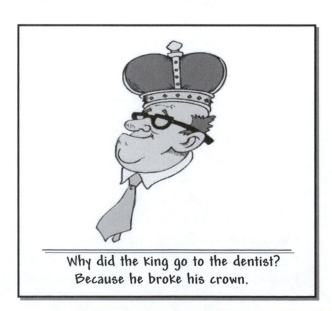

Why did the king go to the dentist?
Because he broke his crown.

**Complete**—The crown that covers the entire clinical crown.

**Dowel**—A complete crown that replaces the entire coronal portion of the natural tooth which is retained by a post extending into the root canal.

**Faced**—A metal crown with a tooth-colored material on the labial or buccal surface.

**Full Veneer**—A dental restoration that covers a tooth in its entirety.

**Jacket**—A term generally used to indicate complete veneer crowns that are made entirely of porcelain or acrylic resin.

**Of a Tooth**—The part covered with enamel.

**Shell**—A metal clasp designed to fit a prepared tooth. It is usually performed and reproduces the natural crown.

**Three-quarter**—A dental restoration that covers all of the exposed tooth except the labial or buccal surface.

**Crozat Appliance**—A removable orthodontic appliance.

**Curettage**—Scraping or removal of diseased tissue with a curette.

**Apical**—Curettement of diseased tissue in the periapical area on the apical portion of the tooth without removal of the root tip.

**Gingival**—Removal of gingival tissue.

**Infrabony Pocket**—The removal of a soft tissue inflammation located within and around an infrabony defect; debridement and cleaning of the root surface of the pocket.

**Root**—Removal of accretions on the root's surface, providing a more suitable environment for development of healthy tissues.

**Subgingival**—Debridement of the entire pocket and epithelial subjacent connective tissues, performed to eliminate the inflammatory process.

**Cusp**—An elevation or point on the surface of a tooth, especially on the occlusal surface.

**Cuspid**—A cuspid or canine tooth with one point or cusp.

**Cyst**—Sac containing fluid.

**DDS**—Doctor of Dental Surgery.

**Debridement**—Removal of diseased or devitalized tissues or foreign materials.

**Debris**—Soft-formed material loosely attached to the surface of a tooth.

**Decalcification**—Withdrawal or acid removal of mineral salts of bone or other calcified substance.

**Decay**—Decomposed structures; caries or other carious lesions of the teeth.

**Deciduous**—Term used to identify primary teeth.

**Def Rate**—Similar to the DMF rate but used for primary dentition (baby teeth). Although lower case letters are used, the symbol (d) standing for decayed primary teeth indicated for filling, and the symbol (f) for filled primary teeth, have the same meaning as DMF. The symbol (e) stands for decayed teeth indicated for extraction. Missing teeth are not counted for this rate.

**Dens in Dente**—A developmental anomaly of a tooth, usually involving the upper lateral incisors. The tooth enamel has the appearance of a tooth within a tooth.

**Dental**—Pertaining to the teeth.

**Dental Floss**—Fine string pulled between the teeth to aid in cleaning the space between the teeth.

**Dental Hygienist**—A person licensed to clean and polish teeth and to instruct in the fundamentals of oral hygiene.

**Dental Laboratory Technician**—A person trained to prepare dental appliances and restorations for placement in the mouth.

**Dental Pulp**—The soft tissue that fills the pulp chamber and the root canals of a tooth and is responsible for its vitality. It consists of connective tissue, blood vessels, and nerves.

**Dental Senescence**—Deterioration of the teeth and associated structures due to the aging process.

**Dentate**—Having teeth.

**Dentifrice**—A substance, as a paste or a powder, used in the cleaning of the teeth.

**Dentin**—The calcified tissue that forms the major part of the tooth. Dentin is related to the bone but differs from it in the absence of included cells.

**Dentinogenesis Imperfecta**—Hereditary disturbance that affects the development of dentin.

**Dentistry**—The profession that is concerned with the prevention, diagnosis, and treatment of diseases of the teeth and adjacent tissues, and the restoration of missing dental and oral structures.

**Operative**—The branch of dentistry concerned with preserving the natural teeth and their supporting structures, and with restoring the teeth.

**Preventive**—The branch of dentistry dealing with prevention of dental diseases by prophylactic and educational methods.

**Prosthetic**—The phase or branch of dentistry that deals with the replacement of missing teeth or oral tissues by artificial means; also called prosthodontics.

**Dentition**—The process of teething; the eruption of teeth in the alveolar ridge; the character and arrangement of the teeth.

**Deciduous**—The 20 teeth which erupt first and are later replaced by the permanent teeth.

**Mixed**—The compliment of teeth in the jaw after eruption of some of the permanent teeth, before all the deciduous teeth are shed.

**Permanent**—The 32 teeth that erupt after the deciduous teeth are lost.

**Dentulous**—Having teeth, as opposed to edentulous, not having teeth.

**Denture**—The natural or artificial teeth of a person considered as a unit.

**Arm**—The portion of the clasp that extends from the body of the clasp out to the end of the clasp.

**Artificial**—The complete artificial replacement of either the upper or lower teeth.

**Butt**—Denture with almost no flange, designed because of full lips, leaving no room for additional thickness of the denture flange.

**Clasp**—The metal part of a partial denture.

**Duplicate**—Usually refers to a second denture that is a copy of the existing denture.

**Duplication**—Usually refers to a jump case or rebasing of the denture; also known as duplicating or re-material. Rebasing is the replacement of the base of the denture because of deterioration or tissue changes. Duplication can be misleading because occasionally the term is used to mean a spare set. Because of its many uses, it is advisable to ask for an explanation of the service.

**Full**—Replacement of the complete dental equipment of either jaw.

**Immediate Full**—Denture constructed to permit some natural teeth to remain in the mouth during its fabrication. When the remaining teeth are removed, the denture is inserted. Hence, the patient is never without teeth of some kind.

**Implant**—A substructure usually made of cast metal which is implanted over the alveolar ridge and under the soft tissues. Posts extend through the gingival tissues to support a denture. There may also be extensions into the bone for support.

**Overlay**—Complete denture that fits over one or more retained natural teeth. Ideally, it provides a more comfortable fit and retention because of the attachment to the teeth. It is used in both the upper and lower jaws but is more frequently placed in the mandible. The preparation consists of performing root canal therapy on the remaining teeth and placing a small gold cap or crown. An alternate method is to perform root canal therapy and then cut the tooth off at the level of the alveolar ridge. Attachments are then inserted into the root canal and used to provide support to a denture.

**Relief**—A recess in a denture to reduce or eliminate pressure from the corresponding area of the mouth.

**Remote**—Denture placed following the healing of an extraction site; may also be the replacement of an existing denture.

**Diagnostic Services**—Procedures such as x-rays, clinical examinations, biopsies, blood tests, study models, and other vitality tests, which assist the dentist in determining the conditions present and the treatment required.

**Die**—An exact reproduction in metal of any object or cast.

**Inlay**—An exact reproduction of a prepared tooth in high-strength dental stone or metal.

**Distal**—Away from the median line of the face following the curve of the dental arch. The surfaces of the teeth most distant from the median line are called *distal surfaces.*

**DMD**—*Dentariae Medicinae Doctor* (Doctor of Dental Medicine).

**DMF Rate**—For an individual, the number of permanent teeth (or for a group, the average number) that are (d) decayed, (m) missing, or indicated for extractions, and (f) filled. A tooth both filled and decayed is counted only as decayed. The DMF rate is a measure of accumulative effects of caries and a useful means for comparing the lifetime of caries experience of a group of comparable age.

**Dolder Bar**—Bar used to connect crowns for stabilization and reduce stress in anterior fixed prosthetics. The bar is attached to the abutments.

**Double Lingual Bar**—A type of lower partial denture that includes a secondary or auxiliary bar in addition to the lingual bar.

**Dowel Post and Pins**—Cast metal or manufactured strengthening device placed in a tooth to provide retention for a crown.

**Duct**—A passage with well-defined walls.

**E Clasp**—A bar-type clasp that is shaped like the letter "E."

**Edentulous**—Without teeth.

**Elongation**—Abnormal elongation of a tooth on a dental x-ray film by improper positioning of the x-ray machine in relation to the x-ray film in the patient's oral cavity.

**Embrasure**—Space between the sloping proximal surfaces of the teeth. The opening may be toward the cheek (buccal), the lips (labial), or the tongue (lingual).

**Enamel**—The vitreous covering tissue of the crowns of the teeth, consisting of enamel rods or prisms and a cementing interrod substance.

> **Mottled**—A defect in the enamel structure of the teeth manifesting as chalky white, yellow-brown, or black discolorations. The enamel may be pitted. The affected areas may vary in size and degree, depending on the severity of the causative factor.

> **Rods**—The calcified column or prism, with an average diameter of 4 mm, extends in a wavy pattern through the entire thickness of the enamel and is generally perpendicular to the surface of the tooth.

**Encirclement**—A clasp that extends more than halfway around a tooth to provide a secure attachment.

**Endodontics**—The branch of dentistry that deals with the diagnosis and treatment of diseases of the dental pulp and periapical tissues.

**Endopost**—A cast post designed to fit into the treated root canal of a tooth to provide strength and stability.

**Epithelium**—Membrane that covers a surface or lines the cavity; the layer of cells forming the epidermis of the skin.

> **Enamel**—Ameloblasts that form the dental enamel of the developing tooth.

> **Gingival**—Epithelial covering of the gingival tissue.

> **Pocket**—Cellular structure that lines the gingival or periodontal pockets.

> **Sulcular**—Stratifying squamous epithelium covering the soft tissue walls of the gingival crevice.

**Epulis**—Solitary tumor-like lesion developing from the periosteum of the maxilla or mandible, appearing clinically as a circumscribed swelling beneath the gum.

**Equilibration**—Maintenance of the balance as a pressure.

> **Occlusal**—Modification of the occlusal form by grinding for equalizing occlusal stress, producing simultaneous occlusion contact or harmonizing cuspal relations.

**Equilibrium**—Perfect balance. The condition made possible by complete synchronization and harmony among all vital factors.

**Erosion**—Wearing away or loss of tooth structure by chemical process without known bacterial action, usually beginning in the enamel at the neck of the tooth.

**Eruption**—The act of breaking up, appearing, or becoming visible; the appearance of a tooth through the gums.

**Esthetics**—Harmony of form, color, and arrangement.

**Etch and Polish**—Removal of portions of enamel, usually performed on primary teeth followed by polishing of the tooth areas.

**Ethical**—Pertaining to standards of right and wrong.

**Ethics**—A system of moral principles and ideas of human behavior.

> **Dental**—The principles of professional conduct; duties a dentist owes to self, colleagues, patients, and fellow man.

**Exfoliation**—A peeling and shedding of a horny layer of skin or tooth.

> **Normal Time**—The time at which a primary tooth is expected to become loose and fall out of a child's mouth.

**Exodontia, Exodontics**—The art and science of extraction of teeth.

**Exostoses**—Bony outgrowths from the surface of a bone.

**Extension of Prevention, Dental**—Extending the margins of a cavity preparation to remove incipient carious lesions to areas of the tooth that are either self-cleansing or readily cleansed. Such extensions are to prevent the recurrence of caries at the edges of the restorations.

**Extracoronal**—The external coronal portion of a natural tooth.

**Extraction**—Removal of a tooth from the oral cavity.

> **Serial**—Extraction of selected teeth over a period of time.
>
> **Simple**—Uncomplicated removal of a tooth.
>
> **Surgical**—Removal by means of surgical methods, usually involving the turning of a flap or removal of bone.

**Extraoral**—Outside the mouth.

**Extrude**—To force a tooth out of its normal occlusal position, possibly due to the absence of opposing teeth.

**Extrusion**—Eruption of a tooth from its socket; movement of the tooth out of the natural occlusal plane.

**Eyetooth**—A canine tooth of the upper jaw; bicuspid.

**Facial**—Pertaining to the face; the surface of the tooth or appliance nearest to the lips or cheeks; used synonymously with the words *buccal* and *labial.*

**Facing**—A manufactured porcelain piece that simulates a natural tooth.

**Festoon**—Carvings in the base material of an artificial denture, simulating contours of the natural tissues being replaced by the denture.

**Fibroblast**—Connective tissue cells found in fibrous tissue, fundamental to all healing processes.

**Filling**—Material used in closing cavities in carious teeth; the process of inserting, condensing, shaping, and finishing a filling.

**Finger Spring**—A small wire attachment soldered to the main arch wire that acts as a spring force to move teeth into an orthodontic appliance.

**Fissure**—A groove or cleft; a fault in the enamel of a tooth caused by imperfect union.

**Flange**—The part of the denture or saddle that extends on the facial or lingual side from the ridge-crest to the periphery.

**Flap**—Mass of tissue partly detached by a knife or blunt instrument in dentistry; the raising of the gingival mucosa from the alveolar bone to access an underlying area. Sometimes a flap procedure is used to remove a broken or retained

root. It is frequently required as a result of periodontal disease.

**FLC**—Full line or finished crown.

**Flipper**—A provisional partial or temporary bridge.

**Fluoridation**—The addition of fluoride to the water supply of a community as an aid to the control of dental caries.

**Fluoride**—A salt of hydrofluoric acid.

**Fluoride, Topical**—The direct application of a solution of fluoride (usually 2% sodium fluoride) to the crowns of the teeth for preventing dental caries; usually carried out at the ages of three, seven, 10, and 13.

**Foramen**—A natural opening in a bone or other structure.

> **Apical**—An opening at or near the apex of the root of a tooth, giving passage to the blood vessels and nerve supply in the pulp.
>
> **Mandibular**—The opening on the medial aspect of the vertical ramus of the lower jaw approximately midway between the mandibular and gonial notches; may be located posterior to the middle of the ramus. It contains inferior alveolar vessels and inferior alveolar nerves.

**Foreshortening**—Term used in dental radiology denoting the abnormal shortening of a tooth or teeth on a dental x-ray film.

**Formocreosol**—A solution used in root canal therapy and in treatment of dental pulp.

**Fossa**—A pit, hollow, or depression.

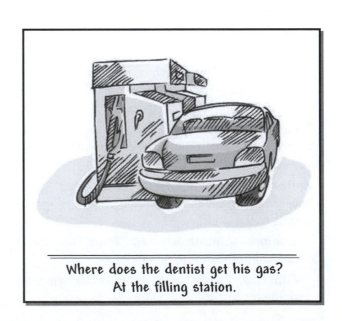

Where does the dentist get his gas?
At the filling station.

**Dental**—A round or angular depression in the surface of a tooth, occurring mostly in the occlusal surfaces of the molar and the lingual surfaces of the incisors.

**Frenectomy**—Excision of the mucous membrane attaching the cheeks and lips to the mucosa of the jawbone; excision of the lingual frenum attaching the tongue to the floor of the mouth and alveolar ridge.

**Frenotomy**—Division of any frenum, especially for tongue-tie.

**Frenum**—A fold of integument or mucous membrane that checks or limits the movements of any organ.

> **Labial**—The fold or tissue that connects the lip with the gingiva at a point normally in the midline.

> **Lingual**—The fold of tissue that connects the tongue to the gingiva and the floor of the mouth in the midline.

**Full Mouth X-ray**—X-ray of the mouth equaling 16 bitewings.

**Furcation**—The tooth area where roots branch out. Bifurcation relates to two roots. Trifurcation relates to three roots.

**Germination**—The division of a single tooth germ or bud that produces double or twin crowns on a single tooth.

**Gerodontics**—Practice of dentistry pertaining to aged patients.

**Gigantism**—Macrosomia; excessive growth.

**Gingiva**—The part of the gum that surrounds the tooth and lies close to the crest of the alveolar ridge.

> **Free**—The part of the gingiva about the neck of a tooth that is not closely opposed or attached to the tooth's surfaces.

**Gingival**—Of or pertaining to the soft tissues of the gum and the tooth.

> **Crevice**—The narrow opening between the circumferential soft tissue of the gum and the tooth.

> **Cuff**—The most coronal portion of the gingival tissue immediately surrounding the tooth to where it attaches to the tooth.

> **Curettage**—Debridement of a diseased gingival attachment to eliminate edema, inflammation, and pocket formations.

> **Margin**—The most coronal portion of the gingiva surrounding the tooth.

> **Morphology**—The form, shape, or profile of gingival tissues.

> **Papillae**—Extensions or projections of gum tissue between the teeth.

> **Stimulation**—Application of frictional activity to the gingival tissue to stimulate circulation and increase keratinization of the surface epithelium.

> **Sulcus**—A crevice, group, or pocket in the gingiva; a trough formed by the attachment of the gingiva to the surface of the tooth.

**Gingivectomy**—The surgical excision from supported gingival tissue to the level where it is attached, creating a new gingival margin, apical and posterior to the old.

**Gingivitis**—Inflammation of the gingival tissue; may be caused by pressure or contact of dentures, metallic poisoning, faulty restorations, dietary deficiency, herpes virus, hormonal imbalances, malopposed teeth, bacterial invasion, organic malfunction, or pregnancy.

> **Desquamative**—Inflammation of the gingiva but not a pathologic entity; may be associated with a biologic stress.

> **Hemorrhagic**—Characterized by bleeding and particularly associated with ascorbic acid deficiency.

> **Herpetic**—Inflammation due to the presence of herpes virus.

> **Hormonal**—Associated with an endocrine imbalance.

> **Necrotizing Ulcerative**—Inflammation with narcosis of the intradental papilla, ulceration of the gingival margins, pain, and offensive odor; an acute gingivitis that is sometimes chronic.

> **Pregnancy**—Gingival enlargement due to hormonal imbalance during pregnancy.

**Gingivoplasty**—The procedure by which gingival deformities are reshaped and reduced to create a normal and functional form; surgical contouring of the gingival tissues.

**Gingivosis**—A degenerative condition of the gingiva and connective tissue of uncertain origin. It is a noninflammatory disease with many phases: edema of the interdental papilla progressing to the marginal and attached gingiva, profuse bleeding progressing to necrosis, recession, and resorption.

**Gingivostomatitis**—A form of oral inflammatory disease that involves both the gingiva and portions of the remaining oral mucosa. Herpetic gingivostomatitis is caused by invasion of the herpes virus, which usually occurs in children.

**Glossitis**—Inflammation of the tongue.

**Gnathology**—The science of the masticatory system, including physiology, functional disturbances, and treatment.

**Gold**—A noble metal used extensively in dentistry, considered superior because of its malleability; may be used in the pure or alloyed state.

**Gold Foil**—Pure gold rolled into a thin sheet compacted into a cavity. The restoration is built to harmonize with the existing tooth. It is a direct gold filling in contrast to an inlay in which an impression is made and an exact form is made and cemented in. The three types are:

> **Gold Dent**—A combination of matte gold and cohesive made into globules.

> **Matte**—Not developed by chemical prescription; a noncohesive form that may be used in combination with cohesive gold.

> **Sheet**—Original type, which was 24-karat gold, rolled into thin sheets and then cut; this is a disappearing art.

**Granuloma**—A small mass of granulated tissue containing bacterial deposits, found on the root of a tooth or in the area of the jaw after the removal of a tooth.

**Groove**—An elongated depression; the portion of a cast that corresponds to the periphery of the impression.

**Gum**—The mucous membrane and underlying connective tissue covering the alveolar processes and necks of erupted teeth.

**Guttering**—Shaping bone to remove dead tissues as a result of osteomyelitis.

**Halitosis**—Bad breath due to poor oral hygiene, periodontal disease, sinusitis, tonsillitis, or bronchopulmonary disease.

**Hard Palate**—Approximately two-thirds of the anterior section of the palate composed of relatively hard and unyielding tissue.

**Hay Rake**—A device used with children, which is fixed temporarily to the upper teeth to break undesirable habits such as thumb or lip sucking.

**Heel-Denture**—The posterior extremities of a denture. It corresponds with the retromolar pad area of a lower denture and the tuberosity area of an upper denture.

**Hemisection**—Surgical dividing of a tooth to make it easier to remove the ensuing fragments or allow salvage of one part of the tooth that is relatively free of disease. Root canal therapy may be necessary on other roots of the tooth before hemisection is performed.

**Herpes**—A blister-like elevation appearing in clusters on the skin; an inflammatory skin disease.

> **Labial (Cold Sore)**—Herpes simplex occurring on the lips caused by the herpes virus.

> **Simplex**—A viral infection appearing on the face or genital regions with resulting itching and localized hyperemia. The lesions dry up and form a yellowish crust that normally disappears in 10 to 14 days depending on care.

> **Zoster**—An acute and painful viral disease that affects the cerebral ganglia and posterior nerve roots. Lesions appear on the skin over the infected area. Oral lesions occur on the tongue, soft palate, cheek, and the gingival tissues.

**Horseshoe Denture**—A partial upper denture from which the palate is omitted. In edentulous cases, a horseshoe denture is termed a *roofless denture*.

**Hutchinson's Teeth**—Congenitally malformed, peg-shaped incisors with incisal edges narrower than the middle part or notching of the incisal edges. Primary dentition is not affected.

**Hygienist**—A person trained and licensed by the state to perform dental prophylaxis under the direction of a licensed dentist.

**Hypercementosis**—Extensive formation of cementum on the roots of the teeth.

**Hyperkeratosis**—The most common white lesion in the oral cavity. A benign lesion that may be elevated or flat and is in the form of a thickened layer of keratin. It may be associated with a cause such as lip biting, or its cause may be obscure. The lesion usually disappears within two to three months if the cause is eliminated.

**Hyperplasia**—Excessive growth of normal cells in the normal tissue arrangement of an organ; may have a hereditary or inflammatory cause.

**Denture**—Enlargement of tissues, caused by trauma to the soft tissues from dentures or other injuries.

**Dilantin**—Caused by the use of dilantin therapy.

**Hypocalcification**—Reduced calcification; a condition that produces opaque white spots on tooth enamel; a possible hereditary anomaly affecting the dentition, both primary and permanent. The enamel peels off, exposing the dentin and giving a yellow appearance to the teeth.

**Hypoplasia**—With dental enamel, it is a defective or incomplete development. When it is a hereditary anomaly, a thin layer of hard enamel covers the dentin, giving a brownish appearance to the teeth.

**I Clasp**—Roach-type clasp shaped like an I.

**Immediate Abutment**—The metal abutment in a three abutment bridge, with a bridge extending from one cuspid to a second molar with a second bicuspid present.

**Immediate Denture**—A complete or partial denture made before the natural teeth are extracted. It is inserted at the time the teeth are extracted.

**Immediate Surgical Splint**—Metal, acrylic resin, or modeling compound fashioned to retain teeth that have been replanted, are unmovable, or have fractured roots; may also be a temporary denture after extraction of teeth. It is an appliance for the protection of a surgical site.

**Impacted Tooth**—Commonly, any tooth that is positioned or wedged against another tooth, bone, or soft tissue, preventing it from erupting normally.

**Impingement**—Over-compaction, displacement, or compression. It may be the result of pressure from a unit of a removable prosthesis or traumatization of the periodontal membrane caused by occlusal force on the tooth.

**Implants**—Dental implants are made of metal or other foreign material and are placed into or on the alveolar bone to provide support.

**Endosseous**—May be a single metal post inserted into the alveolar bone to support an artificial crown that replaces a missing natural tooth; may also be a metal blade to support one or more artificial crowns or to support a metal crown that would serve as an abutment for a fixed bridge. There are many types and shapes of implants.

**Subperiosteal**—Used for support of dentures in which there is sufficient resorption of the alveolar ridge. The gingival tissue is opened along the alveolar ridge, and impressions are made. A metal prosthesis is made from this impression and the tissues opened again to permit placing the implant that creates an artificial ridge. Extensions from the metal saddle extend above the gingival tissue for denture attachments.

**Impressions**—A negative reproduction of the teeth or tissues of the mouth. A positive reproduction is made from the impression and is used in the preparation of restorations such as crowns, fixed and removable prosthetics, and appliances. They are also used for diagnostic purposes.

**Plaginate**—A relationship impression taken in combination of quick-set, plaster, and alginate.

**Relationship**—Impression taken to establish the relationship of abutment teeth.

**Incisal**—Pertaining to the cutting edges of incisors and cuspid teeth.

**Incisor**—A cutting tooth; one of four front teeth of either jaw.

**Infrabulge**—The formation of the crown that is cervical to the clasp guideline, survey line, or height of contour.

**Initial Centric**—A centric determination made by the dentist, usually without the use of mechanical aids, which is fairly accurate and commonly used in the final process in establishing true centric.

**Inlay**—A dental restoration shaped to the form of a cavity and inserted and secured with cement.

**Intercusping**—A correct occlusion of the cusp of the teeth of one jaw with a corresponding impression in the occlusal surfaces of the teeth in the opposite jaw.

**Interdigitation**—Enclosure of the posterior teeth; the striking of the cusp of one denture fairly into the occluding surface of the other denture.

**Interproximal**—Between the proximal surfaces of the adjacent teeth.

**Intraoral**—Inside or within the mouth.

**Ionization**—The process of ionizing; use of an electric current to ionize medication within a root canal; used in treatment of sensitive teeth.

**Jacket**—A term commonly used in reference to an artificial crown composed of fired porcelain or acrylic resin, i.e., porcelain jacket crown, acrylic resin jacket crown.

**Jaw**—Either the maxilla or the mandible.

**Jumpcase**—See Denture Duplication.

**Labial**—Pertaining to the lips. It is the surface of an anterior tooth nearest the lips.

**Labial Bar**—The metal bar (major connector) used to connect the right and left side of a lower partial denture. It is contoured to the labial tissue anterior to the lower teeth.

**Labiolingual**—From the lips toward the tongue.

**Lamina Dura**—The inner bony wall of the tooth socket. It shows up as a fine white line around the root of a tooth in a dental x-ray.

**Lateral (Incisor)**—An anterior tooth located just distal to the central incisors; the second tooth from the midline.

**Ligature Wire**—A fine wire used to tie the main arch wire into the bracket of an orthodontic appliance on the bands or the teeth.

**Lingual**—Pertaining to the tongue; the surface of a tooth or prosthesis next to the tongue.

**Lingual Bar**—The metal bar (major connector) on the lingual surfaces of the teeth connecting the right and left sides of the lower partial denture. It is contoured to the lingual tissue behind and below the anterior teeth.

**Luxation**—Detachment of a tooth from its socket as a result of trauma or disease progress; may be partial or complete.

**Macrodontia**—Abnormally large teeth.

**Macrognathia**—Abnormally large jaws.

**Malalignment**—Displacement; not in normal alignment.

**Malar Process**—The bony extensions of the temporal and maxillary bones that unite with the zygomatic process to form the zygomatic arch; sometimes called the *cheekbone*.

**Malocclusion**—Any deviation from normal occlusion of the teeth, usually associated with abnormal development and growth of the jaws.

**Mandible**—The lower jaw.

**Mandibular**—Pertaining to the mandible.

**Marginal Ridge**—A ridge or elevation of enamel forming the edge of a surface of a tooth; specifically, one of the mesial or distal borders of the lingual surfaces of anterior teeth and the occlusal surfaces of posterior teeth.

**Mastication**—Chewing food at the first stage of digestion.

**Maxilla**—The bone of the skull that supports the upper teeth. Commonly, the term is used to name the upper jaw with its teeth when present, and associated with soft tissues.

**Maxillae**—The bones of the upper jaw.

**Maxillary**—Referring to the maxilla or upper arch.

**Maxillofacial**—Relates to the jaws and the face.

**MDS**—Master of Dental Science.

**Median**—The middle; situated or placed in the middle of the body or in the middle of a part of the body.

**Megadontism**—The condition that results in abnormally large teeth.

**Mental Protuberance**—A triangular elevation forming the prominence of the chin.

**Mesial**—The surface of a tooth which, in normal occlusion, is nearest the midline.

**Mesioclusion**—Occlusion of the teeth in which the mesial buccal cusp of the upper first molar interdigitates between the lower first and second molars.

**Mesiodens**—Accessory or supernumerary tooth which may be erupted or unerupted and located between the maxillary central incisors.

**Mesiodistal**—From mesial (the middle) to distal (farthest from).

**Mesioversion**—In the oral cavity, indicative of a closer than normal position to the median plane or midline of the jaw. When in reference to the maxilla or mandible, the jaw is anterior to its normal position.

**Macrodontia**—Abnormally small teeth.

**Micrognathism**—Abnormal smallness of jaws; lack of normal development.

**Midline**—The imaginary dividing line through the middle of an object or space.

**Migration**—The movement of a tooth or teeth out of the normal position. It is usually caused by loss of supporting structures.

**Milk Teeth**—Primary or deciduous teeth (named for their white or milky appearance).

**Mineralize**—The precipitation of calcium and other salts into an organic matrix to form a hard deposit such as dental calculus.

**Mobility**—The degree of looseness of a tooth as a result of loss of part or all of the attachments and supportive structures.

**Molars**—The three teeth in each quadrant that are located distal to the second bicuspids. They are used for grinding.

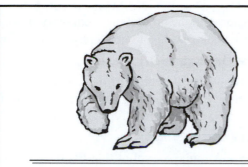

What did the dentist see at the North Pole?
A molar bear.

**Morphology**—The branch of biology that deals with structure and form. It includes the anatomy, histology, and cytology of an organism at any stage of its life history.

**Mottled Enamel**—A dappled condition of the enamel of the teeth caused by ingestion of too high concentrations of fluorides or drugs such as tetracycline during the formative period.

**Mucobuccal Fold**—The junction between the cheek and the mucous membrane of the upper or lower jaw.

**Mucogingivoplastic Surgery**—Procedures designed to correct or modify defects in the morphology and the position of the soft tissues surrounding the teeth.

**Mucoperiosteum (Mucoperiosteal Tissue or Periosteum)**—A layer of connective tissues that covers the outer surfaces of the bone. Periosteum in the oral cavity is covered with gingival tissue and is significant to periodontics.

**Mucositis**—Inflammation of the mucous membrane.

**Mucous Membrane**—The soft tissue covering or lining of the mouth.

**Mulberry Molars**—Congenitally malformed molars. The occlusal surfaces are narrow and there is hypoplasia of the enamel.

**Multirooted**—A tooth with two or more roots.

**Nasion**—The part of the skull located at the midpoint of the nasofrontal suture at the root of the nose; the junction of the nasal bones with the frontal bone. This is a landmark in clinical prosthetics.

**Neutroclusion**—Occlusion of the teeth in which the mesiobuccal cusp of the upper first molar interdigitates with the buccal groove of the lower first molar.

**Nitrous Oxide**—A colorless gas used in dentistry as a general anesthetic with the performance of un-complicated operations; also called *laughing gas and nitrogen monoxide*.

**Nonprecious Metals**—Material developed for use in all types of restorative procedures that are less precious than gold and other precious metals.

**Obturator**—An appliance designed to fill in a cleft palate defect. It is usually held in place with clasps or splinted to the teeth.

**Occlude**—To close, specifically so that the cusps of the posterior teeth fit together.

**Occlusal**—The chewing or masticating surfaces of the bicuspids and molars.

> **Balance**—Contact relationship of the biting surfaces of the teeth; simultaneous contacts; equilibrium of mastication.

> **Equilibration**—The process of refining and perfecting the occlusion.

> **Film**—X-ray exposures made on larger films than those used for the periapical and bite wing exposures. The film is placed in the occlusal plane and held in position by the teeth in occlusion. It is used to augment the other exposures.

> **Guard**—A removable dental appliance usually constructed of acrylic resin, which covers one or both dental arches to protect the teeth from the damaging effects of bruxism and other occlusal habits.

> **Rest**—The part of a clasp that lies on the occlusal surface of the tooth.

> **Surface**—The grinding, chewing, or masticating surface of molars and bicuspids.

**Odontalgia**—Toothache.

**Odontalysis**—Examination of the teeth.

**Odontectomy**—Surgical extraction of a tooth.

**Odontexesis**—Cleaning of the teeth, including thorough scaling.

**Odonthemodia**—Treatment of sensitive teeth.

**Odontinoid**—A tumor composed of tooth substance.

**Odontoblast**—Connective tissue cells that line the surface of the dental pulp adjacent to the dentin. During the tooth development period, these cells have much to do with the formation of dentin.

**Odontoma**—An odontogenic tumor composed of enamel, dentin, cementum, and pulp tissue; an anomaly such as dens in dentes or enamel pearl.

**Odontomy (Prophylactic Odontomy)**—Surgical cutting into a tooth for removal of precarious pits and fissures with subsequent restoration.

**Odontrophia** —Imperfect development of the teeth.

**Onlay**—A cast occlusal restoration that covers the entire incisal or occlusal surface of the tooth, frequently used to restore lost tooth structure and restore vertical dimension.

**Opacity**—The condition of being impervious to light.

**Opaque**—Not transparent; not letting light through.

**Open Bite**—A condition that prevents the anterior mandibular teeth from achieving proper occlusal relationship to the maxilla; more than the correct amount of jaw opening. Cause may be fractures, dislocations, abnormal tongue habits, or genetic or developmental abnormalities.

**Operative Dentistry**—The branch of dentistry primarily concerned with restoring carious, diseased, or damaged natural teeth to a satisfactory state of health.

**Operculum**—Cover or lid, such as a tissue over the crown of a tooth.

**Oral**—Pertaining to the mouth.

> **Habit**—A frequently repeated practice that may produce injury to the teeth and their attachments, the temporal mandibular musculature, or other structures. Oral habits include bruxism, tongue thrust, lip or cheek biting, and biting on hard objects.
>
> **Hygiene**—The laws of health as applied to the mouth.
>
> **Pathology**—The study of diseases of hard and soft tissues of the mouth.
>
> **Surgery**—The branch of surgery dealing with the operative procedures as related to the teeth and jaws.

**Orthodontics**—The branch of dentistry concerned with the detection, prevention, and correction of abnormalities in the positioning of the teeth in relationship to the jaws.

**Orthodontist**—A dentist who has met all the requirements to qualify as a specialist in the practice of orthodontics.

**Orthopantomograph Film**—An extraoral view of the teeth and associated structures on a single, continuous film. It is similar to a panorex film.

**Osseous Tissue**—Bone tissue.

**Osseous Surgery (Periodontal)**—Surgical correction or therapeutic treatment performed to eliminate bone deformities and create a more favorable environment; removal of diseased and defective bone tissue.

**Ostectomy**—The excision of bone; in periodontics, the excision of bone around the teeth or tooth roots to remove pockets or to provide a physiologic form.

**Osteitis**—Inflammation of the bone.

**Overbite**—Vertical overlap of the upper teeth over the lower teeth; overlapping of the mandibular incisors by maxillary incisors.

**Overjet**—See Overbite.

**Overlay**—An inlay or splint that fits over the biting or grinding surface of a tooth.

**Palatal**—Of or pertaining to the roof of the mouth.

**Palatal Bone**—The bone that forms the posterior portion of the hard palate.

**Palate**—The roof of the mouth, consisting of a hard anterior part and a soft moveable part. The palatal structures separate the mouth from the nasal cavity.

**Palatine**—Of or pertaining to the palate.

**Palliative Treatment**—Treatment that relieves pain or prevents a condition from becoming worse but does not cure it.

**Panoramic**—A term applied to any one of several techniques for making an x-ray picture of all the teeth and contiguous structures on a single film.

**Panorex**—See X-ray.

**Pantograph**—An instrument used for occlusal tracing as a part of extensive equilibration.

**Papilla**—A small, nipple-shaped elevation or protuberance.

> **Intradental**—The gingiva filling the intradental spaces between the teeth. It is partly free and partly attached to the gingival tissues.
>
> **Of Tongue**—Finger-like elevations on the surface of the tongue (i.e., taste buds).

**Partial Denture**—A prosthesis replacing one or more, but not all, natural teeth and associated structures; may be removable, fixed, unilateral, or bilateral.

**PCP**—Plaque Control Program.

**Pedodontics**—The specialty of children's dentistry. It includes training the child to accept dentistry, restoring and maintaining the primary, mixed, and permanent dentitions, applying preventive measures for dental caries and periodontal disease, and preventing, intercepting, and correcting various problems of occlusion.

**Peg Laterals**—The lateral incisors that are peg-shaped due to a developmental disturbance.

**Periapical**—The tissues surrounding the apex of a tooth.

**Pericoronal**—The tissues surrounding the crown of a natural tooth.

**Pericoronitis**—Inflammation of the tissues over a partially erupted tooth or the surrounding area of the crown of an erupted tooth. It frequently involves an erupting third molar, and there may be infection in the area.

**Periodontal Membrane**—The fibers between the alveolar bone and the tooth that holds the tooth in its socket; a modified periosteum.

**Periodontics**—The science of examination, diagnosis, and treatment of diseases affecting the periodontium.

**Periodontitis**—Inflammation of the periodontium that may cause alterations of the periodontal process. It may be caused by environmental or systematic factors.

**Periodontium**—Collectively, the tissues that surround and support the tooth.

**Periodontoclasia**—Condition characterized by inflammation accompanied by degenerative and retrogressive changes in the periodontium.

**Periodontosis**—Degeneration of the periodontium; a noninflammatory condition. With resorption of the alveolar bone, loosening and migration of the teeth occur. It is a rare disease, usually occurring in young people.

**Periosteum**—A layer of connective tissue that is a tough, fibrous membrane that covers the outer surface of all bone and varies in thickness in the different areas of the bone.

**Permanent Teeth**—The teeth that replace the primary teeth.

**PFC**—Porcelain face crown.

**Pin Pontic**—A pontic with a long pin porcelain facing. Metal pins are embedded in a porcelain facing and extend out of it lingually. The pins fit into a customized cast metal backing that finishes the occlusal surface.

**Pinlay (Pinledge)**—A thin cast inlay that depends in part on small parallel pins that fit into the prepared tooth for its retention. Pinledge crowns are modified three-quarter crowns gaining retention from cast pins.

**Pit**—An indentation; a depression.

**Pivots**—Elevations, usually artificially developed, on the occlusal surface of natural or artificial posterior teeth to induce mandibular rotation. The term may also be used in reference to dowel pins. Pivots may or may not be adjusted.

**PJC**—Porcelain jacket crown.

**Plane**—A term used to describe an ideal, flat surface which intersects solid body and extends in various directions.

  **Axial**—A hypothetical plane that parallels the long axis of an object.

  **Bite**—An appliance that covers the palate and has an incline or flat plane at the anterior border. It provides resistance to the mandibular incisors when there is contact.

  **Occlusal**—A plane established by the occlusal surfaces of the bicuspids and molars of both the upper and lower jaw in opposition. In orthodontics, a line between two points that represents one-half of the incisal overbite and one-half of the cusp height of the posterior molars.

**Plaque**—An accumulation of bacteria and debris on the tooth's surfaces.

**Plastic**—In dentistry, the capacity to be moved. A restorative material, i.e., amalgam, cement, guttapercha, and resin, which is soft at the time of insertion and may be shaped or molded before it hardens or sets.

**Plastic Fillings**—See restorations.

**Pocket**—A space between the affected tooth and the diseased epithelium; diseased gingival tissues with resulting discoloration, retraction from the root, bleeding, and presence of exudate. Depth of the pocket would be limited by the epithelial attachment at the apex of the root.

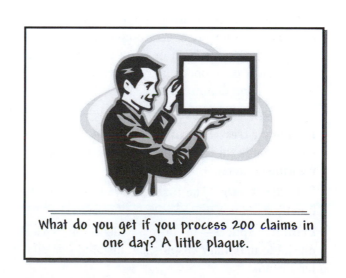

What do you get if you process 200 claims in one day? A little plaque.

**POH**—Personal oral hygiene.

**Polishing**—The act of buffing and shining the teeth.

**Pontic**—The part of a fixed bridge that is suspended between abutments and replaces a missing tooth; an artificial tooth in a removable denture.

**Porcelain**—A tooth-colored, sand-like material used for inlays, facings, crowns, pontics, and denture teeth. It fuses at high temperatures to form a hard substance much like enamel in appearance. Dental porcelain is a fusion mixture that is glass-like.

**Post**—In partial denture work, the minor connector that attaches the clasp body to the framework; an upright, metal device that extends into a tube tooth to retain it; in restorative dentistry, a metal projection in crowns to give strength. It may extend into the root of a pulpless tooth, or it may extend through the root into the alveolar bone.

**Post and Core**—A single cast unit that provides strength and restores lost structure. It is placed into the tooth followed by the permanent exterior restoration, usually a crown.

**Postdam Area**—The soft tissues along the junction of the hard and soft palate where pressures can be applied for retention of a denture. Special provision is designed into the denture for the purpose of sealing against the resilient soft tissue in the palate.

**Posterior Teeth**—All teeth located distal to the cuspids; a tooth having an occlusal surface.

**Postpermanent Dentition**—Teeth that erupt after the loss of permanent dentition. It is a rare condition and these teeth are usually impacted accessory teeth that erupt following the insertion of dentures.

**Predeciduous Dentition**—Teeth that precede the primary dentition. It is a rare condition in which teeth are present at birth or erupt after birth. They are not fully developed and consist only of enamel or enamel and dentin.

**Premolars**—Bicuspids.

**Primary Stress Bearing Area**—The area of the mouth that is suited to withstand heavy stress from wearing dentures.

**Primary Teeth**—The first teeth to erupt in childhood.

**Primate Spaces**—In primary dentition, spaces mesial to maxillary cuspids and distal to mandibular cuspids.

**Process**—In anatomy, a marked prominence or projection of bone. In dentistry, a series of operations that convert a waxed pattern of a dental appliance into a permanent restoration composed of some relatively indestructible material.

    **Alveolar**—The part of the bone that surrounds and supports the teeth in the maxilla and the mandible.

    **Condyloid**—The posterior process on the ramus of the mandible that articulates with the mandibular fossa of the temporal bone.

    **Coronoid**—The anterior part of the upper and ramus of the mandible to which the temporal muscle is attached.

    **Maxillary**—The irregular-shaped bone forming one-half of the upper jaw. The upper jaw is made up of two maxillas.

    **Palatine**—One of four shelf-like extensions of the embryonic upper jaw that gives rest to the premaxillary palate.

**Prognathic**—A protrusive relationship of the jaws to the head.

**Prognathism**—Facial disharmony due to prominence or projection of one or more jaws, occurring most frequently in the mandible.

**Prophylactic Odontotomy**—The technique of opening and filling structural imperfections of the enamel to prevent dental caries.

**Prophylaxis**—Prevention of disease by removal of calculus, stains, and other extraneous material from the teeth; cleaning of the teeth by a dentist or dental hygienist.

**Prosthesis (Plural, Prostheses)**—An artificial replacement of one or more natural teeth or associated structures; replacement of a part of the body.

**Prosthetic**—Pertaining to prostheses.

**Prosthodontics**—The branch of dentistry concerned with restoration and maintenance of function by replacement of natural teeth.

**Provisional Splinting**—A therapeutic appliance placed to assist with healing, repair, or cure. It may serve as a temporary stabilization for mobile teeth.

**Proximal Surface**—The surface of a tooth that is next to another tooth; usually, the mesial or distal surface, unless the tooth is rotated.

**Pulp**—Connective tissues, with nerves and blood vessels which fill the pulp chamber and root canals. "Vitality" of pulp refers to health of the pulp. When there is degeneration or the pulp has been removed, the tooth is termed nonvital.

**Pulp Canal**—See Root Canal.

**Pulp Capping**—See Capping.

**Pulp Chamber**—The space in the coronal portion of the tooth occupied by the pulp.

**Pulpectomy**—Complete removal of either vital or inflamed pulp from the chamber and the root canal. The term is not appropriate in reference to necrotic pulp tissue.

**Pulpotomy**—Removal of dental pulp in the coronal portion of the tooth; removal of exposed vital pulp to retain a healthy pulp in the root. It may be partial or complete.

**Pyogenic**—Pus-producing.

**Pyorrhea**—Flow of pus from the periodontal wound; an outdated term replaced by " periodontitis " or "periodontal disease."

**Quadrant**—One-fourth of the two dental arches; one-half of each arch.

**Radectomy**—Surgical removal of a part of a tooth root.

**Radiculalgia**—Neuralgia of the nerve roots.

**Radicular**—Pertaining to the tooth root.

**Radiograph**—A picture produced on a sensitive surface by a form of radiation other than light; an x-ray or gamma ray photograph. Either one produces a shadow image.

**Ramus**—The ascending part of the mandible from the angle to the condyle.

**Reattachment**—The re-adaptation of the gingival and underlying tissues to the root surface of a tooth.

**Rebase**—Placement of the denture base material without changing the occlusal relations of the teeth; adding to the denture base to compensate for altered tissues.

**Recalcification**—See Remineralization.

**Reline**—Resurface the tissue-borne areas of a denture with new material.

**Remineralization**—The use of calcium hydroxide or similar materials as a treatment prior to placing a temporary restoration.

**Remote Denture**—See Denture.

**Replantation (Reimplantation)**—The replacement of natural teeth that have been dislodged or removed, either accidentally or unintentionally; reinsertion of a natural tooth to the alveolar socket.

**Resin**—A term commonly used to indicate organic substances that may be solid or semi-solid, translucent or transparent. Resins are named according to their chemical composition, physical structure, and means for activation or curing. Examples are acrylic resin, autopolymer resin, synthetic resin, styrene resin, and vinyl resin.

**Resorption**—Loss of substance. Alveolar resorption is loss of substance or structure; reduction in size or residual alveolar ridges; destruction of bone. Primary tooth roots are reabsorbed as a part of normal shedding.

**Rest**—An extension of the prosthesis that provides support.

**Restoration**—Restoring natural or ideal contour and function. The term relates to fillings, inlays, crowns, bridgework, partial and complete dentures, and restoration of contour and function as a result of disease and other factors.

**Retained Root**—A root or part of a root; remaining soft or hard tissue.

**Retainer**—An abutment tooth in a fixed bridge that may be in the form of an inlay or a partial or full crown; a removable prosthesis, a clasp, attachment, or device used for fixation or stabilization. In orthodontics, an appliance to maintain the altered position of the teeth and jaws until they stabilize.

**Retention**—In removable prostheses, a resistance to force or movement. In orthodontics, an appliance used to maintain teeth in the position to which they have been moved for harmonious relationship. The necessary procedure in cavity preparation to prevent loss or displacement of a restoration.

**Retrognathism**—A disharmony as a result of one or both jaws being posterior to normal facial relationships.

**Retrograde Amalgam**—Amalgam filling placed into the apex of a tooth root; also called *retrofilm* or *reverse amalgam*. It would normally follow some form of endodontic therapy.

**Retroversion**—Indicated teeth or associated structures that are posterior to the generally accepted standard.

**Ridge Bar**—A splint or lingual bar that connects abutments.

**Roach Clasp**—See Clasp.

**Root**—The anatomic part of a tooth that is normally within the alveolar bone, and attached to it by the periodontal ligament.

**Root Amputation**—Removal of one or more roots of a multirooted tooth. Also, see Apicoectomy.

**Root Canal**—The space within the root of the tooth containing nerves and blood vessels. They connect the pulp chamber with the apex of the root.

**Root Canal Therapy**—Endodontic therapy; treatment of a tooth having a damaged pulp, or associated with periapical disease. It is normally performed by completely removing the pulp, sterilizing the pulp chamber and root canals, and filling those spaces with a sealing material.

**Root Planing**—The smoothing of roughened root surfaces by the use of scalers and curets.

**Root Resection**—Removal of all or part of the tooth root. See Root Amputation.

**Rotated Teeth**—Teeth rotated out of normal position. The laterals and bicuspids are the most frequently rotated.

**Rugae**—The irregular ridges in the mucous membrane covering the anterior part of the hard palate.

**Saliva**—The digestive secretions from the salivary glands into the mouth. It assists in chewing and preparing the food for digestion by moistening the food and lubricating the mouth. It initiates digestion of starches; it aids in excretion of waste products and regulation of water balance.

**Sanitary Pontic**—A conical-shaped pontic that has been contoured to provide a sanitary environment.

**Scale**—To remove calculus (tartar) and stains from the teeth with a scaler and other special instruments.

**Sealer**—A material used to fill the space around the silver or gutta-percha points as part of root canal therapy.

**Secondary Dentin**—Dentin formed on the inner walls of the pulp cavity after the tooth is fully formed; a protective mechanism whereby the pulp seeks to protect itself from injury. It may be the result of disturbances or irritation and stimulation of the odontoblasts.

**Secondary Stress-Bearing Area**—An area of the mouth not suited for bearing a major part of the pressure under a denture; a relief area in an upper denture.

**Sedative**—Drugs or any other means of producing a calming effect.

**Semiprecious**—Materials developed for dental restorations that have a lesser amount of precious metal.

**Semiridge Bridge (Broken Stress Bridge)**—A fixed bridge in which one of the connections between the units is composed of a male/female joint that reduces the effect of stress.

**Septic Alveolus (Dry Socket)**—Pain from breakdown or loss of the blood clot from a tooth socket following extraction.

**Shell Crowns**—See Crowns.

**Shell Teeth**—Teeth having a form or dentinogenesis imperfecta; lack of root development and wider than normal pulp chambers.

**Sialolithiasis**—Salivary gland or duct stones.

**Sialolithotomy**—Incisions of a salivary gland or duct to remove stones.

**Silica**—One of the three major ingredients in dental porcelain; provides stiffness and hardness.

**Sinus**—A cavity, a canal or passage, recess or hollow space.

> **Alveolar**—A pathologic cavity in the alveolus connecting with either the oral or nasal cavity.

> **Maxillary**—The bony cavity in the body of the maxilla. In dental x-rays, the floor of the sinus may be seen above the alveolar process. Occasionally, the apices of the teeth including the cuspids and posterior teeth may extend into the sinus.

**Sinusotomy**—Incision into a sinus cavity.

**Socket**—An alveolus in the alveolar process that holds the roots of a tooth.

**Sodium Fluoride**—A solution applied topically to the teeth and used in drinking water as a caries preventive agent; also used with kaolin and glycerin as a desensitizing agent for hypersensitive dentin.

**Space Maintainer**—A fixed removable appliance placed to maintain space created by the premature loss of one or more teeth. It may also be used to create space by moving teeth apart while holding the space open.

**Space Obtainer**—An appliance used to increase the space between the two teeth.

**Space Regainer**—A fixed removable appliance to move a displaced tooth into proper position; commonly used for the first premature molar.

**Splint**—An appliance constructed of metal, acrylic resin, or modeling compound, designed to retain teeth in position.

> **Acrylic Resin Biteguard**—An appliance for immobilizing teeth, eliminating the effect of

traumatic oral habits by covering the occlusal and incisal surfaces of the dental arch.

**Cross-arch Bar**—A metal bar that unites one or more teeth from one side of the arch to teeth on the opposite side; also used to stabilize weakened teeth against lateral forces.

**Fixed**—A fixed prosthesis used for treatment of periodontal disease, designed to prevent adverse occlusal forces and maintain good gingival health. It stabilizes and immobilizes the teeth and may also replace missing teeth.

**Gunning's**—A maxillomandibular splint used with maxillofacial surgery.

**Inlay**—A casting to provide retention or support to one or more approximating teeth. This may include two inlays soldered together or a single casting spanning the approximating teeth.

**Intradental**—A splint applied to the teeth on the labial and/or lingual surfaces to provide points for attaching mandibular and/or maxillofacial traction and/or fixation.

**Provisional**—A therapeutic appliance designed to assist in healing, repair, and cure of periodontally involved teeth. It is semifixed and may consist of full crowns to stabilize the teeth during the mandibular movements. Materials used are acrylic resin, metal, and combinations of both.

**Surgical**—A thin acrylic or metal form that fits the contour of the alveolar ridge and is used after surgery. The function is to protect the surgical area during healing.

**Splinting**—Stabilizing or immobilization of periodontally involved teeth. Splinting may be accomplished with acrylic resin biteguards, orthodontic band splints, wire ligation, provisional splints, and fixed prostheses.

**Stannous Acid Fluoride**—A more recently developed form of fluoride, applied topically in a single treatment.

**Stayplate (Flipper)**—An acrylic partial, with or without wire clasps, which replaces one or more teeth; used as a temporary replacement until a more permanent prosthesis is prepared.

**Steele's Facing**—A pontic having a prefabricated backing combined with an acrylic or porcelain grooved facing.

**Stressbreaker**—An attachment that is incorporated into a removable partial denture or fixed bridge work to relieve pressure on the abutment teeth.

**Study Models**—See Diagnostic Casts.

**Subgingival Curettage**—See Gingival Curettage.

**Supernumerary Tooth**—A tooth in excess of the regular or normal number.

**Supraocclusion**—Abnormal overlap of a dental arch or group of teeth over the opposing arch or group of teeth.

**Surfaces**—Tooth surfaces.

    **Buccal**—Pertaining to or adjacent to the cheek.

    **Distal**—Away from the median plane of the face, following the curvature of the dental arch.

    **DLG**—The distal lingual groove, which normally extends to the occlusal.

    **E**—The external gingival surface.

    **Facial**—The same as labial or buccal; the external surface area or next to the face.

    **Incisal**—Cutting surface of the anterior teeth.

    **Labial**—Same as facial but toward the mouth and lips.

    **Lingual**—Pertaining to or adjacent to the tongue.

    **Mesial**—Toward the center of the median line of the dental arch.

    **Occlusal**—The masticating or grinding surfaces of molars and bicuspids.

    **Proximal**—The surface nearest the adjacent tooth.

**Tartar**—See Calculus.

**Temporal Bone**—The irregular-shaped bone at the side and base of the skull.

**Temporomandibular Joint**—The joint formed by the condyles of the mandible and the temporal bone.

**TMJ Syndrome (Costen's Syndrome)**—The symptoms associated with malfunction of the temporomandibular joint, frequently caused by loss of molar support or absence of occlusal balance.

**Three-Quarter Crown**—See Crowns.

**Tinker Bridge**—A fixed bridge involving the use of sanitary pontics.

**Tissue Bar**—A lingual bar connecting crowns for the purpose of stabilizing or reducing stress. They are placed adjacent to the gingival tissues.

**Tissue-borne**—A partial denture is referred to as "tissue-borne" when most or all of the masticatory stresses are borne by the soft tissues of the mouth.

**Tissue Conditioning**—A method of correcting tissue irritation occurring from the wearing of dentures. An impression-type material is placed in the saddle of the denture and, with the denture in place, a displacement of this material indicates any corrections necessary to eliminate distortion from pressure on the tissue. This procedure is more complicated than the usual adjustment.

**Tooth-borne**—A partial denture is referred to as "tooth-borne" when most or all of the masticatory forces are carried by the abutment teeth.

**Traumatogenic Occlusion**—A malocclusion that is injurious to the teeth or associated structures; an injury in the periodontal tissues produced by an occlusal pressure.

**Treatment Partial Denture**—A denture used for a limited time during the transition from normal dentition to complete dentures. It may be the same or similar to a stayplate, thumbplate, splitplate, or butterfly partial, which is also known as a *flipper*. It may be used during a healing period or for aesthetics before a permanent denture is constructed.

**Trial Baseplate**—The temporary foundation used in established maxillomandibular relationship for arrangement of the teeth in a denture, consisting of the baseplate and the occlusal rim.

**Trifurcation**—The area where roots divide into a tri-rooted tooth.

**Truss Bar**—The metal piece placed across the edentulous space between two bridge abutments, on which the pontic is constructed.

**Tube Tooth**—An artificial tooth containing a vertical channel in which a pin or metal post is placed to secure the tooth to a denture base.

**Tuberosity**—The posterior aspect of the maxillary alveolar process. It may appear as a normal bone carving upward, or it may be in the form of a bridge.

**Unerupted Tooth**—A tooth that has not broken through the bone or gingival tissue.

**Vault**—In the oral cavity, the palate or roof of the mouth; a prepared cavity in the bone for placing an implant.

**Veneer Crown**—See Crowns.

**Vertical Dimension**—The vertical height of the face with the teeth in occlusion; vertical relationship; the degree of jaw separation when teeth are in contact. This measurement is usually made from the tip of the chin to the base of the nose.

**Vestibular Space**—Space in the oral cavity bounded by the teeth and gums and externally by the lips and cheeks.

**Vestibule**—The part of the oral cavity that lies between the teeth and the gingiva or between the residual alveolar ridge and the lips and cheeks.

**Vestibuloplasty**—Revision of the vestibule frequently performed to accommodate the placing of dentures.

**Vitality**—Presence of vital dental pulp in the mouth.

**Vitality Test**—A test using thermal electrical or mechanical stimuli to determine the vitality of the dental pulp.

**X-Ray**—Roentgen-ray; called x-ray by the discoverer because of its enigmatic character. It has also been named roentgen-ray to honor Dr. Wilhelm C. Roentgen and to identify this form of radiation. The term x-ray is more commonly used.

    **Bitewing**—Both upper and lower teeth shown on one film.

    **Extraoral**—Film held outside the mouth and recording larger areas than is possible with smaller film; used to detect cysts and tumors and used with orthodontic treatment.

    **Full Mouth**—Usually consists of 14 periapical films plus bitewings.

    **Occlusal**—An intraoral film showing the lingual surfaces of the teeth in a portion of the palate.

    **Panorex**—An extraoral film that provides a continuous view of the teeth and associated structures. It is used for orthodontics and for detection of fractures, temporomandibular joint disease, cysts, and tumors. It is taken with a unit that has a swinging arm that moves from one side of the arch to the other.

    **Periapical**—So named because it records the entire tooth, including the apex of the root and some of the surrounding bone tissues.

**X-ray Film**—A shadowy negative that provides a means of diagnostic evaluation.

**Zinc Phosphate**—Commonly used to seal gold inlays and crowns into place on the teeth and as a base under metallic restorations.

**Zinc Oxide Eugenol**—A sedative cement used as a temporary filling or a base under restorations, where sedative treatment of the tooth is indicated.

Dentists provide services not only for teeth but also for their surrounding and supporting structures. Therefore, it is necessary for the Dental Claims Examiner to understand the structure and formation of the entire oral cavity or mouth.

# On the Job Now

**Directions:** Match each term in each column 1 with the term in column 2 that is closest to its meaning without looking back at the text. Write your answer in the space provided.

| Column 1 | Column 2 | Column 1 | Column 2 |
|---|---|---|---|
| _____ 1. Calculus | A. Gum | _____ 1. fistul- | A. Falling |
| _____ 2. Primary | B. Cleaning | _____ 2. -pexy | B. Tongue |
| _____ 3. Cuspid | C. Composite | _____ 3. retro- | C. In front of, before |
| _____ 4. Radiograph | D. Top | _____ 4. ante- | D. Development |
| _____ 5. Resin | E. Premolar | _____ 5. -ectomy | E. A way of |
| _____ 6. Caries | F. Tartar | _____ 6. pan- | F. Jaw |
| _____ 7. Bridgework | G. Bad Breath | _____ 7. –trophy | G. Duct, tube |
| _____ 8. Bicuspid | H. Groove | _____ 8. cid- | H. Surgical removal |
| _____ 9. Pulp Canal | I. Deciduous | _____ 9. –ology | I. Half |
| _____ 10. Crown | J. X-Ray | _____ 10. lingu- | J. Pipe, tube |
| _____ 11. Prophylaxis | K. Canine | _____ 11. gnath- | K. Study of |
| _____ 12. Gingiva | L. Removal | _____ 12. top- | L. Suspension, fixation |
| _____ 13. Fissure | M. Cavities | _____ 13. doch- | M. All |
| _____ 14. Extraction | N. Root Canal | _____ 14. hemi- | N. Backward |
| _____ 15. Halitosis | O. Partial denture | _____ 15. –ment | O. Place |

If you were unable to match any of the terms, refer back to the text and then fill in the answers.

# On the Job Now

**Directions:** Fill in the correct dental term in the space provided without looking back into the text. Write your answer in the space provided.

_____ 1. A dental restoration shaped to the form of a cavity and then inserted and secured with cement.

_____ 2. Tissues surrounding the apex of a tooth.

_____ 3. Doctor of Dental Medicine.

_____ 4. A collection of pus in a cavity formed within the tissue of the body.

_____ 5. Any deviation from normal occlusion of the teeth, usually associated with abnormal development and growth of the jaws.

_____ 6. Pertaining to the mouth.

_____ 7. The joint formed by the condyles of the mandible and the temporal bone.

_____ 8. The hard, calcified tissue that covers the anatomic root of a tooth. It is formed by cementoblast and arranged in layers that cover the root dentin.

_____ 9. Doctor of Dental Surgery.

_____ 10. An accumulation of bacteria and debris on the tooth's surfaces.

_____ 11. American Dental Association.

_____ 12. Complete removal of either vital or inflamed pulp from the chamber and root canal. The term is not appropriate in reference to necrotic pulp tissue.

_____ 13. The three teeth in each quadrant that are located distal to the second bicuspids and are used for grinding.

_____ 14. The branch of dentistry concerned with restoration and maintenance of function by replacement of natural teeth.

_____ 15. The anatomic part of the tooth that is normally within the alveolar bone, and attached to it by the periodontal ligament.

## The Oral Cavity

The **oral cavity (cavum oris)** is an oval-shaped cavity **(see Figure 11–1)**. Technically, it consists of two parts; the vestibule and the mouth cavity. The **vestibule** is the outer, smaller portion surrounded by the lips, cheeks, gums, and teeth.

The mouth cavity consists of the area surrounded by the alveolar arches and the teeth. In other words, the vestibule is the area between the teeth and the cheek or the teeth and the lips, and the mouth cavity is everything inside the teeth. The oral cavity stops at the lips in front, the palate on the top, the cheeks on the sides, the tongue on the bottom, and the oropharynx at the back. The oral cavity does not include the nose, the sinuses, the palates, the nasopharynx, or the laryngopharynx.

The **mouth** is primarily responsible for the introduction of air, food, and other substances into the body. It is also used for vocalization and speech. The opening of the mouth is connected to the pharynx and the larynx at the back of the mouth.

The process of digestion is begun immediately when food enters the mouth. The teeth break down the food by chewing. In addition, salivary glands secret saliva which helps to chemically break down foods and provide moisture to the mouth.

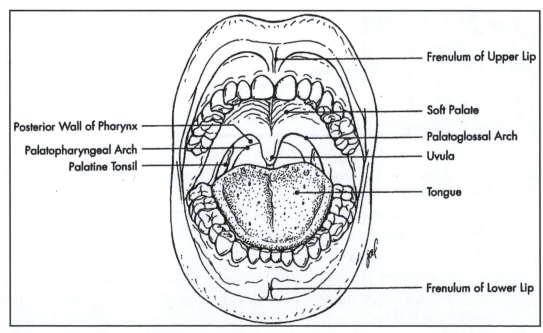

■ **Figure 11–1** The oral cavity

## Saliva and Salivary Glands

**Saliva** consists of salivary amylase and mucus. **Salivary amylase** is an enzyme that helps to break down food molecules. **Mucus** is a liquid containing mucin, leukocytes, inorganic salts, epithelial cells, and water. It is secreted by the mucus membranes and glands that line the mouth. The purpose of mucus is to moisten the food and ease the friction as it passes down the esophagus and into the stomach.

Three main pairs of salivary glands supply saliva to the mouth: the parotids, the submandibulars, and the sublinguals. The parotid gland is located beneath the temporomandibular joint, just in the front of the ear. Saliva is conveyed to the mouth by the parotid duct. The opening of the parotid duct is on the inside of the cheek, across from the second molar; it can be felt with the tongue.

The submandibular glands are located under the mandible, below the bottom molars. The sublingual gland is located below the floor of the mouth. Both the submandibular glands and the sublingual glands secrete saliva through duct openings on the floor of the mouth under the tongue.

## The Palates

The hard and soft palates form the roof of the mouth. The **hard palate** is toward the front and is so named because it is a hard, bony structure. It is formed by portions of the maxillary and palatine bones. The **soft palate** is in the rear portion of the mouth and is composed mostly of muscle. The purpose of the soft palate is to prevent foods or liquids from entering the nasal cavity. The opening of the nasal cavity is directly behind the soft palate. The soft palate is aided in this endeavor by the uvula, the small muscular projection that is suspended in the center, posterior portion of the mouth.

## The Tongue

Although the tongue is generally not treated under dental services, it is helpful to understand its basic function and how it relates to the surrounding structures in the mouth. The **tongue** is a muscular organ that lies on the floor of the mouth and continues partway into the pharynx. The tongue consists of a body and a root. The body of the tongue resides in the mouth, and the root extends down into the pharynx. Its purpose is to assist in the chewing and swallowing of food and the formation of speech and other sounds.

The surface of the tongue is covered with a mucus membrane. A mucus membrane also attaches the tongue to the floor of the mouth, the side walls of the pharynx, and the epiglottis. In addition, the tongue is attached by muscles to the mandibular bone in front, the hyoid bone below, the styloid process behind, and the palate (roof of the mouth) above. A fold (frenulum linguae) runs down the center of the tongue. In addition, the frenulum is a mucous membrane that connects the tongue to the floor of the mouth. There is also a frenulum of the upper and lower lip, which are mucus membranes connecting the lips to the maxilla and mandible.

## Papillae

The surface of the tongue is covered with **papillae** (tiny nipple-like protuberances) which consist of several types:

Filiform papillae are very slender and are situated at the end of the tongue.

Fungiform papillae are broad and flat papillae and resemble a fungus. They are found mostly in the rear central portion of the tongue.

Circumvallate papillae are the large bumps found near the base of the tongue, at the back of the mouth. They are arranged in a V shape.

Gustatory papillae possess a taste bud. They may be either filiform, fungi form, or circumvallate. Not all papillae contain taste buds at any given time.

**Taste buds** are sensory end organs that help carry the sensation of taste to the brain. They are located on the sides of papillae, on the epiglottis, the soft palate, and portions of the pharynx. When chemical stimuli (such as food) come in contact with the taste buds, they produce nervous impulses that are carried by means of the lingual and glossopharyngeal nerves to the brain. This produces one of the four basic taste sensations: sweet, bitter, sour, and salty.

The lingual nerves carry nerve impulses from the taste buds on the front two-thirds of the tongue. The glossopharyngeal nerves carry nerve impulses from the posterior one-third of the tongue. The average life span of a taste bud cell is about 10 days. They are constantly dying off and being replaced by new taste bud cells.

## The Gums

The **gum**, or **gingiva**, is the firm but soft tissue that surrounds the alveolar process and the mandibular and maxillary bones. It also covers the connecting area between the teeth and bone, thus helping to keep out food particles and bacteria as well as to keep the teeth in place. The gingiva is made up of connective tissue that is covered by mucus membrane. Normal healthy gums are pink, but they may become red, white, or black when injured or diseased.

The **alveolar process** is the portion of the mandible or maxilla that contains the tooth socket. The word *alveolar* comes from the Latin word meaning "small hollow" or "cavity."

# On the Job Now

**Directions:** Answer the following questions without looking back at the material just covered. Write your answers in the space provided.

1. Where does the oral cavity stop? _____
_____
_____

2. What is not included in the oral cavity? _____
_____
_____

3. What is the purpose of mucus? _____
_____

## The Jaw

The jaw consists of two bones. The upper fixed (non-movable) bone is the **maxilla**. It is actually made up of two maxillae, which form the skeletal base of most of the upper face, the roof of the mouth, the sides of the nasal cavity, and the floor of the orbit (the portion of the skull that contains and protects the eyeball).

The lower jaw is called the **mandible**. It is non-fixed (movable), which allows for not only biting and chewing food, but for speech, vocalization (speech and sound), and opening and closing of the mouth. The lower jaw is hinged to the upper jaw by a sliding joint called the **temporomandibular joint**. The temporomandibular joint is the only joint in the skull that is synovial, that is, containing synovia.

Synovia is a colorless liquid that lubricates the joints, bursae, and tendon sheaths; it is secreted from synovial membranes. Synovial joints are prone to irritation and inflammation. They are also associated with arthritis, rheumatic fever, and other connective tissue disorders, emotional states, and malocclusional disorders.

Because of the complexity of the problems and the various forms of treatments (many still experimental), disorders of the temporomandibular joint (more often called temporomandibular joint dysfunction or TMJ) are often regarded as a combined medical and dental problem. For further information regarding this disorder, see the **Temporomandibular Joint Disorder** section in the **Dental Services and Coding** chapter.

## Diseases of the Mouth

Following is a list of the more common diseases of the mouth that may require the services of a dentist:

**Gingivitis**—Inflammation of the gums. It may include swelling, redness, pain, bleeding, or difficulty in chewing. Possible causes are improper dental

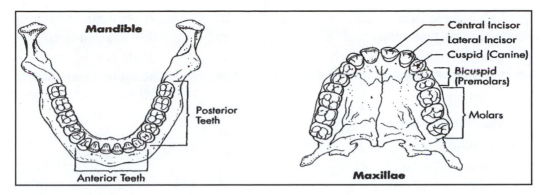

**■ Figure 11–2** Types of Teeth and Positions in Arch

hygiene, dentures or dental appliances that fit improperly, or improper **occlusion** (closure) of the teeth. Occasionally, gingivitis accompanies upper respiratory infections or diseases such as scurvy or metallic poisioning.

**Periodontitis**—Inflammation of the periodontal tissues. It may be caused by bacteria, calcium deposits, or food particles that collect between the tooth and the gum. If not treated, the infection may spread to the bone, possibly causing loss of teeth. Periodontitis is the primary cause of tooth loss in people over the age of 35.

**Periodontosis**—Any degenerative disease of the periodontal tissue.

The following are also diseases of the mouth. However, since they are generally treated by a medical doctor rather than a dentist, they will be given only brief mention here.

**Stomatitis**—Inflammation of the mouth. This can include cold sores, fever blisters, or canker sores.

**Cheilitis**—Inflammation of the lips.

**Cheiloschisis**—A deep groove in the lip. It is also known as a harelip or cleft lip.

**Cleft palate**—A deep fissure of the palate. It may involve the soft palate, the hard palate, the lip, or all three.

**Ankyloglossia**—A shortened frenulum of the tongue, preventing proper movement of the tongue.

**Sialodentitis**—Inflammation of a salivary gland.

# The Teeth

Humans have four types of teeth: incisors, canines, premolars, and molars (**see Figure 11–2**). Canines are referred to as cuspids, with premolars called bicuspids and molars tricuspids. The premolars and molars are considered posterior teeth, and the incisors and canines are anterior teeth.

**Incisors** are located at the front of the mouth and have a sharp edge that is used for biting. The normal adult has eight incisors, four on the top and a matching set of four on the bottom.

Behind the incisors are the cuspids. **Cuspids** or **canines** are used for tearing and piercing, and the normal adult has four, one behind each set of incisors. Behind the cuspids are the **premolars (bicuspids)**, which have two (bi-) cusps or grinding protrusions. Behind those are the **molars (tricuspids)**, which have three cusps. The normal adult has eight premolars (two behind each canine) and 12 molars. However, the third molars, or wisdom teeth, may never appear or erupt.

## Numbering the Teeth

The normal adult has 32 teeth. Accordingly, these teeth are numbered 1 through 32, beginning with the third molar on the upper-right side of the mouth (**see Figure 11–3**). The upper teeth are the maxillary teeth, numbers 1 through 16. The lower teeth are the mandibular teeth, numbers 17 through 32.

| Tooth | Maxillary Teeth |
|-------|-----------------|
| 1 | Right third molar |
| 2 | Right second molar |
| 3 | Right first molar |
| 4 | Right second premolar |
| 5 | Right first premolar |
| 6 | Right canine |
| 7 | Right lateral incisor |
| 8 | Right central incisor |
| 9 | Left central incisor |
| 10 | Left lateral incisor |
| 11 | Left canine |

| 12 | Left first premolar |
| 13 | Left second premolar |
| 14 | Left first molar |
| 15 | Left second molar |
| 16 | Left third molar |

| **Tooth** | **Mandibular Teeth** |
| 17 | Left third molar |
| 18 | Left second molar |
| 19 | Left first molar |
| 20 | Left second premolar |
| 21 | Left first premolar |
| 22 | Left canine |
| 23 | Left lateral incisor |
| 24 | Left central incisor |

| 25 | Right central incisor |
| 26 | Right lateral incisor |
| 27 | Right canine |
| 28 | Right first premolar |
| 29 | Right second premolar |
| 30 | Right first molar |
| 31 | Right second molar |
| 32 | Right third molar |

The primary or **deciduous teeth** number to 20 and apply to children. However, the deciduous teeth are lettered rather than numbered to avoid confusion with the adult numbering system. **Figure 11–4** shows the lettering of the primary teeth, beginning on the maxillary right and ending on the mandibular right. Note that there are no premolars or third molars in the deciduous set of teeth.

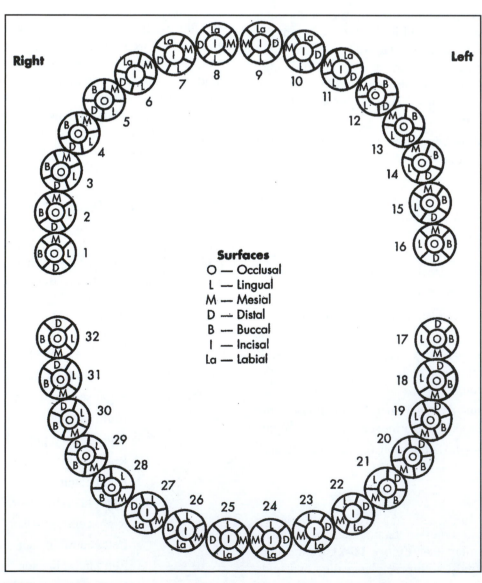

Surfaces
O — Occlusal
L — Lingual
M — Mesial
D — Distal
B — Buccal
I — Incisal
La — Labial

■ **Figure 11–3** Universal System of Tooth Numbers and Surfaces

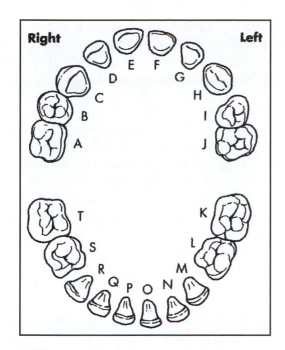

**Figure 11–4** Placement of Primary or Deciduous Teeth

| Tooth | Maxillary Teeth |
|---|---|
| A | Right second molar |
| B | Right first molar |
| C | Right cuspid |
| D | Right lateral incisor |
| E | Right central incisor |
| F | Left central incisor |
| G | Left lateral incisor |
| H | Left cuspid |
| I | Left first molar |
| J | Left second molar |

| Tooth | Mandibular Teeth |
|---|---|
| K | Left second molar |
| L | Left first molar |
| M | Left cuspid |
| N | Left lateral incisor |
| O | Left central incisor |
| P | Right central incisor |
| Q | Right lateral incisor |
| R | Right cuspid |
| S | Right first molar |
| T | Right second molar |

Some dental services are billed according to the section of the mouth that is treated. Most frequently, this involves periodontal (gum) treatment, but it may also apply to the application of sealants. (For more information regarding these procedures, see the **Dental Services and Coding** chapter.)

The mouth may be divided into either quadrants or sextants. A quadrant is one quarter of the two dental arches or one half of each arch. A sextant is one third of a dental arch (**see Figures 11–5 and 11–6**). Quadrants are named and abbreviated in the following manner:

| | |
|---|---|
| URQ | Upper Right Quadrant |
| ULQ | Upper Left Quadrant |
| LRQ | Lower Right Quadrant |
| LLQ | Lower Left Quadrant |

Sextants are named and abbreviated in the following manner:

| | |
|---|---|
| URS | Upper Right Sextant |
| UMS | Upper Middle Sextant |
| ULS | Upper Left Sextant |
| LRS | Lower Right Sextant |
| LMS | Lower Middle Sextant |
| LLS | Lower Left Sextant |

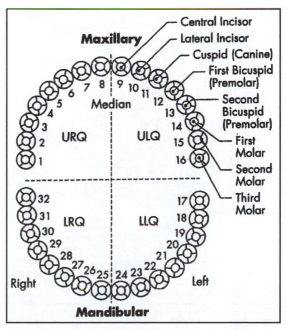

**Figure 11–5** Quadrants

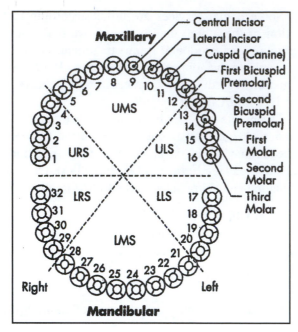

**■ Figure 11–6** Sextants

## The Structure of the Teeth

Each tooth is divided into three parts: the crown, the neck, and the root. The **crown** is the portion of the tooth that shows above the gum. The **neck** is the portion covered by the gum which links the crown to the root. The **root** is the portion that is embedded in the bone (**see Figure 11–7**).

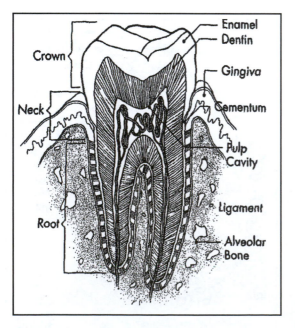

**■ Figure 11–7** Structure of the Tooth

The extreme center of the tooth is called the **pulp cavity**. This cavity contains the tooth nerves, veins, and arteries that allow essential blood flow into the tooth. The **root canal** is the portion of the pulp chamber that carries the blood vessels from the tooth socket to the tooth itself. The **pulp** is made up of connective tissue that contains a network of capillaries. The **capillaries** supply blood nourishment to the tooth. The pulp also contains lymph vessels and nerve fibers. Surrounding the pulp is the **dentin** (sometimes called the ivory), which forms the bulk of the tooth. The **apex** of the tooth is the terminus or end of the root. The root canal connects the pulp chamber with the apex.

In the root and neck of the tooth (the portion below the gum line), the dentin is covered with cementum.

**Cementum** is a bone-like material. Although hard, it is not in the same category as the enamel or the dentin. The cementum forms a junction with the enamel to seal off the exposed portion of the tooth (the crown). The cementum is actually a part of the periodontium or supporting structure of the tooth, since its main function is not biting, chewing, or tooth nourishment.

In the crown of the tooth (the portion above the gum line), the dentin is covered with enamel, which is smooth and white. This is the hardest substance in the human body.

For functional purposes, the tooth is often classified into two parts: the hard part and the soft part. The hard part of the tooth consists of the enamel, the dentin, and the cementum. The main purpose of the hard part is chewing and biting. The soft part of the tooth includes the pulp and the periodontal membrane. The periodontal membrane lines each tooth socket and covers the root of the tooth. The entire periodontal membrane acts as a bond between the cementum and the jawbone (mandible or maxilla). The main purpose of the soft part of the tooth is tooth nourishment.

Cementun, dentin, and enamel are composed chiefly of proteins, calcium carbonate, calcium phosphate, and magnesium phosphate. Calcium and phosphorous are constantly being washed away and replaced. For this reason, the human diet must contain enough calcium and phosphorous to ensure the health of the teeth.

## Surfaces of the Teeth

Each tooth has five surfaces. These surfaces differ, depending on whether the tooth is a posterior tooth (premolar or molar) or an anterior tooth (incisor or canine).

Surfaces that appear on all teeth are the **lingual (Li)**, which is the surface nearest the tongue; the **mesial (M)**, which is the surface nearest the midline (an imaginary line drawn between the maxillary centrals and the mandibular centrals); and the **distal (D)**, which is the surface farthest away from the midline. Posterior teeth have two additional surfaces consisting of the **buccal (B)**, which is the surface nearest the cheek, and the **occlusal (O)**, which is the biting surface. Anterior teeth also have two additional surfaces consisting of the **labial (La, L)**, which is the surface on the anterior teeth nearest the lip, and the **incisal (I)**, which is the biting edge or surface (**see Figure 11–8**).

The surface names of the primary teeth are the same as for adult teeth. Also, note the tooth surfaces shown in **Figure 11–3**.

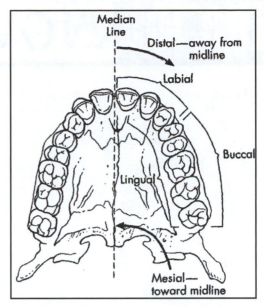

■ **Figure 11–8** Median Line and Tooth Surfaces

# On the Job Now

**Directions:** Label the parts of the tooth in the boxes provided.

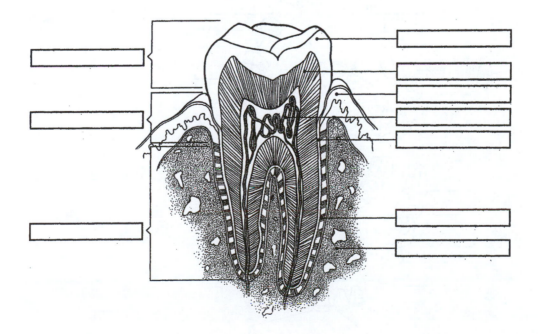

# On the Job Now

**Directions:** Divide the teeth into Quadrants and Sextants.

**Quadrants**

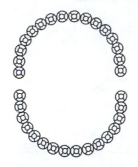

**Sextants**

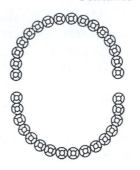

# On the Job Now

**Directions:** Number the Primary and Permanent Teeth.

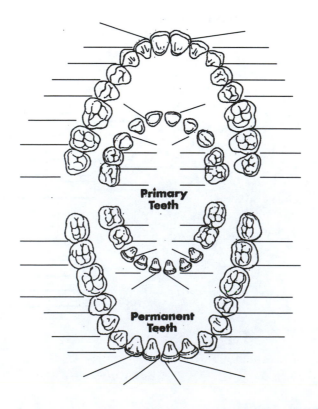

Primary Teeth

Permanent Teeth

# On the Job Now

**Directions:** Place the names of the Permanent and Primary Teeth in the boxes provided.

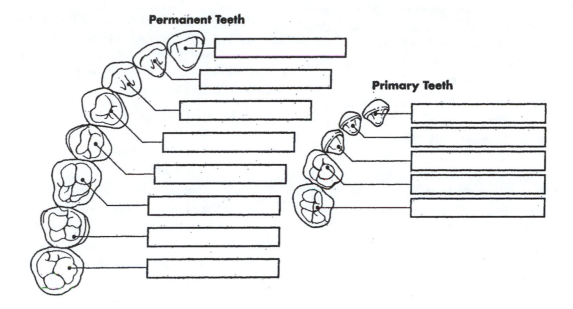

## Growth and Development of Teeth

All teeth, including permanent teeth, begin their development before birth. Calcification of the deciduous teeth takes place just before and after birth. That is why it is important that the mother's diet contain high amounts of calcium, phosphorus, and vitamin D. Without these vital nutrients, the teeth remain soft and are prone to decay. Permanent teeth calcify during infancy and childhood, necessitating the need for high amounts of calcium, phosphorus, and vitamin D in children's diets.

As a general rule, teeth erupt from the midline toward the back. The exception is the first molar, which usually erupts third in the deciduous teeth and first or second in the permanent teeth. The deciduous teeth normally erupt by the time a child is two years old. By the time a person reaches 17 to 24 years of age, the full set of permanent teeth is in place. **Table 11–2** shows the order and general time of eruption.

## Diseases of the Teeth

Following is a list of common diseases and conditions of the teeth that may require the services of a dentist:

| Deciduous Erupts (Months) | |
| --- | --- |
| Central incisor | 6-8 |
| Lateral incisor | 7-12 |
| Canine | 16-20 |
| First molar | 12-16 |
| Second molar | 20-30 |
| | |
| **Permanent Erupts (Years)** | |
| Central incisor | 6-8 |
| Lateral incisor | 7-10 |
| Canine | 9-13 |
| First premolar | 9-12 |
| Second premolar | 10-13 |
| First molar | 5-7 |
| Second molar | 10-13 |
| Third molar (wisdom) | 17-23 |

**Table 11–2  Eruption of Teeth**

**Bruxism**—Grinding of the teeth. It refers to grinding other than chewing and often occurs at night. If it continues, it can cause abnormal wear on the teeth.

**Edentulous**—Without teeth.

**Dentalgia**—A toothache or pain in the tooth. It usually indicates another existing condition such as a dental cavity or a periodontal problem.

**Dental Plaque**—A mass of microorganisms that grows on the exposed portions of the teeth and may spread under the gum line. It is the cause of dental caries and periodontal disease. Calcified dental plaque is called **calculus**. Most dental plaque can be removed by brushing and using dental floss. Calculus may need to be removed by a dentist or a dental hygienist. Such cleaning of the teeth is called prophylaxis.

**Dental Caries or Cavities**—Holes or decayed portions of the tooth. They are caused by the progressive decalcification of the tooth. Decalcification begins when food particles, fluid, or bacteria adhere to the tooth and break down the insoluble calcium salts into soluble salts. The calcium is then washed away and a cavity forms. Proper brushing and use of dental floss can greatly assist in removing food particles and bacteria. Topical application of fluoride while the teeth are still forming (usually prior to age 17 or 18) has also proven effective. After a cavity has begun forming, all bacteria must be removed from the hole and the cavity filled. If the cavity is not treated, it may spread into the pulp of the tooth, causing inflammation and abscess. In such a case, root canal treatment may be necessary, or the tooth may need to be extracted. Following are the three categories of cavities:

1. **Simple Cavities**—Involve only one surface of a tooth.

2. **Compound Cavities**—Involve two surfaces of a tooth.

3. **Complex Cavities**—Involve three or more surfaces of a tooth.

Cavities are classified according to the surface(s) of the tooth, the type of surface (smooth or occurring in a pit or fissure), and a numerical grouping. The most common numerical grouping is Black's Classification System, as follows:

Class 1    Caries beginning in structural defects of the teeth, such as fissures or pits.

Class 2    Caries in the proximal surfaces of (the space between) bicuspids and molars.

Class 3    Caries in the proximal surfaces of cuspids and incisors that do not involve removal or restoration of the incisal angle.

Class 4    Caries in the proximal surfaces of cuspids and incisors that do require removal or restoration of the incisal angle.

Class 5    Caries in the top third (gingival third, not pit cavities) of the labial, buccal, or lingual surfaces of the teeth.

Class 6    Caries of incisal edges and cusp tips of the teeth.

For further information regarding treatment of cavities, refer to the **Dental Services and Coding** chapter.

# CHAPTER REVIEW

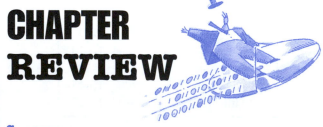

## Summary

- We have covered some of the common prefixes, suffixes, terms, and procedures that you will frequently see when processing dental charges. Familiarize yourself with these. By doing so you will be able to correctly identify dental services and procedures and determine whether the services are a covered dental benefit.

- The primary purpose of the mouth is the ingestion of food, the intake of air, and vocalization.

- The breakdown of food begins as it enters the mouth.

- The teeth aid in the digestive process by chewing and breaking down food particles.

- Further chemical breakdown of food particles is accomplished by the addition of saliva.

- Each tooth consists of a crown, a neck, and a root.

- The tooth itself is made up of dentin, enamel, pulp, and cementum.

- Each tooth is numbered, and each surface of the tooth is labeled. This eliminates confusion and helps to pinpoint the exact tooth and area where procedures have been performed.

- The most common diseases of the teeth are dental caries or cavities. However, teeth can also fall victim to dentalgia, dental plaque, and bruxism.

## Assignments

Complete the Questions for Review.
Complete Exercises 11–1 through 11–6.

## Questions for Review

**Directions:** Define the following prefixes, suffixes, and terms without looking back at the material just covered. Write your answers in the space provided.

**Prefixes and Suffixes**

1. mal- _____

2. apex- _____

3. -itis _____

4. labi- _____

5. arthr- _____

6. -desis _____

7. gloss- _____

8. -antr _____

9. lingu- _____

10. bucc- _____

**Terms:**

11. Anesthetics _____

_____

12. Plane _____

_____

13. Abrasion _____

_____

14. Abutment _____

_____

**15.** Pontic _____

_____

**16.** Rebase _____

_____

**17.** Bridge _____

_____

**18.** Bruxism _____

_____

**19.** Caries _____

_____

**20.** Plaque _____

_____

**21.** Impacted Tooth _____

_____

**22.** Maxilla _____

_____

**23.** Median _____

_____

**24.** Onlay _____

_____

**25.** Splint _____

_____

**Directions:** Answer the following questions without looking back at the material just covered. Write your answers in the space provided.

26. What is the primary purpose of the mouth? _____

_____

27. Are deciduous teeth numbered or lettered? _____

_____

28. In the permanent tooth numbering system, which tooth is number 1? _____

_____

29. What is the palate? _____

_____

30. What are the seven surfaces of the teeth and their abbreviations?

   1. _____

   2. _____

   3. _____

   4. _____

   5. _____

   6. _____

   7. _____

If you were unable to answer any of these questions, refer back to that section and then fill in the answers.

# Exercise 11-1

**Directions:** Define the following prefixes and suffixes without looking back into the text. Write your answer in the space provided.

1. ex- _____

   _____

2. dys- _____

   _____

3. -ostomy _____

   _____

4. infra- _____

   _____

5. -vulse _____

   _____

6. stom- _____

   _____

7. -lysis _____

   _____

8. end- _____

   _____

9. fren- _____

   _____

10. calc- _____

    _____

11. -otomy _____

    _____

12. post- _____

    _____

13. tri- _____

    _____

14. odont- _____

    _____

15. -plasia _____

    _____

If you were unable to answer any of these questions, refer back to that section and then fill in the answers.

# Exercise 11-2

**Directions:** Define the following terms in the space provided without looking back into the text. Write your answer in the space provided.

1. Crown: _____

_____

2. Fluoride: _____

_____

3. Intraoral: _____

_____

4. Prophylaxis: _____

_____

5. Bilateral: _____

_____

6. Amalgam: _____

_____

7. Quadrant: _____

_____

8. Space maintainer: _____

_____

9. Endodontics: _____

_____

10. Full-mouth x-ray: _____

_____

11. Partial denture: _____

_____

12. Root canal: _____

_____

13. Overbite: _____

_____

14. Mucous membrane: _____

_____

15. Primary teeth: _____

_____

If you were unable to answer any of the questions, refer back to that section and then fill in the answers.

# Exercise **11-3**

**Directions:** Label the surfaces of the Anterior Tooth and the Posterior Tooth in the boxes provided. The teeth are shown from the inside of the mouth with the midline being to the left.

**Anterior Tooth**

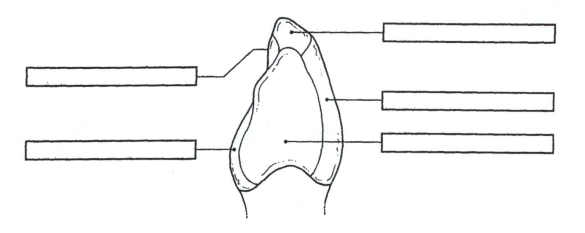

**Posterior Tooth**

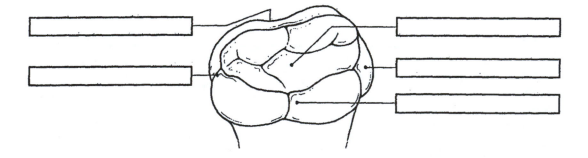

# Exercise 11-4

**Directions:** Find and circle the words listed below. Words can appear horizontally, vertically, diagonally, forward, or backward.

```
S M S R H V M S T U W S F U X X B Q Q E
N R G I H T R I W L E Q X H L Y K T L U
M M A Y T O U Y U I G S R A X O M C S Q
H R Z L S I R O R N O A G R N D A Q A A
M Q G I O G T A M F I N Z D I K X L S L
Q U C I Z M L N T B Z D E P I D I A Y P
A N Z S N L E P O F G P F A B E L V Z L
I R R E I G A R N D L L Z L X Z L B V A
O U N P B L I J P B O W V A Z Q A E E T
L F A U A I Y V Z V N I Z T I Q S Q V N
B C X T D P K H I S Q B R E E L T U C E
R X E T F C V S Y T B B F E L A M Z M D
H T E E T S U O U D I C E D P N U J S B
N T N E A F X S F V D S V X O A G P Q K
Y L J K F I C H P E U G N O T C L H J C
H C C I S I L S B I V N H I J T E R F V
Q Z X R M Z I T E K D S A L F O R E J N
U Z A Q L F W S L R G S K F D O V E F L
E O V B Y S I T I T A M O T S R O W B Y
U C L E F T P A L A T E M A N D I B L E
```

1. Capillaries
2. Cleft Palate
3. Cuspids
4. Deciduous Teeth
5. Dental Plaque
6. Gingivitis
7. Gum
8. Hard Palate
9. Incisors
10. Mandible
11. Maxilla
12. Mouth
13. Periodontitis
14. Premolars
15. Root Canal
16. Soft Palate
17. Stomatitis
18. Suffix
19. Tongue

# Exercise 11-5

**Directions:** Complete the crossword puzzle by filling in a word from the keywords that fits each clue.

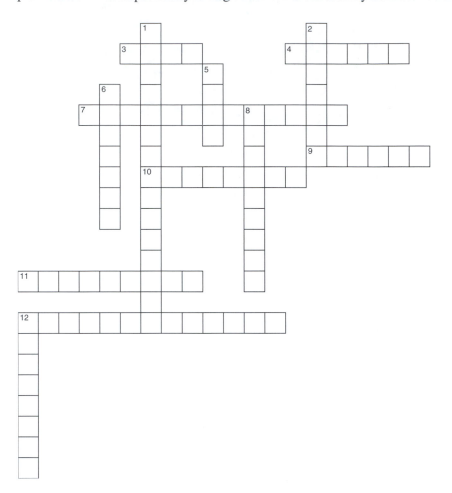

**Across**

3. The portion of the tooth that is embedded in the bone.
4. The beginning portion of a term that modifies the meaning of the root word.
7. Inflammation of a salivary gland.
9. Teeth that are located behind the premolars and have three cusps.
10. A bone-like material that although hard, is not in the same category as the enamel or the dentin.
11. Closure of the teeth.
12. A deep groove in the lip. It is also known as a harelip or cleft lip.

**Down**

1. Cavities that involve three or more surfaces of a tooth.
2. Grinding of the teeth.
5. The terminus or end of the root.
6. The surface nearest to the tongue.
8. Sensory end organs that help carry the sensation of taste to the brain.
12. Calcified dental plaque.

# Exercise 11-6

**Directions:** Match the following terms with the proper definition by writing the letter of the correct definition in the space next to the term.

1. _____ Alveolar Process

2. _____ Ankyloglossia

3. _____ Buccal

4. _____ Cheilitis

5. _____ Compound Cavities

6. _____ Dentin

7. _____ Edentulous

8. _____ Labial

9. _____ Mesial

10. _____ Occlusal

11. _____ Oral Cavity

12. _____ Periodontosis

13. _____ Vestibule

14. _____ Pulp Cavity

15. _____ Root Word

16. _____ Salivary Amylase

17. _____ Simple Cavities

18. _____ Temporomandibular Joint

a. A sliding joint that hinges the lower and upper jaw together.

b. The outer, smaller portion of the mouth surrounded by the lips, cheeks, gums, and teeth.

c. Cavities that involve only one surface of a tooth.

d. The portion of the mandible or maxilla that contains the tooth socket.

e. An oval-shaped cavity.

f. Any degenerative disease of the periodontal tissue.

g. Usually found in the center of a term and identifies the organ or body part involved.

h. The biting surface.

i. An enzyme that helps to break down food molecules.

j. The extreme center of the tooth.

k. Without teeth.

l. The surface nearest the midline. It is an imaginary line drawn between the maxillary centrals and the mandibular centrals.

m. Inflammation of the lips.

n. The surface on the anterior teeth nearest the lip, and the incisal (I).

o. A shortened frenulum of the tongue, preventing proper movement of the tongue.

p. Sometimes called the ivory, which forms the bulk of the tooth.

q. Cavities that involve two surfaces of a tooth.

r. The surface nearest the cheek.

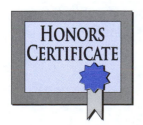

## Honors Certification™

The Honors Certification™ challenge for this chapter consists of a written test of the information contained within this chapter. Each incorrect answer will result in a deduction of up to 5% from your grade. You must achieve a score of 85% or higher to pass this test. If you fail the test on your first attempt, you may retake the test one additional time. The items included in the second test may be different from those in the first test.

# 12
# Dental Plan Provisions
## and Benefit Structures

## After completion of this chapter
**you will be able to:**

- Identify and explain types of dental plans.
- Recognize and define terms related to dental contracts.
- Explain general policy guidelines for processing dental claims.
- Explain benefits and provisions of a given contract.
- Identify and explain common cost containment provisions.
- Identify situations or services that may be covered under major medical provisions.

- Identify the type of treatment as indicated by the provider.
- Identify contract limitations and exclusions.
- List situations or services that often require the requesting of dental x-rays.
- Explain guidelines for using dental x-rays to determine benefits.
- Explain the guidelines for allowance of anesthesia benefits.
- Explain how unspecified or by report procedures are generally handled.

## Keywords and concepts
**you will learn in this chapter:**

- Alternative Benefit Provision (ABP)
- Basic Dental Plan
- Dental Relative Value Study
- Incentive Plans
- Missing and Unreplaced Rule
- Scheduled Dental Plan

The structure of dental plans is similar to the structure of medical plans. The dental portion of a plan may be structured as a Basic plan, a scheduled plan, or an integrated/nonintegrated comprehensive plan.

Initially, Basic medical health plans were developed to cover the most common illnesses or diseases. However, this left the patient without coverage for serious or catastrophic illnesses. To alleviate this problem, Major Medical plans were structured to provide coverage against catastrophic illnesses that were left uncovered by the Basic plans. Finally, dental plans and vision plans were added to cover dental and optometry services.

# Calculating Dental UCR

The allowance for a dental procedure is usually either 100% of a fee schedule or a UCR amount based on the dental relative value study and conversion factors. To determine UCR for a dental procedure, multiply the CDT® code's relative unit value by the appropriate dental conversion factor.

A **dental relative value study** is a scheme used to determine how much a provider should be paid by assessing a unit value to each CDT® code. These values are determined by comparing dental procedure codes to each other in terms of difficulty, time, work, risk, and resources used to perform each procedure. The higher the value assessed, the greater the resources, risk, etc., required to perform the procedure. The dental relative value is multiplied by a conversion factor to determine the allowable amount for a procedure.

A dental conversion factor is a dollar amount based on the geographic area (referred to as region) in which the provider practices. The factors are usually categorized for each class of similar dental procedures. Conversion factors are used to adjust the dental relative value according to geographic locale.

# Types of Dental Plans

Like medical plans, dental plans usually have coinsurance, deductibles, and limitations. However, the major difference between medical plans and dental plans is that dental plans encourage (and therefore, usually cover) preventive care. In addition, many dental plans

pay a higher amount of coinsurance for diagnostic and preventive services than for other services. They may also include an "incentive plan" which encourages participants to make regular visits to their dentist.

## Basic Plans

A **Basic dental plan** pays dental benefits at 100% of either the UCR or a scheduled amount. The UCR can be a set amount, or it can be a sliding scale based on when the service was performed and the geographic area of the provider performing the service. The scheduled amount is a set amount based on the procedure code. It is not contingent on a conversion factor or the location of the provider. As a rule, a Basic dental plan is kept entirely separate from an associated medical plan. That is, if there is a deductible, it is separate from the medical deductible. All dental limitations, exclusions, and maximums are kept separate and unique from the medical provisions. Basic plans are usually easy to process because the exact allowances and procedures are specified in the plan documents.

## Scheduled Dental Plans

In a **scheduled dental plan**, usually no conversion factors are involved. Instead, each CDT® code has a specified dollar amount assigned to it. This dollar allowance applies to the procedure, regardless of where the provider is located or when the procedure is performed. The scheduled allowance never changes unless a plan change is approved to either lower or raise the allowance. Seldom, if ever, are only a few procedures adjusted; usually, there is an overall plan adjustment. Many payers consider a Basic plan and a scheduled plan to be the same and these terms are used interchangeably.

When a scheduled plan is involved, the scheduled allowance is programmed into the computer system so that the examiner simply enters the correct code. For manual claim computation, the examiner would check the schedule listing by code to determine the allowable amount. Deductibles are then subtracted from the scheduled allowances. However, like medical plans, if the scheduled amount exceeds the billed amount, the billed amount is the allowable charge. Generally, scheduled plans allow significantly less than current prevailing charges in most communities.

If a charge is submitted for a procedure that is not listed on the schedule, there are two handling methods:

1. The plan provisions may specify that unlisted procedures are not covered. Consequently, such expenses would be denied as not covered under the plan.

2. Unlisted procedures may be allowable (sometimes based on a dental consultant's review). The amount allowed may be either a specified amount for unlisted procedures or current UCR (or some percentage of current UCR, or the amount billed). The plan provisions must specify which application to use.

Sometimes a Basic dental plan is combined with a scheduled plan, resulting in a scheduled Basic plan. In this case, the variations of the two types of plans will be applied as stipulated by the plan provisions.

## Integrated Dental Plans

The ABC Corporation contract located in Appendix A, is an integrated medical-dental plan. What this means is:

1. There is only one deductible amount for the plan. Any amount applied to the deductible on a dental claim goes towards satisfaction of the one deductible as does any amount applied on a medical claim. In this case, there is a $100 per person deductible, which can include both dental and medical charges.

   a. Notice that the family limit notated on the dental portion of the card is the same as that notated on the medical portion. This is because, as with the individual deductible, the family deductible limit can consist of both medical and dental charges. The first charges processed are the first charges applied toward satisfaction of both the individual and the family deductibles.

   b. The easiest way to think of this type of plan is that limits are considered plan limits, not a medical or dental limit.

2. As with the deductibles, the same logic applies to coinsurance charges. On an integrated plan, the dental coinsurance percentage is usually the same as the medical coinsurance percentage, and amounts applied on dental claims apply toward the plan coinsurance limit as do amounts applied on medical claims.

3. Dental payments apply toward the plan Lifetime Maximum amount. However, the dental portion of the contract usually has a separate calendar year maximum.

4. Benefits are usually based on a UCR basis, with conversion factors, geographic location, and time performed being important.

## Nonintegrated Dental Plans

The XYZ Corporation contract located in Appendix A is a nonintegrated plan. That is, the dental benefits are applied entirely separate from the medical benefits. Each portion of the contract has its own deductible, coinsurance limits, and so on. Only dental charges can be used to satisfy the dental provisions, and only medical charges can be used to satisfy the medical provisions. Therefore, in contrast to an integrated plan, a nonintegrated plan does not have plan limitations; it has dental plan limitations and medical plan limitations with no mixing of the two. Usually, this type of plan uses conversion factors, geographic location, and time performed to determine allowances.

## Preferred Provider Organizations

Some dental insurance plans are administered in a PPO setup. A Preferred Provider Organization (PPO) is a group of healthcare providers who agree to provide services to a specific pool of patients for an agreed fee (contractual). PPOs include doctors, dentists, hospitals, and any provider group that contracts with another entity to provide services at competitive fees. Because the PPO group has agreed to specific benefits, they usually have their own utilization review committees or guidelines to reduce the amount of various services.

## Health Maintenance Organizations

Dental insurance plans are now also available through dental HMOs. These generally operate on the same basic principles as medical HMOs. A Health Maintenance Organization (HMO) is a type of prepayment policy in which the organization bears the responsibility and financial risk of providing agreed-on healthcare services to the members enrolled in its plan, in exchange for a fixed monthly membership fee.

If services are available through the HMO but the insured does not go through the HMO provider, either the benefit will be reduced or the member will be entirely responsible for the payment of care received. Any services provided outside the HMO network must be preapproved by the HMO to be covered. If services are not approved, the HMO usually will not pay the charges.

## Understanding Dental Contracts

The benefits and structure of a dental contract are set up in much the same way as medical contracts with the same types of considerations.

## Covered Expenses

In general, benefits are paid for services that are covered by the plan. The date on which services are rendered is considered the date charges were incurred. Benefits are not payable for services that were performed or begun before the commencement of the plan. In addition, most expenses are subject to an allowable amount based on a table of charges or on what is considered UCR for the time and place of the services.

Most dental contracts specifically list the services that are covered and those that are not covered. They also list the conditions (if any) that must be satisfied for treatment to be covered. These conditions can include:

1. The person who may provide treatment (i.e., licensed dentist, oral surgeon).
2. Coverage of only the least expensive, adequate materials. If other more expensive materials are used, payment will be limited to the allowable amount of the least expensive adequate material.
3. Personalized services or special techniques that are covered at the rate of standard techniques.

## Deductible

Each insured, if applicable, must meet a deductible amount for covered services before any benefits are paid. Any amounts for services that are not covered under the plan or for charges exceeding amounts covered by the plan are not applied toward the deductible.

## Extension of Benefits

As with medical plans, some circumstances allow for an extension of benefits beyond the time when benefits would normally cease or the insured would no longer be eligible for coverage. Extension of benefits can be for the following reasons:

1. An insured is totally disabled at the time coverage would normally end.
2. An insured is confined in a hospital or skilled nursing facility and is considered totally disabled.

In such cases, benefits normally continue until the insured is no longer totally disabled, the maximum benefits have been paid, coverage commences under another plan, or 12 months have elapsed since the time coverage would have ended.

## General Guidelines

Regardless of the method of classification, dental care and treatment provided by most plans is based on the premises covered in the following sections.

### Is Treatment Covered or Excluded?

It is not enough to determine whether a disease or injury requires treatment. It must also be determined that specific services, supplies, or treatment received or planned will correct the condition and restore the mouth to form and function. It must then be determined whether these services, supplies, or treatments are covered under the plan.

Covered services are limited to the listed individual services that will correct or eliminate the specific disease or injury in accordance with recognized professional standards of care. Services not listed or specifically excluded, even when such services are necessary to correct or eliminate disease or injury, may not be considered for coverage.

Covered services vary from plan to plan. For example, periodontal splitting (when specifically excluded), occlusal guards for bruxism (a preventive service not specifically listed), and a crown placed on a tooth with only incipient decay (listed service, but service is not appropriate nor rendered in accordance with recognized professional standards of care for the degree of decay present) may fall into this category.

### Is Treatment Appropriate for the Condition?

The proposed treatment should be appropriate in light of the total existing dental condition. Because so much of what happens in the mouth is interrelated, if part of a disease or injury is left untreated or some of the involved teeth are left untreated, the services provided may be rendered ineffective in a short time. Also, certain treatment approaches may be unrealistic when the total condition of the mouth is considered. Examples are (1) the placement of fixed bridgework where the abutment teeth are diseased and untreated and (2) unreasonable efforts to save teeth, especially for older people who are nearly edentulous.

### Are Services and Supplies of Acceptable Quality?

Materials as well as services are subject to poor quality. Material failure may result from poor laboratory fabrication or poor installation. Service failure may result from improper diagnosis, inadequate preparation, or poor mechanical skills. Examples of substandard quality are root therapy failure due to incomplete extraction of the root pulp and denture or bridgework failure due to poor materials and fabrication.

## What is the Benefit Level?

One of the major problems in providing benefits for dental services is that in dentistry, frequently more than one procedure, material, or technique may be used in accordance with recognized professional standards of care to correct or eliminate a disease or injury. Most dental benefit plans have been designed to provide benefits based on a certain level of care, so that each insured person receives the same benefit level consistent with his or her needs.

The intent of dental plans is to provide benefits for covered services based on a level of dental care that is adequate (when determined in accordance with generally accepted professional standards) for treatment of the existing dental condition. This means that for benefits to be payable, the care and treatment must not be below acceptable standards of quality and appropriateness; it also means that benefits will not be payable for care and treatment that exceeds the level that is adequate and necessary.

Expenses for care above the adequate and necessary level are the patient's responsibility unless specifically listed as payable in the plan provisions.

Moreover, benefits for care above this adequate and necessary level will not be provided, regardless of whether they are provided as a result of the member's or dentist's choice, the limited practice of the dentist, or whether the services have already been provided. The member or dentist is entirely free in the choice of level of care, but this choice will not affect the benefits payable.

## What Treatment Is Required?

Standard dental benefit plans provide benefits for services and supplies that are necessary for the treatment of disease or injury. Following are two examples of some standard wording that may appear in dental plans:

1. "Covered dental expenses are the reasonable charges that a subscriber is required to pay for necessary services received by a covered family member for the treatment of a nonoccupational injury."

2. "Covered dental expenses are the usual charges of a dentist that an employee is required to pay for services and supplies that are necessary for treatment of a dental condition, but only to the extent that such charges are reasonable and customary, as herein defined, for services and supplies customarily used for treatment of that

condition, and only if rendered in accordance with accepted standards of dental practice."

These definitions are supplemented by additional provisions, exclusions, and limitations, both general and specific. Most plans contain provisions similar to one of the following general exclusions:

1. "No insurance is afforded for care, treatment, services, or supplies that are not necessary for the treatment of the injury or disease concerned."

2. "Covered dental expenses do not include and no benefits are payable for charges that are not necessary, according to accepted standards of dental practice."

The intent of dental benefit plans is to provide benefits for covered services and supplies that are necessary to eliminate or correct a dental disease or injury to restore the mouth to reasonable form and function. Not only must there be an existing disease or injury present that requires some treatment, but also the specific service received or planned must be required and the disease or injury must be covered under the plan.

## Prosthetics

Many policies require that the prosthesis replace "natural" teeth. The following are not considered natural teeth:

- Tooth roots, when the condition of the tooth preexisted the effective date of coverage.
- Congenitally missing teeth.
- Diastema (space between two adjacent teeth in the same arch).

The following teeth do not require replacement and are usually not covered:

- Third molars (wisdom teeth) that occupy the third molar position.
- Any tooth that is not in functional occlusion, that is, not opposed by another tooth in the opposite arch.

## Practice
## Pitfalls

**Example:** A denture is replacing teeth #14 and #15, but teeth #18 and #19 (in the opposite arch) are also missing but are not being replaced. Because teeth #14 and #15 will not oppose teeth or prostheses, their replacement will serve no function and thus cannot be considered for coverage.

## Initial Installation

Many plans have a plan limitation called the **"Missing and Unreplaced" rule**. This rule limits coverage for the replacement of teeth that are lost before the patient was covered by the plan. If the prosthesis will replace teeth that were missing prior to coverage and teeth lost while insured, benefits usually are provided for the entire prosthesis unless it represents an unusual attempt to gain benefits for teeth missing prior to coverage. If the plan does not have this limitation, benefits are payable (subject to all other policy limitations) for re-placement of natural teeth whether or not they were extracted while covered. The way this provision works is: If a tooth was missing prior to the effective date of coverage, bridgework, regardless of whether it is permanent or removable, will not be eligible for payment consideration under the plan. This would also include payment for crowns on the abutment teeth, unless the condition of those teeth is such that a crown would be appropriate treatment as covered because of an existing disease condition (decay).

## Practice Pitfalls

For example, suppose that tooth #12 is missing and was extracted before the patient's effective date under the plan. Consequently, if the plan has a Missing and Unreplaced limitation, proceed with the following:

**Step 1.** Determine whether or not the missing tooth is covered.

a. In this case, bridgework to replace tooth #12 would not be allowable (because the tooth was extracted prior to the effective date of coverage).

b. If the tooth was extracted (or lost) after the effective date of coverage, a replacement for that tooth would be covered. If the replacement of a missing tooth is covered, crowning of the abutment teeth (the natural teeth right next to the space where the tooth is missing) is also automatically covered. X-rays are not required to determine whether or not the abutment teeth are decayed.

Remember that if the missing tooth is covered, the abutment teeth are also covered.

**Step 2.** Determine whether or not the abutment teeth are covered.

a. If the missing tooth is not covered, then the abutment teeth need to be evaluated on their own merits. Are these teeth decayed and in need of restoration? X-rays will be required to evaluate this.

b. If restoration is required, is a filling sufficient or is a crown necessary? As a rule, this deter-mination has to be made by a dental consultant or an experienced claims person. If a crown is required, the abutment restorations are covered even though the missing tooth is not covered.

The following represents how these types of claims are generally handled. However, such handling procedures vary greatly from payer to payer:

- If x-rays do not accompany the claim, and no other services reported on the claim would require obtaining x-rays and referring the claim to a dental consultant, then the bridgework should be denied completely as teeth missing prior to coverage. If the claimant or dentist feels that the abutment teeth require crowns for restorative purposes, it is necessary to resubmit for that purpose.

- If x-rays are submitted with the claim or if other procedures would require x-rays and referral to a dental consultant, ask the consultant whether the abutment teeth would require crowns for restorative reasons. If referral to the consultant is not otherwise required and the examiner can tell that a crown would be required, referral is not required. If crowns would be required, they should be benefited as freestanding crowns, not as abutment.

- If x-rays are submitted with the claim and the dental consultant determines that crowns are not needed for restorative reasons, the abutments should be denied along with the pontics.

## Alternative Benefit Plans

Another common dental plan provision that is often applicable to prosthetics is called an **Alternative Benefit Provision (ABP)**. This provision determines the level of care/treatment that can be provided under the plan. Although other restorations are also affected by this provision, it is most frequently associated with prosthetics.

There are two basic types of dental programs that provide benefits based on a specific level of treatment:

1. Plans that have an alternate benefit provision.
2. Plans that do not contain an alternate benefit provision.

**Note:** All plans may not contain the exact wording "alternate benefit provision" or "alternate course treatment;" however; the cumulative wording contained in the provisions indicates the same type of philosophy.

The terminology "alternate benefit" will be used in the following sections when explaining benefit determinations to members and providers. This terminology has been widely misinterpreted by the dental community to mean that the plan is dictating the course of treatment that must be used. That is not the intent. The member or the dentist can choose any method or materials for treatment. However, payment will be based only on what is determined to be the appropriate level of care.

Usually, an Alternative Benefit Provision plan contains wording similar to that indicated in the following:

"Alternate Treatment—If alternate services or supplies may be used to treat a dental condition, covered dental expenses will be limited to the services and supplies that are customarily used nationwide to treat the disease or injury and that are recognized by the profession to be appropriate methods of treatment in accordance with broadly accepted national standards of dental practice, taking into account the family member's total current oral condition."

The "limitations" section may contain examples such as:

"If a cast chrome or acrylic partial denture will restore the dental arch satisfactorily, payment based on the applicable percentage of the reasonable and customary charge for such procedure will be made toward a more elaborate or preci-sion appliance that the patient and dentist may choose to use. The balance of the cost will remain the responsibility of the patient."

The policy may contain a separate section entitled "alternate services," "optional treatment," or "alternate treatment," which details the alternate benefit concept.

The alternate benefit provision has been designed to clearly describe the intent and benefit level of the plans in relation to the various approaches to dental treatment. If an alternate benefit determination is challenged, detailed and conclusive proof from the dentist that an alternate procedure is inadequate would be required. Since professional dental judgment is necessary in such a challenge, the treatment and results of investigations need to be reviewed by a dental consultant.

## Plans Without an Alternate Benefit Provision

The benefit levels for plans that do not contain an alternate benefit provision are controlled by application of the "necessary treatment" provision as well as the "appropriate" provision. As long as the treatment is not inappropriate in light of existing dental conditions, the service will be considered for coverage without regard to the relative costs of the various treatment methods.

## Replacement Provisions

There are normally three provisions in a dental policy, one of which must be satisfied for a replacement prosthesis to qualify for coverage.

1. Additional extractions must occur while the patient is covered under the plan.
2. Five-Year Rule and Unserviceable.
   a. Under the five-year rule, the former prosthesis must be at least five years old and unserviceable. The plan must specify any expectations.
   b. Under some plans, the five-year rule does not apply to replacement of an unserviceable prosthesis under certain conditions (the plan must specify what the conditions are). If the provision is waived, it is usually because the initial prosthesis was not installed under the current dental expense plan.
   c. "Unserviceable" is fairly constant under all policies. The intent of this requirement is that not only is the existing prosthesis unserviceable, but also it cannot "reasonably" be made serviceable by repair, reline, or replacement of specific parts.

"Reasonably" means that the cost of making the prosthesis serviceable versus the cost of replacement makes repair an unreasonable economic choice.

3. Immediate temporary denture and twelve-month rule. For a prosthesis to qualify for replacement under this provision, both of the following requirements must be met:

a. Immediate temporary denture: the existing prosthesis must be constructed of temporary material. Normally, this type of prosthesis is placed until tissue changes have stabilized. The intent of all plans is to provide dentures only once in any five-year period, so usually a temporary is not covered.

b. Twelve-month requirement: this requirement applies without exception whether the immediate temporary denture was installed before or while insured. No exception is usually made under this requirement for replacement that takes place after 12 months have elapsed. When a temporary denture exceeds the 12-month limitation, the denture must meet either the additional extraction or the five-year/unserviceable provision to qualify for replacement benefits.

Any denture constructed of temporary material that is being replaced by a permanent denture can be considered "unserviceable" and in need of replacement. All other policy provisions must be met prior to determining benefits.

## Office Visits

Office visits are generally eligible for coverage if they are for diagnostic purposes. Therefore, these visits are generally paid only when the office visit is billed alone or when it is billed with x-rays or prophylactic treatment. If an office visit is billed (on the same date of service) with any treatment other than prophylaxis or x-rays, it is usually not a covered benefit but is considered part of the normal service. It is presumed that a diagnosis and a plan of treatment were performed prior to the commencement of services.

Any charges for a follow-up review for treatment that occurs on the same day as the procedure is also considered an integral part of the procedure and should be included in the allowance for the procedure itself.

Care should be taken to ensure that this policy limitation is carried out correctly. A patient should not be penalized for failing to delay treatment for which there was no reason for delay. For example, if a cavity is discovered during a patient's routine six-month check-up and the dentist fills the cavity at this time, the office visit should be allowable since it was for diagnostic purposes. Remember that if an office visit is billed with a prophylaxis or with x-rays, generally it is for diagnostic purposes.

Occasionally, the word "Consultation" will appear on a claim. A consultation is the same as an office visit, and the same limitations apply.

## Cost Containment

Containing the costs that the carrier must pay is taken into consideration when writing a plan. Cost containment can include such provisions as predetermination (preauthorization), incentive plans, variable coinsurance, and others listed and explained in the following text.

### Predetermination

Many dental plans stipulate that expenses over a certain amount are not covered unless an estimate of the cost of services is submitted to the insurance carrier prior to the beginning of treatment. Often, this limit is between $100 and $300. Many dental plans also require predetermination for orthodontics and prosthodontics, regardless of the estimated cost.

If predetermination is not obtained, often the plan will not pay more than the predetermination limit, regardless of the amount that would have been allowable for the services.

Predetermination encourages the insured to take an active part in containing the cost of his or her dental care while giving the insured a basis for determining whether the recommended treatment is appropriate. It also discourages dentists from overcharging or prescribing unnecessary treatment because the complete treatment plan and related costs must be submitted prior to the beginning of treatment.

Predetermination is not an authorization to perform the services but merely a statement of what the plan will pay for the listed services. After the predetermination is received, the decision whether or not to authorize treatment is up to the patient. The patient must determine whether the treatment is worth the cost or whether other treatment may be warranted that would cost less money. The determination of benefits usually has a time limit (generally 90 days) during which it is effective. After that time, a new determination of benefits must be requested.

## Practice Pitfalls

**Example:** The plan states that predetermination must be obtained for all services over $300 or a limit of $100 is payable. The amount billed for dental services was $400. The UCR allowance for these services is $430. The coinsurance is 70%, and all deductibles have been satisfied.

If predetermination was obtained, the plan would pay 70% of $400, or $280. The member would be responsible for $120.

If predetermination was not obtained, the plan would pay only the $100 limit. The member would be responsible for $300.

## Incentive Plans

**Incentive plans** encourage regular dental care, thus decreasing the possibility that a minor problem will remain untreated until it becomes a major problem. Incentive plans usually work by increasing the coinsurance percentage for each year in which the insured saw a dentist. For example, during the first year of coverage the coinsurance may be paid at 70%. If the insured visited the dentist during that year, during the second year of coverage the coinsurance would be paid at 80%. If the insured visited the dentist the first and second year, the third year coinsurance would be 90% and so on. Usually, failure to visit a dentist (for any reason) during a given year will cause the loss of the increased coinsurance for the following year. In essence, the increased coinsurance is a reward for taking care of one's teeth.

In addition, the incentive programs may be limited by the type of coverage they provide. For example, many incentive programs apply only to preventive services and not to crowns, inlays, onlays, prosthodontics, and orthodontics.

## Variable Coinsurance

Some dental plans vary the amount paid for different services. For example, they may pay 85% for preventive services, 65% for fillings and routine dentistry, 60% for prosthodontics services, and 50% for orthodontic services. This type of payment situation encourages the insured to seek treatment for a minor problem before it becomes a major one.

Preventive services can include not only regular diagnostic procedures (bi-annual check-ups), but also prophylaxis and even space maintainers to prevent the drifting of teeth.

## Annual Maximums

Dental plans often have an annual maximum rather than a lifetime maximum. Once the "calendar year" limit has been reached, additional services are not covered. Often, dental plan maximums are much lower than major medical maximums. The average dental plan maximum is $1,000, whereas major medical maximums can often be as high as $1,000,000.

There are two exceptions to the annual maximum that are noteworthy:

1. If orthodontic work is covered, there is often a separate lifetime maximum. Some carriers allow only a portion of the lifetime maximum to be paid in any given year. This prevents someone from joining the plan, having expensive orthodontic work done, and then canceling the plan.

2. When dental coverage is integrated with medical coverage, then the dental coverage is often (but not always) considered part of the major medical lifetime maximum. In such a case, annual dental maximums are often eliminated.

## Frequency Limitations

Many dental plans limit the frequency of certain treatments. For example, only one routine oral examination and set of bitewing x-rays may be allowable during a six-month period. The following are other common frequency limitations:

1. Full-mouth x-rays may be allowable only once every 24 to 36 months.
2. Prophylaxis may be limited to twice a year.
3. The five-year and unserviceable rule (see previous text under Replacement Provisions) will be in effect for crowns, jackets, gold or cast restorations, bridgework, and dentures.
4. Appliances to control harmful habits are usually limited to a single appliance with no allowance made for repair or replacement.

## Waiting Period

Many insurers include a waiting period within their contract for certain dental services. This reduces the likelihood that payments will be made for preexisting conditions and that the insured will join the plan just to have expensive treatment covered. The waiting period can be anywhere from three months to one year. Services that may be subject to the waiting period include fixed or removable prosthetics and cast restorations.

## Exclusions

It is not uncommon for dental plans to exclude treatment with a high potential for abuse. The following 17 services are generally not covered by dental plans:

1. Cosmetic dentistry or services for comfort or hygiene.
2. Replacement of lost or stolen appliances.
3. Replacement of teeth that were missing before the insured joined the plan.
4. Treatment started before commencement of coverage under the plan.
5. Tooth implants.
6. Orthodontics may be covered by some plans with the payment of additional premiums.
7. Tooth wear. Over time, the surfaces of the teeth may be worn away due to bruxism or normal wear and tear on the teeth.
8. Charges over the allowable amount.
9. Charges covered by a Workers' Compensation plan.
10. Charges for which the insured would not be obligated to pay or for which there would be no charge if the patient were not insured.
11. Charges for treatment received in a U.S. government hospital or provided by a local, state, or federal government agency.
12. Charges for services that were rendered by a relative (whether by blood or marriage) or by someone who lives in the insured's home.
13. Charges for which a third party is liable or legally responsible.
14. Experimental procedures.
15. Dietary planning or oral hygiene instruction.
16. Wars or acts of God or those for which the underlying cause of the damage was due to nuclear energy.
17. Charges for filling out claim forms.

Some exclusions are listed under the heading "Exclusions" in a contract; however, others may be listed throughout the benefit provisions. It is important to read the contract carefully to determine the proper benefits.

## Second Dental Opinion

Questionable services may need to be evaluated by an independent dentist prior to commencement of treatment. The second dentist is usually selected by the plan, and the patient is referred to this dentist.

The first dentist is usually sent a form to fill out, stating the condition and the proposed treatment. This form is then sent to the second dentist or is taken by the patient. The second dentist will complete the examination and provide a report. These reports help the plan to make a determination of the covered expenses and allowable amounts for the services.

Since the second dental opinion is sought by the plan, the responsibility for payment of the consultation rests solely with the plan. The member is not charged for the consultation.

## Medical Review

Services that have a high abuse rate are often referred to a dental consultant or a prescreener prior to payment. The dental consultant determines the necessity of the procedures and makes recommendation for payment.

Before sending a claim to the dental consultant, the claims examiner should gather all of the necessary information for the dental consultant to make the determination of benefits. These items include the claim, any operative reports, and all x-rays.

Most payers have an itemized list of services that should be sent to the dental consultant before processing. Services on this list can include:

1. Temporomandibular joint procedures or services.
2. By report or relatively not established (RNE) procedures.
3. Multiple fillings (five or more on one claim).
4. Crown restorations, build-ups or posts, or any repairs to crowns.
5. Inlays and onlays.
6. Root canal therapy and apicoectomies.
7. Periodontal services.
8. Prosthodontics (partial dentures and bridges).
9. Multiple extractions (four or more on one claim).
10. Surgical extractions (including impactions).
11. Tests and pathologic exams.
12. Acid-etch restorations.
13. Bonding or sealants.
14. Surgical procedures.
15. Palliative treatments.
16. General anesthesia charges.

After review, the claim is returned to the claims examiner with the determination of benefits included. The claims examiner may then adjudicate the claim.

## Required Participation

Many dental plans require a high participation rate among the eligible insureds in a plan. For example, a dental plan may require that 95% to 100% of the eligible employees in a company must take the dental plan for it to become effective for the entire group. If the participation level drops below the required percentage, dental coverage for all plan members is suspended.

Other dental plans require the employer to contribute 100% of the cost of the plan for their employees. This nearly ensures that 100% of the employees will enroll in the dental plan since there is no cost for coverage.

## Late Enrollment Penalties

Often people delay enrolling in a dental program until they are in need of dental services. This allows them to gain benefits with little or no contribution into the plan. To help discourage this, some plans specify that if an employee enrolls more than 30 days after they are eligible to enroll, many benefits will be limited to 50% of the amounts otherwise payable. In addition, some plans drastically reduce the calendar year maximum during the first year, even to as low as $100.

## Coordination of Benefits

Most dental plans carry a coordination of benefits clause, which states that benefits will be reduced if the member has other coverage (whether dental or medical) for services. Most plans stipulate that total benefits payable by both plans are not to exceed 100% of the charges.

# Major Medical Coverage for Dental Procedures

While most procedures performed on the mouth or teeth are covered under dental plans, some may be covered under Major Medical plans. This holds true even though the services were performed by a dentist or an oral surgeon rather than an M.D. These can include the following services:

1. Accidental injury to the teeth (see section on dental accidents).
2. Surgery to remove impacted, unerupted, or supernumerary teeth. Major Medical benefits are generally paid in the case of tissue-impacted, partly bone-impacted, or totally bone-impacted teeth.

# On the Job Now

**Directions:** Answer the following questions without looking back at the material just covered. Write your answers in the space provided.

1. What services does predetermination authorize a dentist to perform? _____

_____

2. What are the four common frequency limitations? _____

   1. _____

   2. _____

   3. _____

   4. _____

3. Why are services referred to a dental consultant or a prescreener prior to payment? _____

_____

3. Jawbone surgery.
4. Tumors or cysts within the oral cavity.
5. Nasal, auricular, orbital, or ocular prosthesis.
6. Obturators or repair of the cleft palate.
7. Complex, subperiosteal, or endosseous implants.
8. Lab charges such as urinalysis, hemoglobin, hematocrit, and complete blood count.
9. Repair of fractures of the mandible, maxilla, or facial bones.

If a specific service is covered under the Major Medical portion of the plan, then all related services (such as exams and x-rays) are also covered under the Major Medical plan.

Other services that may or may not be covered under a Major Medical policy include:

1. **Emergency room benefits.** If emergency services are necessary and a dentist is not available, benefits may be allowable under the medical plan.

2. **Hospital and anesthesia benefits.** If hospital confinement is necessary for dental services, some plans allow Major Medical coverage for the hospital expense. Anesthesia expenses are usually covered for services that require hospitalization. Anesthesia charges are not usually covered for outpatient services. Hospital confinement may be necessary because of the severity of the condition or because of underlying factors. For example, if a patient has a history of hemophilia or unstable diabetes, because of the possible complications arising from the surgery the hospital benefit is usually paid. When hospital benefits are covered under Major Medical, the physician's or dentist's fees are still covered under the dental plan.

3. **Oral-antral fistulas.** Oral-antral fistulas are unnatural openings between the oral and nasal cavities. If the opening occurs as a result of dental treatment (i.e., tooth extraction where the root has penetrated the sinuses), then the services would be considered dental. However, if the opening is treated after a six-week period, it may be considered a medical expense even though the cause was tooth-related. This occurs because the delayed closure is usually the result of disease or infection. If the fistula is not a result of a dental condition, the cause of the fistula should be indicated (i.e., tumor, disease). In such cases, Major Medical benefits usually cover the services.

4. **Gross misalignment of the jaws.** Often, pretreatment study models and an operative report should be requested to assist in the determination of coverage. If the surgery is a covered expense, it is often covered under both medical and dental plans. The claim usually needs to be referred to a supervisor or a medical review committee for determination of coverage.

5. **Other surgical services.** The following surgeries may be covered under dental or medical benefits, depending on the plan: reduction of fractures to the mandible or maxilla, tumors or cysts of the gums or mouth, alveolectomy (due to a nondental condition), cleft palate or similar medical condition, and nondental bone surgery.

6. **Cobalt therapy-related services.** Cobalt or x-ray therapy causes damage to the teeth and tissues of the oral cavity. Dental services that are necessary due to cobalt or x-ray therapy are generally covered as medical.

7. **Prescriptions and injections.** Prescriptions and injections that are generally covered for nondental services are usually also covered when prescribed by a dentist or oral surgeon.

Occasionally, an orthodontic appliance (i.e., banding, braces) is used immediately before or after surgery. This appliance is often used as a splint. In this case, the appliance would be covered. However, care must be taken to ensure that the appliance is being used for splinting purposes and not for orthodontic purposes. Appliances used for orthodontic purposes would not be covered unless specifically indicated by the contract.

If a dental service is covered under Major Medical, some payers convert the ADA codes into the appropriate CPT® or HCPCS codes and then apply the appropriate UCR conversion. The specific company and plan guidelines vary widely regarding Major Medical coverage for dental services and should be consulted prior to claim processing.

## Dental Accidents

Many carriers cover accidental injury to permanent natural teeth under medical benefits. For the injury to qualify as an accident, you should be able to place the exact date, time, and place at which the accident occurred. However, damage due to chewing or biting is generally not considered accidental.

Under the provisions of most contracts, the teeth must be permanent natural teeth which were in place prior to the accident. Often dentures, partials, or "nonnatural" teeth are excluded. In this case, if there was damage to the pontic and the adjoining abutment teeth, the abutment teeth would be covered but the pontic would not. However, if the teeth were evulsed (knocked out) as the result of an accident, fixed or removable prosthetics may be covered as "required to alleviate the damage." Likewise, deciduous teeth are often not covered since they are not permanent teeth.

Some plans may restrict payment to "sound" natural teeth. The term "sound" natural teeth defines teeth that are in good condition, without substantial restoration, fractures, cracks, extensive decay, or damage due to periodontal disease. The "good condition" clause applies to the crown of the tooth and also to the root structure and the supporting structures of the tooth.

If a plan contains the wording "sound natural teeth," the presence of a fracture, large restorations, and other serious conditions may be grounds for denial of services. It may be necessary to obtain pre-accident x-rays of the tooth or teeth to determine whether or not they would be considered "sound."

# On the Job Now

**Directions:** Answer True or False to the following questions without looking back at the material just covered. Write your answers in the space provided.

1. _____ An M.D. needs to perform services on the mouth or teeth for the services to be covered under Major Medical plans.

2. _____ While a specific service is covered under the Major Medical portion of the plan, all related services (such as exams and x-rays) may not be covered.

3. _____ Prescriptions and injections that are generally covered for nondental services are never covered when prescribed by a dentist or oral surgeon.

4. _____ For the injury to qualify as an accident, you should be able to place the exact date, time, and place at which the accident occurred.

5. _____ Damage due to chewing or biting is generally considered accidental.

## Temporary Restorations

Occasionally, temporary restorations may be needed during the course of dental treatment. The most common reasons for temporary restorations are:

1. When the patient has extensive caries and several treatments may be required. The dentist removes the decay and inserts a temporary filling to seal the hole. This prevents further decay from taking place.

2. When caries are extensive, a temporary filling allows the formation of reparative dentin and seals the hole from exposure to bacteria. In this case, the temporary restoration may prevent the need for more extensive orthodontic treatment.

3. Cavities may need to be sealed during endodontic therapy.

Generally, temporary fillings are not covered. They are considered a necessary part of permanent dental treatment and, therefore, are included in the allowable amount of the covered dental expense. Some dental services (i.e., fixed restorations) normally involve several visits to the dentist over a period of time. Therefore, temporary fillings cover the prepared teeth during the fabrication of the restoration.

## X-Rays

X-rays (also called radiographs) are taken because it is impossible to tell the extent of tooth damage by visual examination alone. X-rays are paid as diagnostic procedures, regardless of the licensure of the person performing the x-rays (i.e., dentist, oral surgeon). X-rays are billed individually according to their type and whether they were intraoral or extraoral (inside the mouth or outside the mouth).

Fourteen or more films that are done on the same day are considered a full-mouth x-ray and should be paid at the full-mouth x-ray rate. In addition, any combination of individual x-rays with a combined RVS unit value greater than that of a full-mouth x-ray should be paid at the full-mouth x-ray rate.

Occasionally, the examiner needs to request x-rays of an insured's teeth from the dentist to aid in determining the extent of damage and the amount of benefits that will be covered.

X-rays may be needed to help determine whether the work is cosmetic, to assist in determination of benefits, to aid in determining preexisting conditions, to aid in determining degrees and types of impactions or supernumerary teeth, to locate and identify tumors, cysts, or abscesses of the mouth, to evaluate the need for orthodontic treatment, and to review damage present as the result of an accident.

## Practice Pitfalls

In general, the following situations or services require the requesting of x-rays:

1. By report or RNE procedures (usually).
2. Multiple fillings (usually five or more billed on the same claim).
3. Crown restorations, buildups or posts.
4. Inlays and onlays.
5. Root canal therapy and apicoectomies.
6. Periodontal services.
7. Prosthodontics (partial dentures and bridges).
8. Multiple extractions (usually four or more billed on one claim).
9. Surgical extractions (including impactions).

The claims examiner is not expected to be able to determine the need for services from the x-rays. Reading x-rays requires extensive training and experience. However, the claims examiner can make a cursory examination of the x-rays and try to determine the benefits payable. In reviewing x-rays, claims personnel, as lay persons, can expect only to see where teeth are missing and to identify impacted teeth (but not the degree of impaction), malposed teeth, supernumerary teeth, mixed dentition, extensive caries, existing restorations, some forms of abscesses, and perhaps evidence of the need for orthodontics. It requires a professional consultant to read and interpret x-rays for other than the most evident condition.

A processor or analyst, on reviewing x-rays, can approve benefits, but a dental consultant's opinion is required for all denials that require a professional opinion. No person other than a dental consultant can recommend that benefits be reduced or denied unless the denial is based on plan limitations or exclusions. The following guidelines will assist in the use of x-rays to determine benefits:

1. If caries appear on x-rays, benefits should be allowable for restorations (fillings).
2. If the caries are deep or extensive, benefits are usually allowable for restorations or crowns.
3. If teeth are missing, benefits should be allowable for prosthetics (fixed or removable).
4. If there are no teeth (the insured is edentulous), benefits are usually payable for full dentures.
5. If several teeth are missing (especially several adjacent teeth), a dental consultant should review any planned bridgework.
6. If there is extensive bone loss, restorative procedures or bridgework near the site of the bone loss should be evaluated by a dental consultant.
7. If treatment is planned and the claims examiner is unable to see the need for treatment, services should be evaluated by the dental consultant.

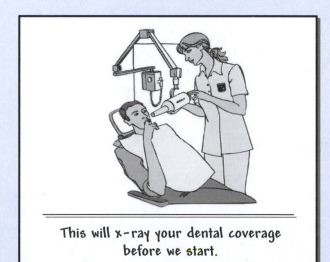

This will x-ray your dental coverage
before we start.

Remember that damage or decay is usually more extensive than that shown on an x-ray. For example, treatment or replacement may be recommended for an existing restoration or crown, but the decay may be hidden beneath the restoration or crown on the x-ray (x-rays do not penetrate many crown and filling materials and therefore, these show up as dark spots on a radiograph).

Some materials do not show up on x-rays. In this case, a tooth that looks as if it needs treatment may already have been treated. As a general rule, if the sides are rough or irregular, restoration has not been done. Smooth sides usually indicate prior treatment.

X-rays belong to the dentist and should be returned as soon as possible, preferably within one week of receiving them. At no time should x-rays be held for longer than two weeks without a letter or call to the dentist to explain the delay and request permission to hold the x-rays for a longer period of time. At all times, x-rays should be handled with care.

## Orthodontic X-Rays

If a general dentist takes x-rays to determine the need for orthodontics, the x-rays would generally be covered if orthodontic treatment is not covered. In this case, x-rays are used as a diagnostic tool to determine the need for orthodontic treatment. Policies that exclude orthodontic treatment would exclude all orthodontic services performed after the need for orthodontic services has been established, regardless of whether they were performed by the originating dentist or whether the insured was referred to an orthodontist for continued treatment.

To determine whether an x-ray is for the diagnosis of orthodontic treatment or a part of the orthodontic service, the following guidelines can be used:

1. If the date of service for the x-rays is prior to the commencement of orthodontic services, x-rays should be allowable as diagnostic.
2. If the date of service for the x-rays is after the commencement of orthodontic services, x-rays should be considered part of the orthodontic services.

## Anesthesia

Anesthesia is usually required for most dental services other than x-rays, prophylaxis, and exams. The four types of anesthesia most commonly used for dental services are:

1. Local anesthesia.
2. Intravenous sedation.
3. Analgesia (nitrous oxide, twilight sleep).
4. General anesthesia.

Local anesthesia is the most commonly used anesthesia and is appropriate for most dental procedures. Local anesthesia can be identified as local anesthesia (D9210 or D9215), regional block anesthesia (D9211), or trigeminal division block anesthesia (D9212). The allowances for local anesthesia are included in the allowance for the basic procedure, so no additional payment is provided for this service.

Intravenous sedation (D9241) and analgesia (D9230) are usually allowable only for surgical extractions or for four or more simple extractions performed during the same visit (intravenous sedation renders the patient semiconscious). Many plans also allow intravenous and analgesic anesthesia for any dental services performed on a patient less than 12 years of age. No permit is required for analgesic or intravenous sedation.

If intravenous sedation or analgesia is performed for other than the previously mentioned services and on a patient above 12 years of age, the allowance for anesthesia (if any) may be awarded.

## Sedative Fillings

Medicated or sedative fillings are considered to be temporary. As a rule, they may not be covered; the final restoration may be the only covered expense. If the medicated or sedative filling is done on the same day as the final restoration, it is usually considered a base and is combined with the charge for the final restoration, since the final should include the base. The combined charge would then be subjected to any UCR limitation based on the coding for the final restoration. If the final restoration is a crown and not a filling, the medicated or sedative filling may be allowable separately. This varies by administrator.

## Cosmetic Services

Remember that even if a particular service is cosmetic and "excluded," the cost of the noncosmetic, less expensive service may be allowable and that amount would be applied toward the cost of the more expensive service. Most plans are subject to the following exclusions:

1. Cosmetic services, such as crowns that are not necessary because of disease or injury. This also includes the use of composite fillings on posterior teeth, bleaching of stains from the teeth, using crowns to straighten or align teeth in an arch, and so on.

2. Precision attachments are usually excluded from consideration. They tend to be significantly more expensive than conventional clasps, with no more usefulness.

3. Characterization or personalization of dentures. Dentures can be custom-designed to include such features as staining or selected duplication of gold restorations that were present prior to the need for dentures.

Procedures that are considered wholly cosmetic include labial veneer (laminate) and bleaching of discolored teeth.

## Unspecified and By Report Procedures

Unspecified procedures are codes that classify services that are not specifically listed in the related section of the CDT® code list. There is an individual code for each section of the CDT® code list. These codes usually end in 99.

### Practice Pitfalls

**For example:**

D0999—unspecified diagnostic procedure

D3999—unspecified endodontic procedure

By report (BR) or relativity not established (RNE) procedures are procedures for which a unit value has not been assigned. This is usually because a procedure is new or not performed often enough for sufficient data to be collected to establish a unit value.

Generally, the payer places a dollar limit on unspecified and BR/RNE procedures. Any claims for unspecified or BR/RNE procedures that fall below this dollar limit are allowed as billed. Any claims above this limit need to be sent to the review board to determine benefits. A common dollar amount is $100 to $150.

# CHAPTER REVIEW

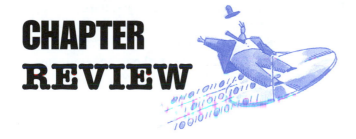

## Summary

- Although there can be multiple variations on all types of dental plans, as a rule, dental plans are easy to understand and apply.

- Missing and Unreplaced, Predetermination of Benefits, Alternate Course of Treatment, and Five-Year Replacement Rule are universal and generally apply to most plans, regardless of whether the plan is basic, scheduled, integrated, or nonintegrated.

- The claims examiner should read the plan provisions to find out how to apply the benefits and what type of plan it is.

## Assignments

Complete the Questions for Review.
Complete Exercise 12–1.
Read through the dental sections of the ABC and XYZ Contracts in Appendix A to be sure you understand them.

## Questions for Review

**Directions:** Answer the following questions without looking back at the material just covered. Write your answers in the space provided.

1. (True or False?) On an integrated plan, dental charges can be applied to the medical calendar year deductible.

_____

2. Usually, on a Basic plan the fees are not dependent on _____ nor _____

**3.** What are the four types of anesthesia most commonly used for dental services?

1. _____

2. _____

3. _____

4. _____

**4.** On a scheduled plan, an unlisted procedure may be handled in the following two ways:

1. _____

2. _____

**5.** (True or False?) The charges for local anesthesia are included in the allowable amount for the procedure. _____

If you were unable to answer any of these questions, refer back to that section and then fill in the answers.

# Exercise 12-1

**Directions:** Match the following terms with the proper definition by writing the letter of the correct definition in the space next to the term.

1. _____ Alternative Benefit Provision

2. _____ Basic Dental Plan

3. _____ Missing and Unreplaced Rule

4. _____ Scheduled Dental Plan

5. _____ Incentive Plans

a. Plans that encourage regular dental care, thus decreasing the possibility that a minor problem will remain untreated until it becomes a major problem.

b. This provision determines the level of care/treatment that can be provided under the plan.

c. Usually no conversion factors are involved. Instead, each CDT® code has a specified dollar amount assigned to it.

d. Pays dental benefits at 100% of either the UCR or a scheduled amount

e. This rule limits coverage for the replacement of teeth that are lost before the patient was covered by the plan.

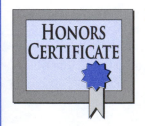

## Honors Certification™

The Honors Certification™ challenge for this chapter consists of a written test of the information contained within this chapter. Each incorrect answer will result in a deduction of up to 5% from your grade. You must achieve a score of 85% or higher to pass this test. If you fail the test on your first attempt, you may retake the test one additional time. The items included in the second test may be different from those in the first test.

# 13

# Dental Services
## and Coding

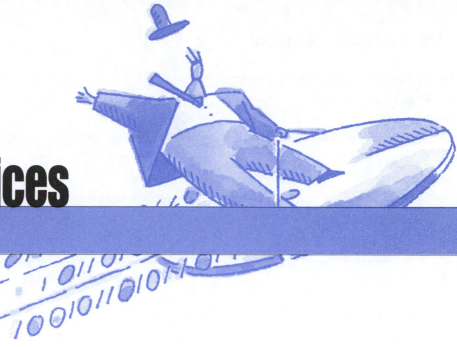

## After completion of this chapter
### you will be able to:

- Identify the four pathologic conditions that require treatment.
- Identify and explain the different types of dental services that are performed.
- Identify services that fall within certain ranges to determine the types of services rendered.
- Identify the common procedures in a given type.
- Explain how codes are broken down and when specific codes should be used.
- Identify the most common types of materials used for fillings.
- State and explain the different types of crowns.
- List the most common materials used for crowns.

- Locate the number of roots in a given tooth.
- Identify types of full and partial dentures.
- Identify different types of dental anesthesia.
- Explain what temporomandibular joint dysfunction is and describe possible treatments for the condition.
- Recognize and define terms related to diagnosis and treatment of TMJ.
- Identify which treatments are accepted and which are not accepted for TMJ dysfunction.
- State the guidelines that generally apply when processing TMJ claims.

## Keywords and concepts
### you will learn in this chapter:

- Abscess
- Abutment
- Adjunctive General Services
- Alveoloplasty
- Apexification
- Appliance
- Banding Fee

- Bitewing X-Rays
- Crown
- Cyst
- Dentistry
- Dentists
- Diagnostic
- Diagnostic Casts

- Diagnostic Photographs
- Distoclusion
- Endodontics
- Extraoral X-Rays
- Filling Restorations
- Fluoride Treatments
- Full Dentures

- Full-mouth X-Ray Limitation
- Impacted Tooth
- Implant
- Inlay
- Intraoral X-Rays
- Jump
- Labial Veneer
- Lingual Bar
- Maxillofacial Prosthetics
- Medicated Filling
- Mesioclusion
- Neoplasm
- Neutroclusion
- Occlusal X-Rays
- Onlay
- Oral Surgery
- Orthodontics

- Ostectomy
- Palatal Bar
- Palliative Treatment
- Periodontics
- Pin Retention
- Pontic
- Preventive Services
- Prophylaxis
- Prosthodontics
- Prosthodontics, Fixed
- Prosthodontics, Removable
- Pulp Capping
- Pulpectomy
- Pulpotomy
- Radiographs
- Rebase
- Removal of Exostosis

- Restoration
- Restorative
- Retainer
- Root Canal
- Sealants
- Seating
- Sequestrectomy for Osteomyelitis
- Space Maintenance
- Surgical Excision
- Temporary Dentures
- Temporomandibular Joint (TMJ) Dysfunction
- Tissue Conditioning
- Tumors
- Vestibuloplasty

---

The terms dentistry and dental are derived from the Latin word *dens*, meaning tooth. **Dentistry** is officially that department of the healing arts that is concerned with the teeth, the oral cavity (mouth), and its associated structures. This includes diagnosis, treatment, restoration, and replacement of missing portions or parts. It also includes surgical procedures performed in and about the inside of the mouth or oral cavity.

## Dental Professionals

**Dentists** are doctors who have received a Doctor of Medical Dentistry (D.M.D) degree. Other recognized titles and degrees include:

D.D.S.    Doctorate in Dental Surgery (DMD and DDS are graduate degrees)

F.A.C.D.  Fellow of American College of Dentists

F.A.G.D.  Fellow of the Academy of General Dentistry

F.I.C.D.  Fellow of the International College of Dentists, an English degree with international recognition

M.D.S.    Master of Dental Science

Diplomas are also awarded to dentists who have met the criteria for certification as a specialist in a chosen field. For the purposes of this book, we will use the term dentist to refer to all of the previous examples.

## Dental Treatment

In dentistry, the following four pathologic conditions require treatment:

1. Tooth decay.
2. Tissue or periodontal disease.
3. Trauma to teeth (including loss of teeth) or supporting structures.
4. Development diseases such as cysts, tumors, and abscesses.

Services are also performed in dentistry for other than existing pathologic conditions. Some of these services (such as prophylaxis, x-rays, fluoride treatments, and repair of dentures and bridgework) are specifically included as covered dental services under most plans but are usually subject to limitations.

Other services may be performed not for pathologic conditions but primarily for cosmetic or similar reasons. They may also be elective procedures of the patient or dentist. Although the particular type or category of service that is received might be covered under the plan, benefits are usually not provided for services performed for cosmetic or similar purposes, or for elective services. An example would be the placing of the crowns on healthy teeth that require no restoration. In other words, the crowns are placed to improve the appearance of the tooth's color or shape.

# Dental Coding

In the late 1960s, the American Dental Association (ADA) created a coding system that served to categorize dental services. This system also established a uniform nomenclature for all dental services. The ADA listing classifies procedures under certain categories. Services (and thus their codes) are defined based on the type of treatment provided. Following is a list of the ADA categories. Most dental plans separate services into similar classifications.

**Diagnostic**—Routine services designed to assist in the diagnosis and planning of required treatment.

**Preventive**—Routine services designed to prevent decay, gum disease, and so on, through the care of the dental structures before disease has occurred.

**Restorative**—Treatment involving the use of fillings or crowns to save or restore dental structures.

**Endodontics**—Treatment of dental pulp or other internal structures of the teeth.

**Periodontics**—Treatment of the tissues surrounding and supporting the teeth.

**Prosthodontics, Removable**—Replacement of the natural teeth through the use of a removable appliance(s).

**Maxillofacial Prosthetics**—Treatment of congenital and acquired defects of the head and neck.

**Implant Services**—An artificial tooth root placed into the jaw to hold a replacement tooth or bridge in place.

**Prosthodontics, Fixed**—Replacement of the natural teeth through the use of a permanent appliance(s).

**Oral and Maxillofacial Surgery**— Treatment of the internal structures of the mouth limited to the dental structures and surrounding tissues.

**Orthodontics**—Correction or prevention of poor or misaligned teeth.

**Adjunctive General Services**—Miscellaneous services, treatments not listed elsewhere.

It is important to know what type of service is being performed in order to code it properly. Not all plans, insurers, or dental offices code claims according to the ADA code list. Many have developed their own version of the list. However, most of these lists are based on the format of the ADA code list.

The main differences that may often be noted include:

1. Dental visits and anesthesia services are given their own section because these services are the most often rendered. Some dental lists also include a section for drugs.

2. Many insurance carrier or plan lists omit codes in areas they do not routinely cover. Such areas usually include orthodontic services, fractures, and dislocations.

Regardless of the differences, it is important for the health claims examiner to become familiar with the types of services since nearly all dental code lists fall under categories similar to the ADA list.

In the following sections we will discuss the treatments covered under each ADA category. It may be helpful to obtain a current ADA Dental Code Listing or a similar listing.

# Diagnostic Services

Diagnostic procedures are those that are necessary to properly determine the most appropriate course of treatment for the patient's condition. The CDT® codes for this category are D0100–D0999.

## Clinical Oral Evaluations (D0120–D0180)

A clinical oral examination is the examination of the mouth by a dentist. Oral examinations are coded by the level of service performed, similar to CPT® coding.

## Radiographs (D0210–D0350)

**Radiographs** are x-rays of the mouth and teeth. The first code is for a full-mouth set of x-rays. Following that are intraoral mouth x-rays and extraoral mouth x-rays. **Intraoral x-rays** are taken with the film placed inside the mouth. **Extraoral x-rays** are taken with the film placed outside the mouth. **Bitewing x-rays** have separate listings for one film, two films, three films, four films, and seven to eight films. Bitewing x-rays show the relationship of the teeth in two opposing dental arches.

In addition, **occlusal x-rays** are larger x-rays (2.5 × 3 inches), which show the floor of the mouth and the palate. An occlusal x-ray shows the lingual (next to the tongue) side of the teeth and a portion of the palate. Its purpose is to aid in locating impacted teeth, bone fractures, cysts, and salivary duct disorders.

In each case, coding is made by the number of films taken. The first film would be coded individually; any additional films taken would be listed under the additional code(s). The exception is for bitewings.

In many plans, there are limitations regarding the number of bitewing or other x-rays that may be taken during a given period of time. The plan should always be checked for such limitations. In addition, many plans have a **full-mouth x-ray limitation**. This means that if the dollar amount payable for the total number of x-rays taken exceeds the dollar amount payable for a set of full-mouth x-rays, the allowable amount would be based on the full-mouth x-ray allowance because the dentist could have taken an entire x-ray series to see all tooth structures.

Certain conditions may require posteroanterior and lateral skull and facial bone survey films. These are usually covered only under orthodontic services or TMJ conditions. These films include the following:

- **Posteroanterior and Lateral Skull and Facial Bone Survey Films.** This set of films shows the architecture, size, density, contouring, and positioning of the skull bones. One film shows height and width, and the second shows height and depth. When used together, they provide a nearly three-dimensional picture. Various views can be selected, including the Towne View, the Waters View, and the Basal View. This is usually covered only under orthodontic services or TMJ conditions.

- **Sialography.** This x-ray allows inspection of the salivary glands and ducts. A radiopaque medium (radioactive dye) is injected and enables the x-ray to show any obstructions or blockages (stones) in the salivary glands or ducts. This examination is most often performed by an otorhinolaryngologist (ear, nose, and throat specialist) in a hospital setting. It is usually performed only for a saliva problem or for a suspected cyst or tumor of the salivary glands.

- **Temporomandibular Joint Film.** The TMJ film allows inspection of the temporomandibular joint and its function. It is usually covered only when TMJ is a covered benefit or when there are orthodontic problems.

- **Panoramic Maxilla and Mandible Film (Panorex).** This is a large x-ray that shows all teeth, the surrounding alveolar bone, the sinuses, and the TMJ all on one film. It helps to show tooth spacing or crowding as well as impacted teeth and jaw fractures. Periodontists use panoramic x-rays to determine the condition of the supporting structures of the teeth. Most plans consider it the same as a full-mouth x-ray and subject to the same guidelines. It is usually covered once every three years.

- **Cephalometric Film.** This is an extraoral x-ray done with a cephalometer. The cephalometer is an instrument that holds the patient's head in position while at the same time measuring the bony structure of the head. The cephalometric film provides the greatest dimensional accuracy. It is used in conjunction with orthodontics or TMJ disorders and is usually covered for orthodontic or TMJ conditions.

- **Intraoral X-rays** include periapicals, bitewings, full-mouth series, and occlusal x-rays.

- **Extraoral X-rays** include Panorex and cephalometrics.

## Tests, Oral Pathology Laboratory, and Other Services (D0415–D0999)

Occasionally, laboratory tests are needed to help determine a specific disease or patient condition. These tests include the following:

- Bacteriologic studies for determination of pathologic agents.
- Caries susceptibility tests.
- Pulp vitality tests.
- Diagnostic casts.

Laboratory tests are often covered under medical plans as well as dental plans. Therefore, specific policy guidelines should be consulted to ensure proper payment.

Diagnostic casts and photographs may need to be taken in order to diagnose the patient's condition. **Diagnostic casts** (models) duplicate the structure of the mouth. They are also called study models and working models. The only difference between a study model and a working model is how they are used. Study models are studied to assist in determining diagnoses and treatments. They are also used by orthodontists to record and evaluate problems or conditions that need treatment. Working models are used to aid in fabricating restorations, crowns, and fixed and removable prosthetics. Since a working model is an integral part of fabricating restorations, normally no additional allowance is given beyond that for the procedure itself. Diagnostic casts are usually covered only for orthodontic services or TMJ conditions.

**Diagnostic photographs** are colored photographs of the oral cavity and are used to show various conditions of the teeth and mouth structures. They are also used to show pre- and postoperative conditions. Diagnostic photographs are generally used in conjunction with orthodontic treatment. Many payers do not cover this procedure because they feel it is merely evidence for the dentist's files, not a diagnostic procedure.

Many plans do not cover any laboratory services or casts and photographs under dental services, with the exception of diagnostic casts and photographs which may be covered if the dental plan covers orthodontic care. Some services may be covered under the medical plan.

# Preventive Services

Preventive services are designed to assist in preventing the development of diseases of the dental structures. If disease is treated in the early stages, it is prevented from spreading to other teeth and structures within the mouth. Dental plans usually cover preventive services because it is less expensive to pay for a small treatment now than for a larger treatment later. The CDT® codes for this category are D1000–D1999.

## Dental Prophylaxis (D1110–D1120)

**Prophylaxis** is the removal of bacterioplaque, calculus, stains, and other potentially harmful materials from the teeth by superficial scaling and polishing as a preventive measure for the control of local irritational factors.

The procedure involves using a scaler to scrape off the built-up calculus (a whitish-yellow chalky substance, also called plaque) from beneath the gum line, then polishing the teeth with an abrasive mixture (a type of pumice).

There are two ADA codes for prophylaxis: one for adults and one for children. Age 14 is usually considered to be the dividing line between adults and children. Many dental plans cover a limited number of prophylaxis treatments (generally no more than two

per year), and some pay for prophylaxis for children, but not for adults.

## Topical Fluoride Treatment (D1201–D1205)

**Fluoride treatments** are the application of a topical fluoride substance to the teeth. The three types of fluoride are stannous, acid, and sodium. All three types can be obtained in either liquid or gel form. Sodium fluoride is usually applied in four treatments. Acid and stannous fluoride are usually applied in a single treatment. Stannous fluoride is the most commonly used. The only difference in the fluoride treatments is in the chemical make-up of the fluoride compound. Stannous fluoride contains tin, acid fluoride contains acid, and sodium fluoride contains salt.

The enamel surface of the teeth is soft in children and grows harder as the teeth mature. Fluorides help to harden the enamel more quickly, thus helping to prevent cavities. When a child reaches about age 14, the enamel has completely hardened. This is one reason why adults usually get fewer cavities than children. Because fluoride is much less effective after the teeth have matured, most plans cover fluoride treatments only up to a certain age, usually ages 14 to 19. While the teeth are immature, the surface is soft and allows for the absorption of the fluoride. After maturity, this is no longer possible. Therefore, fluoride treatment is not usually covered for adults. For children, one treatment every six months is generally allowable.

Fluoride treatments are coded according to the type of fluoride used and whether or not the treatment includes a prophylaxis.

## Other Preventive Services (D1310–D1351)

Occasionally, a dentist provides preventive services other than those already mentioned. These may include dietary planning for the control of dental caries, oral hygiene instruction, and training in preventive dental care. These are considered educational services and thus are generally not covered under most plans.

In addition, a fairly new procedure is the application of **sealants**, which consist of a plastic-like coating that is placed on a healthy tooth to prevent decay. Sealants are coded per quadrant or per tooth. These preventive measures are normally used on children, since the posterior teeth often have fissures (cracks) or pits (holes) during their developmental stage. The application of sealants prevents bacteria, fluids, or food particles from lodging in the fissures or pits, thus preventing cavities. Although the teeth are healthy, the benefits of this type of service are becoming better known and many plans are starting to cover this service.

Note that data indicates that 87% of sealants applied to a tooth are likely to be retained after a period of two years. For this reason, excessive sealant application (more than once every four or five years to the same tooth surface) should be questioned.

## Space Maintenance (D1510–D1550)

**Space maintenance** is the placement of wires or a retainer (either permanent or temporary) in the mouth to prevent the wrongful movement (known as drifting) of teeth into a space where a tooth has been lost. This type of treatment may be covered for children (usually up to age 18) but usually not for adults. Some of the common names for this appliance are stayplate or flipper.

When a deciduous tooth is lost prematurely, space maintainers not only serve to hold the remaining teeth in place, but also prevent the space from being closed and prevent malocclusion with the opposing teeth. Patients with space maintainers should be examined regularly by a dentist. Adjustment of the maintainers or removal may be required. If a space maintainer is left in place longer than necessary, damage to the teeth can occur.

Coding is according to the type (unilateral or bilateral) of maintainer placed and whether or not the appliance is fixed or removable. In many plans, the use of these procedures includes all adjustments and follow-up visits necessary for a specified period of time. Occasionally, it is necessary to recement a space maintainer.

## Restorative Services

A **restoration** is a procedure used to restore a natural tooth. It serves two purposes: to restore the dental structure after removal of the diseased portion, and to make the tooth appear normal. The CDT® codes for this category are D2000–D2999.

Charges/payments for restorations are based on:

- The number of tooth surfaces restored, and
- The type of material used in the restoration.

### Fillings (D2140–D2430)

**Filling restorations**—include a base, polishing, and local anesthetic. The types of materials used for fillings include:

1. **Amalgam**—A silver-colored material composed of a mixture of mercury, silver, tin, copper, and zinc. This is the most durable material but is not aesthetically desirable. It is most appropriate for occlusal surfaces and other surface fillings on posterior teeth. Amalgam is the most inexpensive type of filling material.

2. **Composite**—A plastic white material blended with resin and quartz crystal. This is the second most durable material, about 75% as durable as that of amalgam restorations. Composite is not considered appropriate for occlusal surfaces or for other surfaces of posterior teeth because of its reduced strength. Plans normally consider benefits for placement on anterior teeth and labial and incisal surfaces. Composite fillings should be coded as plastic or acrylic fillings.

3. **Plastics/Acrylics**—Synthetics are not as durable as composites. Many plans limit or exclude payment for plastics. If used, they are appropriate only on the labial surfaces of the anterior teeth. Although plastic or acrylic restorations match natural teeth and are not complicated to perform, they have a tendency to expand with heat, shrink during curing, and discolor. They do not wear well and have a low strength and surface hardness. These restorations are also subject to recurrent decay around the filling.

4. **Silicate**—A synthetic porcelain powder (also called synthetic porcelain or silicate cement) composed of silicate, aluminum, and a flux of either sodium or calcium fluoride. Silicate can be mixed to match existing teeth and therefore is used mainly on the anterior teeth. It is less desirable than other fillers because it is brittle, unable to absorb shock, discolors easily, and has a tendency to shrink or dissolve slowly. Silicate restorations generally last less than five years.

5. **Gold Foil**—A sheet of very thinly pressed gold. Gold restorations are appropriate for cavities covering one, two, or three surfaces. Gold restorations are more time-consuming to perform.

6. **Gold and Metal Alloys**—A combination of one or more different metals. Gold is usually the most desirable filling because of its resistance to corrosion, ability to be adapted closely to cavity walls, extreme density (if properly condensed), maintenance of a high polish and because it does not dissolve in saliva or other mouth fluids. However, gold is generally more expensive than other restorative materials, is less aesthetically

appealing, is difficult to manipulate, can be extremely soft (compared with other fillings), and has a high level of thermal conductivity.

Often gold is mixed with other metals to increase strength. When mixed with copper, it becomes stronger, but it tends to corrode and lose its high polish much faster. Platinum and palladium add strength and hardness to gold and help to whiten the material. Palladium is a less expensive substitute for platinum. Zinc mixed with gold reduces the melting range and helps the gold to combine with any oxides present.

- Miscellaneous synthetic filling materials—May be known under a variety of trade names.
- Acid etch—A procedure, not a filling material. Because of its use during the cavity-filling procedure, it is often lumped together with filling materials. Acid etch is often referred to as an adhesive because it helps to bond the filling material to the tooth. It provides a far more durable bond than regular composites. Acid etch is generally used with acrylics and with composite resins. However, it is usually used on the labial surfaces of the anterior teeth where the adhesion of filling material is difficult and an aesthetic appearance is desired. The acid etch technique (with composite or acrylic resins) has allowed for restoration of teeth that may not previously have been saved or may have required more extensive work (crowns, inlays, or onlays). Such teeth include fractured teeth, those with developmental defects, and with eroded areas among others.

Amalgam, composite, and plastic/acrylic are the most commonly used materials for restorative proce-dures. **Figure 13–1** shows the decay of the tooth and the basic procedure for filling dental cavities or caries. These are caused by insoluble calcium salts being broken down into soluble salts and being washed away. The breakdown of these salts is caused by bacteria that have attached to the tooth or lodged in a hole or fissure. (For further information on dental cavities, see the **Dental Terminology, Anatomy, and Physiology of the Mouth** chapter.)

To treat the cavity, the dentist must first remove all bacteria and diseased material from the teeth to prevent the bacteria from continuing to grow after the cavity has been filled. The hole is then treated with a cavity liner or varnish.

Cavity liners line the outside of the cavity and form a barrier against irritation from the zinc phosphate and silicate cements that are used in the filling material. Cavity liners also reduce the sensitivity of the dentin. Cavity varnishes are applied in several thick layers and help to reduce acid diffusion from the restorative cements into the dentin. They also insulate the pulp from shock due to thermal changes. Finally, the cavity is filled with one of the filling materials previously listed.

Tooth restorations or fillings may involve multiple surfaces. However, only one restoration is generally allowable per tooth.

The following are examples of single restorations (may be multiple surfaces, but only one restoration per tooth):

| | |
|---|---|
| M | one surface |
| MO | two surfaces |
| MOL | three surfaces |
| MODB | four surfaces |
| MODNL | five surfaces |

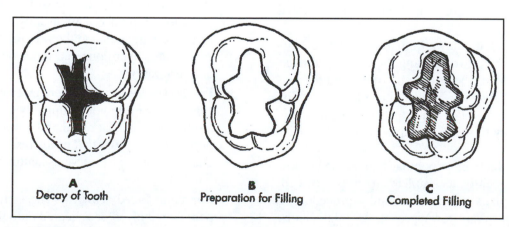

**A**
Decay of Tooth

**B**
Preparation for Filling

**C**
Completed Filling

■ **Figure 13–1** Basic Procedure for Filling Dental Cavities

Examples of multiple restorations:

| | |
|---|---|
| MOD, B | three surfaces and one surface |
| MOD-B | three surfaces and one surface |
| MD | two single surface restorations |
| ML, DL | two single surface restorations if performed on anterior teeth (with the exception of teeth #6 and #11); this is because the anterior teeth are so narrow that an M or a D cannot be performed without going into the L surfaces. An ML or DL filling is really only one surface. In such a case, regardless of how the dentist bills it, only one surface should be allowed. |

Coding for tooth restorations is based on the type of filling used, the number of surfaces, and the type of tooth (primary, permanent, anterior, or posterior).

**Pin retention** is the insertion of a small, thin needle-like pin into the remaining tooth structure to provide extra support for the restoration. Occasionally, a pin retention is done when no restoration was provided. In this case, the pin retention, exclusive of the restoration code, should be used under either the amalgam or acrylic restoration headings.

## Inlays and Onlays (D2510–D2664)

An **inlay** is a gold alloy or porcelain casting that lies on the occlusal surface of the patient's cusps (the pronounced elevation or edge of the tooth). An **onlay** is also a gold alloy casting that lies on the occlusal surface but covers one or more cusps. Inlays and onlays are used to restore lost tooth structure and vertical dimension. Vertical dimension (height) allows for proper occlusion with the opposing teeth. One of the main differences between inlays/onlays and fillings is that fillings are performed within the cavity, whereas inlays and onlays are shaped in a mold and then cemented onto the tooth.

Application of an inlay requires two separate visits to the dentist: the first for drilling the cavity and making an impression of the hole to be filled, and the second for cementing the inlay into place after its manufacture. Inlays also require that enough of the tooth be cut away to make an impression of the cavity to be filled.

Inlays have declined in popularity over the last few years. More frequently, a complete crown is provided. As a rule, most plans require that an inlay procedure be referred to a consultant for approval. An inlay can be applied without an onlay, but an onlay cannot be applied without an inlay. Therefore, if you receive a bill only for an onlay, assume that an inlay was also performed and code accordingly.

## Crowns (D2710–D2799)

A **crown** is a covering that is placed on a tooth. Crowns are required when a tooth has lost so much of its structure that a filling would not be stable. This means that the disease has progressed to the point where there is very little, if any, supporting structure to hold a filling.

Crowns can also be used strictly for cosmetic purposes. For instance, when a tooth may require treatment and a filling would be appropriate, the patient may prefer a crown to a filling because it appears more natural-looking. Perhaps the tooth in question is off-color or crooked. By applying the crown, the color and the position of the tooth can be improved in addition to treating the disease.

The following are the different types of crowns:

- **Full crowns**—These crowns cover the entire top of the tooth and extend to just below the gum line. A cast preparation is formed and then placed over a tooth on which the four outside surfaces (lingual, facial, mesial, distal axial) have been filed toward each other to form a rounded point. Several full crowns connected together and placed over several adjacent teeth can be used to help stabilize those teeth.

- **Full veneer crowns**—These crowns are similar to full crowns, but they have a thin layer of acrylic resin or porcelain bonded to the surface of the crown. They replace nearly the entire tooth and are placed over a "stump" that has been made of the natural tooth.

- **Partial crowns**—Similar to full crowns, partial crowns do not cover all the surfaces of the tooth. The surfaces involved are usually the occlusal or incisal, the lingual, and the proximal. Partial crowns are never done in a series but are single unit restorations.

- **Partial (three-quarter) veneer crowns**—Partial veneer crowns do not completely cover the tooth. They are cast metal and cover only that portion of the tooth that needs restoring. Three-quarter crowns also serve as abutments for a fixed bridge.

- **Porcelain-faced crowns**—These crowns have porcelain inlayed or veneered onto the buccal or labial surface.

- **Seven-eighths crowns**—These crowns are usually placed on the molars to serve as bridge abutments. Their purpose is to strengthen the tooth to help it withstand the added stress of the bridge.
- **Steel crowns**—These crowns are noncast (preformed) crowns that are usually made of stainless steel.

Dental plans cover a crown only when less drastic (and less expensive) methods of treatment are not appropriate. That is, if a filling can correct the problem, then a filling, not a crown, would be the appropriate treatment. Remember that the patient or dentist can use whatever treatment is desired. However, the amount allowed would be based on the necessity of services rendered.

There are permanent crowns and temporary crowns. When a crown is required, the dentist makes a model of the mouth (or arch). Then, a match of the surrounding teeth using a color chart is determined. The patient's natural tooth is then filed down until it resembles a spike. A temporary crown is then placed on the diseased tooth while the model is sent to a dental laboratory for casting (some dental offices perform the casting in-house).

A cast is made from the model from the material ordered by the dentist in a color matching the patient's surrounding teeth. The finished crown is then given to the dentist for application and fitting. The patient usually returns for the "**seating**" (placement) of the finished crown. Normally, the patient has to return to the dentist several times for adjustments to the vertical height of the crown so that it fits comfortably and is properly aligned with the surrounding teeth.

The types of permanent crowns are:

- Full cast (gold).
- Three-quarter gold.
- Porcelain veneer (porcelain outside and a designated metal frame inside, which may be gold, nonprecious metal [alloy], or semiprecious metal).

Temporary crowns are usually constructed of stainless steel. The temporary is precast instead of being made specifically for the patient.

As a rule, porcelain crowns are the most expensive. They may be covered only on the anterior teeth. However, since this material has become the most accepted material for crowns, porcelain crowns may be allowed even on posterior teeth. The semiprecious or gold frame is allowable on anterior

teeth. At one time, most plans were written with the provision that only gold crowns would be covered on posterior teeth. That was because years ago, gold was the least expensive material. Now many plans will allow whatever material is the least expensive on the posterior teeth.

Crowns must be prepped and the natural tooth prepared while the patient is covered under the plan. However, many plans allow the actual seating to take place after the coverage has terminated if it is within 30 days of the termination date. The plan provisions must be checked for this exception.

Stainless-steel crowns are usually covered on deciduous teeth. Regular crowns are not usually covered on deciduous teeth because they will be lost as the child matures.

If properly prepared, a crown should last a minimum of five years. Therefore, if a replacement is requested on a crown that has been in place for less than five years, a review by a consultant is usually required. If the replacement is necessitated because of poor workmanship by the dentist, the original dentist may be expected to redo the restoration at no extra charge. This approach varies greatly by administrator.

Many plans monitor crowns to see whether more than one crown per arch or quadrant is being performed, since the underlying reason may be cosmetic, not functional. In addition, crowns on teeth that are abutments (teeth used to support or stabilize one end of a prosthesis and lie next to an area of a missing tooth) to dentures are also monitored for necessity.

Crowns are coded according to the type of material used in the crown. This may be a single type or a combination of materials.

## Other Restorative Services (D2910–D2999)

It may become necessary to recement a loosened inlay or crown. The codes for recementing are dependent on whether the procedure is for an inlay or a crown.

**Medicated or sedative fillings** are temporary fillings to help relieve pain. As a rule, they may not be covered. The final restoration only may be the covered expense.

Other restorative services include crown buildup (to build up a crown to match the height of other teeth) and a **labial veneer** (a cosmetic procedure that coats the tooth). This can be done to match the color of other teeth or to whiten the teeth and is seldom covered by plans.

# On the Job NOW

**Directions:** Answer the following questions without looking back at the material just covered. Write your answers in the space provided.

1. What two purposes do restorations serve? _____

_____

2. What is the process for filling a cavity? _____

_____

_____

_____

_____

_____

3. Answer the following three part question.

   1. When would a crown be required? _____

   _____

   2. What would this mean in regards to the condition of the tooth? _____

   _____

   3. When would a plan not cover a crown? _____

   _____

## Endodontics

Endodontic treatment deals with the diagnosis and treatment of diseases of the internal structures of the teeth, pulp, and periapical tissues. The most common type of endodontic treatment is a root canal procedure. The CDT® codes for this category are D3000–D3999.

Benefit payments for endodontic procedures include all x-rays and office visits. Additional charges for these services are denied if billed with endodontic procedures.

### Pulp Capping and Pulpotomy (D3110–D3221)

Another type of endodontic treatment is pulp capping. **Pulp capping** is the placing of a covering over an exposed tooth pulp. Pulp capping is performed only on children because the pulp is occluded and becomes a root after a tooth matures. Some dentists bill pulp caps consistently on adults. As a rule, the treatment is considered a sedative filling instead of a pulp cap. A dental consultant needs to review the x-rays to determine the legitimacy of the billing.

There are two types of pulp caps: direct and indirect. A direct pulp cap is directly in contact with the material used (often calcium hydroxide) and the pulp. In an indirect pulp cap, the treatment is placed on the vital or diseased dentin and not directly on the pulp.

Recalcification or remineralization is similar to a pulp cap. In this type of treatment, calcium hydroxide or a similar material is placed in the tooth prior to placing a temporary restoration. If this is done on permanent teeth, a consultant should review the x-rays, since it is usually appropriate only on deciduous teeth.

**Pulpotomy** and **pulpectomy** consist of complete and partial removal of the pulp, respectively, and are appropriate only on deciduous teeth. There are two types of pulpotomies: vital and therapeutic. If the provider does not indicate which type was performed, it is usually safe to assume it was a vital pulpotomy.

### Root Canals (D3230–D3348)

A **root canal** is the removal of the entire root pulp, sterilizing of the chamber, and filling of the chamber with sealing material. This is performed when a tooth has an infected or damaged pulp. There are two types of root canal therapies: conventional (traditional) and Sargenti. Although the Sargenti treatment is done in one seating and the conventional treatment usually takes three treatments, the conventional treatment is preferred since the chamber is sterilized and then allowed to settle before filling. This allows the dentist to be sure that all of the infection is cleared up before the final step—that of placing a crown on the tooth.

Many consultants will question the appropriateness of the Sargenti when submitted because it is essential that the infection be completely cleared before the crown is placed. After the crown is placed, it cannot be removed without ruining it. It is possible to drill through the top of the crown to reach the canal but this is certainly not desirable.

**Table 13–1** will assist in identifying whether or not the dentist is billing correctly. If a root canal is performed, all the roots have to be cleaned and filled even if they are not all infected. This is because the infection will inevitably spread and because, as previously stated, once a crown is placed, it is not desirable to have to remove it for any reason. By treating all the roots, this possibility is minimized.

Root canals are coded according to the type of root canal that is performed. If the Sargenti method is used, the code depends on the number of roots involved in the therapy. A conventional root canal is coded according to the type of tooth (anterior, premolar, or molar).

The process of a root canal leaves a cavity in the tooth that must be filled. All root canal codes do not include the final restoration. Therefore, a corresponding restoration should be billed and coded for each root canal performed. In the Sargenti method, the restoration is done on the same day and should be included on the same billing form. In a non-Sargenti method, the restoration is not completed until a subsequent visit and may be billed on a separate claim form.

| Tooth # | Permanent Tooth Name | # Canals |
|---|---|---|
| 1 | Upper right 3rd molar | 3 |
| 2 | Upper right 2nd molar | 3 |
| 3 | Upper right 1st molar | 3 |
| 4 | Upper right 2nd bicuspid | 1 |
| 5 | Upper right 1st bicuspid | 2 |
| 6 | Upper right cuspid | 1 |
| 7 | Upper right lateral incisor | 1 |
| 8 | Upper right central incisor | 1 |
| 9 | Upper left central incisor | 1 |
| 10 | Upper left lateral incisor | 1 |
| 11 | Upper left cuspid | 1 |
| 12 | Upper left 1st bicuspid | 2 |
| 13 | Upper left 2nd bicuspid | 1 |
| 14 | Upper left 1st molar | 3 |
| 15 | Upper left 2nd molar | 3 |
| 16 | Upper left 3rd molar | 3 |
| 17 | Lower left 3rd molar | 3 |
| 18 | Lower left 2nd molar | 3 |
| 19 | Lower left 1st molar | 3 |
| 20 | Lower left 1st bicuspid | 1 |
| 21 | Lower left 2nd bicuspid | 1 |
| 22 | Lower left cuspid | 1 |
| 23 | Lower left lateral incisor | 1 |
| 24 | Lower left central incisor | 1 |
| 25 | Lower right central incisor | 1 |
| 26 | Lower right lateral incisor | 1 |
| 27 | Lower right cuspid | 1 |
| 28 | Lower right 1st bicuspid | 1 |
| 29 | Lower right 2nd bicuspid | 1 |
| 30 | Lower right 1st molar | 3 |
| 31 | Lower right 2nd molar | 3 |
| 32 | Lower right 3rd molar | 3 |

**Table 13–1  Usual Number of Root Canals for Each Tooth**

## Apexification (D3351–D3353)

**Apexification** is performed on the permanent tooth of a young person when the apex of the tooth is incompletely formed. It is a series of treatments, wherein the pulp is removed and the apex is treated with a solution of calcium hydroxide. This procedure stimulates growth of the cementum and helps to form apical closure.

Often apexification is performed prior to root canal therapy. Apexification treatment occurs in a series of visits and can last from six to 18 months.

## Apicoectomy/Periradicular Services (D3410–D3470)

The common types of treatment to the root surface include the following:

1. **Apicoectomy**—Excision of the apex of a root (usually considered medical, not dental). An apicoectomy is coded depending on whether or not it was performed with other endodontic procedures. The coding method is per root. Therefore, if two or more roots were done, the code (and RVS unit values) should be multiplied accordingly.

2. **Endodontic Implants**—The placement of an implant through the tooth and into the jaw. It is used to stabilize a loose tooth. Because many administrators consider endodontic implants to be experimental, services are referred to a consultant for review.

**3. Retrograde Filling**—Amalgam filling placed into the apex of a root. This usually follows an apicoectomy.

**4. Root Resection**—Cutting off a portion of the root, usually because of disease or decay.

## Other Endodontic Procedures (D3910–D3999)

Other endodontic procedures may include:

**1. Surgical Procedure for Isolation of Tooth with a Rubber Dam**—Use of a thin rubber tissue by the dentist to seal off the tooth from saliva in the mouth. It also protects the patient from dental instruments, assists in the elimination of saliva and other fluids, and helps to keep the gingiva out of the way. Often, payers will not cover this procedure.

**2. Bleaching of Discolored Teeth**—A cosmetic procedure to whiten the teeth. As such, it is not covered by most dental plans.

**3. Canal Preparation and Fitting of Performed Dowel or Post**—The drilling of a canal and the inserting of a post or dowel into the canal.

**4. Hemisection**—Cutting an organ in half.

# On the Job Now

**Directions:** Answer the following questions without looking back at the material just covered. Write your answers in the space provided.

1. What is the most common type of endodontic treatment? _____

2. What do benefit payments for endodontic procedures include? _____

3. How are root canals coded? _____

## Periodontic Services

Periodontal treatment is the diagnosis and treatment of diseases affecting the periodontium, the tissues that surround and support the teeth. This includes the gingiva, cementum, and periodontal membranes. Periodontal procedures are usually performed by a dentist, periodontist, or oral surgeon. The CDT® codes for this category are D4000–D4999.

Periodontal treatment is one of the most highly abused areas of dental care. For this reason, many administrators have very stringent periodontal guidelines together with heavy consultant review. Some periodontal care is considered oral surgery, whereas other treatments are considered strictly dental. To be effective, some periodontal treatments must be used in conjunction with or followed up by other adjunctive treatments.

Such in-depth training is best done at the administrator level instead of in this general training guide.

### Surgical Services (D4210–D4276)

Surgical services to the periodontium include:

**1. Free Soft Tissue Grafts**—Soft tissue grafts that do not involve the use of a pedicle.

**2. Gingival Curettage**—The intentional surgical removal of the inner soft tissue wall of the gingival pocket. It is usually performed with local anesthetic. Access is through the pocket opening and no flap is performed (see item that follows). Many plans consider gingival curettage to be medically necessary if performed by a licensed provider, but limit treatment to one occurrence per year per quadrant.

3. **Gingivectomy**—The surgical removal of diseased gum tissue or gingivoplasty; the surgical correction of the gingival margin or edge.

4. **Gingival Flap Procedure**—The movement of masses of partially detached tissue from one area to an adjacent area  in this case, the gum. The flap is not fully detached so that it retains its own blood supply during transfer. Flap procedures are often used for covering the end of a bone after resection.

5. **Mucogingival Surgery**—Surgery involving the mucous membranes and the gums.

6. **Osseous Grafts**—Transplants involving the bone.

7. **Osseous Surgery**—Surgery involving the bone.

8. **Pedicle Soft Tissue Grafts**—Grafts that involve a pedicle. (A pedicle is a narrow, stem-like projection that attaches the graft to a blood or nutrient supply.)

9. **Periodontal Pulpal Procedures**—Surgical procedures that involve the periodontal pulp.

10. **Vestibuloplasty**—Surgery involving the vestibule of the mouth.

Gingivectomy or gingivoplasty, mucogingival surgery, and osseous surgery can be used for single tooth procedures, multiple tooth procedures, or full quadrant procedures. Check the tooth numbers on the claim to determine how many teeth were affected by the procedure. Benefits will be allowed according to the number of teeth involved.

## NonSurgical Periodontal Services (D4320–D4381)

The following are additional periodontal services:

1. **Athletic Mouth Guard Fabrication**—Making of an appliance that fits over the teeth to protect them from harm during rough athletic activity (i.e., football, boxing). This is not usually covered under the plan.

2. **Occlusional Adjustment**—An adjustment to allow proper occlusion (closing) of the teeth.

3. **Scaling**—Thorough removal of calculus and bacterioplaque from the crowns and all root surfaces of the teeth.

4. **Root Planing**—A more definitive form of scaling to smooth roughened root surfaces (cementum) and to remove deep, heavy plaque. (The ADA describes and codes scaling and root planing as one procedure, since both procedures must be done at the same time.)

For definitive scaling and planing per quadrant per appointment. The entire mouth should be done. This code should be used with a comprehensive approach for a more complicated or advanced case of periodontal disease.

5. **Special Periodontal Appliances (including Occlusal Guards)**—Special appliances that may be required to aid in the treatment of periodontal diseases.

6. **Splinting**—The attaching together of multiple teeth with wire or some other supportive material. In advanced cases of periodontal disease, the teeth become loosened in their sockets due to the loss of supporting tissue. In an effort to salvage the teeth, multiple teeth may be "splinted" together. This provides a wider base so that if one tooth moves, all teeth must move. To move several teeth requires significantly more pressure than to move a single tooth. Consequently, there is less movement in teeth splinted together.

    There are two types of splinting:

    • **Intracoronal** (provisional), in which the teeth are wired together.

    • **Extracoronal,** (a permanent treatment) where crowns or inlays are placed on the subject teeth and soldered together.

    Many plans limit coverage for splinting, and a consultant review should always be provided.

7. **Tooth Movement for Periodontal Purposes**—Allows the teeth to be moved so that the dentist may treat the periodontal tissues underneath.

## Description of Case Patterns

Gingivitis and periodontitis are usually classified under a case pattern section that lists the disease and the appropriate treatment under one ADA code.

• Case pattern modifiers (by report)—For use when extenuating circumstances accompany a specific case pattern.

All the following treatments and procedures are included under one code. If treatment is listed or billed separately, all services should be combined under the single code.

Treatment includes: all necessary diagnostic procedures, training in personal preventive dental care, mouth preparation procedures, occlusal adjustment, surgical procedures (involving flap entry and osseous procedures, and complex procedures), routine finishing procedures, and posttreatment evaluation.

- **Type I Gingivitis**—Shallow pockets, no bone loss.

- **Type II Early Periodontitis**—Moderate pockets, minor to moderate bone loss, satisfactory topography.

- **Type III Moderate Periodontitis**—Moderate to deep pockets, moderate to severe bone loss, unsatisfactory topography.

- **Type IV Advanced Periodontitis**—Deep pockets, severe bone loss, advanced inability patterns (usually cases involving missing teeth and reconstruction).

## Other Periodontal Services (D4910–D4999)

Preventive periodontal procedures (periodontal prophylaxis) include:

1. **Perioprophylaxis (also referred to as a Periorecall or Periodontal Maintenance)**—Performed following the completion of comprehensive periodontal treatment. The patient returns within 12 months (usually at three-month intervals) for posttreatment evaluation and further preventive care. Perioscaling and possibly root planing and polishing of the teeth may be necessary at this time as well as reinstruction in preventive oral hygiene procedures.

2. **Unscheduled Dressing Change**—Used when a dentist other than the treating dentist performs a dressing change.

# Prosthodontic Services (Removable)

**Prosthodontics** is the branch of dentistry concerned with restoration and maintenance of function by the artificial replacement of missing natural teeth. It covers the initial preparation and installation of bridges and dentures. The CDT® codes for this category are D5000–D5899.

On all claims involving prosthodontics, the examiner needs to determine:

- Which teeth, if any, are congenitally missing.

- The tooth number of any and all teeth being replaced, plus the date of extraction or loss of each tooth.

- Whether any other teeth are missing in the arch and whether they are being replaced.

- For a replacement prosthesis, the date of installation of the prior prosthesis.

The charges for all prosthetics (and therefore the coding and billing) include:

- The initial preparation of the teeth for a prosthetic.

- Study models.

- Fitting of the prosthesis.

- Initial installation of the prosthesis.

- All adjustment required within six months of the installation.

## Complete Dentures (D5110–D5140)

These are usually full and partial dentures and appliances. The following sections explain the types of dentures and give general guidelines concerning them.

### Full Dentures

**Full dentures** are appliances that replace all of the patient's natural teeth. The types of complete (full) dentures are (**see Figure 13–2**):

- **Immediate Permanent**—Made before all the natural teeth have been extracted. After extractions, it is placed immediately before the healing is complete.

- **Immediate Temporary**—Constructed of temporary material; has anterior teeth and posterior biting blocks (not true artificial teeth).

- **Overdentures**—Fabricated to fit over the remaining teeth. Usually, two natural teeth per arch remain in the mouth to provide support. Root canals, posts, copings, and crowns are performed on the remaining teeth to provide the necessary strength to support the overdenture.

- **Regular permanent**—Made following all extractions and healing of tissues or for replacement of an existing denture.

Full dentures are coded according to the location (upper or lower) and whether they are complete or immediately placed. Full dentures for patients under age 35 and full bridges on patients under age 16 should normally be reviewed by a consultant for appropriateness.

Relines, tissue conditioning, and adjustments for six months after the initial placement of the dentures are usually considered part of the basic denture procedure. Therefore, additional payments are not allowed.

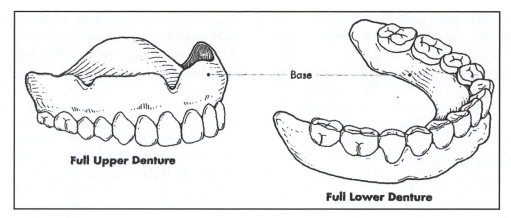

**■ Figure 13–2** Full Dentures

## Partial Dentures (D5211–D5281)

Partial dentures are used to replace missing teeth (**see Figure 13–3**). For a partial denture to be used, enough structurally sound natural teeth must be available to anchor the partial denture. If the patient has advanced periodontal disease, bone disease, or other conditions, a partial denture may not be possible to use. A partial denture may be either fixed or removable. A fixed partial is usually called a bridge.

The types of removable partial dentures are:

**Permanent**—Used when only a few scattered teeth need replacement.

**Temporary**—Temporary replacement. This is usually not covered except after periodontal work. A consultant review is generally required.

**Unilateral Partial**—Replaces only one tooth. A partial is usually constructed "symmetrically," that is, one or two teeth are being replaced in each quadrant of the arch. When teeth are missing in one quadrant, a fixed bridge is usually used, depending on the circumstances of the missing teeth. If only one tooth is missing in one quadrant, a unilateral partial can be used. The charge for a partial denture includes:

- All teeth.
- The base, which is a pink-colored plastic and metal and lies against either the palate or the alveolar ridge (bottom of the mouth).
- Two rests and two clasps.
- All adjustments or relines required during the first six months following seating.

Many dentists routinely itemize their billing for partials, showing a separate charge for each tooth, the base, and the clasps and rests. When processing or billing, all these charges should be combined and coded as one appliance. Additional clasps or rests are coded separately. All the teeth are always included, regardless of the number of teeth involved.

A **palatal bar** is the support that runs across the top of the palate (roof of the mouth). A **lingual bar** is the support that runs along the bottom of the mouth. Different codings reflect different materials used in the construction of the partial. Many plans specify that only certain materials, usually nonprecious or semiprecious materials, can be used in the construction.

Teeth numbers 7 and 10 are often not strong enough to support bridgework or partials. Therefore,

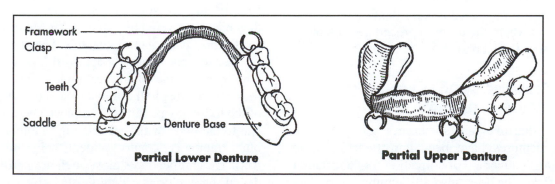

**■ Figure 13–3** Partial Dentures

care should be taken when approving these teeth for use as abutments. A consultant should review the x-rays and treatment plan prior to approval.

Partial dentures are coded according to the type of denture (complete or partial), their location (upper or lower), the materials (i.e., acrylic, chrome), and the number of clasps used.

## Adjustments to Dentures (D5410–D5422)

Occasionally, a dentist has to adjust dentures because of changes in the mouth (often due to aging or disease).

## Repairs to Complete or Partial Dentures (D5510–D5671)

Occasionally, it becomes necessary to repair or add to a denture. These codes are used only when a new denture or partial does not have to be made, when a repair can be made, or when a tooth can just be added on.

## Denture Rebase Procedures (D5710–D5721)

**Jump** or **rebase** is the replacement of the base of the denture because of deterioration or tissue changes. Jump or rebase may be covered depending on the circumstances. Since the teeth from the original denture are being reused and only the base material is being remade, the cost is considerably less than the cost of a completely new denture. However, since these two terms are used interchangeably, it is necessary that an explanation be obtained from the provider that clarifies which service is being performed.

## Denture Relining Procedures (D5730–D5761)

A reline is a soft material placed on top of the base to help prevent tissue damage to the patient's mouth. This makes the partial or denture more comfortable to wear. It is coded according to the type of denture (complete or partial) and where the relining procedure took place (in the office or the laboratory).

## Interim Prosthesis and Other Services (D5810–D5899)

**Temporary dentures** are sometimes used until the permanent dentures have been constructed. **Tissue conditioning** is a method of correcting tissue irritation resulting from the wearing of dentures. First, an impression-making type of material is placed in the saddle of the denture. Then, with the denture in place, displacement of this material will indicate any corrections that are necessary to eliminate distortion from pressure on the tissue. Tissue conditioning is more complicated than the typical adjustment.

As previously indicated, an overdenture is considered a full denture, although it is placed "over" two teeth in each arch left for support. Unlike a partial denture in which clasps are used to grab onto the abutment teeth, an overdenture has two holes left in it to allow it to slide over the two remaining teeth. Overdentures are coded as complete or partial.

# Maxillofacial Prosthetics

**Maxillofacial prosthetics** is the prosthetic rehabilitation of regions of the head and neck that are missing or defective. These deficiencies may be due to surgical treatment, trauma, pathology, or congenital malformation.

Extraoral maxillofacial prostheses may involve the following structures: nose, ear, orbit, or any combination of structures within the head and neck region. Intraoral prostheses are used to reconstruct defects associated with the oral cavity. An obturator prosthesis is used for reconstructing part of the maxilla (upper jaw) and will close oral-nasal openings in the palate. Other prostheses may include mandibular (lower jaw) resection prostheses, feeding appliances, and pediatric and adult speech aid prostheses.

The scope of maxillofacial prosthetics is not limited to reconstruction but also includes treatment appliances such as burn compression stents, radiation carriers and shields, and infant orthopedic appliances used in cleft palate children to properly align the segments of the maxillary dental arch. The CDT® codes for this category are D5900–D5999.

Many of the following services are not performed frequently and therefore have a BR (By Report) or RNE (Relativity Not Established) unit value. However, they may be covered by some Major Medical plans. As a rule, most plans require that this type of procedure be referred to a consultant for approval. The codes are seldom seen by the claims examiner. For this reason, these procedures will not be discussed in depth. Many of the following prostheses are placed because of damage to the bone or tissues relating to either disease or blunt trauma (i.e., auto accident, being hit by an object). These procedures most often are performed by a dental surgeon or an orthodontist.

## Extraoral Prostheses (D5911–D5929)

The following prostheses are actually outside the oral cavity:

1. **Auricular Prosthesis**—A prosthesis in the auricle of the ear.
2. **Composite Facial Prosthesis**—A prosthesis of the facial structure.
3. **Facial Moulage**—The making of a wax model of the face or a portion of the face or mouth. This is usually done in preparation for the making of a prosthesis.
4. **Nasal Prosthesis**—A prosthesis of the nasal cavity or nose.
5. **Ocular Implant**—An implant in the eye.
6. **Ocular Prosthesis**—A prosthesis of the eye (i.e., a glass eye).
7. **Orbital Implant**—An implant to the orbit (the bony structure surrounding the eye).
8. **Orbital Prosthesis**—A prosthesis of the orbit (the bony structure around the eyeball).
9. **Prosthetic Dressing**—The dressing applied to the injured area before, during, or after the insertion of a prosthesis.
10. **Replacement Prosthesis**—Replacement or duplicate of an existing prosthesis. Often much of the measuring of the patient and the formation of molds has been done. Thus, a replacement prosthesis usually costs less than the initial one.

## Intraoral Prostheses (D5931–D5999)

This section is divided into two subheadings, one for acquired defects and one for congenital defects. Congenital defects are those that the patient is born with. Acquired defects are those that develop after birth. Acquired defects in the field of dentistry are most often the result of disease or blunt trauma.

### Acquired Defects

The following are intraoral prosthetics services performed for acquired defects:

1. **Refitting of Obturator**—The refitting or reforming of an obturator to better fit changes in the structure of the patient's palate. An obturator is an appliance designed to fill in the hole created by a cleft palate defect. It is usually held in place with clasps or splinted to the teeth.
2. **Mandibular Resection Prosthesis**—A prosthesis to replace bone that was excised (cut out) during a

mandibular resection. There are two codes depending on whether the prosthesis is a flange (lower, the part of the denture that extends from the embedded teeth to the border of the denture) or a denture (artificial teeth) prosthesis.

### Congenital Defects

The following are intraoral prosthetics services performed for congenital defects:

1. **Feeding Aid**—A prosthesis used to assist in feeding a person with a congenital defect.
2. **Obturator**—A prosthesis to cover the hole created by a cleft palate defect.
3. **Palatal Lift Prosthesis**—A prosthesis that is made to lift the palate.
4. **Speech Aid**—A prosthesis used to help a person's speech. The two codes for speech aids depend on whether the prosthesis is for a child or an adult.
5. **Superimposed Prosthesis**—A prosthesis that is superimposed (placed) over another prosthesis.

## Implant Services

To **implant** means to transfer or to graft something additional onto or into an existing surface. An implant may consist of a piece of tissue or bone, or a pellet of medicine on a tube or needle containing radioactive material. Coding should be for either a single, or a complex implant. The CDT® codes for this category are D6000–D6199.

The following are the various types of implants:

1. **Subperiosteal Implant**—An implant located below the periosteum.
2. **Endosseous Implant**—An implant in the bone.
3. **Endodontic Endosseous Implant**—An implant through the root and into the bone.

## Implant Supported Prosthetics and Other Implant Services (D6010–D6199)

This section is subdivided into two sections: 1) Implant Supported Prosthetics, and 2) Other Implant Services.

The following are prostheses that are generally removed after treatment:

1. **Docket Device**—A device to which something can be anchored or docked during treatment.
2. **Fluoride Applicator**—A plastic receptacle that is filled with fluoride and then fitted around the teeth, allowing fluoride to be absorbed into the

teeth. This is the most common treatment prosthesis used, and it often accompanies billings for fluoride treatments.

3. **Infant Orthopedic Appliance**—An appliance to help preserve and restore the skeletal function in infants.

4. **Mandibular Guide Flange**—An implant below the denture line that helps to guide the mandibular bone.

5. **Radiation Carrier**—A device (usually a tube or needle) that contains a radioactive material.

6. **Radiation Shield**—A shield that protects a portion of the body from radiation.

7. **Splint**—A device that holds a body part rigid or immobile.

8. **Trismus Appliance**—An appliance to aid in trismus. Trismus (often called lockjaw) is a motor disturbance of the trigeminal nerve.

# Prosthodontic Services (Fixed)

The bridge or bridgework is usually used in reference to "fixed" or permanent partials. These are bridges that are permanently attached and seated in the patient's mouth. Whereas a partial is usually removed at night, a fixed bridge is never removed unless required by a dentist for repair. The CDT® codes for this category are D6200–D6999.

Although there are many different types of bridges, the most common is a three-unit bridge. A three-unit bridge is composed of two abutment teeth and one pontic.

## Fixed Partial Denture Pontics (D6205–D6253)

A **pontic** is the part of a bridge that is suspended between abutments and replaces a missing tooth. It is also the artificial tooth in a partial denture. A pontic is the object that is made to look like a natural tooth.

## Fixed Partial Denture Retainers–Inlays/Onlays and Crowns (D6545–D6793)

An **abutment** is a tooth that is used to support or stabilize one end of a prosthetic appliance. A **retainer** is a device used for maintaining the teeth and jaws in an appropriate position. The normal three-unit bridge (the number of units applies to the number of abutments plus the number of pontics involved in a bridge) is:

Abutment – pontic – abutment

Abutments are normally crowned. This is because either a bridge or a partial causes considerable wear and tear on the abutment teeth. Crowns provide the extra strength and support that is needed. The two most common types of bridges are:

1. **Fixed Bridgework**—Made up of pontics (artificial teeth) and abutments (anchors).

2. **Cantilevered Bridge**—Composed of one pontic and one abutment. Cantilevered bridges need to be reviewed by a consultant to determine appropriateness of treatment.

A bridge may also have double abutments. Double abutments are sometimes necessary when the abutting tooth is not very strong (such as lateral incisors seven and 10) or when the bridge is cantilevered. However, some providers consistently bill for double abutments because it significantly increases the cost of the bridge. A bridge is charged and paid for based on the number of units involved. The allowance for an abutment is based on a crown charge. The pontic charge tends to be about the same amount.

If a bridge is covered, the abutments are also automatically covered. If the bridge (replacement of missing teeth) is not covered, the abutment teeth must be evaluated by themselves to see whether they require crowning because of disease. If they are so decayed or diseased that crowning would be appropriate without regard to a bridge, the crowns will be paid for even though the pontic for the missing tooth would not be.

Bridge pontics and crowns (abutments) are coded based on the type of material used in the pontic or crown. Remember that each abutment and each pontic constitute a unit in a bridge. Therefore, a three-unit bridge would be billed as a pontic and two crowns.

Although the crown performed for a bridge is substantially the same as that provided for a stand-alone crown, a different code is used.

## Other Fixed Partial Denture Services (D6920–D6999)

This area includes some of the item needed to prepare or fix a bridge and includes the following:

• **Precision Attachment**—A specially designed attachment used in fixed and removable prosthetics for attachment to the abutment teeth. It usually consists of a tongue and groove or male/female design.

• **Stress Breaker**—A device incorporated into a denture to relieve excess stress on the abutting teeth during chewing.

# On the Job Now

**Directions:** Answer the following questions without looking back at the material just covered. Write your answers in the space provided.

1. What four things should a health claims examiner determine on all claims involving prosthodontics?

    1. _____

    2. _____

    3. _____

    4. _____

2. How are full dentures coded? _____

    _____

3. Answer the following three part question.

    1. What is the most common bridge? _____

    2. What is it composed of? _____

    3. What are bridge charges based on? _____

## Oral and Maxillofacial Surgery

Oral surgery includes the operative procedures related to the teeth and jaws. The CDT® codes for this category are D7000–D7999.

Technically, surgery to the mouth is split into two sections:

1. **Dental Surgery**—For treatment of the teeth and gums, such as extractions.

2. **Oral Surgery**—For treatment of the jaw or parts of the mouth other than the teeth and gums, such as treatment of the joints and bones.

A dentist, oral surgeon, or physician may perform both oral and dental surgery. The type of surgery is defined by the procedure performed, not by the licensure of the person performing the service.

The distinction between oral and dental surgery is important because oral surgery may be covered under the medical portion of the plan, whereas routine extractions are not.

Oral surgery involves cutting into the oral tissues, opening up the area, cutting and removing objects from that area (either teeth or tissues/cysts), and then suturing (sewing) the area. The services that are considered surgical, and are therefore usually covered under the medical portion of the plan, include but are not limited to gingival curettage, gingivectomy, gingivoplasty, osseous surgery, gingival or soft tissue grafts, and osseous grafts. Following are some of the more common oral surgeries and exceptions.

### Extractions (D7111–D7140)

An extraction normally does not involve any cutting (except in a very superficial manner) or suturing. Therefore, extractions are not usually considered oral surgery. Usually, pincers are used to grab the tooth that is to be removed and the tooth is pulled out. The exception may be for impacted wisdom teeth (third molars).

Extractions include local anesthesia and routine postoperative care.

### Surgical Extractions (D7210–D7250)

Surgical extractions include local anesthesia and routine postoperative care. The codes in this section are based on the degree of difficulty for the extraction.

An **impacted tooth** is one that is positioned or wedged against another tooth, bone, or soft tissue and is prevented from erupting normally. When this occurs, the gum must be cut and the tooth removed, often by fracturing into smaller pieces. The gum is then sutured closed. The three molars in each quadrant have a tendency to become impacted.

1. **Root Extraction**—Surgical cutting into the gum and removing the root. This situation may occur when a tooth is extracted and a part of the root breaks off and remains in the gum. This is usually considered a medical procedure.

2. **Oroantral Fistula Closure**—An abnormal opening into the mouth cavity. This code is also used for antral root recovery. Most often, an oroantral fistula occurs when the root of an upper tooth has grown into the nasal cavity. When this tooth is extracted, an unnatural opening occurs between the oral cavity and the nasal cavity. Oroantral fistulas can also occur as a result of infection; however, it is still most often associated with the extraction of a tooth in which bacteria entered the hole left by the root and infection occurred. If an oroantral fistula occurs more than six weeks after the extraction of the tooth, some plans will cover the expense under medical benefits since the cause is usually bacterial.

## Other Surgical Procedures (D7260–D7291)

Following are examples of other surgical procedures:

1. **Tooth Reimplantation**—Stabilization of accidentally evulsed or displaced tooth or alveolus.

2. **Tooth Implantation**—Placement of a tooth back into the same socket after it has been knocked out.

3. **Tooth Transplantation**—Moving a natural tooth from one location to another. As a rule, implantation is covered but transplantation is not. Of course, it depends on the circumstances and the plan provisions.

4. **Surgical Exposure**—The cutting of the gum and sometimes the attachment of wires to the crown of the unerupted tooth to assist in the eruption and proper alignment of the tooth. Often, this is done for orthodontic purposes. In such a case, it would be covered only if the plan has orthodontic provisions.

Biopsy of oral tissue (hard and soft) and surgical re-positioning of the teeth are considered oral surgery and are usually covered under the medical plan.

## Alveoloplasty and Vestibuloplasty (D7310–D7350)

**Alveoloplasty** is surgical preparation of a ridge for dentures. It is coded per quadrant, either in conjunction with extractions or without. Unless otherwise specified in the contract, alveoloplasties are covered under dental, not medical.

A **vestibuloplasty** is a procedure to restore ridge height by lowering muscles attaching to the buccal, labial, and lingual aspects of the jaws.

## Surgical Excision of Soft Tissue Lesions (D7410–D7465)

**Surgical excision** includes excision of reactive inflammatory lesions, scar tissue, or localized congenital lesions. Excision pericoronal gingiva is an excision of the gums around the teeth.

## Surgical Excision of Intra-Osseous Lesions (D7440–D7461)

**Tumors** are abnormal (possibly cancerous) growths in the body. The coding for the removal of tumors depends on their size and whether they are benign or malignant.

A **cyst** is an enclosed pouch that contains fluid, semifluid, or solid material. A **neoplasm** is a new tumor or growth. The code depends on the size of the cyst or neoplasm and whether it is odontogenic (relating to the origin and formation of the teeth) or non-odontogenic. Code D7465 is used for procedures which involve the destruction of lesions by physical methods: electro-surgery, chemotherapy, and cryotherapy.

## Excision of Bone Tissue (D7471–D7490)

**Removal of exostosis** is the removal of a bony growth that arises from either the maxilla or mandible. It often involves the ossification (bone formation) of muscular attachments. An **ostectomy** is the surgical excision of all or part of a bone.

## Surgical Incision (D7510–D7560)

An **abscess** is a collection of pus that results in disintegration or displacement of tissues. In such a case, the abscess needs to be opened and drained of pus, then cleansed and sutured closed.

A **sequestrectomy for osteomyelitis** is isolation of a portion of bone due to inflammation. This procedure prevents the inflammation from spreading to the surrounding bone.

Maxillary sinusotomy for removal of tooth fragment or foreign body is the surgical removal of a tooth fragment or foreign body from the maxilla sinuses.

There are some remaining dental codes used for fractures and dislocations. Some administrators will use these codes, but most will use the codes provided in the *CPT*®. Review all the ADA codes until you are familiar with them.

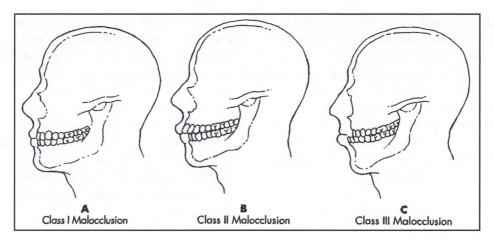

■ **Figure 13–4** Classifications of Malocclusions

Following are additional areas of this section:

**Treatment of Fractures–Simple (D7610–D7680).**

**Treatment of Fractures–Compound (D7710–D7780).**

**Reduction of Dislocation and Management of Other TMJ Dysfunctions (D7810–D7899).**

**Repair of Traumatic Wounds (D7910).**

**Complicated Suturing (D7911–D7912).**

**Other Repair Procedures (D7920–D7999).**

# Orthodontic Services

**Orthodontics** is the branch of dentistry concerned with the detection, prevention, and correction of abnormalities in the positioning of the teeth in relationship to the jaw. The alignment deals with both vertical and horizontal positioning of the teeth. The CDT® codes for this category are D8000–D8999.

The principle of orthodontics is that in order for a person to properly chew food, each tooth must have an aligned opposing tooth. This alignment provides for the proper occlusion.

Many plans do not provide orthodontia benefits. Therefore, if teeth are being extracted (it is common for the bicuspids to be extracted to make sufficient room in the mouth for proper tooth alignment) or if teeth are being crowned (to increase vertical dimension and thus provide proper occlusion) for orthodontic purposes, even though the specific services may be covered by the plan, the services would not be covered because of the purpose of the treatment. Some plans may provide orthodontia benefits but only for children up to a specific age.

Orthodontic treatment is divided into three classifications. The classifications range from the lesser level of misalignment (malocclusion) to the greatest level.

A class I malocclusion is called a **neutroclusion**. This occurs when the upper and lower sets of teeth come together normally, but the teeth themselves do not occlude properly (**see Figure 13–4**). A class II malocclusion is called a **distoclusion**. This occurs when the maxillary arch protrudes out from the mandibular arch. A class III malocclusion is called a **mesioclusion**. This occurs when the mandibular arch protrudes in front of the maxillary arch.

There are other services in which only very slight guidance is required and the level is not even classified. Coding is based on the classification or the type of guidance being provided.

## Comprehensive Orthodontic Treatment (D8070–D8090)

Comprehensive orthodontic treatment is broken into three classifications: D8070–treatment of the transitional dentition (primary teeth), D8080–treatment of the adolescent dentition, and D8090–treatment of the adult dentition.

Auto-reposition appliances are used in temporomandibular joint (TMJ) treatment. Some orthodontic treatment is also done for this reason. TMJ is usually severely limited under most plans but may be allowed if the plan has orthodontic coverage.

The total case fee is the amount charged by the provider for the entire orthodontic treatment program.

This fee should include all diagnostic records, examinations, monthly fees, x-rays, including full-mouth x-rays, cephalometric tracings and photographs, and study models.

Most administrators will pay a portion of the total case fee (called the **banding fee**) upon activation of the orthodontic treatment. The remainder of the total case fee is paid on a monthly basis, and the provider must bill the monthly services charge as treatment is rendered. Some plans have provisions regarding the severity of the malocclusion for orthodontic benefits to be covered. If this is the case, the claim would need to be sent to the dental consultant for review. The average orthodontic case lasts two to three years.

### Minor Treatment to Control Harmful Habits (D8210–D8220)

This area covers appliances that are necessitated because of harmful habits such as tongue thrust, bruxism (grinding of teeth at night), and thumb and lip sucking. These appliances are usually covered only under orthodontics. In each case the coding depends on whether therapy uses a removable or a fixed appliance.

The following is an additional area of this section:

**Other Orthodontic Services (D8660–D8999).**

# Adjunctive General Services

A number of miscellaneous services are necessary for the care and treatment of dental conditions. The CDT® codes for this category are D9000–D9999.

The following are some of the more common services in this area.

### Unclassified Treatment (D9110)

**Palliative treatment** is emergency treatment performed to relieve pain or prevent a condition from worsening. It is not a cure for the disease. Palliative treatment is performed on an emergency basis. After treatment, the patient is directed to go to his or her regular doctor during office hours for treatment of the underlying condition causing the pain.

### Anesthesia (D9210–D9248)

Code D9210 is used for local anesthesia (not in conjunction with the operative or surgical procedures). If another service is being performed, a local anesthesia is normally combined with the procedure and not allowed separately.

General anesthesia is usually allowed for limited services. Usually by administration or through plan provisions, it will be allowed only on procedures that are more definitive (such as oral surgery). Many people have an anxiety about going to a dentist. In such cases, the provider may administer either general, intravenous (IV) sedation, or "twilight sleep." Twilight sleep is a type of relaxation induced by the patient breathing gas. This may also be referred to as "laughing gas." IV sedation is usually allowed on the same basis as general anesthesia. Commonly, it is nitrous oxide. Many plans handle this on the same basis as a local anesthetic; no additional allowance is provided and it may be combined with other procedures performed.

### Professional Consultation (D9310)

This code is used for diagnostic service(s) provided by a physician or dentist other than the practitioner providing the treatment. This code is also used for a second opinion. Often, the consulting provider is a specialist.

### Professional Visits (D9410–D9450)

These codes are used when a dentist visits a patient at the patient's home, at the hospital, at the office during regularly scheduled hours, or at the office outside of regularly scheduled hours.

### Drugs (D9610–D9630)

All drugs are coded as therapeutic drug injections or other drugs or medications.

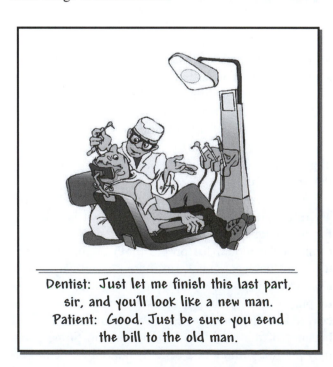

Dentist: Just let me finish this last part, sir, and you'll look like a new man.
Patient: Good. Just be sure you send the bill to the old man.

## Miscellaneous Services (D9910–D9999)

These codes are used for services that do not fall into any other category. They are used to denote the application of desensitizing medications, any complications or unusual circumstances, the performance of an occlusion analysis, and the completion of a claim form.

Code D9999 is used for any services or procedures that do not have a code listed in the ADA code listing. It is classified as "unspecified" and usually requires the addition of a medical report describing the procedure.

# Coverage for TMJ

**Temporomandibular joint (TMJ) dysfunction** is a manifestation of an abnormality of the joint where the lower jaw hinges to the upper jaw (the temporomandibular joint; **see Figure 13–5**). This manifestation can result from various conditions: a disease of the bones such as arthritis, an injury to the TMJ joint, a disintegrative wearing down of the joint socket (the hollow area where the lower joint actually fits into the upper jaw), rheumatic fever or other connective tissue disorders, malocclusion, and even anxiety, emotional problems, and stress.

Symptoms of TMJ dysfunction can include tenderness and pain of the TMJ and surrounding areas, muscle spasms, limitation of movement, and clicking or grating sounds during chewing or speaking.

Because of the variety of causes of TMJ dysfunction, confusion often exists regarding how payment should be handled. If the disorder is caused by arthritis or rheumatic fever, it is due to illness and should fall under medical benefits. If it is caused by anxiety, stress, or emotional problems, it is a psychological problem and should be handled under psychological benefits. If the cause of TMJ dysfunction is malocclusion, it is a dental problem and falls under the dental benefits.

Even under dental benefits, categorizing TMJ dysfunction is confusing because some plans consider it to be a dental problem and some an orthodontic problem. If orthodontic services are not covered, TMJ benefits may then be denied for this reason. Add to all this confusion the knowledge that some dental providers have overutilized the concept (often a patient has malalignment of the teeth, not TMJ dysfunction) in an effort to make the charges eligible under medical benefits rather than dental. Such an arrangement usually results in greater benefit payments because most medical plans have higher allowances and do not have the typical calendar year maximums that dental plans have.

As a result, most payers have adopted stringent guidelines regarding the payment of TMJ claims. Since treatment of TMJ is a very controversial subject, the following list shows some of the more common handling procedures. This is designed to provide guidance only. Remember that the handling of services varies greatly by payer. Therefore, the examiner needs to be aware of

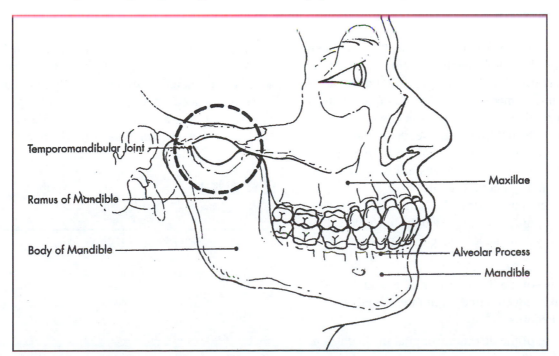

**■ Figure 13–5** Dental Skeletal Structures

these differences and to recognize that special handling or guidelines may apply. Often, services and supplies must meet the following criteria to be payable:

1. They must be recognized by the medical or dental profession as effective and appropriate treatment for TMJ dysfunction and its symptoms.
2. They cannot be self-administered by the patient except with guidance by a licensed physician or dentist.

The following guidelines generally apply when processing TMJ claims:

1. Services or supplies covered under medical plans when provided or prescribed by a dentist for TMJ dysfunction would be recognized as covered medical expenses if they were provided or prescribed by a physician for treatment of comparable forms of intractable pain not involving TMJ dysfunction.
2. Services or supplies covered under dental plans with separate orthodontic benefits are those that are primarily or exclusively used to alter occlusion or reposition the lower jaw.
3. Services or supplies not covered under medical plans or dental plans without separate orthodontic benefits are those specifically excluded under the contract or used to alter occlusion or reposition the lower jaw.

In other words, look at the services that have been rendered, not the TMJ diagnosis. For example, if surgery is performed and the surgery would normally be covered under medical benefits for other than a TMJ diagnosis, then the surgery is covered. If onlays or crowns are used to build up the teeth and reduce the malocclusion, these benefits would be covered under dental benefits if onlays or crowns are normally covered for other noncosmetic reasons.

If the exact cause of the TMJ disorder is proved, the following guidelines are used (often medical or dental review will be necessary before processing the claim):

1. If the cause of the disorder is an accident, treatment is covered under both the dental and medical benefits.
2. If the cause of the disorder is dental malocclusion (decayed, worn, or missing teeth), services are covered under dental benefits (if there is no exclusion for coverage of worn or missing teeth).

3. If the cause of the disorder is congenital malocclusion (hereditary) or developmental (supernumerary teeth, teeth too large for the jaw), the plan should be consulted. If there is an exclusion for congenital or developmental problems, no benefits would be provided. If there is no exclusion, the services would be considered dental.

Some plans eliminate the confusion entirely by excluding TMJ services. In such a case, no benefits would be payable, regardless of the services rendered.

## Appliances

An **appliance** is defined as any device or brace that includes banding or wiring used to reposition teeth, a jaw joint, or the lower jaw to restore normal occlusion. Appliances are often used in restoring normal occlusion to those with TMJ disorders.

### Claims Handling

Claims for appliances are usually referred to a dental consultant for review. The referral must include study models and all current x-rays that support the diagnosis.

If the consultant determines that current occlusion/malocclusion contributes to the patient's condition, benefits are usually paid only under orthodontic coverage unless the plan provides special TMJ coverage. If the plan does not have either type of coverage, benefits under medical or dental provisions (without orthodontic) are usually denied as excluded. If the consultant determines that occlusion is not contributing to the patient's condition and there is radiographic evidence of degenerative joint changes, an appliance may be recommended and covered as an eligible medical expense. Of course, if the plan specifically disallows TMJ treatment, the services still will not be covered.

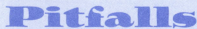

### Practice Pitfalls

Examples of appliances include:

- Auto-repositioning appliance.
- Bite splint.
- Bite guard.
- Orthopedic appliance.
- Orthodontic appliance.
- Mandibular orthopedic reposition appliance.

TMJ handling procedures should always be discussed with your supervisor prior to processing.

## Services and Supplies

The following is a list of services and supplies often associated with the treatment of TMJ disorders, their descriptions, and general dental and medical benefit guidelines to be used in the processing of claims for these types of services and supplies. This list is intended as a general guideline only, and specific payer policies should be consulted.

**Acupuncture**—Insertion of needles into designated areas of the body to relieve or prevent pain. Dental benefits: Allowable only in lieu of general anesthesia for a covered surgical procedure. Acupuncture is covered under the dental plan if medical coverage is not available, and is subject to applicable frequency limits. Medical benefits: Allowable only in lieu of general anesthesia for a covered surgical procedure.

**Behavior Modification and Relaxation Therapy**—Educational training to modify behavior patterns and teach relaxation techniques. Dental benefits: Deny, not usually allowable. Medical benefits: Deny, not for the treatment of a disease or injury.

**Biofeedback**—Electronic devices used to monitor and control automatic body functions such as blood pressure and respiration. Dental benefits: Deny, not usually allowable. Medical benefits: Apply biofeedback guidelines.

**Cranial Manipulation**—Chiropractic adjustment technique involving manipulation and realignment of skull bones. Dental benefits: Deny, not usually allowable. Medical benefits: Deny, not broadly accepted or recognized as effective or necessary treatment of TMJ.

**Diagnostic Examinations**—Oral examination not including or related to a prophylaxis. Dental benefits: Cover under dental plans if no medical coverage available. Medical benefits: Cover as a medical expense.

**Diagnostic X-ray**—Dental x-rays, x-ray of the jaw joint. Dental benefits: Cover under dental plans if no medical coverage available; subject to applicable frequency limits. Medical benefits: Cover as a medical expense.

**Dry Needling**—See Acupuncture.

**Electro Galvanic Nerve Stimulation/ Stimulators (EGS)**—Same as transcutaneous electrical nerve stimulation (TENS) except that a different type of electrical current is used. Refer to discussions on TENS.

**Holistic Therapy**—Hair analysis, fingernail analysis, vitamin therapy. Dental benefits: Deny, usually not listed as a covered expense. Medical benefits: Deny, not broadly accepted or recognized as effective treatment for TMJ.

**Injections of Muscle Relaxants or other Drugs**—Any prescription item to treat muscle spasms; local anesthesia to relieve pain; or steroids to reduce inflammation. Dental benefits: Cover under dental plan if no medical coverage, unless specifically excluded. Medical benefits: Cover when prescribed or administered by a physician or dentist and not excluded by the plan.

**Kinesiographic Analysis**—Measurement and analysis of muscle movement. Dental benefits: Deny, not necessary. Malfunctioning or spastic muscles can be recognized by direct observation or examination. Medical benefits: Deny, not necessary. Malfunctioning or spastic muscles can be recognized by direct observation or examination.

**Mandibular Repositioners**—Stabilizing appliance to reposition the mandible. Dental benefits: Cover if orthodontic services are covered. Medical benefits: Deny, not covered.

**Occlusal Equilibration**—Corrects minor malocclusion by selective grinding of teeth. This balances the bite and allows the lower jaw to relocate into proper position. Dental benefits: Considered orthodontic treatment; cover only under plans with orthodontic benefits. Medical benefits: Deny. Adjustments, correction, or altering of occlusion by any means including appliances are included as covered expenses only under plans that provide orthodontic benefits.

**Occlusal Rehabilitation**—Full-mouth reconstruction using crowns, fixed bridgework, or dentures to restore occlusion and proper relationship between the upper and lower jaw. Dental benefits: Considered orthodontic treatment. Cover only under plans with orthodontic benefits and only for noncosmetic purposes. Medical benefits: Deny. Adjustments, correction, or altering of occlusion by any means, including appliances, are included as covered expenses only under plans that provide orthodontic benefits.

**Oral Surgery**—Any surgical procedure necessary to remove, repair, revise, or reposition the TMJ; such as

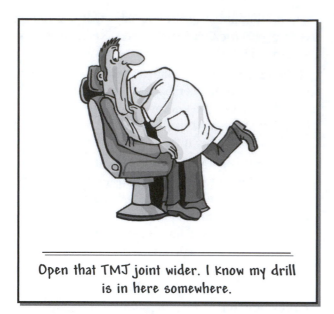

Open that TMJ joint wider. I know my drill is in here somewhere.

meniscectomy, condylectomy, arthrectomy, high condylar shave, or joint implant. Dental benefits: Cover only when no medical coverage is available and oral surgery is listed as a covered dental expense. Medical benefits: Cover as a medical expense.

**Physical therapy**—Vapocoolant sprays, moist heat, massage, cold packs, exercise. Dental benefits: Deny, usually not considered a covered expense. Medical benefits: Deny. Physical therapy can be self-administered by the patient with instruction by a physician or dentist. Physical therapy does not require professional administration.

**Prescription Drugs**—Any prescription item to treat muscle spasms. Dental benefits: Cover if benefits are payable for other prescription drugs. Medical benefits: Cover, payable as treatment of a physical condition, not a mental/nervous disorder.

**Prosthetic Appliances**—Fixed or removable appliances (bridges, dentures, space maintainers). Dental benefits: Cover if prosthetic appliances are covered for other conditions. Medical benefits: Deny, not covered.

**Splinting**—Joining or tying the teeth for stabilization and immobilization or control of bad habits. Dental benefits: Cover if benefits are generally payable for splinting. Medical benefits: Deny, not covered.

**Transcutaneous Electrical Nerve Stimulation/Stimulators (TENS)**—Device used to apply electrical nerve stimulation to relieve TMJ pain. Dental benefits: Deny, usually not considered a covered expense. Medical benefits: Cover charges of a physician or dentist for office visits to administer or supervise TENS therapy for a maximum of one month for intractable pain only (eight to 12 visits, based on two to three visits per week, are reasonable). If TENS therapy is effective during the one-month period, purchase or rental may be recommended. Allow benefits by following normal TENS guidelines limiting rental charges up to usual and customary purchase price of TENS unit.

# On the Job Now

**Directions:** Answer the following questions without looking back at the material just covered. Write your answers in the space provided.

1. Why does confusion often exist regarding how payments should be handled for TMJ dysfunction? _____
_____

2. Why is categorizing TMJ dysfunction confusing under dental benefits? _____
_____

3. What must be included in a claim for appliances that is referred to a dental consultant for review? _____
_____

# CHAPTER REVIEW

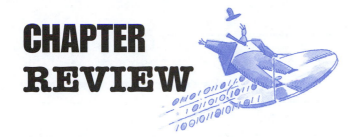

## Summary

- Dentistry is officially that department of the healing arts that is concerned with the teeth, the oral (mouth) cavity, and its associated structures. This includes diagnosis, treatment, restoration, and replacement of missing portions or parts.
- Dentistry also includes surgical procedures performed in and about the inside of the mouth or oral cavity.
- There are services in dentistry that are performed for other than existing pathologic conditions. Some of these existing services (such as prophylaxis, x-rays, fluoride treatments, and repair of dentures and bridgework) are specifically included as covered dental services under most plans, but are usually subject to limitations.
- Other services can be performed not for a pathologic condition but primarily for cosmetic or similar reasons. Although the particular type or category of service that is received might be covered under the plan, benefits are usually not provided for services that are performed for cosmetic or similar purposes, or for elective services.
- In the late 1960s, the American Dental Association (ADA) created a coding system that served to categorize dental services. This established a uniform nomenclature for all dental services.
- The ADA list classifies procedures under certain categories.
- Services (and thus their codes) are defined based on the type of treatment provided. It is important to know what type of service is being performed to code it properly. Familiarity with the different types of dental services and their codes will help to ensure accurate dental coding.
- Temporomandibular joint dysfunction is a manifestation of an abnormality of the TMJ joint. Since the causes of TMJ dysfunction can be many and varied, the treatment can also take a variety of forms. Some treatments fall under coverage for dental services; others are covered as medical services.
- Because of the variety of payment options (and the past history of provider abuse in TMJ services), care should be taken to fully understand the terms of the contract and the TMJ policies of the payer.

## Assignments

Complete the Questions for Review.
Complete Exercises 13–1 through 13–3.

## Questions for Review

**Directions:** Answer the following questions without looking back at the material just covered. Write your answers in the space provided.

1. List the 12 ADA classifications of dental services.

1. _____

2. _____

3. _____

4. _____

5. _____

6. _____

7. _____

8. _____

9. _____

10. _____

11. _____

12. _____

2. What are diagnostic procedures? _____

_____

3. What are preventive services? _____

_____

4. What are orthodontic services? _____

_____

5. What is prosthodontics? _____

_____

6. What are restorative services? _____

_____

7. What are endodontic services? _____

_____

8. What are periodontic services? _____

_____

9. Under what ADA category do routine fillings fall? _____

10. What are inlays and onlays and under what ADA category do they fall? _____

_____

_____

11. What is TMJ dysfunction? _____

_____

**12.** Why have some dental providers overutilized the concept of TMJ? _____

_____

_____

**13.** What are the claims handling procedures for TMJ appliances? _____

_____

_____

**14.** What is the description for diagnostic examinations? _____

_____

**15.** Is holistic therapy usually a covered expense for TMJ? _____

_____

If you were unable to answer any of these questions, refer back to that section and then fill in the answers.

# Exercise **13-1**

**Directions:**    Find and circle the words listed below. Words can appear horizontally, vertically, diagonally, forward, or backward.

```
S H N L S D S W D E V L I Q W G N E Q E
M E H E R I E E H A H O P N E O V C A
P P R P U Q X F E B S S O I V T I I W U
O U N U X T G A I C T M L H W O S T D J
U P L T T N R A L E S I R F I M I A E X
Q H N P I N L O C Y F B J F X A C R N A
C P E D E V E T C D H Z A W Q T X O T N
Z H N I E C O D E L R P C L R O E T I M
K A I N S M T T Y O U U O U Z P L S S F
B R E R Y X A O X R L S G R U L A E T G
O E T V V C L H M P A K I G P A C R R N
R T X R I N L A Y Y E R Z O L S I M Y I
O M C D J L A N A C T O O R N T G S S T
A P E X I F I C A T I O N P B Y R S W A
S M S C I T N O D O D N E W M O U E D E
X L B D I A G N O S T I C I M E S K Z S
Y J X Q O Z V X B V S H A U U L T M L T
X H Z S T T L V Y Q U F T X X B L H S U
T B Q P E Q U X D F T D G Q I A G I R A
F J S M H D V J G U Q U O K H N S D Q V
```

1. Abscess
2. Apexification
3. Banding Fee
4. Dentistry
5. Diagnostic
6. Endodontics
7. Inlay
8. Labial Veneer
9. Neutroclusion
10. Ostectomy
11. Prophylaxis
12. Pulpectomy
13. Restorative
14. Root Canal
15. Seating
16. Surgical Excision
17. Temporary Dentures
18. Tumors

# Exercise 13-2

**Directions:** Complete the crossword puzzle by filling in a word from the keywords that fits each clue.

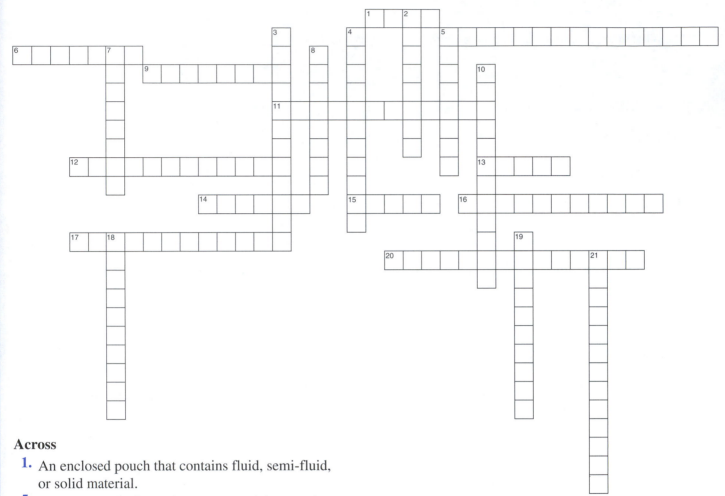

**Across**

1. An enclosed pouch that contains fluid, semi-fluid, or solid material.
5. Models that duplicate the structure of the mouth.
6. To transfer or to graft something additional onto or into an existing surface.
9. A device used for maintaining the teeth and jaws in an appropriate position.
11. Correction or prevention of poor or misaligned teeth.
12. Occurs when the maxillary arch protrudes out from the mandibular arch.
13. A covering that is placed on a tooth.
14. The part of a bridge that is suspended between abutments and replaces a missing tooth.
15. A gold alloy casting that lies on the occlusal surface but covers one or more cusps.
16. The placing of a covering over an exposed tooth pulp.
17. Appliances that replace all of the patient's natural teeth.
20. Rays taken with the film placed outside the mouth.

**Down**

2. Plastic-like coating placed on healthy teeth to prevent decay.
3. Treatment of the tissues surrounding and supporting the teeth.
4. Procedures used to restore a natural tooth.
5. Doctors who have received a Doctor of Medical Dentistry (D. M. D) degree.
7. A new tumor or growth.
8. A tooth that is used to support or stabilize one end of a prosthetic appliance.
10. Occurs when the mandibular arch protrudes in front of the maxillary arch.
18. The support that runs along the bottom of the mouth.
19. The support that runs across the top of the palate (roof of the mouth).
21. Surgical preparation of a ridge for dentures.

# Exercise 13-3

**Directions:** Match the following terms with the proper definition by writing the letter of the correct definition in the space next to the term.

1. _____ Adjunctive General Services

2. _____ Appliance

3. _____ Bitewing X-rays

4. _____ Diagnostic Photographs

5. _____ Fluoride Treatments

6. _____ Full-mouth X-ray Limitation

7. _____ Impacted Tooth

8. _____ Intraoral X-rays

9. _____ Occlusal X-rays

10. _____ Oral Surgery

11. _____ Palliative Treatment

12. _____ Pin Retention

13. _____ Preventive Services

14. _____ Prosthodontics, Removable

15. _____ Prosthodontics, Fixed

16. _____ Removal of Exostosis

17. _____ Sequestrectomy for Osteomyelitis

18. _____ Space Maintenance

19. _____ Temporomandibular Joint (TMJ) Dysfunction

20. _____ Tissue Conditioning

a. A manifestation of an abnormality of the joint where the lower jaw hinges to the upper jaw.

b. The placement of wires or a retainer in the mouth to prevent the wrongful movement of teeth into a space where a tooth has been lost.

c. A method of correcting tissue irritation resulting from the wearing of dentures.

d. The isolation of a portion of bone due to inflammation.

e. A tooth that is positioned or wedged against another tooth, bone, or soft tissue and is prevented from erupting normally.

f. Replacement of the natural teeth through the use of a permanent appliance.

g. X-rays which show the floor of the mouth and the palate.

h. An emergency treatment performed to relieve pain or prevent a condition from worsening.

i. Treatment of the internal structures of the mouth limited to the dental structures and surrounding tissues.

j. X-rays taken with the film placed inside the mouth.

k. The insertion of a small, thin needle-like pin into the remaining tooth structure to provide extra support for the restoration.

l. Routine services designed to prevent decay, gum disease, etc., through the care of the dental structures before disease has occurred.

m. Colored photographs of the oral cavity.

n. If the dollar amount payable for the total number of x-rays taken exceeds the dollar amount payable for a set of full-mouth x-rays, the allowable amount would be based on the full-mouth x-ray allowance because the dentist could have taken an entire x-ray series to see all tooth structures.

o. The application of a topical fluoride substance to the teeth.

p. X-rays that show the relationship of the teeth in two opposing dental arches.

q. The removal of a bony growth that arises from either the maxilla or mandible.

r. Replacement of the natural teeth through the use of a removable appliance.

s. Miscellaneous services, treatments not listed elsewhere on a dental code listing.

t. Any device or brace that includes banding or wiring used to reposition teeth, jaw joint, or lower jaw to restore normal occlusion.

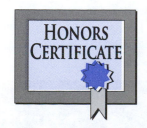

## Honors Certification™

The Honors Certification™ challenge for this chapter consists of a written test of the information contained within this chapter. Each incorrect answer will result in a deduction of up to 5% from your grade. You must achieve a score of 85% or higher to pass this test. If you fail the test on your first attempt, you may retake the test one additional time. The items included in the second test may be different from those in the first test.

# 14

# Dental Claims
## Administration

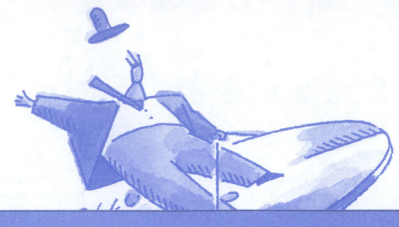

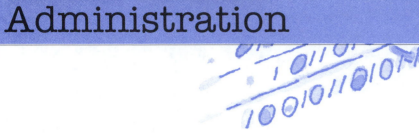

## After completion of this chapter
**you will be able to:**

- Explain the dental claim form and its proper use.
- Identify the minimum data requirements on a dental claim form.
- Properly complete a dental claim form using a given scenario.
- Explain the differences between the medical Patient Information Sheet and the dental Patient Information Sheet.
- Properly complete a dental Patient Information Sheet using a given scenario.

- Calculate dental conversion factors for a given procedure.
- Process dental claims, applying all contract provisions and limitations.
- Complete all necessary information on a claim Payment Worksheet.
- Identify and explain the use of common dental form letters used by health claims examiners.
- Identify the most common fraudulent claim situations.

## Keywords and concepts
**you will learn in this chapter:**

- Claim Payment Worksheet
- Dental Claim Form
- Patient Claim Form
- Request for Additional Information Form

There are two basic forms that dental providers use to bill claims. These forms are the American Dental Association (ADA) claim form and the Patient Information Sheet. The ADA **Dental Claim Form** lists specific information regarding the patient and the services that have been or are going to be performed. The **Patient Claim Form** contains basically the same information as the ADA Dental Claim Form.

When a claim for dental services is received, it is the responsibility of the claims examiner to determine whether the claim received is eligible for payment. This entails several steps including verifying eligibility, determining whether services rendered are covered, and identifying any coverage limitations that may exist. After a preliminary investigation is performed, the processing of the claim can be completed.

Processing of dental claims occurs in much the same manner as the processing of medical claims. Basic steps should be followed in each instance for the processing to be properly completed.

## The ADA Dental Claim Form

There are several versions of the ADA Dental Claim Form currently in use; however, there is little difference among each of the versions (see **Figures 14–1** and **14–2**). This claim form can be used as a billing statement for services performed and also for a pretreatment estimate of services to be performed. However, at no time should services already performed be included with those for which the dentist or patient is seeking a pretreatment estimate.

Following is a list of items, their descriptions, and uses. The word "Same" as a description indicates that the description of the item is the same as the item name.

### Item # Item Name/Description

Following are the numbers, titles, and descriptions of the items found on the ADA Dental Claim form.

1 **Type of transaction.** The appropriate box would be checked depending on whether services have been performed yet or not. Only one box should be checked. Therefore, services previously performed and services to be performed should not be combined on the same form.

2 **Predetermination or preauthorization number.** Enter the number provided by the payer when submitting a claim for services that have been predetermined or preauthorized.

3 **Carrier name and address.** The name and address of the payer to whom this bill is being sent.

### Secondary insurance coverage items

Leave items 4–11 blank if there is no other coverage.

4 **Other dental or medical coverage?** Indicate "yes" or "no". Items 5 through 11 should be answered only if the patient has coverage by a second carrier.

5 **Subscriber name.** If the employee or subscriber indicated in item 5 is not the patient, list the employee's/subscriber's name here.

6 **Date of birth.** If the employee or subscriber indicated in item 5 is not the patient, list the birthdate here.

7 **Gender.** Check the box indicating the gender of the subscriber.

8 **Subscriber identifier (SSN or ID#).** If the employee or subscriber listed in item 5 is not the patient, list the social security number here.

9 **Plan/group number.** Indicate the group numbers of the policies indicated in item 5.

10 **Relationship to primary subscriber.** Indicate the relationship of the patient to the employee/subscriber listed in item 5.

11 **Other carrier name, address, city, state, zip code.** Indicate the name and address of the carrier indicated in item 5.

### Primary subscriber information items

12 **Name, address, city, state, zip code.** Enter the name as last name, first name, middle initial, and suffix.

13 **Date of birth.** Enter birthdate as month, date, and year.

14 **Gender.** Check the box indicating the gender of the subscriber.

15 **Subscriber identifier (SSN or ID#).** Same.

## ADA Dental Claim Form

SAMPLE

### HEADER INFORMATION

**1. Type of Transaction (Check all applicable boxes)**

[X] Statement of Actual Services  – OR –  [ ] Request for Predetermination / Preauthorization

[ ] EPSDT / Title XIX

**2. Predetermination/Preauthorization Number**

### PRIMARY PAYER INFORMATION

**3. Name, Address, City, State, Zip Code**

BALL INSURANCE CARRIERS
3895 BUBBLE BLVD STE 283
BOXWOOD CO 85926

### OTHER COVERAGE

**4. Other Dental or Medical Coverage?**  [X] No (Skip 5-11)   [ ] Yes (Complete 5-11)

**5. Subscriber Name (Last, First, Middle Initial, Suffix)**

**6. Date of Birth (MM/DD/CCYY)**   **7. Gender** [ ] M [ ] F   **8. Subscriber Identifier (SSN or ID#)**

**9. Plan/Group Number**   **10. Relationship to Primary Subscriber (Check applicable box)** [ ] Self [ ] Spouse [ ] Dependent [ ] Other

**11. Other Carrier Name, Address, City, State, Zip Code**

### PRIMARY SUBSCRIBER INFORMATION

**12. Name (Last, First, Middle Initial, Suffix), Address, City, State, Zip Code**

PATIENT PATTY P
655 PAIN LANE
PEN PA 15522

**13. Date of Birth (MM/DD/CCYY)** 05/15/CCYY-35   **14. Gender** [ ] M [X] F   **15. Subscriber Identifier (SSN or ID#)** 555 55 XYZ

**16. Plan/Group Number** 62958XYZ   **17. Employer Name** XYZ CORPORATION

### PATIENT INFORMATION

**18. Relationship to Primary Subscriber (Check applicable box)** [X] Self [ ] Spouse [ ] Dependent Child [ ] Other   **19. Student Status** [ ] FTS [ ] PTS

**20. Name (Last, First, Middle Initial, Suffix), Address, City, State, Zip Code**

PATIENT PATTY P
655 PAIN LANE
PEN PA 15522

**21. Date of Birth (MM/DD/CCYY)** 05/15/CCYY-35   **22. Gender** [ ] M [X] F   **23. Patient ID/Account # (Assigned by Dentist)**

### RECORD OF SERVICES PROVIDED

| | 24. Procedure Date (MM/DD/CCYY) | 25. Area of Oral Cavity | 26. Tooth System | 27. Tooth Number(s) or Letter(s) | 28. Tooth Surface | 29. Procedure Code | 30. Description | 31. Fee |
|---|---|---|---|---|---|---|---|---|
| 1 | 2/8/CCYY | | | | | D1110 | PROPHYLAXIS | 80 00 |
| 2 | 2/8/CCYY | | | | | D0140 | LIMITED ORAL EVAL | 20 00 |
| 3 | 2/8/CCYY | | | 4 | B | D2140 | AMALGAM – ONE SURFACE | 65 00 |
| 4 | | | | | | | | |
| 5 | | | | | | | | |
| 6 | | | | | | | | |
| 7 | | | | | | | | |
| 8 | | | | | | | | |
| 9 | | | | | | | | |
| 10 | | | | | | | | |

### MISSING TEETH INFORMATION

Permanent                                          Primary                      **32. Other Fee(s)**

**34. (Place an 'X' on each missing tooth)**

| 1 | 2 | 3 | 4 | 5 | 6 | 7 | 8 | 9 | 10 | 11 | 12 | 13 | 14 | 15 | 16 | A | B | C | D | E | F | G | H | I | J |
|---|---|---|---|---|---|---|---|---|---|---|---|---|---|---|---|---|---|---|---|---|---|---|---|---|---|
| 32 | 31 | 30 | 29 | 28 | 27 | 26 | 25 | 24 | 23 | 22 | 21 | 20 | 19 | 18 | 17 | T | S | R | Q | P | O | N | M | L | K |

**33. Total Fee** 165 00

**35. Remarks**

### AUTHORIZATIONS

**36.** I have been informed of the treatment plan and associated fees. I agree to be responsible for all charges for dental services and materials not paid by my dental benefit plan, unless prohibited by law, or the treating dentist or dental practice has a contractual agreement with my plan prohibiting all or a portion of such charges. To the extent permitted by law, I consent to your use and disclosure of my protected health information to carry out payment activities in connection with this claim.

X *Patient Patty*                   02/08/CCYY
Patient/Guardian signature              Date

**37.** I hereby authorize and direct payment of the dental benefits otherwise payable to me, directly to the below named dentist or dental entity.

X _____
Subscriber signature              Date

### BILLING DENTIST OR DENTAL ENTITY (Leave blank if dentist or dental entity is not submitting claim on behalf of the patient or insured/subscriber)

**48. Name, Address, City, State, Zip Code**

OSCAR ORTIZ DDS
4444 OLSEN BLVD
OLIVER PA 15555

| 49. Provider ID | 50. License Number M94732 | 51. SSN or TIN 70-3333333 |
|---|---|---|

**52. Phone Number** ( 000 ) 555 - 3333

©American Dental Association, 2002
J515 (Same as ADA Dental Claim Form) – J516, J517, J518, J519

### ANCILLARY CLAIM/TREATMENT INFORMATION

**38. Place of Treatment (Check applicable box)** [X] Provider's Office [ ] Hospital [ ] ECF [ ] Other

**39. Number of Enclosures (00 to 99)** Radiograph(s) 0  Oral Image(s) 0  Model(s) 0

**40. Is Treatment for Orthodontics?** [X] No (Skip 41-42) [ ] Yes (Complete 41-42)

**41. Date Appliance Placed (MM/DD/CCYY)**

**42. Months of Treatment Remaining**   **43. Replacement of Prosthesis?** [X] No [ ] Yes (Complete 44)   **44. Date Prior Placement (MM/DD/CCYY)**

**45. Treatment Resulting from (Check applicable box)** [ ] Occupational illness/injury [ ] Auto accident [ ] Other accident

**46. Date of Accident (MM/DD/CCYY)**   **47. Auto Accident State**

### TREATING DENTIST AND TREATMENT LOCATION INFORMATION

**53.** I hereby certify that the procedures as indicated by date are in progress (for procedures that require multiple visits) or have been completed and that the fees submitted are the actual fees I have charged and intend to collect for those procedures.

X *Oscar Ortiz*                   02/08/ccyy
Signed (Treating Dentist)              Date

**54. Provider ID**   **55. License Number** 13331

**56. Address, City, State, Zip Code**

4444 OLSEN BLVD
OLIVER PA 15555

**57. Phone Number** ( 000 ) 555 -3333   **58. Treating Provider Specialty**

**Figure 14–1**  Front of the ADA Dental Claim Form

General Instructions:

The form is designed so that the Primary Payer's name and address (Item 3) is visible in a standard #10 window envelope. Please fold the form using the 'tick-marks' printed in the left and right margins. The upper-right blank space is provided for insertion of the third-party payer's claim or control number.

a)   All data elements are required unless noted to the contrary on the face of the form, or in the Data Element Specific Instructions that follow.
b)   When a name and address field is required, the full entity or individual name, address and zip code must be entered (i.e., Items 3, 11, 12, 20 and 48).
c)   All dates must include the four-digit year (i.e., Items 6, 13, 21, 24, 36, 37, 41, 44, and 53).
d)   If the number of procedures being reported exceeds the number of lines available on one claim form the remaining procedures must be listed on a separate, fully completed claim form. Both claim forms are submitted to the third-party payer.

Data Element Specific Instructions

1.    **EPSDT / Title XIX** -- Mark box if patient is covered by state Medicaid's **E**arly and **P**eriodic **S**creening, **D**iagnosis and **T**reatment program for persons under age 21.
2.    Enter number provided by the payer when submitting a claim for services that have been predetermined or preauthorized.
4-11. Leave blank if no other coverage.
8.    The subscriber's Social Security Number (SSN) or other identifier (ID#) assigned by the payer.
15.   The subscriber's Social Security Number (SSN) or other identifier (ID#) assigned by the payer.
16.   Subscriber's or employer group's Plan or Policy Number. May also be known as the Certificate Number. [Not the subscriber's identification number.]
19-23. Complete only if the patient is **not** the Primary Subscriber. (i.e., "Self" not checked in Item 18)
19.   Check "FTS" if patient is a dependent and full-time student; "PTS" if a part-time student. Otherwise, leave blank.
23.   Enter if dentist's office assigns a unique number to identify the patient that is **not** the same as the Subscriber Identifier number assigned by the payer (e.g., Chart #).
25.   Designate tooth number or letter when procedure code directly involves a tooth. Use area of the oral cavity code set from ANSI/ADA/ISO Specification No. 3950 'Designation System for Teeth and Areas of the Oral Cavity'.
26.   Enter applicable ANSI ASC X12 code list qualifier: Use "**JP**" when designating teeth using the ADA's Universal/National Tooth Designation System. Use "**JO**" when using the ANSI/ADA/ISO Specification No. 3950.
27.   Designate tooth number when procedure code reported directly involves a tooth. If a range of teeth is being reported use a hyphen ('-') to separate the first and last tooth in the range. Commas are used to separate individual tooth numbers or ranges applicable to the procedure code reported.
28.   Designate tooth surface(s) when procedure code reported directly involves one or more tooth surfaces. Enter up to five of the following codes, without spaces: **B** = Buccal; **D** = Distal; **F** = Facial; **L** = Lingual; **M** = Mesial; and **O** = Occlusal.
29.   Use appropriate dental procedure code from current version of *Code on Dental Procedures and Nomenclature*.
31.   Dentist's full fee for the dental procedure reported.
32.   Used when other fees applicable to dental services provided must be recorded. Such fees include state taxes, where applicable, and other fees imposed by regulatory bodies.
33.   Total of all fees listed on the claim form.
34.   Report missing teeth on each claim submission.
35.   Use "Remarks" space for additional information such as 'reports' for '999' codes or multiple supernumerary teeth.
36.   Patient Signature: The patient is defined as an individual who has established a professional relationship with the dentist for the delivery of dental health care. For matters relating to communication of information and consent, this term includes the patient's parent, caretaker, guardian, or other individual as appropriate under state law and the circumstances of the case.
37.   Subscriber Signature: Necessary when the patient/insured and dentist wish to have benefits paid directly to the provider. This is an authorization of payment. It does not create a contractual relationship between the dentist and the payer.
38.   ECF is the acronym for Extended Care Facility (e.g., nursing home).
48-52. Leave blank if dentist or dental entity is **not** submitting claim on behalf of the patient or insured/subscriber.
48.   The individual dentist's name or the name of the group practice/corporation responsible for billing and other pertinent information. This may differ from the actual treating dentist's name. This is the information that should appear on any payments or correspondence that will be remitted to the billing dentist.
49.   Identifier assigned to Billing Dentist or Dental Entity other than the SSN or TIN. Necessary when assigned by carrier receiving the claim.
50.   Refers to the license number of the billing dentist. This may differ from that of the treating (rendering) dentist that appears in the treating dentist's signature block.
52.   The Internal Revenue Service requires that either the Social Security Number (SSN) or Tax Identification Number (TIN) of the billing dentist or dental entity be supplied **only** if the provider accepts payment directly from the third-party payer.
      When the payment is being accepted directly report the: 1) SSN if the billing dentist in unincorporated; 2) Corporation TIN if the billing dentist is incorporated; or 3) Entity TIN when the billing entity is a group practice or clinic.
53.   The treating, or rendering, dentist's signature and date the claim form was signed. Dentists should be aware that they have ethical and legal obligations to refund fees for services that are paid in advance but not completed.
56.   Full address, including city, state and zip code, where treatment performed by treating (rendering) dentist.
58.   Enter the code that indicates the type of dental professional rendering the service from the 'Dental Service Providers' section of the *Healthcare Providers Taxonomy* code list. The current list is posted at: http://www.wpc-edi.com/codes/codes.asp. The available taxonomy codes, as of the first printing of this claim form, follow printed in **boldface**.

122300000X Dentist -- A dentist is a person qualified by a doctorate in dental surgery (D.D.S.) or dental medicine (D.M.D.) licensed by the state to practice dentistry, and practicing within the scope of that license.

Many dentists are general practitioners who handle a wide variety of dental needs.
**1223G0001X** General Practice

Other dentists practice in one of nine specialty areas recognized by the American Dental Association:
**1223D0001X** Dental Public Health
**1223E0200X** Endodontics
**1223P0106X** Oral & Maxillofacial Pathology
**1223D0008X** Oral and Maxillofacial Radiology
**1223S0112X** Oral & Maxillofacial Surgery
**1223X0400X** Orthodontics
**1223P0221X** Pediatric Dentistry (Pedodontics)
**1223P0300X** Periodontics
**1223P0700X** Prosthodontics

■ **Figure 14–2**  Back of the ADA Dental Claim Form

**16**  **Plan/group number.** Indicate the group or policy number.

**17**  **Employer name.** Indicate the full name of the company for which the employee/subscriber works.

**Patient information items**

**18**  **Relationship to primary subscriber.** Check the appropriate box of self, spouse, child, or other. If other is checked, indicate the relationship of the patient to the employee or insured.

**19**  **Student status.** If the patient is a full-time student, enter the name of the school and the location (city) of the school.

**20**  **Patient name, address, city, state, zip code.** Enter the name as last name, first name, middle initial, and suffix.

**21**  **Date of birth.** Enter birthdate as month, date, and year.

**22**  **Gender.** Check the box indicating the gender of the patient.

**23**  **Patient ID/account #.** Same.

## Record of services provided items

**24**  **Procedure dates.** Same.

**25**  **Area of oral cavity.** Designate tooth number or letter when procedure code directly involves a tooth.

**26**  **Tooth system.** Enter the applicable tooth system used for coding.

**27**  **Tooth number(s) or letter number(s).** Enter the tooth letter or number for the treatment described.

**28**  **Tooth surface.** The surface letter for each surface of the tooth affected by the treatment.

**29**  **Procedure code.** Enter the ADA procedure code for the service.

**30**  **Description.** Include all x-rays, prophylaxis, materials used, and so on.

**31**  **Fee.** Enter the amount billed for the service. Remember to total the fees and place this amount in the "Total fee charged" item at the bottom of the column.

**32**  **Other fee(s).** Used when other fees applicable to dental services provided must be recorded. Such fees include state taxes, where applicable, and other fees imposed by regulatory bodies.

**33**  **Total fee.** Total of all fees listed on the claim form.

Note: If the patient made partial payment for the services rendered, the words "Patient paid" should appear at the bottom of the description item and the amount paid should appear at the bottom of the fee column. This payment should then be subtracted from the above fees and the balance due placed in the item labeled "Total fee."

**34**  **Missing teeth information (Place an "X" on each missing tooth).** Report missing teeth on each claim submission.

**35**  **Remarks.** Enter any remarks that clarify the services or use of materials in services above.

Indicate tooth number or procedure code if necessary for clarification of the procedure being remarked upon. Any additional description needed for items 24 through 29 can also be added here.

**36**  **Patient/guardian signature.** A patient must sign and date this item to authorize the provider (dentist) to release information to the payer.

**37**  **Subscriber signature.** Necessary when the patient/insured and dentist wish to have benefits paid directly to the provider. This is an authorization of payment. It does not create a contractual relationship between the dentist and the payer.

## Ancillary claim or treatment information items

**38**  **Place of treatment.** Check the appropriate box for whether treatment was rendered at an office, a hospital, an Extended Care Facility (ECF), or other.

**39**  **Number of enclosures (00–99).** Indicate "yes" or "no" and the number of radiographs (x-rays) or models enclosed with the claim. These are generally enclosed to allow the claims examiner or review board to determine the necessity of services rendered. Radiographs or models will more often accompany a pretreatment estimate to assist the claims examiner in determining appropriate benefits.

**40**  **Is treatment for orthodontics?** If your answer is "no", skip items 41–42. If the answer is "yes", complete items 41–42.

**41**  **Date appliance placed.** Same.

**42**  **Months of treatment remaining.** Same.

**43**  **Replacement of prosthesis?** If your answer is no, skip item 44. If your answer is yes, complete item 44.

**44**  **Date of prior placement.** Same.

**45**  **Treatment resulting from?** Check the appropriate box of occupational illness or injury, auto accident, or other accident. If treatment is the result of an auto accident, answer items 46 and 47.

**46**  **Date of accident.** Same.

**47**  **Auto accident state.** Same.

## Billing dentist or dental entity items

Leave items 48–52 blank if dentist or dental entity is not submitting the claim on behalf of the patient or insured/subscriber.

**48  Billing dentist or dental entity name, address, city, state, zip code.** Enter the dentist's mailing address. Payments will be sent to this address.

**49  Provider ID.** Same.

**50  License number.** Same.

**51  SSN or TIN.** Enter the dentist's social security number or taxpayer identification number.

**52  Phone number.** Same.

### Treating dentist and treatment location information items

**53  Treating dentist's signature and date the claim form was signed.** By signing this form, the dentist indicates that those fees that have a date of service have been performed, and that the charges are the actual charges for the services.

**54  Provider ID.** Same.

**55  License number.** Same.

**56  Address, city, state, zip code.** Same.

**57  Phone number.** Same.

**58  Treating provider specialty.** Enter the code that indicates the type of dental professional rendering the service from the "Dental Service Providers" section of the *Health Providers Taxonomy* code list. The current list is posted at: http://www.wpc-edi.com/codes.asp.

## Patient Claim Form

In addition to the ADA Dental Claim Form, a dental claims examiner may occasionally receive a Patient Claim Form (see **Figures 14–3** and **14–4**). This form is usually provided by self-funded plans; therefore, the format varies widely from one plan to another. However, the information contained on the form is generally the same.

The information on the form is self-explanatory. The member should complete the information entitled "To Be Completed by Member," and the provider of services should complete the information entitled "To Be Completed by Physician."

At the bottom of most Patient Claim Forms, there is a space for the dental claims examiner to indicate the maximum allowable amount for the services, the deductible applied to the claim, the coinsurance percentage that the payer is responsible for, the amount the payer is responsible for, and the amount the patient is responsible for.

## Predetermination and Preauthorization

As a claims examiner, if you receive a dental claim form, be sure to check whether it is for services that have been rendered or if it is a request for a pretreatment estimate. If the pretreatment estimate box is checked and there is no date of when services were rendered, the claim is for a pretreatment estimate. Be sure not to issue a check for these services. Simply process the claim as you normally would according to the benefit guidelines, and complete the information at the bottom of the claim form. A copy of the claim form and the EOB should be kept in the member's file.

## Claim Analysis

A good claims examiner must have a thorough and systematic process for analyzing claims. The same process is used on each claim no matter how simple or complex. This is how consistency and accuracy are developed. The following steps may be used in the development of a systematic approach to performing a uniform initial claim analysis:

Perform an initial claim analysis by answering the following questions:

1. Was the correct claim form used for the services provided?
2. Has the claim form been properly filled out?
3. Is all the information complete?
4. Did the member authorize the release of information?

If the answer to any of the above questions is no, deny the claim or pend it and request additional information.

If the initial claim analysis warrants, proceed to the next step, evaluating the eligibility of the claimant.

## Eligibility

A member must be eligible for benefits at the time services are rendered; otherwise, no benefits will be payable. Therefore, performing a complete eligibility analysis is critical. The following steps may be helpful in performing a thorough eligibility check.

# Dental Patient Claim Form

- This [DENTAL PLAN] is administered by [COMPANY]
- Please provide complete information and print clearly.

| Part 1: To be completed by Dentist | | Unique Number | Spec. | Patient's Office Account No. | I hereby assign my benefits payable from this claim to the named dentist and authorize payment directly to him/her. |
|---|---|---|---|---|---|
| PATIENT | Last Name        First Name | DENTIST | | | |
| | | | | | Signature of Subsrciber |

| For Dentist's Use Only – For additional information, diagnosis, procedures, or special consideration. | I understand that the fees listed in this claim may not be covered by or may exceed my plan benefits. I understand that I am financially responsible to my dentist for the entire treatment. I acknowledge that the total fee of $ _____ is accurate and has been charged to me for services rendered. I authorize release of the information in this claim form to my insuring company/plan administrator. |
|---|---|
| | Signature of Patient (Parent/Guardian) |
| Duplicate Form ☐ | Office Verification/Dentist's Signature |

| Date of Service | | | Procedure Code | Intl. Tooth Code | Tooth Surfaces | Dentists's Fee | Laboratory Charge | Total Charges | For Plan Administrator Use Only |
|---|---|---|---|---|---|---|---|---|---|
| Month | Day | Year | | | | | | | |
| | | | | | | | | | |
| | | | | | | | | | |
| | | | | | | | | | |
| | | | | | | | | | |
| | | | | | | | | | |
| | | | | | | | | | |
| | | | | | | | | | |
| | | | | | | | | | |
| | | | | | | | | | |
| | | | | | | | | | |
| | | | | | | **TOTAL FEE SUBMITTED** | | | INDICATE MISSING TEETH WITH AN 'X' |

## Part 2: To be completed by member

### Member Information

| Contract Number | Certificate Number | Date of Birth | Month | Day | Year |
|---|---|---|---|---|---|
| | | | / | / | |

| Last Name | First Name | Language of Preference |
|---|---|---|
| | | |

| Street Address | Apt. Number | Telephone No. |
|---|---|---|
| | | |

| City | State or Province | Postal Code | Country |
|---|---|---|---|
| | | | |

### Family Member Covered by this Claim

| Full Name of Spouse or Common Law Partner | Date of Birth | Month | Day | Year |
|---|---|---|---|---|
| | | / | / | |

| Name of Dependent Child | Relationship to Insured | | Date of Birth | | | If child is 21 or over, check whether child is: | |
|---|---|---|---|---|---|---|---|
| | Son | Daughter | Day | Month | Year | Disabled | Full-time Student |
| | ☐ | ☐ | / | / | | ☐ | ☐ |

**■ Figure 14–3** Patient Claim Form Side 1

## Details of Claim

1. Major restorative or prosthodontic claims (e.g. crowns, inlays, bridges, dentures, etc.)

| Is this the initial placement? | No ☐ | Yes ☐ | |
|---|---|---|---|
| If No,<br>Date of prior placement:<br>• Reason for replacement | • : | | Date dentist took impression for this treatment: |
| Please ask your dentist to include the following to facilitate handling of your claim: | | • | Pre-treatment x-rays (for crowns, inlays, onlays, veneers, and bridges only). |

2. Are any expenses the result of an accident?

| When and where did the accident occur? | Month     Day     Year<br>/        / |
|---|---|
| How did the accident occur? | |
| Are any expenses the result of a condition covered by Worker's Compensation/Workplace Safety and Insurance Board?    No ☐      Yes ☐ | |

3. Orthodontics

| Is this treatment for orthodontic purposes?    No ☐    Yes ☐ ▶ | Date initial appliance was installed: | /        /<br>Month     Day     Year |
|---|---|---|

## Coverage Under Other Benefit Plans

Are **you** covered for any of these expenses under any other benefit plan as an active employee?

No ☐      Yes ☐ ▶        If yes: You must submit a claim to your employee plan **first**; then attach the original Explanation of Benefits (EOB) from that plan and complete this form.

Are **you** covered for any of these expenses under any other benefit plan as a pensioner?

No ☐      Yes ☐ ▶

Please indicate:    Name of Insurer: _____

Contract Number: _____    Certificate Number: _____

Is **your spouse, common law partner, or child** covered for any of these expenses under any other benefit plan?

No ☐      Yes ☐ ▶        Spouse or common law partner's date of birth:        /        /
Month     Day     Year

**If yes:**

• You must submit a claim for your spouse or common law partner to their plan **first**.

• You must submit a claim for your child **first** under the plan of the parent with the earliest birthday (month and day) in the calendar year.

• Once the other plan processes the claim, attach the original Explanation of Benefits (EOB) from that plan and complete this claim form.

## Member Certification & Authorization

I certify that the statements in this claim are true and complete and do not contain a claim for any expenses previously paid for by this or any other plan. I also certify that my covered family members, if applicable, meet the plan eligibility requirements. I authorize release of any information or record requested in respect of this claim to the Plan Administrator to be used for the limited and sole purposes of underwriting, administering, and paying claims under the PDSP. The Plan Administrator may check the accuracy of the information given in support of this claim.

| Member Signature<br><br>x | Date | Month     Day     Year<br>/        / |
|---|---|---|

## Mail the completed form to:

Insurance Company Name
Company Address
PO Box if Necessary                    (555) 555-5555 or
City, State  Zip Code                  (800) 555-5555

■ **Figure 14–4**  Patient Claim Form Side 2

Determine the eligibility of the member by answering the following questions:

1. At the time of service, was the member currently enrolled under the plan (check each listed date of service)?
2. If a dependent, is the member within the proper age limit? If not within the proper age limit, is the member a full-time student and within the extended age limit?
3. Is the plan currently in force (i.e., have all premiums been paid)?
4. Have all eligibility requirements set forth in the contract been met?

If the answer to any of the previous questions is no, the claim is automatically denied since the member was not insured at the time of service.

If it is determined that the member is eligible, then proceed to the next step, evaluating whether there is other insurance.

## Other Insurance

The purpose of COB is to allow coverage and usually payment of 100% of allowable expenses without the covered member or members "making" money over and above the total costs for care. Therefore, it is necessary to perform a complete investigation to determine if there is other insurance that may be liable for payment of the presented services.

To determine whether the member has other insurance answer the following questions:

1. Does the member have other insurance that might cover these services?
2. Is the claim related to Workers' Compensation?
3. Is the claim related to an accident? If yes, is there a third party that could be held legally responsible for the payment of the claim?

If the answer to any of the above questions is yes, it is necessary to determine the benefits that were paid by the other party.

If it is determined that there is no other insurance then proceed to the next step, evaluating whether the provider has authority to render the services indicated.

## Provider Authority

The provider that renders the services must have the required qualifications and licensure from the proper authorities. Each state has its own requirements for the licensing of dentists.

To determine whether the provider has the authority to render the indicated services answer the following questions:

1. Who is the provider of service?
2. What is the medical degree of the provider of service? Is this a recognized medical degree for the type of treatment provided?
3. Is the provider's license number included on the form?
4. Is the place of treatment appropriate for the services rendered?

If it is determined that the provider has authority to render the services indicated, then proceed to the next step, determining if there is coverage for the services.

## Coverage of Services

One of the most important parts of processing a claim is to determine whether services are covered. To determine whether services are covered answer the following questions:

1. Are any of the services listed as excluded by the plan?
2. Was prior work done on the tooth that would exclude services?
3. Was there prior damage to the tooth that would exclude services (i.e., is the tooth previously listed as missing)?
4. If there are limitations to the number of times that a service can be provided, has that limitation been met previously?
5. If the service was an office visit, was there an exam, prophylaxis, or x-rays, or was the service in conjunction with a treatment procedure?
6. Does the missing and unreplaced provision apply?
7. Does the five-year limitation apply for prosthodontics?
8. Does the less than six-month limitation apply for adjustments to appliances, prosthetics, or dentures?
9. Have calendar year or lifetime maximums already been reached for this member?

If it is determined that the services are covered, then proceed to the next step, evaluating the services that were performed.

## Evaluating the Services

Evaluating the services that were performed must be done in order to ascertain the types of benefits that may be allowable, and to ensure that the services performed were appropriate for the situation presented.

To perform a thorough evaluation of services answer the following questions:

1. Are tooth numbers consistent with surfaces (anterior and posterior teeth with anterior and posterior surfaces)?
2. Do the services match the codes?
3. Were any services performed on the same day as another service that would disallow one of the other services (i.e., consultation/office visit billed with treatment)?
4. Do any other limitations apply (i.e., for multiple x-rays, full-mouth series)?
5. Does the contract list specific provisions for the services provided (i.e., orthodontic treatment is paid at 50%; second opinions are paid at 100%, and so on)?
6. Is a second opinion required for the services? If so, was a second opinion obtained? If a second opinion was required but not obtained, what are the ramifications to the processing of the claim? Are benefits reduced or denied?

After performing an evaluation of the services, if warranted proceed to the next step, processing the claim.

## Processing the Claim

After it has been determined that the claim is correctly filled out, the member is covered, the provider is appropriate, there is no other insurance, and the services are covered, begin processing the claim.

The first step is to determine the allowable amount for the service or procedure. Using the ADA Dental Code List in Appendix B determine the type of service or conversion factor code (CFC). Types of service fall under three categories, and each is listed next to the unit value on the Dental Code list. The three types of services are:

A. Diagnostic and preventive services.
B. Gold restorations, crowns, and prosthetics.
C. All other services.

Next, determine the appropriate unit value for the service or procedure. The unit value is listed on the Dental Code List next to the codes.

Then, using the first three digits of the provider's zip code, look up the conversion factor in Appendix B Dental Prevailing Conversion Factors. Be sure to use the correct conversion factor according to the type of service or conversion factor code.

Multiply the conversion factor by the unit value for the procedure. This will give you the allowable amount. However, remember that if the billed amount is less than the allowable amount, the billed amount is considered to be the allowable amount.

# On the Job Now

**Directions:** Using the Dental Conversion Factor chart and the ADA Dental RVS Units in Appendix B calculate UCR for the following procedures. Use conversion factor for zip code **94325**.

| Description | Proc. Code | Units | Conv. Factor | Amount |
|---|---|---|---|---|
| 1. Adult prophylaxis | ___ | ___ | ___ | ___ |
| 2. Gold inlay, two surfaces | ___ | ___ | ___ | ___ |
| 3. Complete upper denture | ___ | ___ | ___ | ___ |
| 4. Composite filling, tooth #28, two surfaces | ___ | ___ | ___ | ___ |
| 5. Excise benign tumor, odontogenic, 1.45 cm | ___ | ___ | ___ | ___ |
| 6. Bitewing x-rays, four films | ___ | ___ | ___ | ___ |

| Description | Proc. Code | Units | Conv. Factor | Amount |
|---|---|---|---|---|
| 7. Sodium fluoride treatment only, child | _____ | _____ | _____ | _____ |
| 8. Apicoectomy, anterior | _____ | _____ | _____ | _____ |
| 9. Upper bridge w/two chromo clasps w/rests, acrylic base | _____ | _____ | _____ | _____ |
| 10. Pulp vitality test | _____ | _____ | _____ | _____ |
| 11. Amalgam filling, primary tooth #F, three surfaces | _____ | _____ | _____ | _____ |
| 12. Single x-ray film, periapical | _____ | _____ | _____ | _____ |
| 13. Extraction, tooth #21 | _____ | _____ | _____ | _____ |
| 14. Comprehensive oral exam | _____ | _____ | _____ | _____ |
| 15. Porcelain base-metal crown | _____ | _____ | _____ | _____ |

# On the Job Now

**Directions:** Using the Dental Conversion Factor chart and the ADA Dental RVS Units in Appendix B calculate UCR for the following procedures. Use conversion factor for zip code **90020**.

| Description | Proc. Code | Units | Conv. Factor | Amount |
|---|---|---|---|---|
| 1. Adult prophylaxis | _____ | _____ | _____ | _____ |
| 2. Gold inlay, two surfaces | _____ | _____ | _____ | _____ |
| 3. Complete upper denture | _____ | _____ | _____ | _____ |
| 4. Composite filling, tooth #28, two surfaces | _____ | _____ | _____ | _____ |
| 5. Excise benign tumor, odontogenic, 1.45 cm | _____ | _____ | _____ | _____ |
| 6. Bitewing x-rays, four films | _____ | _____ | _____ | _____ |
| 7. Sodium fluoride treatment only, child | _____ | _____ | _____ | _____ |
| 8. Apicoectomy, anterior | _____ | _____ | _____ | _____ |
| 9. Upper bridge w/two chromo clasps w/rests, acrylic base | _____ | _____ | _____ | _____ |
| 10. Pulp vitality test | _____ | _____ | _____ | _____ |
| 11. Amalgam filling, primary tooth #F, three surfaces | _____ | _____ | _____ | _____ |
| 12. Single x-ray film, periapical | _____ | _____ | _____ | _____ |
| 13. Extraction, tooth #21 | _____ | _____ | _____ | _____ |
| 14. Comprehensive oral exam | _____ | _____ | _____ | _____ |
| 15. Porcelain base-metal crown | _____ | _____ | _____ | _____ |

## Completing the Claim Payment Worksheet

The **claim Payment Worksheet (see Figure 14–5)** is equivalent to an explanation of benefits. A copy of this form will be sent to the insured to explain the benefit payment for the claim. Therefore, it is important that each section be filled out completely to reduce the likelihood of confusing the insured. The claim Payment Worksheet is the same for dental benefits as for medical benefits.

The claim Payment Worksheet used for this book is intended to be an example only. It contains the information in much the same format as other insurance carrier payment forms. The Payment Worksheet and the guidelines for completing it are to be used for training and reference purposes only, since the individual company or plan worksheets may differ.

# Payment Worksheet

| | | | | |
|---|---|---|---|---|
| **Eligible Employee:** | Patty P. Patient | **Accident Benefit:** | $ 0.00 | (CCYY) |
| **Company:** | XYZ Corporation | **Lifetime Max:** | $ NA | |
| **Insured's ID Number:** | 555-55-XYZ | **Deductible:** | $ 50.00 | (CCYY) |
| **Patient:** | Patty P. Patient | **Carryover Ded:** | $ 0.00 | (CCNY) |
| **Relationship:** | Self | **Coinsurance:** | $ 7.13 | (CCYY) |
| **Provider's Zip Code:** | 15555 | **Date of Injury:** | NA | |

| Procedure Type of Service | Dates of Service | Billed Amount | Excluded Amounts* | Allowed | Basic/ Accident 100% | Maj. Med. ___% | DNT 80% | UCR Calculations |
|---|---|---|---|---|---|---|---|---|
| 1. D1110 | 02/08/CCYY | $80.00 | $45.00 | $35.00 | $ | | $35.00 | 1.0 X 35.0 |
| 2. D0140 | 02/08/CCYY | 20.00 | 9.50 | 10.50 | | | 10.50 | 0.3 X 35.0 |
| 3. D2140/4 | 02/08/CCYY | 65.00 | 24.85 | 40.15 | | | 40.15 | 1.1 X 36.5 |
| 4. | | | | | | | | |
| 5. | | | | | | | | |
| 6. | | | | | | | | |
| **Remarks:** Totals: | | $165.00 | $ 79.35 | $ 85.65 | $ | | 85.65 | |
| Deductible: | | | | | $ | | $50.00 | |
| Amount Subject to Coinsurance: | | | | | $ | | $35.65 | |
| Coinsurance: | | | | | $ | | $7.13 | |
| Amount Subject to Adjustment: | | | | | $ | | $28.52 | |
| Adjustment (See Remarks): | | | | | $ | | $0.00 | |
| **Payment Amount:** | | $28.52 | | | $ | | $28.52 | |

| *Denial Reasons |
|---|
| 1. $45.00 not covered — charge exceeds amount allowed by your plan. |
| 2. $9.50 not covered — charge exceeds amount allowed by your plan. |
| 3. $24.85 not covered — charge exceeds amount allowed by your plan. |
| 4. |
| 5. |
| 6. |

| Payees |
|---|
| 1. $28.52— Patty P. Patient |
| 2. |
| 3. |
| 4. |
| 5. |
| 6. |

If you disagree with our decision on your claim, you have the right by law to request that your claim be reviewed by your plan administrator. This request must be made in writing within 60 days of receipt of this notice. If you wish, you may submit your written comments and views. Please consult your plan's claim review procedures. See your employer regarding any other ERISA questions.

**■ Figure 14–5** Payment Worksheet

**Step 1.** Complete the information regarding the patient and insured first. This information is contained in the box in the upper-left-hand corner of the Payment Worksheet.

| Payment Worksheet Field | ADA Dental Claim Form | ADA Dental Claim Form Item Number |
|---|---|---|
| Eligible Employee | Patty P. Patient | Item 12 |
| Company | XYZ Corporation | Item 17 |
| Insured's Identification Number | 555-55-XYZ | Item 15 |
| Patient | Patty P. Patient | Item 20 |
| Relationship | Self | Item 18 |
| Provider's Zip Code | 15555 | Item 56 |

**Step 2.** Next, each CDT® code should be listed in the "Procedure Type of Service" column. Only codes that are the same should be combined together, otherwise list one code per line, regardless of whether this means using more than one payment worksheet. Procedures which have a tooth number listed in Field 27 should have the procedure code listed along with the tooth number, ex: D2140/4 (4 is the number of the tooth this procedure was performed on).

| Procedure Type of Service | 1. D1110 | Item 29, 27 |
|---|---|---|
| | 2. D0140 | |
| | 3. D2140/4 | |

**Step 3.** List the date(s) of service in the "Dates of Service" column.

| Dates of Service | 1. 02/08/CCYY | Item 24 |
|---|---|---|
| | 2. 02/08/CCYY | |
| | 3. 02/08/CCYY | |

**Step 4.** Enter the amount the provider billed in "Billed Amount" column.

| Billed Amount | 1. $80.00 | Item 31 |
|---|---|---|
| | 2. $20.00 | |
| | 3. $65.00 | |

**Step 5.** Determine the allowed amount for the service or procedure. Using the Relative Value Study shown in Appendix B, locate the unit value for the CDT® code assigned to each service provided. The unit value for the procedure is located in the column titled "unit value." Next, determine the conversion factor for the procedure from the UCR Conversion Factor Report (see Appendix B).

Using the first three numbers of the provider's zip code, locate the type of service. Three categories are listed next to the zip code location. The categories are:

1. Diagnostic and Preventive
2. All Other Excl. Gold Restorations Crowns, Prosthetics
3. Gold Rest. Crowns, Prosthetics

Multiply the appropriate conversion factor by the unit value for the procedure. The appropriate category is determined by the CDT® code, not the description of service. This total is the allowed amount. If the billed amount is less than the allowed amount, the billed amount is considered to be the allowed amount.

Thus, you will have: (35.00, 10.50, and 40.15) (1.0 [RVS] x 35.00 [Dental Conversion factor for zip codes starting 155] = 35.00), (0.3 [RVS] x 35.00 [conversion factor] = 10.50), (1.1 [RVS] x 36.50 [conversion factor] = 40.15).

Skip to the Allowed column and enter the allowed amounts as figured above.

| Payment Worksheet Field | Calculation |
|---|---|
| Allowed | 1. $35.00 <br> 2. $10.50 <br> 3. $40.15 |

**Step 6.** Next, subtract the allowed amount from the billed amount. The resulting figure is the excluded amount that should be placed in the Excluded Amounts column. Remember, if the allowed amount is greater than the billed amount, the billed amount will be the allowed amount. Therefore, the excluded amount will be: ($45.00, $9.50, $24.85) ($80.00 [billed amount] – $35.00 [allowed amount] = $45.00, $20.00 – $10.50 = $9.50, $65.00 – $40.15 = $24.85)

| | |
|---|---|
| Excluded Amounts | 1. $45.00 <br> 2. $9.50 <br> 3. $24.85 |

**Step 7.** Each explanation of benefits must list any amounts that are denied and the reason for the denial. Skip to the Denial Reasons section and enter a denial reason on the corresponding line in the denial reasons section. Usually, a brief explanation such as "$45.00 not covered — charge exceeds amount covered by your plan" is sufficient. If the service is not covered, the corresponding code (or description) and an explanation should be listed in the same manner (i.e., $300.00 not covered— orthodontic services are not covered by your plan). See Appendix B for a list of denial reasons to use.

| | |
|---|---|
| Denial Reasons | 1. $45.00 not covered—charge exceeds amount allowed by your plan. <br> 2. $9.50 not covered—charge exceeds amount allowed by your plan. <br> 3. $24.85 not covered—charge exceeds amount allowed by your plan. |

**Step 8.** If the plan has a basic allowance, the unit value should be multiplied by the basic allowance listed in the contract. For example, if the contract stipulates that the basic allowance for a dental visit is $7.00 and the service has a unit value of 1.0, then the basic allowance would be $7.00. The basic allowance amount would be placed in the Basic/Accident 100% column. Note that if the contract is part of a medical contract, the medical basic allowances do not transfer to the dental plan. If basic allowances are not listed in the dental contract, they do not apply.

| | |
|---|---|
| Basic/Accident 100% | 1. N/A <br> 2. N/A <br> 3. N/A |

**Step 9.** The basic allowance is subtracted from the allowed amount and the remainder is placed in the Untitled column (which should be marked 'DNT'). ($35.00, $10.50, $40.15)

| | |
|---|---|
| Untitled (DNT) | 1. $35.00 <br> 2. $10.50 <br> 3. $40.15 |

**Step 10.** After all the charges have been figured individually, the total for each column is added up and placed at the bottom of the column in the "Totals" row. ($165.00, $79.35, $85.65, $85.65)

Check your totals for accuracy by adding the DNT amount to the Basic amount. These two figures should total the Allowed Amount. Then add the Allowed Amount to the Excluded Amount. The total of these two figures should match the Billed Amount column and the total amount of the claim.

If the contract allows different percentages based on the type of service (i.e., diagnostic services at 80%, restorative at 75%, etc.), then each different type of benefit should be placed in a different column. If there are not enough columns on the Payment Worksheet, all services paid at the same percent may be placed together in a single column. There is also an additional untitled column to allow for varying percentages.

| Totals | 1. $165.00 |
|---|---|
| | 2. $79.35 |
| | 3. $85.65 |
| | 4. $85.65 |

**Step 11.** Now it is time to calculate the actual benefit payment. At the top of each payment column (columns six through eight), place the coinsurance percentage amount that applies to the figures in that column if it is not indicated (i.e., 100%, 80%). If it is necessary to pay items at 100%, use the Basic/Accident column and re-mark it as 'DNT'.

**Step 12.** Check the contract for the deductible amount and the Beginning Financials if applicable, for any previously paid deductible amounts. The following questions should also be answered.

- Is there a deductible amount for basic benefits?
- Has the deductible for this individual been satisfied?
- Does the deductible combine the medical plan with the dental plan (the plans are integrated)?
- If so, has the deductible been satisfied under the medical or dental portion of the contract?
- Has the family deductible been satisfied?
- Is there any carryover deductible from the previous year that should be applied?

Using the above questions and information, calculate the deductible that should be applied to this claim. The deductible amount on the basic portion of a plan will only usually be for hospital services. Place the amount of the deductible across from the word deductible in the first column in which benefits are payable at less than 100%. If the deductible remaining is more than the amount of the column, place the amount of the column in the deductible column and carry over any remaining amounts to additional columns with less than a 100% coinsurance amount.

| Deductible | 1. $50.00 |
|---|---|

**Step 13.** To calculate the Basic Benefits, first, enter the amount of the deductible in "Deductible" row in the basic benefits column. In this case there is no basic deductible on the services for Patty P. Patient.

| Deductible | N/A |
|---|---|

**Step 14.** Next, subtract the deductible amount from the total of the column and place the resulting amount in the "Amount Subject to Coinsurance" row. Since there is no Basic dental benefit, this does not need to be calculated for Patty P. Patient's claim.

| Amount Subject to Coinsurance | N/A |
|---|---|

**Step 15.** Next, multiply the amount subject to coinsurance by the insured's portion of the coinsurance amount (the remaining amount needed to reach 100%). For example, if the plan's coinsurance amount is 80%, then the insured's responsibility is 20%. For this column, the payment amount is 100%, so there is no coinsurance amount for the patient.

| Coinsurance | N/A |
|---|---|

**Step 16.** Finally, subtract the coinsurance amount from the amount subject to coinsurance. The remaining balance is the amount subject to adjustment and goes in the next column.

We will cover the rows "Adjustment (See Remarks)," and "Payment Amount" in Steps 22 and 23.

| Amount Subject to Adjustment | N/A |
|---|---|

**Step 17.** To calculate the Dental (DNT) benefits, first, calculate the Dental deductible that should be applied on this claim. Since this treatment is for a new patient visit at the beginning of the year, we will conclude that Patty P. Patient has not yet paid any of her deductible. Therefore, we will place $50.00 in the "Deductible" row of the DNT column.

**Note:** If any individual or family deductible or coinsurance amounts are met on this claim, an asterisk should be placed beside the deductible or coinsurance amount and a notation made in the remarks box (i.e., CCYY individual deductible has now been met).

| Deductible | $50.00 |
|---|---|

**Step 18.** Next, subtract the deductible amount from the total of the column and place the resulting amount in the "Amount Subject to Coinsurance" row. ($35.65) [$85.65 − $50.00 = $35.65]

If the amount in the "Deductible" field equals the amount in the "Totals" field, then the "Amount Subject to Coinsurance would be $0, and no payment will be made on the claim.

| Amount Subject to Coinsurance | $35.65 |
|---|---|

**Step 19.** Next, multiply the amount subject to coinsurance by the insured's portion of the coinsurance amount (the remaining amount needed to reach 100%). For example, if the plan's coinsurance amount is 80%, then the insured's responsibility is 20%. ($7.13) [$35.65 x .2 = $7.13]

| Coinsurance | $7.13 |
|---|---|

**Step 20.** Next, ask the following questions:

* What is the maximum coinsurance amount listed in the contract?

* Has this coinsurance limit been met?

* If the individual coinsurance limit has not been met, has the family coinsurance limit been met?

If any coinsurance limits have been met, the coinsurance amount should be adjusted accordingly. For example, if the individual coinsurance limit is $1,500 and $1,495 has been paid by the individual, the coinsurance amount would be $5.

**Step 21.** Finally, subtract the coinsurance amount from the amount subject to coinsurance. The remaining balance is the amount subject to adjustment and goes in that row. ($28.52) [$35.65 − $7.13 = $28.52]

| Amount Subject to Adjustment | $28.52 |
|---|---|

**Step 22.** Ask the following questions:

* If there is other insurance, what is the amount paid by the other insurance company?

* Are there any other reasons why there would be an adjustment to this claim?

* If so, what is the proper adjustment amount?

If there is an adjustment, the amount of the adjustment should be placed in the row "Adjustment (See Remarks)," and an explanation should be placed in the "Remarks" box to the left. See Appendix B for a list of remarks to use. Many claims will not have an adjustment amount. If there is an adjustment amount, the amount of the adjustment cannot be more than the amount shown in the "Amount Subject to Adjustment." For example, if there was an adjustment of $100 on Nancy's claim, $62.75 would be placed in the first column and $37.25 would be placed in the second column. Since there is no adjustment on this claim, we will place 0.00 in this box for the DNT column.

| Adjustment (See Remarks) | $0.00 |
|---|---|
| Remarks | |

**Step 23.** The adjustment amount if any, should then be subtracted from the amount subject to adjustment, and the resulting amount would be placed in the "Payment Amount" row. For the DNT column this amount is $28.52.

| Payment Amount | $28.52 |
|---|---|

**Step 24.** Add up the payment amount from all columns. The resulting payment amount should be placed in the box immediately to the right of the words "Payment Amount." This is the amount of the benefits being paid by the insurance carrier for this claim. ($28.52)

| Payment Amount | $28.52 |
|---|---|

**Step 25.** In this case, Patty has paid on the claim. Since she did not sign an assignment of benefits, she is the payee. The $28.52 will therefore be reimbursed to Patty. This information is placed in the "Payees" section.

| Payees | $28.52—Patty P. Patient |
|---|---|

**Step 26.** In this case, this is the first claim for Patty. Thus, the following amounts are listed in her updated history:

Accident Benefit: $0.00 (CCYY) [This was not an accident claim, so no accident benefits were paid.]

Lifetime Max: N/A [This is the total amount of all claims paid on Patty during her lifetime. Since this is her first claim, it is just the amount from this claim.]

Deductible: $50.00 (CCYY) Patty paid $50 in deductible on this claim. She has now met the CCYY year deductible.

Carryover Ded: $0.00 (CCNY) [This claim was not paid in the last three months of the year so there is no carryover deductible.]

Coinsurance: $7.13 (CCYY) [This is the amount of Patty's copayment on this claim.]

Date of Injury: [This would not apply since this claim is not an accident.]

You have now finished processing this claim!

| Accident Benefit | $0.00 |
|---|---|
| Lifetime Max | N/A |
| Deductible | $50.00 |
| Carryover Ded | $0.00 |
| Coinsurance | $7.13 |
| Date of Injury | N/A |

## Practice Pitfalls

**Example:** An exam and x-ray were performed on 9/18. Two cavities were found and an appointment was made for filling them on 10/10. The billed amount for the exam and x-ray was $40, and all of it was allowable (the UCR amount was higher than the billed amount). The allowable amount for the filling was $120.

The member had satisfied $75 of the $150 deductible. The total paid deductible amount would be $75 on this claim. Forty dollars of the deductible would be for the first two services and $35 would be for the two fillings. Therefore, $35 would be considered the carryover deductible amount.

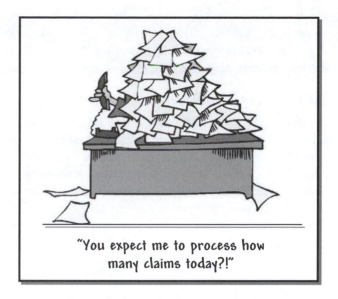

"You expect me to process how many claims today?!"

# On the Job Now

**Directions:** Answer the following questions without looking back at the material just covered. Write your answers in the space provided.

1. What is the first step when figuring the benefit payment? _____

_____

_____

2. After you calculate the amount subject to adjustment, what three questions should you ask?

1. _____

2. _____

3. _____

## Dental Form Letters

Occasionally, certain form letters are used during the processing of dental claims. These form letters are the same as those used for medical claims processing and thus have not been duplicated here.

## Request for Additional Information

A **Request for Additional Information Form** is used when more information is needed from the provider of services or the member regarding the services that were performed or the necessity for those services. If there is any question on the claim, especially regarding the services, the member identification, or other insurance that might be applicable, a Request for Additional Information form should be completed and mailed out.

## Third Party Liability

If the services were performed as the result of a work-related situation, the Workers' Compensation carrier should be paying the bill, not the member's insurance carrier. In addition, if the member was involved in an accident (especially an auto accident), another insurance carrier may be responsible for all or part of the bill. In this case, this would be the insurance carrier of the driver who caused the accident. In an accident that is not auto-related, negligence may be cited as a reason for another carrier to incur responsibility (i.e., the member fell through a rotted stair at a grocery store and broke his leg).

If any of the latter cases apply, the member's payer may make payment on the claim; however, the payer usually requires the insured to sign a third party liability statement. In effect, this statement provides that if any monies are paid by a third party on the claim(s), the patient's insurance carrier will receive the money. After the carrier has been reimbursed for all monies paid out, additional monies revert to the patient or the insured.

## Authorization to Release Information

Occasionally, no patient or insured signature is on file, nor on the claim, that authorizes the release of information to the payer. This authorization must be completed before a claim is sent in. Often, an insurance carrier has a copy of an authorization to release information on file. This allows the carrier to receive requested claim information without delay.

## Handling Fraudulent Dental Claims

Occasionally, dentists and insureds submit fraudulent claims for processing. These fraudulent claims can include the following:

- Claims that have been submitted twice, either to the same insurer or to different insurers.
- Claims that have been submitted for services that were not actually rendered.
- Claims that have been altered to make it appear that services were performed on a different date or patient.

The various types of fraudulent dental claim situations are as follows:

- Duplicate charges.
- Duplicate services.
- Altering dates of treatment.
- Reporting services other than the ones actually performed.
- False information or rationale about diagnosis, treatment, or condition of dentures.
- Submission of incorrect x-rays.

Fraud or mistakes are usually detected during the usual processing or review procedures prior to payment by the following:

1. Review of prior treatment against present treatment.
2. Completion or review of dental charts, checking prior work, existing work, and present or proposed work.
3. Verification of tooth numbers and positions.
4. Verification of dates of services and charges.
5. Checking for date of first visit and age of claimant.
6. Checking for erasures and changes of pen color and other indications of changes.
7. Reviewing post-treatment x-rays.
8. Evaluating treatment plan by use of x-rays rather than rationale or facts supplied by the dentist. Rationale should be used to supplement x-rays and not as the sole determinant of benefits.
9. Verifying services with claimant.

There are several methods of determining if misrepresentation has occurred. Before any steps are taken, the file should be reviewed by the supervisor and the dental consultant.

Postoperative x-rays should be obtained to show satisfactory completion of the work. This is not conclusive evidence one way or the other since the wrong x-rays can be submitted.

Oral exams by outside dentists are the best method of determining what work has actually been performed. In cases involving large amounts, it may be helpful to request the examining dentist to take x-rays as a record of any discrepancies. It may also be wise to duplicate the preoperative x-rays before returning them to the attending dentist.

In a few instances, an on-site claim representative may examine the dentist's records. This method should be used judiciously and only for the purpose of verifying dates of treatment and whether duplicate services were rendered.

In all dealings of potential fraud with either claimants or dentists, it is important not to accuse anyone without adequate proof. Mistakes can easily be made in completing a claim form, and every effort should be made to rule this out. The supervisor or administrator should always be advised prior to taking any action.

The rules regarding documentation of the claim file, which were previously discussed in relation to medical claims, apply to dental claims also. Basically, if the information was not written down, the services are deemed not to have happened.

# CHAPTER REVIEW

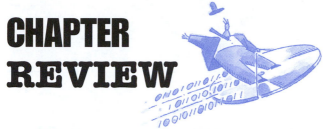

## Summary

- The two forms used for billing dental services are the ADA Dental Claim Form and the dentist's Patient Claim Form.
- The ADA Dental Claim Form and Patient Claim Form allows the dentist to either request a benefit determination on a proposed treatment plan or to report services already performed and request payment for those services.

- When a claim for dental services is received, it is the responsibility of the claims examiner to determine whether the claim received is eligible for payment. This entails several steps, including verifying eligibility, determining whether services rendered are covered, and identifying any limitations that may exist on coverage.
- After all preliminary investigation is completed, the processing of the claim can be completed.
- The basic steps just covered should enable you to process claims with the highest degree of accuracy and in the least amount of time.

## Assignments

Complete the Questions for Review.
Complete Exercises 14–1 through 14–6.

## Questions for Review

**Directions:** Answer the following questions without looking back at the material just covered. Write your answers in the space provided.

1. What is the purpose of the Patient Claim Form? _____

_____

2. On the Dental Claim Form, how would you indicate that the member had made a partial payment for the services rendered? _____

_____

3. What does a signature in the "Payment of benefits to provider" box mean? _____

_____

4. What does the box "Month to Month" denote on the Information Sheet? _____

_____

5. What does a dentist's signature on a dental claim form mean? _____

_____

6. What is the first thing that the claims examiner should check upon receipt of a claim form? _____

_____

7. The claim Payment Worksheet is equivalent to an _____

8. How do you determine the appropriate unit value for a dental service? _____

_____

9. How do you determine the allowable amount for a procedure? _____

_____

10. (True or False?) The Dental Claim Form can be used as a billing statement for services performed and also for a pretreatment estimate of services to be performed. _____

If you were unable to answer any of these questions, refer back to that section and then fill in the answers.

# Exercise **14-1**

**Directions:** Using the Dental Conversion Factor chart and the ADA Dental RVS Units in Appendix B calculate UCR for the following procedures. Use conversion factor for zip code **93504**.

| Description | Proc. Code | Units | Conv. Factor | Amount |
|---|---|---|---|---|
| 1.  Adult prophylaxis | _____ | _____ | _____ | _____ |
| 2.  Gold inlay, two surfaces | _____ | _____ | _____ | _____ |
| 3.  Complete upper denture | _____ | _____ | _____ | _____ |
| 4.  Composite filling, tooth #28, two surfaces | _____ | _____ | _____ | _____ |
| 5.  Excise benign tumor, odontogenic, 1.45 cm | _____ | _____ | _____ | _____ |
| 6.  Bitewing x-rays, four films | _____ | _____ | _____ | _____ |
| 7.  Sodium fluoride treatment only, child | _____ | _____ | _____ | _____ |
| 8.  Apicoectomy, anterior | _____ | _____ | _____ | _____ |
| 9.  Upper bridge w/two chromo clasps w/rests, acrylic base | _____ | _____ | _____ | _____ |
| 10.  Pulp vitality test | _____ | _____ | _____ | _____ |
| 11.  Amalgam filling, primary tooth #F, three surfaces | _____ | _____ | _____ | _____ |
| 12.  Single x-ray film, periapical | _____ | _____ | _____ | _____ |
| 13.  Extraction, tooth #21 | _____ | _____ | _____ | _____ |
| 14.  Comprehensive oral exam | _____ | _____ | _____ | _____ |
| 15.  Porcelain base-metal crown | _____ | _____ | _____ | _____ |

# Exercise 14-2

**Directions:** Complete the crossword puzzle by filling in a word from the keywords that fits each clue.

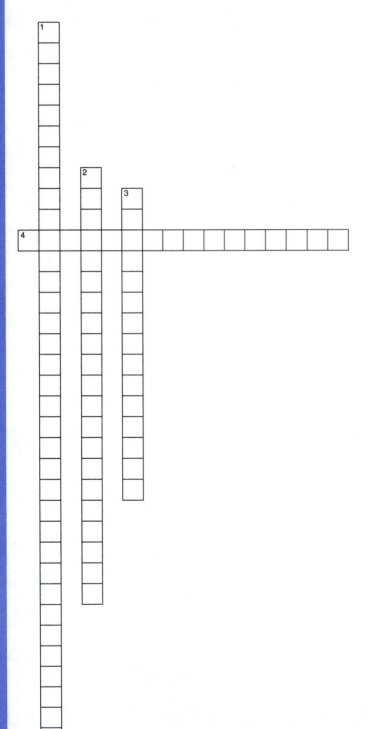

**Across**

4. A form that contains basically the same information as the ADA Dental Claim Form, but is usually provided by self-funded plans.

**Down**

1. A form used when more information is needed from the provider of services or the patient regarding the services that were performed or the necessity for those services.

2. A form that is equivalent to an explanation of benefits. A copy of this form will be sent to the insured to explain the benefit payment for the claim.

3. A form that lists specific information regarding the patient and the services that have been or are going to be performed.

# Exercises **14-3** through **14-6**

**Directions:** Process on a Payment Worksheet each of the dental service claims found on the following pages. Refer to Appendices A and B for contracts and additional information.

All insureds are eligible for coverage under their respective plans. There are no beginning financials for members. Amounts paid for each claim should be accumulated and carried forward to subsequent claims.

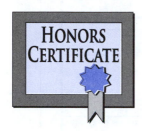

### Honors Certification™

The Honors Certification™ challenge for this chapter consists of a written test of the information contained within this chapter. Each incorrect answer will result in a deduction of up to 5% from your grade. You must achieve a score of 85% or higher to pass this test. If you fail the test on your first attempt, you may retake the test one additional time. The items included in the second test may be different from those in the first test.

## ADA Dental Claim Form

SAMPLE

### HEADER INFORMATION

**1. Type of Transaction (Check all applicable boxes)**

☐ Statement of Actual Services – OR – ☒ Request for Predetermination/Preauthorization

☐ EPSDT/Title XIX

**2. Predetermination/Preauthorization Number**

### PRIMARY PAYER INFORMATION

**3. Name, Address, City, State, Zip Code**

BALL INSURANCE CARRIERS
3895 BUBBLE BLVD STE 283
BOXWOOD CO 85926

### OTHER COVERAGE

**4. Other Dental or Medical Coverage?** ☒ No (Skip 5-11) ☐ Yes (Complete 5-11)

**5. Subscriber Name (Last, First, Middle Initial, Suffix)**

**6. Date of Birth (MM/DD/CCYY)** | **7. Gender** ☐ M ☐ F | **8. Subscriber Identifier (SSN or ID#)**

**9. Plan/Group Number** | **10. Relationship to Primary Subscriber (Check applicable box)** ☐ Self ☐ Spouse ☐ Dependent ☐ Other

**11. Other Carrier Name, Address, City, State, Zip Code**

### PRIMARY SUBSCRIBER INFORMATION

**12. Name (Last, First, Middle Initial, Suffix), Address, City, State, Zip Code**

MURDOCK MARIA
9876 MARABAN LANE
MONTROSE CA 92318

**13. Date of Birth (MM/DD/CCYY)** 08/23/CCYY-51 | **14. Gender** ☐ M ☒ F | **15. Subscriber Identifier (SSN or ID#)** 111 22 XYZ

**16. Plan/Group Number** 62958 | **17. Employer Name** XYZ CORPORATION

### PATIENT INFORMATION

**18. Relationship to Primary Subscriber (Check applicable box)** ☐ Self ☐ Spouse ☒ Dependent Child ☐ Other | **19. Student Status** ☒ FTS ☐ PTS

**20. Name (Last, First, Middle Initial, Suffix), Address, City, State, Zip Code**

MURDOCK MAGGIE
9876 MARABAN LANE
MONTROSE CA 92318

**21. Date of Birth (MM/DD/CCYY)** 02/16/CCYY-13 | **22. Gender** ☐ M ☒ F | **23. Patient ID/Account # (Assigned by Dentist)**

### RECORD OF SERVICES PROVIDED

| | 24. Procedure Date (MM/DD/CCYY) | 25. Area of Oral Cavity | 26. Tooth System | 27. Tooth Number(s) or Letter(s) | 28. Tooth Surface | 29. Procedure Code | 30. Description | 31. Fee |
|---|---|---|---|---|---|---|---|---|
| 1 | 02/02/CCYY | | | | | D0220 | 1 SINGLE FILM | 13 00 |
| 2 | 02/02/CCYY | | | | | D0230 | 1 ADDTL X-RAY | 7 00 |
| 3 | 03/13/CCYY | | | 3 | | D3330 | ROOT CANAL TREATMENT | 390 00 |
| 4 | 02/02/CCYY | | | | | D1120 | PROPHYLAXIS | 50 00 |
| 5 | | | | | | | | |
| 6 | | | | | | | | |
| 7 | | | | | | | | |
| 8 | | | | | | | | |
| 9 | | | | | | | | |
| 10 | | | | | | | | |

### MISSING TEETH INFORMATION

**34. (Place an 'X' on each missing tooth)**

Permanent: 1 2 3 4 5 6 7 8 9 10 11 12 13 14 15 16 / 32 31 30 29 28 27 26 25 24 23 22 21 20 19 18 17

Primary: A B C D E F G H I J / T S R Q P O N M L K

**32. Other Fee(s)**

**33. Total Fee** 460 00

**35. Remarks**

### AUTHORIZATIONS

**36.** I have been informed of the treatment plan and associated fees. I agree to be responsible for all charges for dental services and materials not paid by my dental benefit plan, unless prohibited by law, or the treating dentist or dental practice has a contractual agreement with my plan prohibiting all or a portion of such charges. To the extent permitted by law, I consent to your use and disclosure of my protected health information to carry out payment activities in connection with this claim.

X *Maria Murdock*     03/13/CCYY
Patient/Guardian signature     Date

**37.** I hereby authorize and direct payment of the dental benefits otherwise payable to me, directly to the below named dentist or dental entity.

X _____
Subscriber signature     Date

### ANCILLARY CLAIM/TREATMENT INFORMATION

**38. Place of Treatment (Check applicable box)** ☒ Provider's Office ☐ Hospital ☐ ECF ☐ Other

**39. Number of Enclosures (00 to 99)** Radiograph(s) 0 Oral Image(s) 0 Model(s) 0

**40. Is Treatment for Orthodontics?** ☒ No (Skip 41-42) ☐ Yes (Complete 41-42)

**41. Date Appliance Placed (MM/DD/CCYY)**

**42. Months of Treatment Remaining** | **43. Replacement of Prosthesis?** ☒ No ☐ Yes (Complete 44) | **44. Date Prior Placement (MM/DD/CCYY)**

**45. Treatment Resulting from (Check applicable box)** ☐ Occupational illness/injury ☐ Auto accident ☐ Other accident

**46. Date of Accident (MM/DD/CCYY)** | **47. Auto Accident State**

### BILLING DENTIST OR DENTAL ENTITY (Leave blank if dentist or dental entity is not submitting claim on behalf of the patient or insured/subscriber)

**48. Name, Address, City, State, Zip Code**

MABLE MILLER DDS
1895 MYRTLE ROAD
MONTROSE CA 92309

**49. Provider ID** | **50. License Number** D49542 | **51. SSN or TIN** 70-9823478

**52. Phone Number** ( 000 ) 555 - 3478

### TREATING DENTIST AND TREATMENT LOCATION INFORMATION

**53.** I hereby certify that the procedures as indicated by date are in progress (for procedures that require multiple visits) or have been completed and that the fees submitted are the actual fees I have charged and intend to collect for those procedures.

X *Mable Miller*     03/14/ccyy
Signed (Treating Dentist)     Date

**54. Provider ID** | **55. License Number** D49542

**56. Address, City, State, Zip Code**

1895 MYRTLE ROAD
MONTROSE CA 92309

**57. Phone Number** ( 000 ) 555 -3478 | **58. Treating Provider Specialty**

**Exercise 14–3**

## ADA Dental Claim Form

**HEADER INFORMATION**

1. Type of Transaction (Check all applicable boxes)

☐ Statement of Actual Services  – OR –  ☒ Request for Predetermination/Preauthorization
☐ EPSDT/Title XIX

2. Predetermination/Preauthorization Number

SAMPLE

**PRIMARY PAYER INFORMATION**

3. Name, Address, City, State, Zip Code

BALL INSURANCE CARRIERS
3895 BUBBLE BLVD STE 283
BOXWOOD CO 85926

**PRIMARY SUBSCRIBER INFORMATION**

12. Name (Last, First, Middle Initial, Suffix), Address, City, State, Zip Code

MURDOCK MARIA
9876 MARABAN LANE
MONTROSE CA  92318

13. Date of Birth (MM/DD/CCYY)  08/23/CCYY-51
14. Gender  ☐M ☒F
15. Subscriber Identifier (SSN or ID#)  111 22 XYZ

**OTHER COVERAGE**

4. Other Dental or Medical Coverage?  ☒ No (Skip 5-11)  ☐ Yes (Complete 5-11)

5. Subscriber Name (Last, First, Middle Initial, Suffix)

6. Date of Birth (MM/DD/CCYY)
7. Gender  ☐M ☐F
8. Subscriber Identifier (SSN or ID#)

9. Plan/Group Number
10. Relationship to Primary Subscriber (Check applicable box)  ☐ Self  ☐ Spouse  ☐ Dependent  ☐ Other

11. Other Carrier Name, Address, City, State, Zip Code

16. Plan/Group Number  62958
17. Employer Name  XYZ CORPORATION

**PATIENT INFORMATION**

18. Relationship to Primary Subscriber (Check applicable box)  ☐ Self  ☐ Spouse  ☒ Dependent Child  ☐ Other
19. Student Status  ☒ FTS  ☐ PTS

20. Name (Last, First, Middle Initial, Suffix), Address, City, State, Zip Code

MURDOCK MADEAN
9876 MARABAN LANE
MONTROSE CA  92318

21. Date of Birth (MM/DD/CCYY)  02/16/CCYY-18
22. Gender  ☐M ☒F
23. Patient ID/Account # (Assigned by Dentist)

**RECORD OF SERVICES PROVIDED**

| | 24. Procedure Date (MM/DD/CCYY) | 25. Area of Oral Cavity | 26. Tooth System | 27. Tooth Number(s) or Letter(s) | 28. Tooth Surface | 29. Procedure Code | 30. Description | 31. Fee |
|---|---|---|---|---|---|---|---|---|
| 1 | 02/28/CCYY | | | | | D0270 | 4 BW X-RAY & EXAM | 25 00 |
| 2 | 02/28/CCYY | | | | | D1110 | PROPHY | 24 00 |
| 3 | 03/11/CCYY | | | | BOL | D2394 | COMPOSITE | 74 00 |
| 4 | 03/11/CCYY | | | | MOD | D2394 | COMPOSITE | 74 00 |
| 5 | 03/11/CCYY | | | | DO | D2393 | COMPOSITE | 64 00 |
| 6 | 03/06/CCYY | | | | BOL | D2394 | COMPOSITE | 74 00 |
| 7 | 03/06/CCYY | | | | BO | D2393 | COMPOSITE | 64 00 |
| 8 | 03/06/CCYY | | | | BO | D2393 | COMPOSITE | 64 00 |
| 9 | | | | | | | | |
| 10 | | | | | | | | |

**MISSING TEETH INFORMATION**

34. (Place an 'X' on each missing tooth)

Permanent: 1 2 3 4 5 6 7 8 9 10 11 12 13 14 15 16
32 31 30 29 28 27 26 25 24 23 22 21 20 19 18 17

Primary: A B C D E F G H I J
T S R Q P O N M L K

32. Other Fee(s)

33. Total Fee  463 00

35. Remarks

**AUTHORIZATIONS**

36. I have been informed of the treatment plan and associated fees. I agree to be responsible for all charges for dental services and materials not paid by my dental benefit plan, unless prohibited by law, or the treating dentist or dental practice has a contractual agreement with my plan prohibiting all or a portion of such charges. To the extent permitted by law, I consent to your use and disclosure of my protected health information to carry out payment activities in connection with this claim.

X  *Maria Murdock*    03/11/CCYY
Patient/Guardian signature          Date

37. I hereby authorize and direct payment of the dental benefits otherwise payable to me, directly to the below named dentist or dental entity.

X
Subscriber signature          Date

**ANCILLARY CLAIM/TREATMENT INFORMATION**

38. Place of Treatment (Check applicable box)  ☒ Provider's Office  ☐ Hospital  ☐ ECF  ☐ Other
39. Number of Enclosures (00 to 99)  Radiograph(s) 0  Oral Image(s) 0  Model(s) 0

40. Is Treatment for Orthodontics?  ☒ No (Skip 41-42)  ☐ Yes (Complete 41-42)
41. Date Appliance Placed (MM/DD/CCYY)

42. Months of Treatment Remaining
43. Replacement of Prosthesis?  ☒ No  ☐ Yes (Complete 44)
44. Date Prior Placement (MM/DD/CCYY)

45. Treatment Resulting from (Check applicable box)  ☐ Occupational illness/injury  ☐ Auto accident  ☐ Other accident

46. Date of Accident (MM/DD/CCYY)
47. Auto Accident State

**BILLING DENTIST OR DENTAL ENTITY** (Leave blank if dentist or dental entity is not submitting claim on behalf of the patient or insured/subscriber)

48. Name, Address, City, State, Zip Code

MABLE MILLER DDS
1895 MYRTLE ROAD
MONTROSE CA  92309

49. Provider ID
50. License Number  D49542
51. SSN or TIN  70-9823478

52. Phone Number  ( 000 ) 555 - 3478

**TREATING DENTIST AND TREATMENT LOCATION INFORMATION**

53. I hereby certify that the procedures as indicated by date are in progress (for procedures that require multiple visits) or have been completed and that the fees submitted are the actual fees I have charged and intend to collect for those procedures.

X  *Mable Miller*    03/11/ccyy
Signed (Treating Dentist)          Date

54. Provider ID
55. License Number  D49542

56. Address, City, State, Zip Code

1895 MYRTLE ROAD
MONTROSE CA  92309

57. Phone Number  ( 000 ) 555 -3478
58. Treating Provider Specialty

©American Dental Association, 2002
J515 (Same as ADA Dental Claim Form) – J516, J517, J518, J519

**Exercise 14–4**

## ADA Dental Claim Form

### HEADER INFORMATION

1. Type of Transaction (Check all applicable boxes)

☐ Statement of Actual Services – OR – ☒ Request for Predetermination/Preauthorization

☐ EPSDT/Title XIX

2. Predetermination/Preauthorization Number

SAMPLE

### PRIMARY PAYER INFORMATION

3. Name, Address, City, State, Zip Code

WINTER INSURANCE CO
9763 WESTERN WAY
WHITTIER CO  82963

### OTHER COVERAGE

4. Other Dental or Medical Coverage?  ☒ No (Skip 5-11)  ☐ Yes (Complete 5-11)

5. Subscriber Name (Last, First, Middle Initial, Suffix)

6. Date of Birth (MM/DD/CCYY)   7. Gender ☐ M ☐ F   8. Subscriber Identifier (SSN or ID#)

9. Plan/Group Number   10. Relationship to Primary Subscriber (Check applicable box) ☐ Self ☐ Spouse ☐ Dependent ☐ Other

11. Other Carrier Name, Address, City, State, Zip Code

### PRIMARY SUBSCRIBER INFORMATION

12. Name (Last, First, Middle Initial, Suffix), Address, City, State, Zip Code

OWEN ORVILLE
1000 OSWALD STREET
OJAI CA  93051

13. Date of Birth (MM/DD/CCYY)  08/23/CCYY-51
14. Gender  ☒ M ☐ F
15. Subscriber Identifier (SSN or ID#)  000 55 ABC

16. Plan/Group Number  36928
17. Employer Name  ABC CORPORATION

### PATIENT INFORMATION

18. Relationship to Primary Subscriber (Check applicable box)  ☐ Self ☐ Spouse ☒ Dependent Child ☐ Other
19. Student Status  ☒ FTS ☐ PTS

20. Name (Last, First, Middle Initial, Suffix), Address, City, State, Zip Code

OWEN ODELL
1000 OSWALD STREET
OJAI CA  93051

21. Date of Birth (MM/DD/CCYY)  02/28/CCYY-11
22. Gender  ☒ M ☐ F
23. Patient ID/Account # (Assigned by Dentist)

### RECORD OF SERVICES PROVIDED

| | 24. Procedure Date (MM/DD/CCYY) | 25. Area of Oral Cavity | 26. Tooth System | 27. Tooth Number(s) or Letter(s) | 28. Tooth Surface | 29. Procedure Code | 30. Description | 31. Fee |
|---|---|---|---|---|---|---|---|---|
| 1 | 02/12/CCYY | | | | | D0220 | 1 SINGLE FILM | 13 00 |
| 2 | 02/12/CCYY | | | | | D0230 | 4 ADDITIONAL X-RAYS | 28 00 |
| 3 | 02/12/CCYY | | | | | D4211 | 1 GINGIVAL CURETTAGE U/R | 90 00 |
| 4 | 03/09/CCYY | | | | | D1120 | PROPHYLAXIS | 50 00 |
| 5 | 03/09/CCYY | | | | | D0120 | COMPLETE ORAL EXAM | 30 00 |
| 6 | | | | | | | | |
| 7 | | | | | | | | |
| 8 | | | | | | | | |
| 9 | | | | | | | | |
| 10 | | | | | | | | |

### MISSING TEETH INFORMATION

34. (Place an "X" on each missing tooth)

Permanent: 1 2 3 4 5 6 7 8 9 10 11 12 13 14 15 16 / 32 31 30 29 28 27 26 25 24 23 22 21 20 19 18 17

Primary: A B C D E F G H I J / T S R Q P O N M L K

32. Other Fee(s)

33. Total Fee  211 00

35. Remarks

### AUTHORIZATIONS

36. I have been informed of the treatment plan and associated fees. I agree to be responsible for all charges for dental services and materials not paid by my dental benefit plan, unless prohibited by law, or the treating dentist or dental practice has a contractual agreement with my plan prohibiting all or a portion of such charges. To the extent permitted by law, I consent to your use and disclosure of my protected health information to carry out payment activities in connection with this claim.

X  _Orville Owen_   03/09/CCYY
Patient/Guardian signature   Date

37. I hereby authorize and direct payment of the dental benefits otherwise payable to me, directly to the below named dentist or dental entity.

X _____
Subscriber signature   Date

### BILLING DENTIST OR DENTAL ENTITY (Leave blank if dentist or dental entity is not submitting claim on behalf of the patient or insured/subscriber)

48. Name, Address, City, State, Zip Code

OLIVER OSHEA DDS
2711 ORNATE BLVD
OJAI CA  93055

49. Provider ID
50. License Number  G00100
51. SSN or TIN  70-0000002
52. Phone Number ( 000 ) 555 - 0002

### ANCILLARY CLAIM/TREATMENT INFORMATION

38. Place of Treatment (Check applicable box)  ☒ Provider's Office ☐ Hospital ☐ ECF ☐ Other

39. Number of Enclosures (00 to 99)  Radiograph(s) 0  Oral Image(s) 0  Model(s) 0

40. Is Treatment for Orthodontics?  ☒ No (Skip 41-42)  ☐ Yes (Complete 41-42)

41. Date Appliance Placed (MM/DD/CCYY)

42. Months of Treatment Remaining
43. Replacement of Prosthesis?  ☒ No ☐ Yes (Complete 44)
44. Date Prior Placement (MM/DD/CCYY)

45. Treatment Resulting from (Check applicable box)  ☐ Occupational illness/injury ☐ Auto accident ☐ Other accident

46. Date of Accident (MM/DD/CCYY)
47. Auto Accident State

### TREATING DENTIST AND TREATMENT LOCATION INFORMATION

53. I hereby certify that the procedures as indicated by date are in progress (for procedures that require multiple visits) or have been completed and that the fees submitted are the actual fees I have charged and intend to collect for those procedures.

X  _Oliver O'Shea_   03/09/ccyy
Signed (Treating Dentist)   Date

54. Provider ID
55. License Number  G00100

56. Address, City, State, Zip Code

1895 MYRTLE ROAD
MONTROSE CA  92309

57. Phone Number ( 000 ) 555 -0002
58. Treating Provider Specialty

## Exercise 14-5

## ADA Dental Claim Form

### HEADER INFORMATION

1. Type of Transaction (Check all applicable boxes)

☐ Statement of Actual Services  – OR –  ☒ Request for Predetermination/Preauthorization

☐ EPSDT/Title XIX

2. Predetermination/Preauthorization Number

SAMPLE

### PRIMARY PAYER INFORMATION

3. Name, Address, City, State, Zip Code

WINTER INSURANCE CO
9763 WESTERN WAY
WHITTIER CO  82963

### OTHER COVERAGE

4. Other Dental or Medical Coverage?  ☒ No (Skip 5-11)  ☐ Yes (Complete 5-11)

5. Subscriber Name (Last, First, Middle Initial, Suffix)

6. Date of Birth (MM/DD/CCYY)  |  7. Gender ☐ M ☐ F  |  8. Subscriber Identifier (SSN or ID#)

9. Plan/Group Number  |  10. Relationship to Primary Subscriber (Check applicable box) ☐ Self ☐ Spouse ☐ Dependent ☐ Other

11. Other Carrier Name, Address, City, State, Zip Code

### PRIMARY SUBSCRIBER INFORMATION

12. Name (Last, First, Middle Initial, Suffix), Address, City, State, Zip Code

OWEN ORVILLE
1000 OSWALD STREET
OJAI CA  93051

13. Date of Birth (MM/DD/CCYY)  08/23/CCYY-51  |  14. Gender ☒ M ☐ F  |  15. Subscriber Identifier (SSN or ID#)  000 55 ABC

16. Plan/Group Number  36928  |  17. Employer Name  ABC CORPORATION

### PATIENT INFORMATION

18. Relationship to Primary Subscriber (Check applicable box)  ☒ Self ☐ Spouse ☐ Dependent Child ☐ Other  |  19. Student Status  ☐ FTS ☐ PTS

20. Name (Last, First, Middle Initial, Suffix), Address, City, State, Zip Code

OWEN ORVILLE
1000 OSWALD STREET
OJAI CA  93051

21. Date of Birth (MM/DD/CCYY)  02/28/CCYY-51  |  22. Gender ☒ M ☐ F  |  23. Patient ID/Account # (Assigned by Dentist)

### RECORD OF SERVICES PROVIDED

| | 24. Procedure Date (MM/DD/CCYY) | 25. Area of Oral Cavity | 26. Tooth System | 27. Tooth Number(s) or Letter(s) | 28. Tooth Surface | 29. Procedure Code | 30. Description | 31. Fee |
|---|---|---|---|---|---|---|---|---|
| 1 | 01/02/CCYY | | | | | D0210 | FULL MOUTH X-RAY | 45 00 |
| 2 | 01/06/CCYY | | | 17 | | D7230 | EXT. – PART BONE | 175 00 |
| 3 | 01/06/CCYY | | | 18 | | D2140 | AMALGAM | 40 00 |
| 4 | 01/20/CCYY | | | | | D4341 | PERIO ROOT PLANNING | 38 00 |
| 5 | 01/20/CCYY | | | | | D4341 | PERIO ROOT PLANNING | 38 00 |
| 6 | 01/25/CCYY | | | | | D4341 | PERIO ROOT PLANNING | 38 00 |
| 7 | 01/25/CCYY | | | | | D4341 | PERIO ROOT PLANNING | 38 00 |
| 8 | 02/03/CCYY | | | | | D1110 | PROPHY | 45 00 |
| 9 | | | | | | | | |
| 10 | | | | | | | | |

### MISSING TEETH INFORMATION

34. (Place an 'X' on each missing tooth)

Permanent: 1 2 3 4 5 6 7 8 9 10 11 12 13 14 15 16 / 32 31 30 29 28 27 26 25 24 23 22 21 20 19 18 17

Primary: A B C D E F G H I J / T S R Q P O N M L K

32. Other Fee(s)

30. Total Fee  457 00

35. Remarks

### AUTHORIZATIONS

36. I have been informed of the treatment plan and associated fees. I agree to be responsible for all charges for dental services and materials not paid by my dental benefit plan, unless prohibited by law, or the treating dentist or dental practice has a contractual agreement with my plan prohibiting all or a portion of such charges. To the extent permitted by law, I consent to your use and disclosure of my protected health information to carry out payment activities in connection with this claim.

X  _Orville Owen_  02/03/CCYY

Patient/Guardian signature  Date

37. I hereby authorize and direct payment of the dental benefits otherwise payable to me, directly to the below named dentist or dental entity.

X _____

Subscriber signature  Date

### BILLING DENTIST OR DENTAL ENTITY (Leave blank if dentist or dental entity is not submitting claim on behalf of the patient or insured/subscriber)

48. Name, Address, City, State, Zip Code

OSCAR ORTIZ DDS
4444 OLSEN BLVD
ORANGE CA  92711

49. Provider ID | 50. License Number  M94732 | 51. SSN or TIN  70-3333333

52. Phone Number ( 000 ) 555 – 3333

### ANCILLARY CLAIM/TREATMENT INFORMATION

38. Place of Treatment (Check applicable box)  ☒ Provider's Office ☐ Hospital ☐ ECF ☐ Other

39. Number of Enclosures (00 to 99)  Radiograph(s) 0  Oral Image(s) 0  Model(s) 0

40. Is Treatment for Orthodontics?  ☒ No (Skip 41-42)  ☐ Yes (Complete 41-42)

41. Date Appliance Placed (MM/DD/CCYY)

42. Months of Treatment Remaining  |  43. Replacement of Prosthesis? ☒ No ☐ Yes (Complete 44)  |  44. Date Prior Placement (MM/DD/CCYY)

45. Treatment Resulting from (Check applicable box)  ☐ Occupational illness/injury  ☐ Auto accident  ☐ Other accident

46. Date of Accident (MM/DD/CCYY)  |  47. Auto Accident State

### TREATING DENTIST AND TREATMENT LOCATION INFORMATION

53. I hereby certify that the procedures as indicated by date are in progress (for procedures that require multiple visits) or have been completed and that the fees submitted are the actual fees I have charged and intend to collect for those procedures.

X  _Oscar Ortiz_  02/03/ccyy

Signed (Treating Dentist)  Date

54. Provider ID  |  55. License Number  M94732

56. Address, City, State, Zip Code

1895 MYRTLE ROAD
MONTROSE CA  92309

57. Phone Number ( 000 ) 555 -3333  |  58. Treating Provider Specialty

**Exercise 14–6**

**CHAPTER 15** BASIC OFFICE FUNCTIONS AND EFFECTIVE COMMUNICATION

# 15

# Basic Office Functions
## and Effective Communication

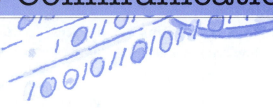

## After completion of this chapter
**you will be able to:**

- Draft a letter using proper letter format.
- Use proper terminology in written and verbal communications when given a scenario to respond to.
- State specific guidelines for writing to claimants and physicians.
- List the standards that denial communications must meet.
- State the ERISA requirements for communications regarding claim payments or dispositions.
- Write a letter requesting repayment of an overpayment amount on a claim.
- Explain how to handle incoming mail.

- Explain how to handle outgoing mail.
- Explain special shipping services that are available.
- List the main types of office equipment and explain their use.
- Describe a tickler file and explain its use.
- List the basic components of effective written communications.
- Write an effective letter and memo.
- Discuss how to properly handle correspondence containing negative content.
- List and explain proper telephone techniques.
- Describe items important to proper telephone etiquette.

## Keywords and concepts
**you will learn in this chapter:**

- Binding Machines
- Body
- Certified Mail
- Clarity in Writing
- Coherence in Writing
- Collate
- Complimentary Close
- Correspondence
- Effectiveness in Writing

- Enclosures
- ERISA Right of Review Statement
- Etiquette
- Facsimile Machine (more commonly referred to as the fax machine)
- Garnishment
- Heading

- Inside Address
- Memo
- Multiline Phones
- Reservation of Rights
- Return Receipt Requested
- Salutation
- Signature
- Tickler Files

Most communication with claim contacts will be by letter or through telephone conversations. These contacts will include claimants, attorneys, physicians, hospital personnel, and employers. These contacts will be with people of different educational and socio-economic backgrounds. Therefore, it is important to be able to adapt to any situation and to be understood.

Health claims examiners at times communicate with someone who has lost a loved one, or with someone who is experiencing stress due to severe illness. Although professionalism is required, so is compassion.

Many ideas can be transmitted through effective communication. Communication is relevant in the functioning of any organization. Communication can be used to influence, to show cooperation, but most importantly to give and obtain information. The more effective the communication medium is, the greater the chances of giving understandable answers or receiving the information being sought.

# Verbal Communication

The most commonly used mode of communication is verbal (speech). We speak so others may listen. When you speak to someone, it is a stimuli which produces a response. The manner in which you speak to someone usually has an influence on the response received.

# Telephone Communication

The majority of a health claims examiner's communication with a claimant will be over the telephone. Rarely will a claimant come into the office. When dealing with an Employer Group Plan, contact will usually be with the employer, and contact with the claimant rarely occurs.

Telephone conversations may be judged by the listener and are subject to interpretation. Therefore, being tactful and professional when speaking is essential.

Be very careful about giving out information which may be contradicted at a later date. For example, unless a request is already in process for a check to be sent, do not say a check will be sent unless it is a certainty that it will. A situation may arise where a claim may appear to be payable, however after consulting with a superior it may not be payable, or a piece of correspondence may be received that sheds a different light on the claim. Therefore, be very careful about any commitment you make.

When speaking on the telephone, speak slowly and distinctly. Keep in mind that you will usually be speaking to someone who has no knowledge of claims procedures and in most cases little or no understanding of insurance terminology. Also, the claimant may have little knowledge of requirements necessary to claim benefits under the policy.

Be sure to thank people for complying with the plan requirements. Remember also to preface any requests for additional information with a "please."

The tone of one's voice is very important. Our words can sometimes be helpful but condescending. Avoid getting into arguments with others, even if they are irate. Try to understand the other person's viewpoint.

When taking a message for a coworker, always read the message back or ask for the spelling of names. Repeat telephone numbers and ask for area codes. It is very frustrating for a person to get a message they cannot return. Also, never commit a coworker to returning a call at or by a specific time or date, because your coworker may not be able to comply with the commitment made. Instead of saying "I'll have her call you back at 11:15," say "I'll have her call you at her earliest convenience."

Being an effective speaker is more important than being an effective writer. A letter can always be rewritten, but once words are spoken, they cannot be taken back.

# Telephone Techniques

Because claims examiners conduct a large amount of their business over the telephone, proper telephone skills are very important.

## Answer Promptly

When the telephone rings, make a point of answering it before the third ring, whenever possible. Prompt answering helps avoid irritation and builds a reputation for efficiency.

## Identify Yourself

Let the caller know with whom he or she is speaking. It establishes a rapport and lets the caller know that you are a person, as opposed to a computer, and are willing to work to resolve their problem or concern.

## Be Friendly

Your tone of voice should convey willingness to help, and make the caller feel that their call is important. A pleasant sounding voice and words spoken at a moderate pace are ideal. Make the caller feel that you are eager to be of assistance. To accomplish this:

1. Be a good listener so that the caller will not have to repeat things.
2. Indicate that you are interested. Use the caller's name whenever possible (but use the last name, not the first name).
3. Be sincere and genuine, and let this come through in your voice.
4. Give your full attention to the caller. A discussion with others while a caller is waiting on the line is inconsiderate and irritating.
5. Avoid interrupting the caller.

## Returning to the Line

When you must leave the line to get information, be courteous. Ask if the caller is able to hold or if it would be more convenient to call back. Do not automatically assume that the caller has the time or inclination to wait on the line. Here are some suggestions:

1. If the caller agrees to hold, use the hold button. If this is unavailable on your phone, set the phone down gently. Bear in mind that the caller can overhear conversation when the phone is not placed on hold. Be careful not to say anything that might be overheard or misunderstood.
2. If it takes longer than anticipated to obtain the information, update the caller on your progress. If it is going to be more than a couple of minutes, tell the caller that you will contact him as soon as you can get the information. Give the caller an estimate of how long it will take, and keep your promise to call back.
3. When you return to the line, let the caller know you have returned. For example, say, "Thank you for waiting."

## Transferring Calls

Try to take care of the caller's concern yourself. It is irritating for the caller to be transferred from one person to another. If the caller has a simple problem that is not your responsibility (i.e., change of address, request for an application or material), write the information and give it to the person who is responsible for that function. When it is necessary to transfer a call, take the following four steps:

1. Explain why you need to transfer the call ("I'm unable to assist you with that. However, Mr. Gonzales can help you. May I transfer you?").
2. Wait for the caller's response. If the person does not wish to be transferred, write down her name and phone number and tell the caller that someone will call them back ("I'll have Ms. Smith call you back with the information.").
3. If the caller agrees to be transferred, be careful not to disconnect the call. To be safe, always give the caller the name of the person you are transferring them to and their extension or phone number. Then if the caller is accidentally disconnected, they can call that person directly.
4. Finally, briefly explain the situation or problem to the person to whom you are transferring the call, along with the caller's name. Be concise, but convey enough information that the caller will not need to repeat everything a second time.

## Closing the Call

Summarize the conversation to be sure it is closed and to note any follow-up action required of either party. Try your best to say good-bye in a way that will leave the caller feeling satisfied that their problem will be properly handled. Let the calling party hang up first.

# Phone Calls

The following are general guidelines regarding phone usage. Since these guidelines may vary from company to company or even between departments in a company, be sure to understand the company's phone policies prior to making or receiving phone calls.

1. **Collect call policy:** Some companies accept collect calls from customers; however, others do not. If you are going to be handling inquiry calls, it is important to know the company's policy prior to accepting collect calls, not after.

## Practice
# Pitfalls

In addition to the previous points, here are more suggestions that may be helpful:

1. If the call is going to be lengthy, make an appointment with the caller for a date and time for the extended call. In this way, the call will have a better chance of being answered, and the person will have a better chance of having the time needed to resolve the situation.

2. Outline the topics to be discussed before placing the call; then stick to the list of topics.

3. Before placing the call try to mentally picture the other person, and smile at that person. This will provide a friendlier frame of mind.

4. Be kind to whomever answers the phone, even if it is not the person with whom you wish to speak. This person may be the only link to the person requested.

5. If the person called cannot be reached, leave a message and make sure the messenger also takes down your phone number. This increases the chances for a returned phone call.

6. Make sure the person has a few minutes to speak. A simple, "Do you have a moment to speak with me?" can help a lot. If the answer is "no," ask when the best time would be to call back.

7. Most callers find it unnerving to be asked what their call is about. If you are unable to answer your own phone, instruct those who answer it not to ask this question.

8. Avoid doing other things (i.e., writing or typing) while on the phone.

9. Complex information is best handled in person or in writing, especially if it contains critical information or details.

10. Make sure that the caller is satisfied and fully understands before closing a conversation. A confused expression cannot be seen over the phone, so listen for it in the caller's voice.

11. When taking a message for someone else, do not tell the caller when this person will call back. If the caller is unable to reach the person at that time, he may become upset.

12. Never slam down the receiver, no matter how upset you may be with the caller.

13. Do not eat, drink, chew, or smoke while on the phone. The telephone receiver can magnify these sounds, and they can be very annoying to the caller.

14. Always terminate a call pleasantly and politely.

2. **Long distance:** Long distance calls to customers are usually permitted if the information requested in the call is necessary for business purposes. You should organize your thoughts and write down your questions prior to making the call, so that as little time as possible is spent on the call. This will drastically reduce the overhead costs of the company.

3. **Telephone system:** Telephone systems can vary greatly from one company to another. It is essential to know how to properly answer a call, transfer a call, and place a caller on hold. Nothing is more irritating to a caller than to be disconnected after being on hold for a long period of time.

## Telephone Etiquette

It is important to use proper etiquette on the phone. The word **etiquette** is defined as the practices and forms prescribed by convention or by authority. In essence, etiquette is manners.

While using the telephone, etiquette includes your tone of voice, some basic telephone manners, speaking on the level of the caller, controlling the conversation, and making the appropriate verbal responses.

### Tone of Voice

One's tone of voice is the single most important factor in conveying willingness to help others. Be pleasant and professional. Pay attention to the other person and respond to their questions in a sincere manner. If you smile while on the phone, this smile will usually come across in your voice.

Customer service can be demanding, frustrating work. Many callers are angry, irritated, or tired. But the difference between providing good customer service and poor customer service is that good customer service is always provided in a pleasant and kind manner to every caller, no matter how the person comes across. You cannot allow the person's feelings to influence your own.

Be natural and use simple straightforward language. Use a normal volume that can be heard easily, but is not too loud. Talk at a moderate rate, neither too fast nor too slow.

In many geographic areas there are high concentrations of non-English-speaking or English-as-a-second-language speaking persons. If you do not speak the caller's language and they do not speak English well, it is important to speak slowly and to pronounce words correctly. Do not yell. These callers are not deaf; they just have difficulty with the language. If possible, find someone in your office who speaks the caller's language. If that is not possible, take the time to work with the caller. If necessary, spell out words. Many people have a higher understanding of written language than of spoken language. Above all else, be patient and do not try to rush the situation.

## Telephone Manners

Every call is important to the caller and should be treated as such. When the caller feels that they are receiving individual attention, rather than routine consideration, he or she will have more confidence in you and the company.

Be tactful. When a request must be denied because of company policy, give a full and sympathetic explanation. A comment such as "If you will submit your request in writing, we will be glad to give it consideration" sounds more tactful than, "You have to send it to us in writing to get an answer."

Apologize for errors or delays, even if they are not your fault. Things may not always go right, but a little courtesy can help defuse anger. However, be sure your apologies are genuine; otherwise they will sound insincere.

Take time to be helpful. It only takes a little more effort to make your phone contacts pleasant, and it can brighten your day as well as the caller's. Remember that it is better to spend a few minutes trying to keep a member happy than months trying to regain her business.

If you are having a bad day and all the customers seem to be angry or defensive, consider that the problem might be you. People respond to what they think they hear in someone's voice. If there is irritation, it may make them irritated and can begin a downward spiral. Turn things around by changing the way you are talking or your tone of voice. This simple change may turn your day around.

## Speak at the Caller's Level

You will receive calls from people with varying degrees of education and knowledge. Listen to the way the caller pronounces words and the type of words they use. Then use words on a similar level that the caller can understand. Regardless of the level of the caller, avoid the use of technical words that the caller may not understand.

## Controlling the Conversation

Your primary goal should be to give the client complete satisfaction in the least amount of time. The following suggestions may be helpful in accomplishing this:

1. Find out as soon as possible what the question or problem is. Have the caller tell you exactly what they want. Do not try to guess. You may guess wrong and provide unwanted or incorrect information or could bring up questions the caller may not have thought of.

2. Obtain specific information immediately. This may include information such as:
   * What is the member's ID number?
   * What is the member's name?
   * What was the date of the claim?
   * What was the name of the doctor who provided the services?

3. Answer all questions and make sure the caller understands the issues. Before closing the call, ask whether there are other questions.

4. Do not bring up issues or claims unrelated to the caller's questions.

5. Do not chitchat with the caller. Be polite, but keep the conversation centered on the business at hand.

6. Choose your words and tone of voice carefully. If the caller becomes angry or irritated, the call may take longer.

7. After the caller's questions have been answered or the requested information has been given, politely close the conversation.

## Appropriate Verbal Responses

If a question requires a simple yes or no, it is appropriate to answer as such. However, be aware of questions with which disclaimers should be used. These can involve questions such as, "Does the payer cover this type of surgery?" or "Does my insurance provide surgical coverage?" Answers to these questions should include disclaimers such as, "Yes, if the services are medically necessary" or "Yes, with certain restrictions. Cosmetic surgery is not covered, or a second opinion may be needed to verify the need for some surgeries." Explain that without proper information from the doctor or medical documentation, you cannot tell the caller whether her particular procedure will be performed or covered and whether other conditions might need to be taken into consideration.

Many insurance companies have a preauthorization process, which allows the provider of service to submit documentation regarding the case and suggested procedures prior to the performance of these procedures. This information is reviewed and a qualified approval may be given. This is similar to obtaining an estimate before car repair work is done, but here the estimate covers not how much it will cost, but how much the insurance carrier will cover. If the procedure falls into a gray area, the claims examiner should suggest that a preauthorization review be performed prior to the services being rendered.

If the caller is presenting a hypothetical question, the variables may range too widely to provide an answer. Without documented facts it is difficult to make a decision regarding any situation. If the caller insists that you give an answer, explain that your reply is based on the information given and that the answer could vary greatly when the written documentation is received.

If you are unsure about the answer to a question, do not guess. Inform the caller that you are not sure but that you will find out the answer and call them back.

When verifying benefits, all facts of coverage should be checked. This includes the diagnosis, the eligibility status, current coverage, dependent eligibility, age limits, and others.

Most calls can be handled using your knowledge, common sense, and patience. Remember never to make any promises you cannot guarantee. Actually, the only promise you should ever make is to follow through in handling the situation.

# On the Job Now

**Directions:** Successful people know their strengths as well as the areas that need improvement. Complete the following questions.

1. Identify three strengths you currently possess which contribute to positive customer service relations.

    1. _____

    2. _____

    3. _____

2. Identify three areas that you would like to grow in to be more effective in customer service relations.

    1. _____

    2. _____

    3. _____

3. Specifically, what actions or steps can you take to improve in the previous three areas?

    1. _____

    2. _____

    3. _____

# On the Job Now

**Directions:**  Read the following statements and rate yourself on how you feel you handle customers. Be honest. This is the only way you can recognize your strengths and weaknesses and work toward improving your weaknesses. Use the following numbers to answer the questions:

1 = Never, 2 = Seldom, 3 = Sometimes, 4 = Often, 5 = Always.

1. _____ I want the service I provide to leave an excellent impression, so I constantly look for ways to improve it.
2. _____ I put the customer's needs first since (s)he is my ultimate boss.
3. _____ I accept people without judging them.
4. _____ I am aware that my attitudes and moods affect the way I respond to customers.
5. _____ I show patience and courtesy regardless of the customer's behavior.
6. _____ I do not allow myself to become irritated or lose my composure when dealing with angry customers.
7. _____ I have developed the habit of following up on all complaints that are brought to my attention.
8. _____ I understand the customer and see his/her problem as most important, and I do all I can to resolve it.
9. _____ I treat all customers equally, regardless of their position, rank, color, clothes, accent or other distinguishing features.
10. _____ I recognize it is perceptions that count when dealing with customers, so I do not allow my frustrations or irritations to show.
11. _____ If something the customer says offends me, I focus on what the client is feeling, not on getting even.
12. _____ I use professional language in my dealings with customers.
13. _____ I use proper telephone techniques and always identify myself to the caller.
14. _____ I make sure the customer is satisfied before terminating the conversation.
15. _____ I do not transfer a call unless it is absolutely necessary to resolve the customer's problem.
_____ Total

**Scoring:**  Add the total for each question and then compute your score. The following scale gives an analysis of your client service quotient.

| | |
|---|---|
| 68–75 | Excellent! Your behavior and attitudes set examples for others to follow. |
| 59–67 | Good. You have a high awareness of how important your role is in customer service. |
| 50–58 | Moderate. You may be allowing your own biases and feelings to affect your customer service. |
| 41–49 | Needs definite improvement. Time to get in touch with the obstacles between you and the quality service you should be providing. |
| Below 40 | Poor. You need to make a concentrated effort to turn your attitudes and values around. Change may be slow. |

## Written Communication

**Correspondence** is written communication between two people, and it has become an integral part of the business world. Without effective written communication it is almost impossible for a company to succeed. Written communications have permeated every aspect of the business world, from interoffice memos to letters, and from filed reports to e-mail messages.

Therefore, one of the most important skills that a claims examiner can have is the ability to write clearly and effectively. No one wants to read a dull, boring letter, no matter how short. The dullest subject can be made inviting and exciting with effective writing techniques. Remember that the reader will judge you and your company by the type of correspondence received. Learn to use effective language that is clear, concise, and interesting. Correspondence should also be grammatically correct and properly punctuated.

Before beginning to write think of who the audience is going to be. Are you writing a personal letter to a single person or a newsletter that will be distributed to many people? It will be easier to tailor your writing when you have a clear picture of the reader.

**Effectiveness in writing** means being able to evoke the type of response you want your reader to have, whether you want the reader to call, to send back a request for additional information, or send in an EOB.

## Letter Writing

Letters written to others have a primary purpose: to give or request information. Each letter also influences your public image. Clients perceive a company's reliability and personality from its letters. Are they curt or friendly, threatening or helpful?

The key to a good letter is organization. Present the information in a manner which is understandable. A letter should be readable and project a professional image. This can be achieved through the use of basic letter structure and clear, concise language.

Many insurance carriers use form letters. Be sure that when filling in information on these letters, you write clearly and carefully convey what you want the person to do.

When composing a letter you should initially determine to whom you are writing, in order to use the proper language and tone to convey your meaning.

### Language

When writing, consider the message you want to deliver. Choose words which will convey your message clearly and concisely. Keep in mind that business letters should be written in formal language, not colloquial everyday language. However, remember that writing too formal can alienate readers, and an overly obvious attempt to be casual and informal may strike the reader as insincere or unprofessional.

## Practice Pitfalls

Before beginning to compose a letter, ask yourself the following questions:

1. Is this correspondence really necessary? If the answer is no, eliminate it.
2. Could this information be easily expressed over the phone? Would it save time? If the answer is yes, pick up the phone and call.
3. Has this information been expressed in previous correspondence? If so, perhaps a copy of the previous material or a short note referencing it will suffice.
4. Is it vital that the information be written "for the record?" If so, it must be written.

No one wants to waste time reading through information that is not necessary or that has already been covered. Too many communications of this sort may cause your reader to pay less attention when an important piece of correspondence arrives. If the information must be written, follow these points:

1. Determine what you want to say before you begin to write.
2. Determine what action or response you are seeking from the reader.
3. After the correspondence has been written, proofread it carefully for clarity, proper spelling, and proper grammar.
4. Finally, make sure that the correspondence conveys the message you intended.

### Tone

Build goodwill by writing letters with a friendly tone. Cold, stiff letters often create the wrong impression. Keynote each letter with courtesy. If the occasion warrants, be sympathetic, but not overly apologetic. Always show respect to the reader.

Be positive. Some people would write: "We are sorry that we shall be unable to compile this information for you in less than one week." Good writers would say it this way: "We shall be glad to compile this information for you and we could have it ready in one week." Avoid using negative words such as "cannot," "unable," and "impossible."

## Voice

Whenever possible, write in the active voice rather than the passive voice. Instead of "the enclosed form should be returned within 30 days," try using "please return the enclosed form in 30 days."

# Parts of a Business Letter

As you are probably aware, a letter consists of certain elements. A typical business letter consists of six main parts as follows: the heading, inside address, salutation, body, complimentary close, and signature. While the body of the letter contains the "significant information", the opening, which is the initial part of the body, "sets the scene," and the closing leaves the "lasting impression."

## Heading

The **heading** contains the return address, date, and a reference line and other notations if applicable. Sometimes it may be necessary to include a line after the address and before the date for a phone number, fax number, or email address. It is not necessary to type the return address if you are using stationery with the return address already imprinted. The date line is used to indicate the date the letter was written.

## Inside Address

The **inside address** is the address to which the letter is being sent. An inside address helps the recipient to route the letter properly and can help should the envelope be damaged and the address become unreadable.

Make the address as complete as possible. It is always best to write to a specific individual. Include titles such as Ms., Mrs., Mr., or Dr. If you are unsure of a woman's preference in being addressed, use Ms.

## Salutation

The **salutation** is a form of greeting the letter recipient. It normally begins with the word "Dear" and always includes the person's last name (i.e., Dear Dr. Suess:). However, if you know the person and typically address them by their first name, it is acceptable to use only the first name in the salutation (i.e., Dear Theodor:). The salutation in a business letter always ends with a colon.

If you cannot determine a recipient's gender, use a nonsexist salutation, such as "To Whom it May Con-cern:" It is also acceptable to use the full name in a salutation if you cannot determine gender (i.e., Dear Presley Taylor:).

## Body

The **body** of the letter contains the main text or message. The first paragraph and the first sentence of your correspondence are critical. You must gain your reader's attention, interest him in reading further, and make the reader receptive to your ideas. Without the reader's attention, you cannot hope to gain the response you are seeking.

Remember that your reader's first interest is usually himself. The reader automatically defines the correspondence according to the personal benefits it will bring. Therefore, you must involve the reader or you run the risk of losing him. When writing letters, it is important to be personable but direct. The reader should be able to understand the reason for your letter by reading the first paragraph. Get your reader's attention by appealing to their interests. Think of the subject from the reader's point of view.

The two principal purposes of the **opening** (which is a subpart of the body) are to attract attention and to develop interest. Therefore, do not try to say too much in the opening. To be successful, the opening must invite sufficient interest to draw the reader into the body of the correspondence. Do not give all the information in the first paragraph. Briefly explain your reason for writing (i.e., "a complete review has been made of your claim as you requested..."). Then, explain the details of the situation.

The body of the correspondence is where you present the purpose of the communication. Here, you let the reader know what you wish to obtain, if anything. If it is succinct enough, any additional information that is needed to verify the request or purpose should also be included here. If it is not, a copy of the information should be attached and a reference should be included in the body of the letter (i.e., see accompanying account statement). Details you want to impart should be included in this section. Often, a brief review of claim facts, an explanation of the policy provisions that apply, and relevant statements pertaining to the situation should be included.

Lead the reader step-by-step toward an objective. First try to clear their mind of any preconceived notions. Respect their opinions and views while proceeding to help them understand and accept the principles you advocate. Be sure to provide enough information for the reader to understand your purpose, but not so much that it is overwhelming. Keep the information concise and move the correspondence forward.

The closing paragraph is the final chance to make your point. It should be a brief summary of the major points contained in the body of the correspondence. Also include a congratulatory or consolatory note if the body of the letter contains good or bad news. Your closing should be fresh, and state in a new and interesting way what the recipient should do, thus enticing them to carry out your wishes. The closing paragraph of your letter should be friendly but decisive. It serves any or all of the following purposes:

- Requests action on the part of the reader.

- Leaves the door open for future action.

- Ends the correspondence.

If you are requesting action, be sure to let the reader know the following:

- What you want done ("send," "contact," etc.).

- When you want it done (be specific; not "A.S.A.P.," but "within 14 days," etc.).

- How to complete your request ("call me at (XXX) 555-1212," etc.).

## Complimentary Close

The **complimentary close** is where you bring your letter to an end in a short polite manner, and always begins with a capital letter and ends with a comma (i.e., Sincerely yours,).

## Signature

The **signature** is the name of the person writing the letter or for whom the letter has been written. Spell out the name to be signed. The signature customarily includes a middle initial. The signature line may also include a second line for a title, if appropriate.

## Enclosures

**Enclosures** are anything that you are sending along with the letter, such as x-rays or forms. To indicate that there are enclosures included, type the word "Enclosures" one line below the signature. You may also list the name of the document(s) that is being included.

Business letters should not contain postscripts.

## Terminology

The words chosen to express an idea can greatly impact a reader's interpretation. Clarity can be achieved with conciseness. Generally, short words are better than long ones. For example, "begin" is better than "initiate," "try" is better than "endeavor." Also, break complex sentences down into several simple ones. However, because business let-

# On the Job Now

Name the six parts of a business letter and what each part consists of.

1. _____

2. _____

3. _____

4. _____

5. _____

6. _____

| When you Mean | Use |
|---|---|
| Addition | And, also, again, besides, plus, finally, then, too, furthermore. |
| Contrast | However, though, although, but, nevertheless, yet, rather, than, otherwise, instead. |
| Result | It, consequently, therefore, thus, since, so, hence, accordingly. |
| Concession | Naturally, of course, perhaps, admittedly, granted. |

**Table 15–1**  **Examples of everyday terminology**

ters should not be an endless series of short, choppy sentences, do not be so concise that you become blunt.

When writing to an insured, it is helpful to use everyday terminology rather than insurance jargon. Use words that everyone can understand. However, be extremely careful in paraphrasing the policy or certificate. Quote the policy verbatim whenever possible.

There are other phrases that are overused or abused, such as the following:

1. "N/A" – Try not to use this abbreviation. It may not be understood by the reader.

2. "Above named insured," "Above captioned insured" – A better way is to state the insured's name, "Mr. Jones."

3. "Enclosed is an envelope" – The insured can see the envelope and will usually realize from the rest of your letter its intended use.

4. "Please be advised" – These are wasted words. Try writing your sentence then cross out these words. Usually the sentence is complete without them.

5. "Thank you in advance for your anticipated cooperation" – Can easily be reworded into a much shorter phrase, as "Thank you for your cooperation."

The use of connectives can be a valuable tool. However, make sure that you use a connective that conveys your intended meaning.

# Content Structure

A letter is useful only when it clearly states the message that is being conveyed. While wordiness is not recommended, extreme shortness can create a poor impression. Use words sparingly, but not sparsely.

When writing, keep the reader in mind. Tailor your letters for effectiveness and readability. Get all of the facts, do your homework, and do not guess.

## Clarity and Coherence

**Clarity in writing** means exactness of language. It results in the reader understanding what you intended to say. If the meaning is not clear, the entire message has failed, no matter how eloquently it was stated. Remember that your reader cannot respond appropriately if he cannot figure out what you want.

After writing a piece of correspondence, take a moment to put yourself in the reader's place and read the letter as if you were seeing it for the first time. Ask yourself, "Does this say what I intended it to say?" If not, it needs to be rewritten.

Coherence means "sticking together." **Coherence in writing** means that the letter or information flows logically from one idea to the next. Being coherent requires that you do not cram too many ideas into a single piece of correspondence. Eliminate any ideas that are not necessary.

If all the information is necessary and the correspondence is still lengthy, consider inserting headings to help the reader determine when you are moving from one thought to another. If your document is not clear and coherent, you will have failed in your attempt to get a message across to your reader and it is not worth sending.

## Grammar, Sentence Structure, and Paragraphs

Make sure your grammar and sentence structure are accurate. The impression your letter creates will be a reflection of you and the company for which you work. The last thing you want is your members thinking that they are signed up with an unprofessional company.

Paragraphs should be kept short and to the point. A paragraph should end when a thought is complete. The only exception is when you add a transitional thought to the end of the final sentence. A transitional thought segues into the topic of the next paragraph.

# Correspondence Containing Negative Content

When writing letters that contain negative content (i.e., letters of denial), say "no" as graciously as possible. Your success in keeping this person as a client depends on your saying "no" nicely. Use positive words and phrases to develop a positive feeling within your reader.

Never give bad news in the first paragraph. The reader may stop reading without understanding the reasoning behind the decision. You will have lost the reader without getting the reasons and rationale across in a manner that creates mutual understanding.

Clearly state the reasons for the decision and, if possible, refer the reader to any applicable information to support the provider's decision (i.e., a copy of the contract provisions, a copy of the EOB). If appeals procedures are applicable, include all the necessary information regarding appeals in your correspondence. This will eliminate unnecessary phone calls at a later date.

Because of time constraints and financial considerations, it may be necessary to respond to your client with a form letter. If the form letter is written in a pleasing tone and uses specific references, you reduce the chances that your reader will think of it as just another form letter. If the letter has been photocopied and is obviously a form letter, consider adding a personal note to the margin that will soften the message.

# Proofreading

Never send a letter you have not proofread. Check for errors as well as readability. Since many of the letters you write will deal with benefits, it is especially important to check any dollar amounts that are included.

Check the remainder of the letter as well, because just one letter can make a difference between "unit" and "unite," "owning" and "owing."

When corrections are necessary, indicate changes to be made at the point in the text where they occur. Make corrections in red ink so that they stand out from the rest of the letter and can be located easily by the typist. Always have a corrected letter retyped – sloppy, handwritten corrections leave a poor impression.

# Format of the Letter

For correspondence to be taken seriously, it is important for it to look professional. There are numerous books available that show various styles and formats for letters. Each company has a preferred style, and this style should be used for all correspondence.

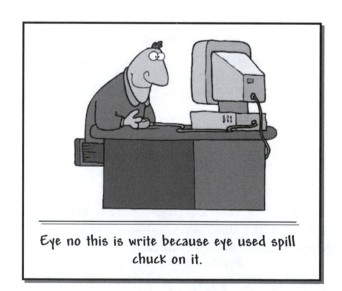

Eye no this is write because eye used spill chuck on it.

Listed below are the three main styles of letters: block style, modified block style, and semiblock style **(see Figures 15–1 through 15–3)**. Each of these styles has specific rules regarding formatting of the letter. It is not considered acceptable to mix two or more styles in a single letter or communication.

[Your Name]
[Address]
[City, State, Zip]
[Phone]
[Date Today]
[Re: To What This Letter Refers]

[CERTIFIED MAIL]
[PERSONAL]

[Recipient's Name]
[Company Name]
[Address]
[City, State, Zip]

Dear [Recipient's Name]

[Subject]

The main characteristic of a full block letter is that all typed information is flush with the left-hand margin. The margins are 1.5 inches on the left and the right. The letter is centered up and down, with at least a 1.5 inch margin. There is a double space between paragraphs.

If there is more than one page, the complimentary closing, typist's initials, enclosures, and cc's are placed only on the last page.

Full block is considered to be the most formal style of letters.

Sincerely,

[Signature]

[Your Name]
[Title]

[Typist Initials]
Enclosures: [#]

Cc: [Name of Copy Recipient]
[Name of Copy Recipient]

**■ Figure 15–1** Block Style Letter

1. **Return Address:** If your stationery has a letterhead, skip this. Otherwise, type your name, address, and (optionally) phone number. These days, it is common to also include an email address.

2. **Date:** Type the date of your letter two to six lines below the letterhead. Three lines are standard. If there is no letterhead, type it where shown.

3. **Reference Line:** If the recipient specifically requests information, such as a job reference or invoice number, type it on one or two lines, immediately below the **Date (2)**. If you are replying to a letter, refer to it here. For example:
   - Re: Job # 625-01
   - Re: Your letter dated 1/1/CCYY

4. **Special Mailing Notations:** Type in all uppercase characters, if appropriate. Examples include:
   - SPECIAL DELIVERY
   - CERTIFIED MAIL
   - AIRMAIL

5. **On-Arrival Notations:** Type in all uppercase characters, if appropriate. You might want to include a notation on private correspondence, such as a resignation letter. Include the same on the envelope. Examples are:
   - PERSONAL
   - CONFIDENTIAL

6. **Recipient's Address:** Type the name and address of the person and/or company to whom you are sending the letter, three to eight lines below the last component you typed. Four lines are standard.

7. **Salutation:** Type the recipient's name here. Type Mr. or Ms. [Last Name] to show respect, but do not guess spelling or gender. Some common salutations are:
   - Ladies:
   - Gentlemen:
   - Dear Sir:
   - Dear Sir or Madam:
   - Dear [Full Name]:
   - To Whom it May Concern:

8. **Subject Line:** Type the gist of your letter in all uppercase characters, either flush left or centered. Be concise and only use one line. If you type a **Reference Line (3)**, consider if you really need this line. While it is not really necessary for most employment-related letters, examples are below.
   - SUBJECT: RESIGNATION
   - LETTER OF REFERENCE
   - JOB INQUIRY

9. **Body:** Type two spaces between sentences. Keep it brief and to the point.

10. **Complimentary Close:** What you type here depends on the tone and degree of formality. For example:
    - Respectfully yours (very formal)
    - Sincerely (typical, less formal)
    - Very truly yours (polite, neutral)
    - Cordially yours (friendly, informal)

11. **Signature Block:** Leave four blank lines after the **Complimentary Close (10)** to sign your name. Sign your name exactly as you type it below your signature. Title is optional depending on relevancy and degree of formality. Examples are:
    - John Doe, Manager
    - S. Smith
    - Director, Technical Support
    - J. J. Jones – Sr. Field Engineer

12. **Identification Initials:** If someone typed the letter for you, he would typically include three of your initials in all uppercase characters, then two of his in all lowercase characters. If you typed your own letter, just skip it since your name is already in the **Signature Block (11)**. Common styles are below.
    - AAA/dd
    - AAA:dd
    - Ddd

13. **Enclosure Notation:** This line tells the reader to look in the envelope for more items. Type the singular for only one enclosure, plural for more. If you do not enclose anything, skip it. Common styles are below.
    - Enclosure
    - Enclosures: 3
    - Enclosures (3)

14. **cc:** Stands for **courtesy copies** (formerly **carbon copies**). List the names of people here to who you distribute copies, in alphabetical order. If addresses would be useful to the recipient of the letter, include them. If you do not copy your letter to anyone, skip it.

[Your Name]
[Address]
[City, State, Zip]
[Phone]
[Date Today]
[Re: To What This Letter Refers]

[CERTIFIED MAIL]
[PERSONAL]

[Recipient's Name]
[Company Name]
[Address]
[City, State, Zip]

Attention [Recipient's Name]

Dear [Recipient' Name]

[Subject]

The main characteristic of a modified block letter is that all typed information is flush with the left-hand margin. The margins are 1.5 inches on the left and the right. The letter is centered up and down, with at least a 1.5 inch margin. There is a double space between paragraphs.

If there is more than one page, the complimentary closing, typist's initials, enclosures, and cc's are placed only on the last page.

Modified block letter is not as formal as full block letter.

　　　　Sincerely,

　　　　[Signature]

　　　　[Your Name, Title]

[Typist Initials]
Enclosures: [#]

Cc: [Name of Copy Recipient]
　　[Name of Copy Recipient]

**■ Figure 15–2** Modified Block Style Letter

1. **Return Address:** If your stationery has a letterhead, skip this. Otherwise, type your name, address, and (optionally) phone number, five spaces to the right of center or flush with the right margin. Five spaces to the right of center is common. These days, it is also common to include an email address.

2. **Date:** Type the date five spaces to the right of the center or flush with the right margin, two to six lines below the letterhead. Five spaces to the right of the center and three lines below the letterhead are common. If there is no letterhead, type it where shown.

3. **Reference Line:** Same as Block Style

4. **Special Mailing Notations:** Same as Block Style

5. **On-Arrival Notations:** Same as Block Style

6. **Inside Address:** Same as Block Style

7. **Attention Line:** Same as Block Style

8. **Salutation:** Same as Block Style

9. **Subject Line:** Same as Block Style

10. **Body:** Same as Block Style

11. **Complimentary Close:** Type this aligned with the **Date (2)** Same as Block Style

12. **Signature Block:** Align this with the **Complimentary Close (11)**. Same as Block Style

13. **Identification Initials:** Same as Block Style

14. **Enclosure Notation:** Same as Block Style

15. **cc:** Same as Block Style

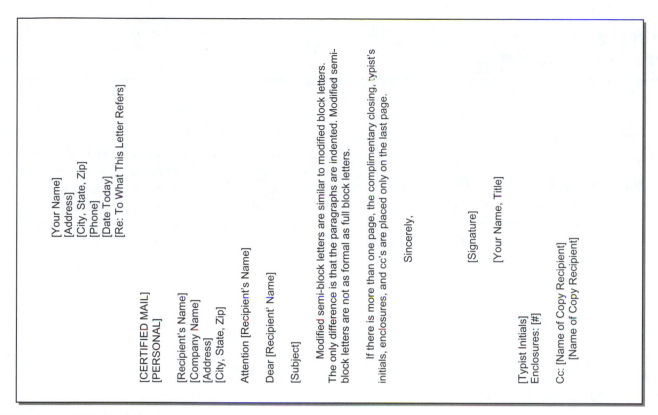

**■ Figure 15–3** Semiblock Style Letter

1. **Return Address:** If your stationery has a letterhead, skip this. Otherwise, type your name, address and (optionally) phone number, five spaces to the right of center or flush with the right margin. Five spaces to the right of center is common. These days, it is also common to include an email address.

2. **Date:** Type the date five spaces to the right of the center or flush with the right margin, two to six lines below the letterhead. Five spaces to the right of the center and three lines below the letterhead are common. If there is no letterhead, type it where shown.

3. **Reference Line:** Same as Block Style

4. **Special Mailing Notations:** Same as Block Style

5. **On-Arrival Notations:** Same as Block Style

6. **Inside Address:** Same as Block Style

7. **Attention Line:** Same as Block Style

8. **Salutation:** Same as Block Style

9. **Subject Line:** Same as Block Style

10. **Body:** Same as Block Style

11. **Complimentary Close:** Type this aligned with the **Date (2)**. Same as Block Style

12. **Signature Block:** Align this block with the **Complimentary Close (11)**. Same as Block Style

13. **Identification Initials:** Same as Block Style

14. **Enclosure Notation:** Same as Block Style

15. **cc:** Same as Block Style

## Business Letter Envelope Components

This sample business letter envelope (**see Figure 15–4**), includes formal components, some of which are optional for typical, employment-related business letters.

The graphic below represents the U. S. Postal Service automation guidelines for a standard business envelope that is 4-1/8 × 9-1/2 inches.

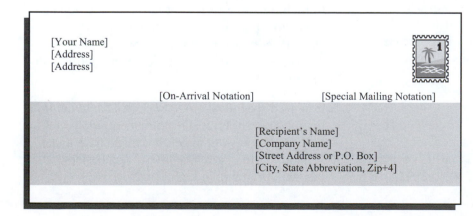

**■ Figure 15–4** Sample Business Letter Envelope

## Practice
# Pitfalls

Use the following tips when writing letters:

1. Replace the text in brackets [ ] with the component indicated. Do not type the brackets.

2. Try to keep your letters to one page.

3. How many blank lines you add between lines that require more than one depends on how much space is available on the page.

4. The same applies for margins. The standard for margins is one and one-half inch (108 points) for short letters and one inch (72 points) for longer letters. If there is a letterhead, its position determines the top margin.

5. If you do not type one of the more formal components, do not leave space for them. For example, if you do not type the **Reference Line (3)**, **Special Mailing Notations (4)**, and **On-Arrival Notations (5)**, type the **Inside Address (6)** four lines below the **Date (2)**

## Practice
# Pitfalls

Use the following tips when creating envelopes:

1. Replace the text in brackets [ ] with the component indicated. Do not type the brackets.

2. If your envelope does not have a preprinted return address, type it in the upper left-hand corner, in an area not to exceed 50% of the length and 33% of the height of the envelope. Leave a little space between your return address and the top and left edges. How much space will depend on the margin limitations of your printer or typewriter. For example, laser printers typically require margins of at least 1/8 inch (9 points). However, 1/4 inch (18 points) to 1/2 inch (36 points) looks good.

3. Type the **Special Mailing Notation** under the postage area. It does not have to line up perfectly with the stamp as shown, but it looks professional. Type the notation in all uppercase characters, if appropriate. Examples include:

   - SPECIAL DELIVERY
   - CERTIFIED MAIL
   - AIRMAIL

4. Type the **On-Arrival Notation** so that its right edge lines up with the left edge of the recipient's address. This is not a post office requirement but, rather, standard formatting. Type the notation in all uppercase characters, if appropriate. You might want to include a notation on private correspondence, such as when mailing a resignation letter. Examples include:

   - PERSONAL
   - CONFIDENTIAL

5. The gray shaded area is where the OCR (optical character reader) at the post office scans for the recipient's address. Type the recipient's address within the shaded area, below other information. Do not type anything to the left, right or below the recipient's address. It is a good idea to include a line or two of space below nonaddress information (such as the notations shown), before typing the recipient's address. This makes it easier for the OCR to distinguish the address.

6. You need special software to print a bar code. It is not required for typical, employment-related letters, but if you want to get fancy, and have a later version of Microsoft Word® or WordPerfect®, they will print bar codes.

# On the Job Now

**Directions:** Write a letter and prepare an envelope for each of the following scenarios. Be sure to use appropriate style, structure, and grammar.

1. Write a block style letter to Patty Patient at 655 Pain Lane, Pen, PA 15522, to inquire as to whether she has other medical or dental insurance coverage.

2. Write a semiblock style letter to Dana D. Dingbat at 404 Doorway Drive, Denver, ND 58444 to request that she send a copy of Danny's birth certificate.

3. Write a letter to Nancy Normal at 707 National Street, Nando, NV 89577, to let her know that her claim for date of service 5/2/CCYY in the amount of $215.00 from Dr. Bombay has been pended until the information requested from the provider is received.

## Memos

If a message needs to be communicated to a number of people within a company, a memo is often written. A **memo** (short for memorandum) is a letter intended for distribution within a company **(see Figure 15–5)**.

Companies often write memos to share information internally, such as a change of office policy or a new method of performing a task. However, memos can be written about any subject.

There are usually three main reasons for disseminating a memo:

COMPANY LETTERHEAD

TO: ALL EMPLOYEES

FROM: ANNA ABLEBODY

RE: COMPANY DINNER

DATE: JANUARY 2, 2005

*****************************************************************************************

I would like to take this opportunity to express my appreciation to all those who helped put together a wonderful New Year's Eve party for the company.

I'm sure you all agree that the Food Committee, consisting of Ginny Gourmet and Terri Tidbit did an excellent job of finding a superb caterer and choosing a wonderful menu.

The decorations created by Winnie Wallpaper, Daniel Décor and Orville Ornaments made the lunchroom an enticing place to be and create a festive atmosphere that set the tone for a wonderful party.

The exciting program, which I'm sure we all enjoyed, was prepared and performed by Rita Recital, Patty Presentation, Peter Performance, Annie Appearance and Sally Staging.

And of course we can't forget the much-appreciated efforts of the cleanup crew: Wally Wiper, Betty Broom and Tracy Trash.

Without the efforts of each and every one of these people we would not have enjoyed such a wonderful party. Please take a moment to thank each of these people personally.

■ **Figure 15–5** Sample Memo

1. It is easier to reach a large number of people with a memo, especially if some of them are out of the office. A memo can be left on a desk, ensuring that more people will see it, rather than relying on word of mouth.

2. A memo contains information that a number of recipients need to read (such as a policy change), or information that they may need to refer to at a later time.

3. A memo provides a tangible medium of communication in a documented form.

Although typing a memo may seem like a minor part of a claims examiner's day, memos can be an important part of keeping a company running smoothly.

Many companies will set or change company policies, then notify the personnel by creating a memo and circulating it among the office employees. Employees are then expected to read and follow the new guidelines. If necessary, the memo should be filed with other important papers so the employee may refer to it at a later date.

For these reasons it is important that memos be written in a clear and easy to understand manner. Be careful of the tone you use when writing a memo, as memos often become a permanent part of a company's or an individual's record.

Additionally, morale can be boosted by a well-written, positive memo, or significantly lowered by a negative one. In fact, a memo praising a certain group of employees and sent to all other employees in the company is one of the easiest and least expensive ways to make people feel important.

Writing a memo of praise lets people know you appreciate their work. It can also motivate others to become involved in future projects.

## Memo Format

Most companies have a specific format for their memos. This usually consists of printing them on company letterhead, beginning with a header, then the body of the memo.

### The Header

The header usually consists of four items: TO, FROM, SUBJECT, and DATE.

**TO:** The TO header is usually typed in capital letters. The name of the recipients may also be in capital letters, or may be in upper and lower case, depending on the policy of the company. Often company memos are addressed to groups of people rather than to individuals. For example, a memo may be designated "TO: All Managers." When a memo is for several people who are not of a designated group (i.e., all managers), the names of the recipients are typed one after another with a comma and space separating the names. Often these people are listed in order of rank (i.e., partners, managers, general staff), or in alphabetical order.

**FROM:** The FROM header is also typed in capital letters, with the name of the person creating the memo in either all uppercase or uppercase and lowercase letters, depending on company policy. Usually if one item (i.e., TO, FROM, or SUBJECT) is in all uppercase, then all items will be in all uppercase letters. As with the TO field, this field may also be from a single person or from a group of people (i.e., The Partners).

**SUBJECT:** The SUBJECT header is typed in all capital letters (also written as RE, short for regarding) and is a one-line sentence or topic for the memo. Since memos are often filed among other company papers, two or more subjects of importance are not often covered in the same memo. Instead two (or more) separate memos are issued. This allows people to file the memo according to the subject matter, which then makes it much easier to locate and retrieve when necessary.

**DATE:** The DATE header is also typed in all capital letters. The date should be given as the date the memo will be distributed. This allows people to track the memos and determine which is the most recent. This can be especially important with memos that alter a company policy or institute a new company policy.

### The Body

On most memos, a line or a row of asterisks follows the header information. This separates the header from the body of the memo.

The body of the memo is then typed without a salutation (i.e., Dear Managers), or closing (i.e., Sincerely, The Partners).

Be sure to write clearly and concisely, including all pertinent information. However, extraneous information, which is often included in a formal letter, is not included (i.e., How are you?). Memos usually state the important facts in as few lines as possible. It is very rare for a memo to be longer than one page unless it covers a major policy change.

Once the memo has been typed the person who initiated the memo should approve it. Their approval is usually given by having them initial the original next to their name in the header section. This initialed original is then photocopied and copies are given to each person to whom the memo is addressed. If you issue two or more conflicting memos regarding the same subject on a single day, the subject line should include information that this memo changes or alters the previous memo issued.

In addition, if more than two memos are issued in a single day with conflicting instructions or changes, the time of the second memo should be placed next to the date. For example, if you issue a memo, and later realize you forgot the word "not" in the sentence "On Thursday you should park in the parking garage," then the second memo should include the time next to the date. Additionally, the subject line should read something like "Correction of memo re: Parking" to indicate that something on the original memo has been changed.

# Specialized Letter Writing

The remainder of this section will discuss various guidelines to consider when writing to certain individuals.

## Claimant

When writing to a claimant, remember that he is not usually an insurance company employee and may not understand certain terminology (i.e., preexisting, proceeds, EOB, transfer, etc.).

It is important to use courtesy and tact when corresponding with claimants. When dealing with sensitive issues (i.e., medical status), choose your words carefully. Review the following paragraph:

"In reviewing the operative report for your surgery, we note that while cancer was removed from your lung, the entire lung did not have to be removed. So, we can only pay $1,200 as the customary and reasonable fee, rather than the $2,200 charged by the doctor."

This claimant may not have known about the cancer and it is not your responsibility to relay this information. More appropriate wording is as follows:

"The operative report for the surgery that Dr. Jones performed describes a procedure which suggests a benefit based on $1,200 as a reasonable fee, rather than the $2,200 charged by the doctor."

## Physician

Correspondence with the claimant, physician, or hospital can facilitate or prolong the claim evaluation process, depending upon the manner in which requests are presented.

In your opening paragraph, state your reason for writing (i.e., "evaluating Mrs. Smith's claim for medical benefits"). Include any policy requirements that the physician may need to take into consideration. Be careful not to use insurance jargon that may not be readily understood.

State your request as clearly and concisely as possible. Present your questions in either paragraph or list form, whichever is clearer. Try to keep in mind the intended use of the reply. Word your questions carefully so that the answers you obtain will be of use in the claim evaluation. Anticipate all the information needed, then write asking for everything early and at one time. Doctors and hospitals do not easily cooperate when three or four letters are sent requesting additional information about the claimant.

## Other Contacts

There are other parties with which you may communicate during the processing of claims (i.e., collection agencies, attorneys, and other insurance carriers).

Remember that courtesy and professionalism go a long way towards gaining the cooperation of those involved in the claim process.

# Denial Letters

All denials must meet the following standards:

- A prompt and complete investigation is needed before a claim can be denied. The file must maintain and document the basis for denial. This means that the facts substantiated by the claim material and investigations are appropriate to the policy provisions related to the denial. Denial letters, which are required for all denied claims, must state all defenses available.

- A reasonable, written explanation of a denial which quotes or provides reference to the proper policy provisions is required. Investigations need to be complete and documented.

- Determining eligibility is considered the first line of defense. Any complete investigation starts with a proper determination of eligibility.

It should be standard practice to write a letter when a relatively low payment is made compared to the total expense submitted, or compared to total benefits claimed.

Sensitive denial categories requiring letters include, but are not limited to, the following:

- Preexisting conditions.
- Extension of benefits requirements not met.
- Questionable medical necessity.
- Questionable eligibility.
- Distinction between accident and illness.

For medical claims, not every small disallowed charge has to have a denial letter. Explanation of Benefits form (EOB) messages are often used, but they may not always adequately meet denial requirements outlined by some regulatory authorities. When small, noncovered charges are included on a bill where essentially everything is payable, use of an EOB message is adequate. Also, when numerous services are submitted with a few expenses incurred before insurance became effective, or which occurred after termination, an EOB message is usually sufficient. Although telephone calls do not meet the policy definition of "Notice Claim," when a claimant does notify you of a claim or loss and if the claimant is advised the claim is not covered, a follow-up, written confirmation of the denial should be given. This requirement does not apply to hypothetical, "what if" questions or to general questions about coverages.

### Getting Your Point Across

If you are writing to the claimant or any claimant contacts such as the attorney or employer, denying benefits, the notification to them should contain elements such as:

- What was required to be eligible for benefits (i.e., "bodily injury caused by an accident…").
- What happened (i.e., "death was caused by conditions more properly classified as a sickness").
- What is the result (i.e., "no benefits are payable").
- What alternatives are available (i.e., "we will be glad to review any additional information you may wish to submit").

Each aspect of the denial should contain certain key information. The requirements should be quoted or carefully paraphrased from the certificate. All reasons for denials should be included and clearly stated, referencing medical terms when appropriate. However, terms should be simplified when possible. For example, use broken arm instead of fractured arm, or refer to heart condition instead of myocardial infarction.

Be very careful about giving the claimant information that the physician has submitted. You do not want to start a conflict between the doctor and the patient, nor violate the confidentiality of sensitive medical information. Instead of saying "your doctor said," consider using wording such as "medical information received." If additional details are requested, you may then be in a position to be more specific or refer the person to her doctor to clarify medical information.

### Conclusions and Alternatives

The final paragraph(s) of the denial letter should inform the insured of any alternatives that are available (i.e., submit additional information, ERISA, etc.). If a reservation of rights is appropriate, it should also be stated here. A **reservation of rights** allows the payer to assert a general denial, but to also retain the authority to suspend or pend the claim if so warranted.

### Notice of Availability

Where all or a part of a claim is denied and the claimant is a resident of a state requiring a Notice of Availability by the State Insurance Department, all denial letters and EOBs must contain the appropriately worded notice, as required by the state of residence. Contact your state's insurance commissioner for more information and to determine if your state requires such notice.

### Right of Review/ERISA

Federal ERISA requirements affect all claim denials. The **ERISA Right of Review Statement** must be included with every claim denial letter and on every EOB when all or part of a claim is denied: the wording to be used is as follows:

If you disagree with the decision on your claim, you have the right by law to request that your claim be reviewed by your Plan Administrator (or your plan's claim reviewer). This request must be made in writing within sixty (60) days of receipt of this notice. If you wish, you may submit your written comments and views. Please consult your Plan's claim review procedures. See your employer on any other ERISA questions.

# Adjustments

Special guidelines apply when contacting claimants or providers regarding an adjustment on a claim. This is especially true when there was an overpayment on the claim and you are requesting reimbursement.

## Overpayments

Overpayments usually fall into the three categories listed below:

1. A simple calculation error when all the necessary information was available in the claim file.
2. Professional or claimant errors which, because of misunderstanding, are unavoidable.
3. Deliberate misstatement or fraudulent acts by the insured or others.

## Overpayment Reimbursement Requests

When forwarding a request for reimbursement of an overpayment to an insured or other party, the following should be included:

- A statement of the facts as to why an overpayment of insurance benefits has been made, including a reference to an EOB and the relevant policy provisions.
- The amount of the overpayment.
- A request for reimbursement of the overpayment.
- A statement to the effect that if a lump sum repayment is not feasible, you are willing to discuss an alternative method of repayment, (i.e., monthly installment payments).
- A statement informing the insured or other party that you will be happy to answer any questions or consider any comments or additional facts which the insured may have with regard to the matter, but that in any event you wish to hear from him within a reasonable amount of time regarding reimbursement (usually two weeks).

The claims examiner should retain a copy of all outgoing correspondence in case the need arises to clarify any misunderstandings resulting from the correspondence.

When contacting an insured regarding reimbursement for an overpayment of benefits, you should not:

- State or threaten that if reimbursement is not made, you will garnish the insured's wages. (**Garnishment** is a method of collecting an unpaid debt, which may only be utilized after a lawsuit has been filed, and a judgment is obtained).
- Threaten independent legal action.
- Threaten that if reimbursement is not made, you will turn the matter over to a collection agency.

A follow-up to an overpayment letter should be sent to the insured, with a copy to the provider if it was an assigned claim, every two weeks, and these attempts should continue for a reasonable period of time.

If no acknowledgment of the overpayment is received from the claimant or provider after a six-week period, the case should be referred to the legal department or to supervisory personnel.

# Mail

Mail can be separated into two types: incoming mail and outgoing mail. Each has its own set of procedures.

## Incoming Mail

In any office, it is imperative that the mail be handled properly and routed to the correct person. Generally, one person is designated to handle the incoming mail. Of course, every office has its own preferences, so check with your supervisor to see what handling procedures have been established for the company where you are employed.

1. Separate mail according to the department or person to whom it is addressed. When separating mail, take note of any mail that was delivered incorrectly to your address. Separating the mail before opening it will allow you to return incorrectly delivered mail in the same condition in which it arrived.
2. If mail is to be opened before it is distributed, slit the envelope neatly across the top. Do not tear or destroy the envelope, so that any needed information can be preserved. This may include

**1.** Overpayments usually fall into what three categories?

   **1.** _____

   **2.** _____

   **3.** _____

**2.** What five items should be included when requesting reimbursement of an overpayment?

   **1.** _____

   **2.** _____

   **3.** _____

   **4.** _____

   **5.** _____

**3.** What three things should you not do when contacting an insured regarding reimbursement for an overpayment of benefits?

   **1.** _____

   **2.** _____

   **3.** _____

the postmark date, return address, or the city from which the envelope was mailed.

**3.** Many offices date stamp their mail on receipt. If this is the case with your company or organization, there are several steps that you should follow:

**a.** Be sure the date on the stamp is accurate. This may be very important when certain pieces of correspondence need to arrive in a timely manner (i.e., billing department mail when interest or late fees are charged on overdue accounts).

**b.** Stamp the date stamp on a piece of scratch paper to ensure that it has enough ink and that the impression is clear. If the impression is faint, stamp several more times on the ink pad (if it is used) or on a piece of paper (if the stamp is self-inking). This should start the ink flowing again.

**c.** When you stamp a piece of correspondence, place the date in an area where it will not cover any writing.

**d.** Stamp down once, firmly and securely. Wiggling the stamp back and forth can cause an unclear impression.

**e.** Do not stamp checks, business cards, legal documents, or order forms unless your office specifically requests it. Date stamping such items can result in difficultly processing checks, ordering, or complying with legal requirements.

**f.** If you have a choice of ink colors, black is best. Other colors are more difficult to photocopy or may cause a negative impression. This is especially true of red, as most people associate red ink with a warning.

**4.** If you receive checks in the mail, be sure they are securely attached to any additional papers (i.e., invoices, statements) that are included. These papers may be the only clue as to which account the check should be credited. Some offices prefer that the account number be immediately written on the check. This ensures that the check will be credited to the proper account even if it is separated from its attached documentation.

If no documentation is attached, check the envelope for additional clues. If the name and address on the check does not match the name and address on the envelope, attach the envelope to the check. This may assist the billing department in locating the correct account.

Some offices request that the person who opens the checks make an adding machine tape and total the day's receipts. You should always run the tape twice, ensuring that the total is the same each time. Then, take an extra minute to double-check your figures. Often numbers will become transposed, and once a number is in your mind, it is easy for the transposition to occur a second time.

5. When distributing the mail, put urgent-looking correspondence on top of the stack. Also be sure to put the mail in a place where the recipient will be sure to see it.

6. If correspondence is received that is marked "Personal and Confidential," leave the envelope sealed and deliver it to the intended recipient unopened.

7. If you receive a document in a "next day" or "urgent" envelope, it should be delivered immediately. This type of document should never sit on your desk for more than five minutes.

Although handling mail may seem like a minor task, it is important to do it properly and efficiently. Mail is the lifeblood of many offices. Without it, checks and revenues may be lost, clients may not be served, and communication usually breaks down.

## Signing for Mail

Some incoming mail requires a signature on delivery. Before signing, know exactly what you are signing for. Most shipping companies include a notation in fine print stating that your signature is verification that the package was received in good condition and that the contents were not damaged. Also note the number of packages you are signing for. Your signature across four lines of the receipt column is stating that you received four packages. Be sure that the order is complete before

signing for it or you or your company may be held liable for any merchandise or shipments not received.

It is impossible to tell if the contents are undamaged without opening the box. Take the time to look at the boxes before signing. If the box appears to be damaged, insist on opening it and checking the contents before signing. The delivery person will attempt to have you sign immediately so that he or she can get to the next delivery, but if you do sign, the damaged goods will often not be replaced or paid for by the shipper.

If the contents of the package appear to be damaged, you should note this on the receipt right next to your signature.

Be sure you are authorized to sign for a package. In many offices, the authority to sign for packages is limited to a few people, not to anyone in the office.

## Returned Mailings

In any company there will be mail that is returned because of improper addressing, lack of postage, or the inability of the postal service to locate the intended recipient.

Mail will usually only be forwarded for one year from the date of the recipient's move. After that time, a sticker will be placed on the envelope indicating the new address and the article will be returned to the sender. If a piece of mail is returned because a forwarding address has expired, and the postal service has indicated the new address, the mail should be placed in a new envelope, addressed with the new address, and remailed. Be sure to keep the old envelope so that you can update your records.

If a piece of mail is returned with no forwarding address indicated, be sure to delete the name and address from your records. If there is an outstanding balance on an account that has mail returned, be sure the member's records are also updated. If an outstanding balance or a current member history does not exist, do not delete the record. Take the time to contact the member by phone and attempt to locate their new address.

## Outgoing Mail

The condition of your outgoing mail is a direct reflection on your office. Therefore, it is imperative that your mail be handled properly. You can imagine the response of a client who receives a letter bearing bad news that has also been stamped by the postal service "Postage Due."

The first thing is to make sure the mail has been packaged properly. Be sure that the envelope is of adequate size for the material. If there are more than five pages in a document, a #10 (standard-sized) envelope should not be used. The thickness of the pages can cause the envelope to become jammed in the postal service's automated equipment. This may result in tearing and loss of the contents. To ensure that envelopes mailed in larger packages arrive in good condition, a thin sheet of cardboard can be placed in the envelope to add resilience.

Before sealing a box, place a letter or other item inside that lists the company's and the recipient's address. This will allow the package to be delivered even if the address shown on the outside is removed or becomes obliterated. Boxes should be sealed with strong packing tape, not with string.

All shipping companies, including the postal service, have weight and size limits for the packages they will ship. Most will have a weight limit of 70 pounds per box. The combined length and girth should not exceed 108 inches. To determine the measurement, wrap a tape measure once around the box, then add to the resulting measurement the length of the box. Before shipping, contact the carrier and be sure that you know the exact weight and measurement limits they will allow.

## Special Shipping Services

Most companies offer numerous shipping services. These include certification (proof of delivery), return receipt requested, COD (cash on delivery), insurance, overnight delivery, and two- or three-day delivery. Additional charges, above and beyond the normal shipping charges, are added for each of these services. Keep any receipts issued to you by the shipper. Without these documents, it is very difficult to trace lost articles or to make a claim for services not delivered.

**Certified mail** (see Appendix D) is a package or envelope that must be signed for on delivery. This provides you with a record of when the item was delivered and the name of the person who signed for it. To send an envelope by certified mail, fill out the certified mail slip provided by the shipping company. The basic information requested is the name and address of the recipient, and postage must be paid. Calculate the total postage for the item being sent. The total postage amount will include two components, the regular postage fee and the certified mailing fee. The regular postage fee will vary depending on the size and weight of the item being sent. The certified postage fee can be obtained by contacting the U. S. Postal Office. This tag is attached to the envelope or package to the right of the return address. The tag has a tracking number printed on it. The top portion of the tag is torn off at the perforation and kept as a receipt. If the envelope or package does not arrive, a tracer can be put on it by using the tracking number.

With **return receipt requested** (see Appendix D), on delivery, a receipt is issued and mailed back to the sender of the package. This allows the sender to have proof of the delivery and the name of the person who signed for it. This procedure is usually used with certified mail. The recipient's name and address are placed on one side of the card. The sender's name and address are placed on the reverse of the card. The card is then attached to the envelope or package on the front, or, if there is not sufficient room, on the back. When the article is delivered, the recipient signs the card and the date of delivery is listed. If requested (and if an additional fee is paid), the recipient's address will be provided. The sender may also choose to restrict delivery only to the person or persons to whom the article is addressed.

# On the Job Now

Ms. Minnie Claims, the office supervisor, hands you a letter. She indicates that she needs to have the letter sent to Nancy Normal at 707 National Street, Nando, NV 89577, by certified mail. You work for Any Insurance Carrier, Inc. at 123 Any Drive, Anywhere, USA 12345, phone # (800) 555 1234.

Please fill out the necessary forms to send the letter to Ms. Normal by certified mail.

When mailing a shipment of merchandise that the recipient must pay for, COD is often requested. This means that the shipper will collect payment for the item at the time of delivery. When shipping COD (see Appendix D), you must specify whether cash, check, or either is acceptable, and the amount to be collected. Add any shipping charges to the amount if the recipient is to pay for shipping.

# On the Job Now

Dana Dingbat calls and requests a copy of her insurance policy be sent to her at 404 Doorway Drive, Denver, ND 58444, phone # (701) 555 3344. She indicates that she needs it immediately for a court custody hearing, and says she will pay for the shipping cost, just bill her the costs COD.

Please fill out the necessary PPS Express COD forms to ship a copy of the insurance policy to Dana Dingbat. Ship the policy PPS Priority overnight; PPS Pak; Any Insurance Carrier's account number is 4434-5556-7; the COD amount to be collected by the carrier is $14.80.

You may wish to purchase insurance for items being shipped. This insurance will pay for lost or damaged items. Many shippers include the first $100 of insurance in the cost of shipping a package. Any amount over this must be requested and paid for before shipping. The fee is usually nominal, between $.50 and $.75 for every $100 of insurance.

If you need an envelope or package to arrive overnight, it is possible to request this service. Articles can be scheduled for either an afternoon delivery or, for an additional charge, a morning delivery. The delivery area is limited, usually to within the continental United States. In addition, articles must be picked up or delivered to the shipper before a specified time to qualify for next-day delivery. This time varies according to your location and the shipper. You must also complete special address labels that request the sender's and receiver's name, address, and phone number, as well as the specific services requested. Many carriers require you to use special packaging and may provide this packaging free of charge on request.

There is also a special charge for two- or three-day delivery, and delivery is usually limited to the continental United States. There are also similar labels and packaging requirements. Check with your shipper for specific details.

In large cities, it is possible to have a package delivered by courier or messenger. The courier comes to your office, picks up the article, and hand-delivers it to the recipient. These services are expensive and are used only for important documents.

# On the Job Now

Patty Patient came to the claims office to drop off some claims. After she left the office, the receptionist noticed that Ms. Patient had left her insurance cards in the reception area. Ms. Minnie Claims, the office supervisor, asks you to send the insurance cards to Ms. Patient at 655 Pain Lane, Pen, PA 15522, phone # (878) 555 3355.

Please fill out the necessary forms to ship this item back to Ms. Patient using PPS Ground; PPS Standard Overnight; PPS Pak; bill to Any Insurance Carrier at 123 Any Drive, Anywhere, USA 12345, account number 4434-5556-7.

# Office Machines

In every office, you will use a number of machines nearly every day. These include the telephone, facsimile (fax) machine, and copy machine.

## The Telephone

Virtually every company in existence has a telephone and uses it extensively during the working day. The telephone is often more important than the mail in communicating with customers and helping with the running of the office. Therefore, it is important that you understand how to properly use the telephone.

Most companies have **multiline phones**. This means that there is more than one telephone line into the office. However, the number of these phone lines is limited. If all of the lines are being used, the customer or caller will hear a busy signal and their call will not be connected. For this reason, you should keep your call as brief as possible.

Multiline phones often work similarly to single-line phones, with a few exceptions. Most multiline phones have a single number (i.e., 555-1234), with each additional line numerically increased by one (i.e., line two is 555-1235; line three is 555-1236). The caller needs only to dial the original number (555-1234) and, if that line is busy, the call will automatically roll over to the first available line.

When placing an outgoing call on a multiline phone, many times you will need to choose a line by pushing a button. Before picking up a line, make sure that it is available. Usually, a small lighted button indicates whether the line is currently in use.

Multiline phones often give you the option of placing callers on hold by depressing a hold button. When transferring a call, speaking with a coworker or interrupting a conversation for any reason, it is best to put the caller on hold rather than to hold your hand over the mouthpiece or set the phone down.

Different types of phones and phone systems have different ways of transferring calls and returning to a held call. These procedures will need to be described to you by someone who is familiar with the phone or system. It is important to know these procedures before needing them so that you do not delay or disconnect a caller.

## The Facsimile Machine

The **facsimile machine (more commonly referred to as the fax machine)** is a machine that transmits pictures over the phone lines by transmitting a series of dot messages. This allows for nearly instantaneous transmission of a letter, picture, or other document from one place to another.

The invention of the fax machine has made life easier in offices and has taken some of the stress out of having to mail documents early so that they can be received on time. Although the fax machine is a wonderful invention, it is not perfect. Documents can be lost in transmission and they are generally not as clear as printed material. The special paper used in many fax machines is thinner than normal paper, and an imprint can be left on it. For these reasons, it is important that you always follow up a faxed copy with a hard copy of the document sent through the mail.

The ease of transmitting using the fax machine has led to using it for nonessential situations. Always remember that a fax transmission is not as clear, and, therefore, not as professional-looking as something that is printed directly from a typewriter or printer. Also, remember that when transmitting long distances, you are using a phone line. Therefore, a charge will appear on the telephone bill just as if you had spoken over the phone.

If the company you are faxing to has several different departments, there may be several fax machines. A fax cover sheet should always be included with the fax. A cover sheet should include the following information:

- The date and time the fax is being sent.
- The name and telephone number of the person sending the fax.
- The name of the person to whom the fax is directed and his/her department or company.
- The number of pages being sent.
- Sufficient space for messages to be conveyed to the receiver.

## The Copy Machine

The copy machine is possibly one of the most widely used office machines. There are always numerous reasons for needing a second copy of a document.

Copy machines can be one of the easiest machines to operate if you understand the basic principles. The first item of importance is the placement of the original. The original should be placed face down on the glass. The exact placement is usually indicated by markings running along the left-hand side of the glass or the bottom. The cover should be closed before making a copy.

To begin the copy process, push the button marked start. Do not lift the cover or remove the original until the copying is complete. To do so will cause a blurred or darkened image on the copy.

Many copiers have special features, such as reduction or enlargement of the original, special paper sizes or types, and collation of the copies. To **collate** copies means to place them in order. For example, if you are making two copies of a document that is three pages long, the machine will turn the pages out in the order of 1, 2, 3, 1, 2, 3. In documents that are not collated, the pages would be done in order of 1, 1, 2, 2, 3, 3.

These special features are usually selected by the push of a button.

Because copiers vary according to style and brand name, it is important that you be shown the exact features and the correct operating procedures for the copier that your company uses.

## Other Office Machines

A number of other machines may be used in a medical office setting. These can include the postage meter, postage scale, binding machines, folding machines, coffee makers, and vending machines.

**Binding machines** bind several pages of a document together, often with a strip down the left-hand side of the document. There are numerous types of binding machines, and numerous brands for each type. Generally, the bindings fall into one of three categories: comb binders (have a plastic strip with projecting teeth), spiral binders (have a curved plastic strip with rounded teeth forming an enclosed circle), and spiral wire binders (have a single continuous piece of wire wound through successive holes from top to bottom of the document).

Folding machines are used to fold numerous pieces of paper. The folding guides can be adjusted to various lengths to handle different sizes of paper and different folds. Because of the strength and speed of most folding machines, care should be taken that jewelry, loose clothing, and long hair are not allowed to enter the machine.

Many offices provide free or low-cost cups of coffee to their employees. However, the responsibility often falls to one or more of the employees to keep the pots filled. All coffee machines require the addition of fresh coffee grounds, and some require the addition of water. Care should be taken to keep the pots cleaned on a regular basis. Also, never set an empty or near-empty glass pot on a heated burner. The glass will shatter when it reaches a certain temperature.

Vending machines are available in many offices. Most are stocked and serviced by outside vending companies that are also in charge of handling the monies received. Many vending companies return a portion of the proceeds to the company that has allowed space for the machine, and the vending company should be called if the machine has run out of items or if service is needed.

## Tickler Files

The tickler file system is used by a number of people in numerous office settings. **Tickler files** are often expanding file folders that help you remember items that need to occur on a specific date. Basically a tickler file helps tickle your memory.

A tickler file usually consists of the following folders:

- 12 folders labeled with each month of the year.
- 31 folders labeled with the numbers 1 through 31.

To use a tickler file, place the folders numbered 1 through 31 into the folder for the current month (i.e., if today's date is May 5th, place all the numbered folders inside the May folder). Place all folders in front of the current month (i.e., January through April) behind the December folder at the back of the group. Then place all numbered folders for the days before the current one into the folder following the current month (i.e., if the date is May 5th, the numbered files for days 5–31 would be in the May folder and the folders for days 1–4 would be in the June folder). Now your tickler file is ready to use.

To use your tickler file, simply file each item into the folder for the day when it needs to occur. For example, if you need to send a follow-up for a request for information by June 1, then place the information for the follow-up request in the folder numbered 1, which should be in the June folder.

On each day, simply look in the folder for that day. Those are the items that you need to accomplish before the day is out.

If you have items that require your attention several months in the future, simply place them in the folder for that month. At the beginning of each month, take the items in that month's folder and insert them into the proper folder for the day of the month they need to be taken care of.

As each day passes, place the folder for that day into the folder for the next month.

By using a tickler file, you can always remember to accomplish the things that require your attention in the future. You will always be reminded of that call you were supposed to return when someone returned from vacation or that conference to sign up for, and so on.

## Postal Abbreviations

There are a number of official abbreviations which the United States Postal Service uses. The State Abbreviations table in Appendix C contains abbreviations for the most common states and territories.

# CHAPTER REVIEW

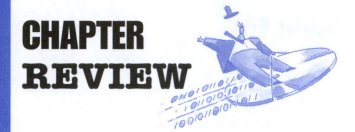

## Summary

- Most communication with claim contacts will be through letters (often form letters) and telephone conversations.

- It is important to use tact and careful wording when speaking since the listeners will often judge their experience with the company by their conversations with a claims examiner.

- When creating letters or completing form letters, it is important to be sure that you convey the correct intent of the letter. Be sure it is clear as to what you want the reader to do or how you want them to respond.

- When communicating with others, it is important to remember that they may not be familiar with all the terminology used in insurance communications.

- Abbreviations should be avoided, and terminology which can be misunderstood should be fully explained.

- ERISA requirements state that any claim that is denied must contain the ERISA Right of Review Statement. This statement must appear on each letter or EOB associated with the denied claim.

- Although each office has its own procedures to follow, it is important to understand the basic procedures that govern incoming mail, outgoing mail, special shipping services, and dealing with office machines. Without basic knowledge of the equipment and how to use it, it is impossible for the claims examiner to do their job properly.

- Correspondence is written communication between two people. Regardless of the content of the letter or the response you wish to evoke, the main purpose of correspondence is to communicate your thoughts, ideas, and desires to another person. To achieve this, be sure that the correspondence is necessary, formulate your ideas before beginning to write, and determine the action you wish the recipient to take.

- Written business correspondence should contain a heading, inside address, salutation, body, complimentary close, and a signature. It should also be clear, concise, coherent, and grammatically correct. Combining all these elements will help to achieve effective written communications.

- A memo is a way of communicating important information within a company as quickly and easily as possible. Memos usually follow a specified format, with a header including TO, FROM, SUBJECT, and DATE headings.

## Assignments

Complete the Questions for Review.
Complete Exercises 15–1 through 15–4.

## Questions for Review

**Directions:** Answer the following questions without looking back at the material just covered. Write your answers in the space provided.

1. What is the most commonly used mode of communication? _____

2. What is a heading? _____

   _____

3. What details does the body of a letter often contain? _____

   _____

4. Instead of the wording "Above named insured" what should you use in a letter? _____

   _____

**5.** There are several sensitive denial categories which require letters. List them. _____

_____

**6.** What is the Right of Review Statement? _____

_____

**7.** What is the best ink color to use when date stamping incoming mail? _____

**8.** (True or False?) When signing for receipt of a package, your signature certifies that the contents were received undamaged and in good condition. _____

**9.** Name five special shipping services that you can purchase.

1. _____

2. _____

3. _____

4. _____

5. _____

**10.** When dialing out on a multiline phone, what is the first thing you should check before picking up the phone?

_____

**11.** Before you begin writing a piece of correspondence you should _____

_____

**12.** What is the purpose of the opening in a letter? _____

_____

**13.** The body of the letter explains the _____

**14.** If information must be written in the form of a letter, what four points should be followed?

1. _____

2. _____

3. _____

4. _____

**15.** If you are writing a letter of denial, should you give the bad news in the first paragraph? _____

**16.** What are the three main reasons for disseminating a memo? _____

_____

_____

_____

**17.** What is the usual format for a memo? _____

_____

**18.** What four items does the header section usually consist of? _____

_____

**19.** (True or False?) Headers are usually typed in lowercase letters. _____

**20.** (True or False?) Approval of a memo is given by signing one's name at the bottom of the memo. _____

If you were unable to answer any of these questions, refer back to that section and then fill in the answers.

# Exercise 15-1

**Directions:** Write a letter to handle the following situations.

**1.** To the insured: A surgery claim is denied because the patient was not covered under the insurance plan when the surgery was performed.

**2.** To a physician: You need the operative report on a surgery before you can process the claim.

**3.** To a claimant: The claim was overpaid due to a clerical error at the insurance company (the wrong code was entered). You need the insured to reimburse the company $135.78.

# Exercise 15-2

**Directions:** Find and circle the words listed below. Words can appear horizontally, vertically, diagonally, forward, or backward.

```
U W U N H Z X E O N J S O G H
X M S B I S K J M G Y W A Z G
M I M E M E R Q H A P N T K D
T U P L L S T O J J T H W L U
N K F H V I L I S J H K B X C
E Y X I C G F D Q K B X R L G
M Y Z N F M F R K U Y M D F B
H S Y Q O B M J E O E B V O I
S E N O H P E N I L I T L U M
I P V B T Z C F S E K I T J E
N J N P Y Q A O J C B C M E N
R A J T J P O S T S C R I P T
A L H O R Z S N H R X D Y T M
G U B T N I R Q D F B I Q Z C
H T A Y E C D N F X N K B Z N
```

**1.** Etiquette

**2.** Garnishment

**3.** Multiline Phones

**4.** Tickler Files

# Exercise 15-3

**Directions:** Complete the crossword puzzle by filling in a word from the keywords that fits each clue.

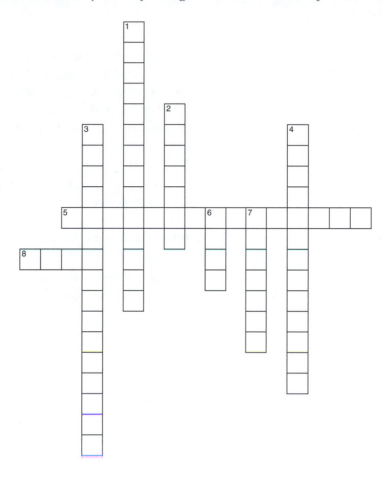

**Across**

5. Bind several pages of a document together, often with a strip down the left-hand side of the document.

8. This part of the letter contains the main text or message.

**Down**

1. Written communication between two people.

2. The part of a business letter that contains the return address, date, and a reference line and other notations if applicable.

3. Exactness of language.

4. A package or envelope that must be signed for upon delivery.

6. Short for memorandum, it is a letter intended for distribution within a company.

7. To put photocopies in the original order of the pages.

# Exercise 15-4

**Directions:** Match the following terms with the proper definition by writing the letter of the correct definition in the space next to the term.

1. _____ Coherence in Writing

    a. Upon delivery, a receipt is issued and mailed back to the sender of the package. This allows the sender to have proof of the delivery and the name of the person who signed for it.

2. _____ Effectiveness in Writing

    b. A statement which must be included on all denied claims.

3. _____ ERISA Right of Review Statement

    c. Being able to evoke the type of response you want your reader to have, whether you want the reader to subscribe to a magazine or to purchase a product or service.

4. _____ Facsimile Machine

    d. Information that follows logically flow from one idea to the next.

5. _____ Return Receipt Requested

    e. More commonly known as a fax machine. It sends pictures over the phone lines by transmitting a series of dot messages.

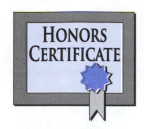

## Honors Certification™

The Honors Certification™ for this section constitutes a written test on the information covered in this chapter. Additionally, students will be asked to write a letter and a memo, and also be tested on address abbreviations.

## Letters

The certification challenge for this section consists of a written test. The instructor will give you a topic along with sender and receiver addresses and ask you to compose a letter in block, modified block, or semiblock style. You must create and print out a letter in the correct style, as well as create an envelope. Spelling, grammar, and punctuation count, as well as correct style. The letter should have no errors in it. Each error will result in a deduction of up to 5% from your grade, depending on the type of error. You must receive a score of 85% or higher to pass this test. You are not allowed to use any reference materials when taking the test.

If you fail the test on your first attempt you may retake the test one additional time. The addresses, subject matter, and style may be changed for the second test.

## Memos

The certification challenge for this section consists of a written test. You will be required to create a memo in the correct format using the header information and topic supplied to you by your instructor. Spelling, grammar and punctuation count, as well as correct style. The memo should have no errors in it. Each error will result in a deduction of up to 5% from your grade, depending on the type of error. You must receive a score of 85% or higher to pass this test. You are not allowed to use any reference materials when taking the test.

If you fail the test on your first attempt you may retake the test one additional time. The items included in the second test may be different from those in the first test.

## Address Abbreviations

You will be given a list of states or other address indicators. You must provide the correct abbreviation for each item. You must score 85% or higher to pass this test. If you fail the test on your first attempt you may retake the test one additional time. The items included in the second test may be different from those in the first test.

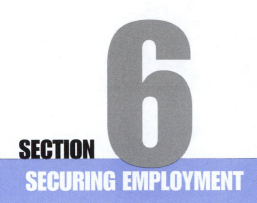

CHAPTER 16   JOB SEARCH PREPARATION

# 16
# Job Search
## Preparation

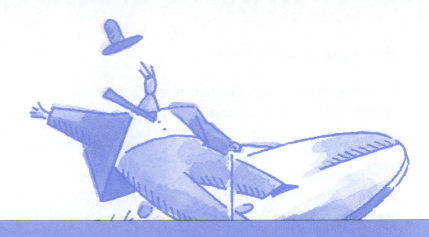

## After completion of this chapter
**you will be able to:**

- Explain the keys and functions of the calculator.
- Properly use the calculator to add, subtract, multiply, and divide numbers.
- Gain speed and accuracy in using the calculator.
- List and describe the items that will help to make you faster and more accurate when using the computer.
- Describe the three different machines that make up a computer.
- Describe the keyboard and its five components: Typewriter Keys, Numeric Keys, Editing and Cursor Control Keys, Function Keys, and Status Lights.
- List and describe the eight techniques that can help you achieve frustration-free computing.

- Recognize and define computer terms.
- List the tips for properly maintaining your computer files.
- Determine your marketing objectives.
- List and discuss the five items that should be included on a résumé.
- Prepare a top-notch résumé.
- List and describe the five things to avoid when preparing a résumé.
- Exhibit proper interviewing techniques and appropriate mannerisms and dress.
- Write an effective cover letter requesting a job.
- List and describe the four basic components to the interview process.
- Describe the most common misconceptions regarding how a salary should be determined.

## Keywords and concepts
**you will learn in this chapter:**

- Brightness Control
- Calculator
- Central Processing Unit (CPU)
- Computer Disk Drive

- Computer Monitor
- Contrast Control
- Cover Letter
- Cursor

- Hard Drive
- Keyboard
- Power Switch
- Résumé

After having learned the necessary information to work in your chosen field, it is time to look for employment. In order to get the job you want, it is essential to have the job-hunting skills that will allow you to find the best position for you, and then to successfully get hired. As part of the job search preparation, it is important to become proficient in the use of calculators and computers. These tools are widely used in most businesses, and health claims examiners use them to do much of their work.

## Calculator Basics

A **calculator** is a machine that computes numbers. It is used to add, subtract, multiply, and divide numbers, as well as compute percentages, square roots, and other mathematical calculations.

Working as a claims examiner, you will probably use a calculator every day. Often, there are charges that need to be totaled and amounts that need to be figured. Calculating these sums manually would take many hours. Therefore, it is vital that a claims examiner master the use of the calculator.

## Key Descriptions

Following are the keys most commonly found on a calculator and a description of their functions.

 **PAPER ADVANCE KEY** — Advances the paper tape without affecting your calculations.

 **CLEAR KEY** — Clears the display and the independent add register, pending operations and error/overflow conditions. Reactivates the calculator after an automatic power down.

 **PERCENT KEY** — Completes multiplication and division operations and shows the result as a decimal.

 **CLEAR ENTRY KEY** — Clears the last entry only, thus enabling you to enter another number in its place without clearing out all previously entered numbers.

 **DIVIDE KEY** — Instructs the calculator to divide the number in the display by the next value entered.

 **EQUAL KEY** — Completes any pending operation.

 **MULTIPLY KEY** — Instructs the calculator to multiply the number in the display by the next value entered.

 **BACKSPACE KEY** — Deletes the right-most digit in the display and shifts the remaining digits one place to the right.

 **NUMBER KEYS** — Enter numbers containing up to 10 digits. For numbers between one and negative one, a zero automatically precedes the decimal, allowing a maximum of nine digits to the right of the decimal.

 **DECIMAL POINT KEY** — Enters a decimal point. Most calculators have a floating decimal point which allows you to automatically set the decimal point at a given location in the number.

 **SUBTRACT KEY** — Subtracts the number in the display from the independent add register.

 **ADD KEY** — Adds the number in the display to the independent add register.

 **DATE/NON-ADD KEY** — Prints a reference number or date without affecting calculations in progress.

**SUBTOTAL KEY** — Displays and prints the subtotal in the independent add register. Pressing this key does not affect the contents of the add register.

**\*/T** — **TOTAL KEY** — Displays and prints the total in the independent add register, then clears the register.

**M** — **MEMORY TOTAL KEY** — Displays and prints the value in memory, then clears the memory.

**MS** — **MEMORY SUBTOTAL KEY** — Displays and prints the value in memory without clearing the memory.

**M-** — **SUBTRACT FROM MEMORY KEY** — Prints the number in the display and subtracts it from the value in memory. If a pending multiplication or division operation has been entered, this key completes the operation and subtracts the result from memory.

**M+** — **ADD TO MEMORY KEY** — Prints the number in the display and adds it to the value in memory. If a pending multiplication or division operation has been entered, this key completes the operation and then adds the result into memory.

# On the Job Now

**Directions:** Fill in the blank spaces without looking back at the text just covered.

1. The _____ instructs the calculator to divide the number in the display by the next value entered.

2. The Percent Key completes _____ and division operations and shows the result as a decimal.

3. The Backspace Key deletes the _____ digit in the display and shifts the remaining digits one place to the right.

4. The _____ prints a reference number or date without affecting calculations in progress.

5. The Memory Subtotal Key _____ and prints the value in memory without clearing the memory.

## Printer Tape Symbols

Multiple symbols may be printed on printer tapes during calculations. Usually, these symbols will appear to the right of tape entries. Symbols not indicated should be explained in the specific calculator manual.

| Symbol | Meaning or Explanation |
|---|---|
| + | Addition operation |
| – | Subtraction operation |
| <> | Subtotal of additions and subtractions |
| * | Total after "=," "%," or "*/T" is pressed |
| × | Multiplication operation |
| ÷ | Division operation |
| = | Completion of an operation |
| % | Percentage |
| + * | Percentage add-on |
| – * | Percentage discount |
| # | Reference number or date printed in the center of the printer tape |
| C | Clear key erases all entries |
| M * | Addition to memory |
| M– | Subtraction from memory |
| M <> | Memory subtotal |
| M * | Memory total |
| E | Error/overflow condition |
| IC | **Item Counter Symbol.** When the printer switch is in the IC position, the number of additions to and subtractions from the independent add register is printed above each total or subtotal. The item counter for the independent add register is reset when " */T" is pressed. |

# On the Job Now

**Directions:** Add each of the following columns of numbers, then subtract the numbers from your total to arrive at zero. Clear the entries from your calculator and subtract the following columns of numbers and total, then add the numbers to your total to arrive at zero. Use the printer tape to check accuracy.

| | | | |
|---|---|---|---|
| 54659 | 46181 | 645.25 | 54.65 |
| 54165 | 35164 | 618.46 | .12 |
| 41579 | 87319 | 614.79 | 2.76 |
| 45126 | 63453 | 641.76 | 78.11 |
| 56421 | 34150 | 123.08 | 457.12 |
| 20131 | 78455 | 469.61 | 3894.94 |
| 78991 | 23459 | 849.25 | 845.79 |
| 54164 | 89925 | 456.57 | 209.46 |
| 77986 | 24875 | 172.85 | 568.78 |
| 12094 | 23459 | 501.36 | 1056.23 |
| 12323 | 57847 | 841.43 | 347.51 |
| 71014 | 56748 | 051.65 | 351.91 |
| 71952 | 80893 | 540.71 | 6519.19 |
| 13671 | 10781 | 211.65 | 5056.20 |
| 24563 | 80974 | 549.93 | 645.51 |
| 63541 | 43729 | 635.45 | 345.48 |
| 0.168 | 89174 | 333.01 | 470.00 |
| 48567 | 39874 | 514.45 | 456.47 |

## Computer Basics

As with most other industries, the majority of businesses are automated. The computer has, therefore, become an indispensable tool.

Only time and usage will make the claims examiner accurate and fast on the computer. However, the following information may assist you when entering data:

**Familiarity**—Become familiar with the processing program you are using. If you know the fields (spots where specific information is entered), input rates will significantly increase because less verification and decision making will be required.

**Visual Coordination**—When learning to use the computer, watch either the video screen or the document you are inputting. Every effort should be made not to watch your fingers, as it is a difficult habit to break.

**Preparation**—Prepare your documents so that less shuffling of papers is required (i.e., unstaple, arrange by date).

**Comfort**—A comfortable chair that is adjusted to the correct height decreases fatigue.

**Hands Free of Objects**—Both hands should be free for typing in data. Pens, pencils, and other tools should not be held when entering data.

The computer is actually a combination of three different machines; the central processing unit (CPU), the monitor, and the keyboard.

# The Computer

The **central processing unit (CPU)** is the rectangular box that houses the memory and functional components of the computer. A tremendous amount of studying is required to understand all the inner workings of the computer. However, you should become familiar with a few components, such as the power switch, the reset button, and the disk drives.

The power switch is the on/off switch for the computer. It can be located anywhere on the computer, but it is often found toward the back.

The reset button is often found on the front of the computer. Pressing this button clears the screen and "reboots" or restarts the system. In other words, it achieves the same function as turning the computer off and then on again. Use caution with this button. If you do not save your data before pressing this button, it may be lost.

A **computer disk drive** is simply a place for the storage of information. Usually, a computer contains a "hard drive" within it. The **hard drive** provides space (memory) for information to be stored within the computer itself.

If there is insufficient memory in the hard drive or if there is a need to make data transportable to another computer or to make a copy of the data, you may record the information on disks.

In the front of most computers is a slot (or several slots). These are alternate floppy disk drives. If the data you are using is stored on a disk, slide the disk into the slot to retrieve it.

At no time should a claims examiner be required to repair the computer (unless this is part of their job). If something is wrong with the equipment, a computer repair technician should be called for on-site repair or the computer should be returned or taken to a computer service center. However, first make sure that all connections are in place at the back of the unit. This is similar to making sure that a television set is plugged in before calling a repairman.

There are a number of connections between the computer and its various components, the power source, and peripheral units (i.e., modems, fax machines). To ensure that all connections are in place, turn off the computer, and simply look at the back of the computer. If any cords or cables are disconnected, they may be the source of the problem. However, be sure that you know where to plug in the cable before attempting to slide it into any of the slots. Plugging in a cord or cable incorrectly can destroy your machine, your programs, or the machines and programs of others whose computers are attached to yours.

# The Monitor

The **computer monitor** is the screen that is connected to the computer. It is this screen that allows you to see the programs and the data you are working with. There are four items you should be familiar with on the computer monitor: the power switch, the contrast control, the brightness control, and the cursor.

There is a **power switch** on the monitor like the one on the computer, which turns the monitor on and off. When the monitor is not in use for an extended period of time, the power switch should be turned off to prevent the image from burning into the screen. Be aware that turning off the monitor does not turn off the computer. Therefore, the data and information you were working on are still there. You simply cannot see it.

The **contrast control** turns the contrast up and down between varying fields. This control is usually used to provide more or less contrast between those sections in a document that have been bolded or highlighted and those that have not.

The **brightness control** changes the brightness of the image on the screen. Adjust this knob so that you can read the screen without difficulty or glare.

The **cursor** is the small lighted symbol on the monitor screen that indicates where you are in the program or document. Depending on the system, this symbol may look like a bright straight line, a bright blinking line, or a blinking or solid box.

# The Keyboard

The **keyboard** is your primary means of communicating with your computer. The input commands and data are typed in through the keyboard. Its layout roughly resembles that of an ordinary typewriter. To describe the keyboard more clearly, we will divide it into six parts, each with its own function:

- Keyboard angle adjustment.
- Typewriter keypad with control keys.
- Numeric keypad.
- Editing and cursor control keys.
- Function keys.
- Three status lights.

## Keyboard Angle Adjustment

You can adjust your keyboard to two different positions for your typing comfort. To adjust, push on the adjustable leg handles on both sides and turn them to the desired position.

# On the Job Now

**Directions:** Fill in the blank spaces with the correct word without looking at the material just covered.

1. There are four items you should be familiar with on the computer monitor: the power switch, the _____, the brightness control, and the cursor.

2. There is a _____ on the monitor like the one on the computer that turns the monitor on and off.

3. The cursor is a _____ symbol on the monitor screen that indicates where you are in the program or document.

4. The keyboard is your _____ means of communicating with your computer.

5. The _____ changes the brightness of the images on the screen.

## Typewriter Keypad with Control Keys

The typewriter area of the keyboard looks and behaves a lot like a standard typewriter keyboard. Like a typewriter, the Shift key produces capital letters. To type the special characters shown above the numbers on the number keys, hold down the Shift key and press the appropriate number key. For example, the Shift key with the number 1 produces an exclamation mark (!).

The computer keyboard also includes several special control keys specifically associated with computer operations, including Esc, Ctrl, Alt, and Enter. Here is a brief explanation of some important keyboard and control key functions:

**CAPS LOCK—**With this key, you can type uppercase letters without holding down the Shift key. When Caps Lock is engaged, the indicator light in the upper-right-hand corner of the keyboard lights up. The Caps Lock key only affects the 26 letters of the alphabet. To type special symbols, you still need to press the Shift key.

**ENTER—**This key acts as both the Return key and the Enter key. As the Return key, it ends the line being typed and advances the cursor to the next line. As the Enter key, it is used to execute commands you have typed.

**SHIFT—**For uppercase letters, punctuation, or symbols, either one of the two Shift keys can be pressed. When the Caps Lock key is engaged, the Shift key acts as an "Un-Shift" key, allowing you to type lowercase letters.

**SPACE BAR—**Moves the cursor one position to the right. It will also erase characters to the right, replacing them with blanks if the computer is in the typeover mode instead of insert mode.

**BACKSPACE—**This key erases one character to the left of the cursor.

**TAB—**Moves the cursor to the next tab stop. In some programs the Tab key will act as a margin release to the left if the Shift key is depressed, or will move the cursor one tab spot to the left.

**ESC—**The Escape key has different functions depending on the program.

**ALT—**Like the Shift key, Alt performs no function on its own. It is used in combination with other keys. The function of Alt varies depending on the application being used.

**CTRL—**This key performs no function on its own. Like the Shift and Alt keys, the control key (Ctrl) is used only in combination with other keys. Ctrl performs many different functions depending on the application being used.

Pressing two or three keys simultaneously can be used to perform a series of unique program control and screen control functions as shown in the following:

| KEYS | FUNCTION DESCRIPTION |
|------|---------------------|
| Ctrl/Break | Terminates the execution of a program and identifies the line where it stops. |
| Ctrl/Alt/Del | This function resets the computer. |
| Shift/Print | Causes all data on the screen only to be printed. |

To produce the function indicated, press and hold down the first (and second if it is a series of three) key(s) and press the last key. This is by no means a comprehensive list of the functions available.

## Numeric Keypad

The numeric keypad is located separately from the alphabetic keys. It is usually on the right-hand side of a computer keyboard. The keypad performs a dual function.

With the Num Lock key engaged (indicated by the status light in the upper-right-hand corner of some keyboards), the keypad can be used for the rapid data entry of numbers. With Num Lock disengaged, the keypad can be used to move the cursor or to perform special editing features.

A 101-key-enhanced keyboard provides a separate keypad for cursor control and editing (located immediately to the left of the numeric keypad). For this reason, most users will find it convenient to leave the Num Lock key on, thus allowing for the rapid entry of numbers. If your keyboard is not a 101-enhanced keyboard, you will probably not want to leave the Num Lock key on.

The following keys operate the same regardless of whether or not the Num Lock key is on or off:

| ENTER | Works the same as the Enter key on the typewriter keypad. |
|-------|----------------------------------------------------------|
| + | Displays the Plus symbol. |
| – | Displays the Minus symbol. |
| * | Displays the Asterisk, used for multiplication. |
| / | Displays the Slash, used for division. |

The following keys perform differently depending on whether the Num Lock key is turned on or off:

| KEY | NUM LOCK ON | NUM LOCK OFF |
|-----|-------------|--------------|
| 1 End | 1 | END—Moves the cursor to the end of the line. |
| 2 ↓ | 2 | ↓—Moves the cursor down. |
| 3 Pg Dn | 3 | Pg Dn—Moves the cursor down one page, or 25 lines. |
| 4 ← | 4 | ←—Moves the cursor to the left. |
| 5 | 5 | No function. |
| 6 → | 6 | →—Moves the cursor to the right. |
| 7 Home | 7 | HOME—Moves the cursor to the beginning of the line. |
| 8 ↑ | 8 | ↑—Moves the cursor up. |
| 9 Pg Up | 9 | Pg Up—Moves the cursor up one page, or 25 lines. |
| 0 Ins | 0 | INS—This key toggles (turns on and off) between Insert and Typeover mode. |
| . Del | Decimal | DEL—(Delete) Erases one character at the position of the cursor. |

## Editing and Cursor Control Keys

The 101-key-enhanced keyboard contains a separate set of editing keys usually located between the Typewriter and Numeric keypads.

**HOME**—Moves the cursor to the first character of the line.

**CURSOR UP**—Moves the cursor up one line for each keystroke.

**CURSOR DOWN**—Moves the cursor down one line for each keystroke.

**CURSOR RIGHT**—Moves the cursor to the right one character position for each keystroke.

**CURSOR LEFT**—Moves the cursor to the left one character position for each keystroke.

**END**—Moves the cursor to the right of the last character on the current line.

**DELETE**—Deletes characters at the cursor. All characters to the right will be moved left. If this key is held down, it will erase each character as it reaches the cursor.

**INSERT/TYPEOVER**—On "Insert", characters typed will be inserted before previously typed text, pushing the existing text to the right. On "Typeover", existing characters will be typed over.

**PAGE UP**—Moves the cursor up one page, or 25 lines.

**PAGE DN**—Moves the cursor down one page, or 25 lines.

**SCROLL LOCK**—When the Scroll Lock key is pressed, the Scroll Lock light will be illuminated on the keyboard. Once the Scroll Lock light is on, it can be turned off by pressing the Scroll Lock key again, which will also turn off the Scroll Lock mode of operation. Refer to the computer application program manual for more details on this key.

**PRINT SCREEN**—When the Print Screen key is pressed, the data displayed on the screen will be printed (if the computer is connected to a printer). If the Ctrl key is pressed and held while this key is pressed, the printer function will be disabled or enabled.

**PAUSE BREAK**—This key suspends the program execution until another key is pressed. When used with the Ctrl key, the program being run will be terminated.

## Function Keys

Along the top half of the keyboard or on the left side of some keyboards are 12 function keys that allow complex program commands to be performed with a single keystroke.

Different software programs use function keys for different purposes. Therefore, to properly use these keys, the program-specific user's guide must be referred to. It is highly advisable not to use the function keys without referring to the program instructions, as they may delete data or cancel parts of a program.

## Three Status Lights

The three status lights are usually located in the upper right-hand corner of the keyboard. They are labeled NUM LOCK, CAPS LOCK, and SCROLL LOCK. The **Num Lock** light, when lit, signifies the Num Lock function is engaged, thus causing the keys on the numeric keypad to act as numbers rather than cursor movement keys.

When the **Caps Lock** light is on, it signifies that all letters typed on the keyboard will appear as capital letters.

Scroll Lock is a feature that only works with some computer programs. When the **Scroll Lock** is used in these applications, the cursor is locked onto whatever line it is on when the Scroll Lock button is pushed, and the entire page will move around it. For example, if your cursor is halfway down the page when you hit the Scroll Lock button, your cursor will remain halfway down the page. When you hit the arrow down key, the entire document will move up one line, but the cursor will remain in the center of the screen.

## Practice Pitfalls

According to Murphy's Law, anything that can go wrong will go wrong. However, a number of techniques will help to eliminate the frustration of losing computer-stored information. The following eight techniques should be learned and should become a daily part of your computer life:

1. Save your data often and make backup copies while working on it. A second copy of the data should be saved to a second file when you are finished. A power surge or brief break in the power supply can erase your entries in less than one second.

2. Keep a backup copy in a different location. A second copy of important data should be stored in a different room or, if possible, a different building. This preserves the data in case of fire, destruction of the building, or water damage.

3. Always date the copies of your files so that you can retrieve the latest disk easily.

4. Use permanent disks or tapes to store copies of financial and confidential records and keep them in a secure, fireproof location.

5. Maintain a notebook or log that shows what you have stored in the computer and the file name it is located under.

6. Set up a system for naming documents so that they will be easily accessible even if you do not have the log.

7. Handle data diskettes properly. This includes:

   a. Never touch the magnetic media housed inside the plastic cover. There is a hole in the plastic through which the computer reads the information. On the 3.5-inch disk, this hole is covered by a piece of sliding metal.

**b.** Store all disks inside plastic or paper covers to protect them from damage. Insert and remove the disk carefully from the cover to prevent scratching the magnetic media.

**c.** Never fold, spindle, or mutilate your disk.

**d.** Keep diskettes stored at temperatures between 50° and 125° F. Never leave a data disk exposed to sunlight.

**e.** Keep all magnets away from your data disks. Information stored on a magnetic medium can be erased when it comes in contact with a magnet. This includes the magnet contained in office supplies, such as paper clip holders.

**f.** Before touching a data disk, discharge any static electricity you may have picked up by touching a piece of metal or an antistatic mat. Static electricity also demagnetizes and can erase the data contained on a disk.

**g.** When carrying disks across a carpeted area, place the disk inside its protective sleeve and inside another object such as a disk storage box or between the pages of a book. This will prevent erasure by any static electricity that you may pick up by walking across the carpet.

**h.** To prevent any changes to information stored on a data disk, slide the button on the disk designed for this purpose. To change the data at a later date, simply slide the button back to the original position.

**i.** Do not write on a disk label with a ballpoint pen or pencil; use a felt-tip marker. The pressure applied when writing with a pen or pencil may cause indentations on the magnetic media, which may damage the diskette.

**8.** If you accidentally delete or are unable to retrieve information, immediately remove the disk from the computer. Do not save anything on the disk. Many computer files can be reconstructed with the proper programs but only if the information has not been written over.

Remember that it is far easier to retrieve data that has been stored properly than to recreate it. Taking proper care of your data will ensure that it will be retrievable when you need it.

# Computer Terms

There are a number of terms used in the computer industry that can be confusing to those who have never dealt with computers. The following terms are those most commonly used by claims examiners and other computer users.

**Bit**—(Contraction for binary digit) a single binary digit, either 0 or 1. A bit is the smallest unit of data stored in a computer; all other data must be coded into a pattern of individual bits.

**Boot (or bootstrap)**—the process of starting up a computer.

**CD-ROM**—a compact disc format used to hold text, graphics and hi-fi stereo. Basically, it is like an audio CD, but it uses a different format for data. You will need a CD-ROM drive for most new software, as it is a lot easier and quicker for developers to distribute and for you to install software in this format.

**Chip or Silicon Chip**—another name for an integrated circuit, a complete electronic circuit on a slice of silicon crystal only a few millimeters square.

**Computer Graphics**—use of computers to display and manipulate information in pictorial form.

**Central Processing Unit (CPU)**—the CPU or processor is considered the brain of the computer. The CPU makes everything else perform, and it is one of the major factors that determine the computer's overall speed. The faster the CPU, the faster the computer can execute your instructions.

**Data**—facts, figures, and symbols, especially as stored in computers. The term is often used to mean raw, unprocessed facts, as distinct from information, to which a meaning or interpretation has been applied.

**Database**—a structured collection of data, which may be manipulated to select and sort desired items of information.

**Desktop Publishing**—use of microcomputers for small-scale typesetting and page makeup.

**Disk**—a common medium for storing large volumes of data. A magnetic disk is rotated at high speed in a disk-drive unit as a read-write (playback or record) head passes over its surfaces to record or read magnetic variations that encode the data.

**Download**—to load a file from the Internet or another source onto your computer.

**DOS**—acronym for disk operating system, a computer operating system specifically designed for use with disk storage; also used as an alternate name for a particular system, MS-DOS.

**Electronic Mail**—or e-mail, is a system that enables the users of a computer network to send messages to other users.

**Gigabyte**—a measure of memory capacity, equal to one billion bytes. It is also used, less precisely, to mean 1,000 megabytes.

**Hacking**—unauthorized access to a computer, either for fun or for malicious or fraudulent purposes.

**Hard Drive**—the storage place on a computer. It stores information in your computer. You will need a lot of hard drive space to hold all the information you want on your computer.

**Hardware**—the mechanical, electrical, and electronic components of a computer system, as opposed to the various programs that constitute software.

**Interface**—the point of contact between two programs or pieces of equipment.

**Joystick**—an input device that signals to a computer the direction and extent of displacement of a hand-held lever.

**Keyboard**—an input device resembling a typewriter keyboard, used to enter instructions and data.

**Laptop Computer**—a portable microcomputer, small enough to be used on the operator's lap.

**Light Pen**—a device resembling an ordinary pen, used to indicate locations on a computer screen.

**Megabyte**—a unit of memory equal to 1,024 kilobytes. It is sometimes used, less precisely, to mean one million bytes.

**Memory**—the part of a system used to store data and programs either permanently or temporarily. There are two main types: immediate access memory and backing storage. Random Access Memory (RAM) is what your computer and operating system uses to perform functions. RAM is considered a temporary storage area for particular pieces of information required by the computer at any given moment. The more RAM you have, the faster your computer will perform.

**Microprocessor**—complete computer central processing unit contained on a single integrated circuit, or chip.

**Modem**—(acronym for modulator/demodulator) device for transmitting computer data over telephone lines.

**Mouse**—an input device used to control a pointer on a computer screen.

**Operating System**—a program that controls the basic operation of a computer.

**Printer**—an output device for producing printed copies of text or graphics.

**Procedure**—a small part of a computer program that performs a specific task, such as clearing the screen or sorting a file.

**Screen or Monitor**—an output device on which the computer displays information for the benefit of the operator.

**Software**—a collection of programs and procedures for making a computer perform a specific task, as opposed to hardware, the physical components of a computer system.

**Speech Recognition**—or voice input, any technique by which a computer can understand ordinary speech.

**Spreadsheet**—a program that mimics a sheet of ruled paper, divided into columns and rows.

**Touch Screen**—an input device allowing the user to communicate with the computer by touching a display screen.

**Virtual Memory**—a technique whereby a portion of the computer-backing storage memory is used as an extension of its immediate-access memory.

**Virtual Reality**—advanced form of computer simulation, in which a participant has the illusion of being part of an artificial environment.

**Virus**—a piece of software that can replicate itself and transfer itself from one computer to another without the user being aware of it. Some viruses are relatively harmless, but others can damage or destroy data.

**Word**—a group of bits that a computer's central processing unit treats as a single working unit.

**Word Processing**—storage and retrieval of written text by computer. Word processing software packages enable the writer to key in text and amend it in a number of ways.

**Workstation**—high-performance desktop computer with strong graphics capabilities, traditionally used for engineering, scientific research, and desktop publishing.

**Zip Drives**—like floppy disk drives, except they hold the equivalent of about 80 floppy disks. You could also use a zip drive for backup purposes.

## Practice Pitfalls

Following are several tips for maintaining your computer files:

1. Make sure your paper systems are uncluttered and well structured by adhering to the following:

   a. Throw out old or marginally useful information.

   b. Divide remaining paper files into three classes: working, reference, and archives. Arrange the working files to be nearest you, and the archives to be out of your office.

   c. Create a subject filing structure for each of these classes of paper by mapping out your key functions.

2. Now go into your computer system and set up the same filing structure for your electronic documents. The closer your paper and electronic systems parallel each other, the easier it will be to remember where to file things and where to search for them.

3. If you use e-mail, especially in a corporate environment, you may have hundreds, or in extreme cases even thousands, of messages in your inbox. Begin deleting messages that are no longer needed, starting with the oldest.

4. Messages you want to save should be put into the electronic folders or directories you set up in step 2.

5. Now do the same with word processing or spreadsheet files.

6. If you need to recapture space on your hard drive, organize your electronic archive system with the same categories you established in step 1 and transfer your files from your hard drive to floppies or another storage medium.

7. Go through your hard drive and determine if there are any programs you are not using. If so, delete or transfer these to another storage medium.

8. If you are in a corporate environment, or on the Internet and are being swamped with messages, remove yourself from these distribution lists.

9. Go through your documentation and clear out manuals for programs you are no longer using.

10. In the future, establish a certain time each day to process both your paper and e-mail. Do it daily so that your files do not build up in your system.

## Job Search Basics

Regardless of the career path you have chosen, all the education in the world is worthless if you do not have good job-hunting skills. Without them, you may never gain employment.

Gaining successful employment requires you to look for a job, and also to market yourself. This works for direct mail advertising companies around the world, and it can work for you, too. It is important to start with a set of written objectives, know what separates you from the competition, and familiarize yourself with your target audience.

## Job Search Objectives

First, determine your job search objectives. What responsibilities do you want in the position you are looking for? Is there a specific title for such responsibilities? What type of work environment do you desire (i.e., office, hospital, restaurant, outdoor work)? What can you reasonably expect, both in the way of title and salary? Writing down your objectives can help to solidify them in your mind and help you formulate a plan of action.

## Uniqueness

Most available job openings have numerous people applying for the position. You need to emphasize your uniqueness and the talents that you can bring to the job. What sets you apart from your competitors? Do you have a special talent or area of expertise? Call attention to it. What about a skill you can share with other employees? Highlight it. Let prospective employers know how you can help to train co-workers, saving the company time and money while helping the operation run smoothly. Do you have contacts in a particular industry that might allow your employer to expand? Tell prospective employers these details to set you apart from the competition.

## Target Audience

Success at finding the right job depends not only on the previous two areas discussed but also on looking in the right place. You would not go to a restaurant to find a job as a typist. Likewise, you would not go to a typing pool to find a job as a waiter. Much depends on where you look for a job.

After deciding on the particular organizations offering the best opportunities, find out who the decision makers are. Who would be the best person for you to contact regarding employment? Get the person's title and name. Find out as much as you can about the person who makes the decisions at the companies you are targeting. What are their professional affiliations (i.e., AFL-CIO, AMA)? What is their career background? What are their job-related concerns and corporate responsibilities? The answers to these questions will help you establish rapport with the person and help you bring out your commonalities.

## Build Your Database

Once you have established your target audience, make an organized collection of information about the companies and possible job prospects. Your collection needs to keep track of potential employers, professional contacts, and resources.

Keep detailed and well-organized notes on everyone you speak with who can help you reach your objectives. Always write down the person's name, title, the company or organization name, address, phone and fax numbers, any professional affiliations, the date you spoke or met, how you reached them, what follow-up you should make, and any other relevant information.

Build a file on each company from all the resources available to you. This can include job banks, trade publications, executive search firms, civic groups, alumni associations, social networks, colleagues or coworkers, former employers, and anyone else who can help you. You will be surprised at how many people you know when you start to write them down.

## The Résumé

Now you are ready to develop your résumé and cover letter. Think of these items as sales materials for your career. The cover letter should invite and interest your target audience enough that they will read your résumé. Your **résumé** is a summary of employment experience and qualifications, essentially the marketing brochure that gets you in the door. Both need to proclaim the benefits you offer to an employer. Sample résumés can be found at the end of this chapter.

## A First-Class Résumé

A résumé can be your best friend or your worst enemy. A first-class résumé is one of the most important items you can have in your job search and can open doors for you. A bad résumé will slam them shut. In essence, a résumé is your personal representative. It tells the company not only who you are but also the type of person you are. No one would welcome an employee who is sloppy and disorganized. Likewise, your résumé should not be full of errors or difficult to read. Your résumé is a direct reflection of you. Its goal is to get you an interview and help you to land that great job.

The initial screening of a résumé occurs very quickly; sometimes it is merely scanned for a few seconds. Your format should keep this in mind. The purpose of this quick scan is to weed out the résumés that have obvious typographic errors, are poorly organized, or are substandard in reproduction. If the author of a résumé was not careful enough to proofread and correct his own résumé, why should an employer think the person would be any more conscientious at work? If your résumé is hard to read or difficult to file (because of odd-shaped paper), it will undoubtedly end up in file 13, also known as the trash can.

Before you write your résumé, do a little research. Find a current book on résumé writing. This type of book will give you a wealth of information and good résumé samples.

### The Basics

Your résumé should typically be no longer than one page. It should be printed on white or off-white 8.5 × 11 inch paper. Do not use bright or fancy colors. Professionals in the Human Resources area prefer one-page résumés. One-page résumés are easier to read and yet provide enough information to introduce you and your experience. Do not jeopardize your job opportunities by being long-winded or by listing every minute detail about your professional history.

Always be concise and do not abbreviate any words. The chance of being misunderstood is not worth saving the space.

The following five items should be included on your résumé:

1. **Name, address, and telephone number:** you would be surprised at how many people leave off one or more pieces of this vital information. Make sure that all the information is correct. Do not cut corners. Your address should include an apartment number and the zip code, and your phone number

should include the area code. The easier it is for an employer to contact you, the better.

2. **Objective statement:** some employers and résumé writers consider an objective statement to be optional. However, if you have a specific direction, include it. It lets the prospective employer know what your goals are. If you are interested in several different jobs, you might want to replace the objective statement with a qualifying statement. In this way, you will not have to prepare separate objective statements (and résumés) for each job title. Make sure that your résumé shows that you have some direction. Your cover letter should also reinforce this.

3. **Qualifying statement:** a qualifying statement is a way to toot your own horn. It sells you as a potential employee and lists your abilities and experiences. You can get ideas for your qualifying statement in the want ads. See what skills and characteristics are desired (i.e., excellent written and verbal communication skills, ability to handle a variety of tasks, and excellent organizational ability). These are exactly the types of statements that should go into your qualifying statement.

4. **Work experience:** there are a variety of ways to state your experience. The most common approach is to list your employment history in reverse chronological order, putting your most recent job first. However, if you have had numerous job changes or a gap in employment, you do not necessarily want to emphasize this. Therefore, you might consider using the functional format résumé. This lists together all related experiences rather than listing according to date.

5. **Education:** if you have education or training beyond the high school level you will want this fact to stand out. Find a way to highlight this so that, even when your résumé is scanned quickly, additional education can be noticed. The simplest format is to list the degree or certificate, followed by your major or course of study. Follow this with the name and location of the school and year in which you graduated (i.e., Certificate of Completion, Medical Billing, Los Angeles College, Los Angeles, CA, 2001). Education and training should be listed in reverse chronological order. See sample résumés at the end of this chapter.

Optional information, if you have room at the bottom, should include special skills, personal notes, hobbies, and references.

## Professional Services

If you need additional help, a number of professional résumé services are available. It is essential that your résumé look professional. This includes the use of a word processor and a letter-quality printer. If you do not have access to this type of equipment, it may be a good investment to hire someone to type and print it for you.

## Edit and Proofread

You must edit and proofread your résumé very carefully. Remember that this single sheet of paper can either help or hurt you in getting a job. It is a direct reflection of you. Before you send it to a potential employer, get a friend to check it for errors and content. Another person can often spot things that you have missed.

## What to Avoid

Some of these items may seem obvious, but a surprising number of people make these errors on their résumés. The following seven items are things to avoid when you are composing your résumé:

1. Never send a carbon copy or an inferior quality copy of your résumé to a prospective employer.

2. Never use abbreviations; this includes the term "etc." Anything important enough to be stated should be written out. Write it out or leave it out.

3. Do not waste time and space detailing mundane, entry-level jobs that have no bearing on your present job search.

4. Do not list a desired salary. Discussions of this sort should be saved for the interview. If you ask for too high of a salary, you may not be granted an interview. If you ask for too little, a prospective employer may wonder what you are worth.

5. Consider the importance of salary, job location, and position desired before you limit yourself. Ask yourself if any of these are more important than a chance for advancement.

6. Do not include information on your age, marital status, religion, or race.

7. Do not put "References available on request," as this just annoys prospective employers.

## Words to Use in Your Résumé

Use an active voice in your résumé. Action verbs and specific nouns are best when describing your job duties and accomplishments. Following are words to use in your résumé:

| | | |
|---|---|---|
| Accomplish | Achieve | Act |
| Adapt | Administer | Advertise |
| Advise | Aid | Analyze |
| Apply | Approach | Approve |
| Arrange | Assemble | Assess |
| Assign | Assist | Attain |
| Budget | Build | Calculate |
| Catalog | Chair | Clarify |
| Collaborate | Communicate | Compare |
| Compile | Complete | Conceive |
| Conciliate | Conduct | Consult |
| Contract | Control | Cooperate |
| Coordinate | Correct | Counsel |
| Create | Decide | Define |
| Delegate | Demonstrate | Design |
| Detail | Determine | Develop |
| Devise | Direct | Distribute |
| Draft | Edit | Employ |
| Encourage | Enlarge | Enlist |
| Establish | Estimate | Evaluate |
| Examine | Exchange | Execute |
| Exhibit | Expand | Expedite |
| Facilitate | Familiarize | Forecast |
| Formulate | Generate | Govern |
| Guide | Handle | Head |
| Hire | Identify | Implement |
| Improve | Increase | Index |
| Influence | Inform | Initiate |
| Innovate | Inspect | Install |
| Institute | Instruct | Integrate |
| Interpret | Interview | Introduce |
| Invent | Investigate | Lead |
| Maintain | Manage | Manipulate |
| Market | Mediate | Moderate |
| Modify | Monitor | Motivate |
| Negotiate | Obtain | Operate |
| Order | Organize | Originate |

| | | |
|---|---|---|
| Oversee | Perceive | Perform |
| Persuade | Plan | Prepare |
| Present | Preside | Process |
| Produce | Program | Promote |
| Propose | Provide | Publicize |
| Publish | Qualify | Raise |
| Recommend | Reconcile | Record |
| Recruit | Rectify | Redesign |
| Reduce | Regulate | Relate |
| Renew | Report | Represent |
| Reorganize | Research | Resolve |
| Review | Revise | Scan |
| Schedule | Screen | Select |
| Sell | Serve | Settle |
| Solve | Speak | Staff |
| Standardize | Stimulate | Summarize |
| Supervise | Support | Survey |
| Synthesize | Systematize | Teach |
| Train | Transmit | Update |
| Write | | |

## Practice

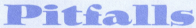

The following tips will help you to create a top-notch résumé:

**Put a brief description of yourself at the top that highlights your strengths.** For example, "A seasoned veteran responsible for overseeing three branch offices in three states." Most employers spend only a few seconds on each résumé, so get your selling points up front.

**Try several different formats.** Do not limit yourself to a standard chronological format. Experiment with a functional format, grouping your past activities under headings such as "Team Coordination" or "Supervisory Activities" with applicable experience listed under each. If you have a strong specialty that a prospective employer may need, this format may highlight that trait more effectively than a list of jobs held.

**Stick to one or two fonts.** Do not try to show off your computer skills by including a multitude of fonts in your résumé. This often ends up looking messy and disjointed.

# On the Job Now

**Directions:** Answer the following questions without looking back at the material just covered. Write your answers in the space provided.

1. Why should you make sure that your résumé is no longer than one page? _____

_____

_____

2. List the five items that should be included on your résumé.

    1. _____

    2. _____

    3. _____

    4. _____

    5. _____

3. List the seven items to avoid when you are composing your résumé.

    1. _____

    2. _____

    3. _____

    4. _____

    5. _____

    6. _____

    7. _____

## The Cover Letter

Your résumé provides a potential employer with your qualifications. The **cover letter** is an introduction to your résumé. It invites the potential employer to read further. Your cover letter should be concise and to the point. What you are really trying to say with the cover letter is that you are enclosing your résumé and are available for an interview at the prospective employer's convenience. The cover letter should be neatly typed on white or off-white 8.5 × 11 inch paper. See a sample cover letter at the end of this chapter.

### Letter Writing Do Nots

The following are items you should avoid when writing your cover letter:

1. Do not include anything in your letter that cannot be substantiated in your interview.

2. Do not try to force an interview by using sympathy or any sense of urgency.

3. Do not load your cover letter with unnecessary information; just present the important facts. The cover letter should be an addendum to your résumé.

4. Do not address your letter to a company or a title. Find out the name of the person who holds that title and address it to that person. If you cannot, address it to the department or division that will supervise your work.

5. Do not mail a résumé without a cover letter.

6. Do not forget to request an interview in your cover letter.

7. Do not forget to proofread your cover letter, checking for appearance, grammar, and spelling errors.

# Marketing Yourself

When marketing your skills, keep in mind the following things:

- Segment your audience.
- Prepare your portfolio.
- Professionally market yourself.

Let's discuss each item individually.

People respond to various things differently. Salespeople know this and segment their audience accordingly. You also need to segment your audience to be sure you are presenting the right benefit (talent) to the right market in the right tone. This often means you have to write several different résumés and cover letters. It is worth it if you want to get the right job. Just be sure your objectives, experience, and message are appropriate to the segment you are trying to sell.

You might also consider creating a portfolio on yourself. This portfolio could include your résumé, letters of reference, graphs or charts supporting your accomplishments, samples of previous work, and other informational material. Present the information neatly. A handsome presentation folder conveys a stronger impact than a cover letter and résumé alone. Its very size commands more attention. Be careful to not overload it with too much extraneous information. Present only the best of what you have to offer.

Depending on the situation, it can often be best to present your portfolio during the interview rather than including it with your résumé.

Searching for a job is not enough. Instead, you must professionally market yourself. Take charge of the situation and of your career. Job hunters take what comes along; marketing yourself means more. It means going out and searching for the job you want, then selling yourself until you get it.

Develop a plan that will make things happen. Assemble your resources. Present yourself with purpose, professionalism, and positive energy. Not only is this more effective, but it is better for your morale than just starting another dreaded job search!

# The Job Interview

The job interview can be one of the most frightening experiences a potential employee faces. Add to this the knowledge that most working adults make an average of 10 career changes in their lifetime, each requiring a number of job interviews. That is a lot of stress to go through, but with knowledge can come the power to take control of the interview and turn fear into success.

Part of being prepared for an interview is having your directions, questions, interview agenda, and information about the company before the interview, so do your homework! If prepared properly, you (the applicant) will know exactly where you stand and how you did by the end of the interview.

Keep in mind that the key to getting hired is chemistry. If someone likes you, they will go out of their way to make you fit.

Your goal should be to get a job offer or at the very least get to the next step, which is another interview. Remember you can turn any offer down but not if you do not have it!

## Dress

How you dress and present yourself is also very important. Men should wear a gray or dark blue suit, a white shirt with contrast tie, and polished black shoes. Women should wear a conservative suit with a plain blouse that has a conservative neckline, and low-heeled shoes. Both men and women should make sure their hair is neat and trimmed, and that their hands and nails are clean. Wear little or no jewelry, and no perfume or cologne; you never know what the interviewer might be sensitive to. Give a firm handshake, smile, and make eye contact. Display interest, energy, and confidence.

## The Application

When you arrive, you may be given an application to fill out. This application is very important because whatever information you put on it is what the employer will be verifying (i.e., salary, reasons for leaving, education). Remember, keep it simple. Take a black pen to fill out your application. This color of ink photocopies well.

In the section for "Salary Desired" write the word "open" or "negotiable." NEVER write a dollar amount!

Remember when filling out the area "Reasons for Leaving" that once you put this information on an application it becomes a permanent record. You have signed to have this information verified by the potential employer. Companies do not typically give information beyond salary, start and end dates, and voluntary or involuntary termination (involuntary could be layoff or fired). Whatever you write should be as positive as possible. Employers look for patterns (i.e., job changes due to disagreement with boss, laid off more than once, conflict with other employees, disagreements with management decisions, etc.). When found, good or bad, they feel they get the picture of the applicant. Although you want to be honest, you also want to keep these reasons neutral if possible.

Be accurate with your education. State the correct degree you earned and the year you received it. This is the easiest information on your application to verify.

## Interviewing

Interviewing research indicates that there are four basic components to the interview process:

- The first four seconds.
- The next five minutes.
- The main portion.
- The end or closing.

It is important to fully understand each of these components so that you can control them and reap the best rewards from the interview process.

### The First Four Seconds

First impressions are very important. They can put you off to a good start, or they can strike a mark against you that will be hard to erase if an interviewer forms a negative impression.

Eighty percent of a first impression is based on your appearance. For that reason, it is suggested that you dress more formally than you might dress on the job. Keep your appearance conservative; flashy styles can be risky.

The handshake is a symbolic gesture of trust. A firm, brief handshake and direct eye contact indicate self-confidence and trustworthiness.

### The Next Five Minutes

The next five minutes of an interview can often determine whether you get a job offer or not. Studies reveal that interviewers often form an opinion within this five-minute period. They then seek information that will validate this initial impression. Thus, their opinion influences their decision to either hire or reject the candidate. If the impression was negative, one study reveals, 90% of the time the applicant was not hired. If the opinion was positive, the candidate received a job offer 75% of the time.

Therefore, your primary goal during this time should be to make sure the initial impression is positive. The following suggestions have been found to be the most important:

1. Keep the tone of your voice calm but interested. You should be careful to speak clearly in a voice that is loud enough to be heard, but not so loud that it is annoying.

2. Make direct eye contact with the interviewer. It gives the impression that you are open and honest and have nothing to hide. Eye contact can actually be equal in power to the sound and tone of the voice.

3. Your posture conveys a large message when you are sitting as well as standing. Remaining straight and tall with shoulders back will convey confidence. Leaning forward slightly in your chair will convey interest.

4. Never underestimate the power of a smile for opening the lines of communication.

### The Main Portion

After the important amenities have been taken care of, the general questioning will begin. Listen carefully to the questions and focus your answers on the job requirements and on highlighting your strengths. Look for any specific problems that the organization may have. Highlight your skills and work history as they relate to the employer's needs. Remember that if they did not have a need, they would not be interviewing you. Make them believe they need you.

Try to find out as much as possible about the company, the job, and the people. A good interview is a two-way, give-and-take situation. Interviewers expect you to ask questions. Therefore, strong well-directed questions help to create a positive impression. Be sure to listen carefully to the response, and use the information to strengthen your position.

The personality trait that attracts an interviewer the most is enthusiasm. If you like what you have heard about this company, or what you are hearing in the interview, do not be afraid to let the interviewer know. Be comfortable about revealing your personality and the kind of person you are, but do it with interest, awareness, and energy. Many studies have indicated that individuals are often hired based more on their personality than on their skills.

The middle portion of the interview can present some of your greatest difficulty. Be aware of the hidden agenda behind each question. Is the interviewer trying to find out about your skills, your education, or your background?

If an interviewer continually returns to a specific topic, especially in your past, they are unconsciously telling you that they are questioning the response or that they discern a weakness. Remember to control your responses. Frame your experiences in a positive light and focus on the positive aspects that will most benefit the company.

There is probably at least one situation in your history that you would rather not have come out in the open. This may be a termination, a misdemeanor or felony conviction, or a similar problem.

First, determine whether the information will come up during the normal course of the interview, or during the background check. Most companies run a preliminary check on their prospective employees. This may include a brief phone call to previous employers and a check of police records.

Research has shown that negative aspects are seen much more negatively when they are revealed bit by bit. The impression is that you may have other things wrong if they ask the right questions to bring them out.

Take control of this situation by disclosing any negative information briefly and forthrightly before you are asked. In this way you can place the best possible light on the situation. Even a termination can be turned from a negative into a positive by sincerely and honestly discussing what you have learned from the experience and what you will do differently, if you are given the opportunity.

### The End or Closing

Finally, you have reached the closing moments of the interview. Many people begin to lose concentration and relax at this point. Do not! Keep yourself focused. A strong finish may be the difference between you and someone else in a tight race. Show the interviewer you are still excited about the job, especially now that you know more about it and the company.

Make a strong final note by succinctly summarizing your positive points as they relate to the job. There is nothing wrong with asking when a decision on the candidates will be made. When you have the answer, show your enthusiasm by letting the interviewer know that you will call back the afternoon of the decision.

Interviewing is much like a game. If you make all the right moves, you will win the job. If you make errors, you will not. In the end, it is all up to you and the way you play.

# On the Job Now

**Directions:** Answer the following questions without looking back at the material just covered. Write your answers in the space provided.

**1.** List four items you will need to be prepared for an interview.

   **1.** _____

   **2.** _____

   **3.** _____

   **4.** _____

**2.** List the four basic components to the interview process.

   **1.** _____

   **2.** _____

   **3.** _____

   **4.** _____

**3.** What portion of the interview can be the most difficult and why? _____

_____

_____

# Getting Paid What You Are Worth

The issue of salary will undoubtedly come up, either during the interview or before. Salary is probably the most important issue among workers today. Nevertheless, the way in which salary is determined is often one of the least understood aspects when it comes to evaluating your worth. Far too many people see their salary as an extension of themselves and how much they are worth. Often, their point of view is totally unrealistic according to the marketplace.

Let's review four of the most common misconceptions regarding how a salary should be determined:

**1. Seeing your monetary compensation as a reflection of your worth as a person.** It is not. Your salary is based on your objective value in the marketplace. If your skills are in high demand, you will be paid more than if they are not. This is perhaps the single most common mistake employees make. Their pride tells them that they are too good to work for such meager pay. If you are one of these people, you need to face the fact that the laws of supply and demand determine your market worth, not you. If everyone were able to set their own salary, inflation would increase drastically. You would be making $450 per hour, but a loaf of bread would cost $50.

Bear in mind that when supply and demand chooses a market value for your work, at least it is an objective value, not a subjective one determined by others. So do not take it personally.

**2. Expecting your pay to be determined by your needs.** This is the second most common complaint, and we have all heard it. Employees making comments like: "My partner is out of work, and we cannot pay our bills on my salary alone." "I'm a single parent with children to feed." "I have to put my children in private school." "This salary barely covers the cost of rent and bills every month. What am I supposed to eat on?"

The fact is that no employer can afford to pay an employee based on their needs. People are funny characters. When they have money, they tend to spend it. In the end, you will probably always need more money than you earn. Keep your professional dignity by never basing a request for a raise on these types of appeals.

**3. Expecting the length of your employment to determine your market value.** No matter how long you have worked at a particular position, if you can offer nothing more than the person who has worked at the job for a year, then both of you will be paid at approx-

imately the same level. Many employees expect automatic annual raises. This works fine until a company decides that it is less expensive to terminate the older employee and hire a new one at a lower salary. Then the policy does not sound so good anymore.

Recognize that your pay reflects the value of the work you do. Granted, more experience usually leads to a higher quality of employee, and often the pay reflects this. However, the box boy in the supermarket, no matter how great a box boy he is, will never earn as much as the supervisor of a department.

**4. Expecting your pay to go up as the company's profits go up.** This idea ignores a fundamental concept: Employees are not shareholders. They are not taking risks with their money. Those who expect their pay to increase when the company's profits increase almost never suggest that they should take a pay cut when the company has a bad year. Yet, one is exactly the same as the other. If an employee wishes to share in a company's profits and if the company is publicly held, the employee should purchase company stock. However, these employees, like the current shareholders, will then run the risk of losing their money if profits fall.

If you, as an employee, recognize these misconceptions about salary, you are less likely to base your request for a raise on unsound reasons. Take into consideration what would be a valid reason for requesting a raise.

First and fundamentally, you need to make some personal decisions. Ask yourself: "Am I in the right job?" "Do I enjoy what I am doing?" Regardless of your answer, the next question should be, "Is it more important for me to have money or to be happy?" The truth is that it takes a lot of money to compensate someone for being miserable. And if you are miserable in your job, you are probably not putting forth your best effort. Lack of effort is definitely not going to get you the raises you would like. So what do you do? First, find the right job.

The next important principle is that the laws of supply and demand will prevail. If you want to increase your market value, you must increase your worth to the company, usually by increasing your skills and abilities.

The following suggestions can help you increase your value to the company:

1. Adopt an active mentality, not a passive one. No one is going to increase your skills and abilities for you; you have to do it yourself and it takes work.

2. Never stop learning. Do not be satisfied with knowing your job inside and out. After you have mastered that, begin learning the other jobs in the company, preferably those of the next step up the ladder. Ask questions, read books, or take classes. Make sure that you become a valuable asset to the company and that you are ready for advancement and promotion when the opportunity arises.

3. Make long-range plans rather than waiting for life to just happen to you. Those who sit around rarely go anywhere.

4. Finally, realize that very often a significant change in salary comes from changing jobs, either within your present company or by moving to a different employer. We have all heard comments such as, "If I were working at the company down the street, I could make more than this!" The obvious response is, "If that is true, then why don't you go work at that company?" If the bosses hear you make such a comment, they may assist your transfer to the company down the street by firing you.

Many employees cannot accept the fact that it is either true that their current pay is below market, or it is not. If it is true, why not move on? If it is not, change your market value.

# CHAPTER REVIEW

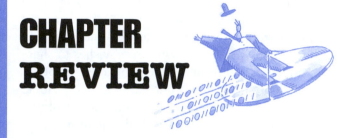

## Summary

- Proficient use of the calculator is essential for the claims examiner. Learning the functions of each of the keys and how to use the calculator to achieve the desired results takes practice.

- Computers have infiltrated all aspects of business life. Using the computer saves time and produces neater and cleaner reports, reduces errors, and allows for the electronic submission of data.

- Learning to use a computer program quickly and accurately and learning the proper means of storing information will provide the claims examiner with a valuable skill.

- To find the right job takes more than just a passive look at the classified ads. You must first determine your objectives, your uniqueness, and your target audience. With these topics firmly in mind, write an effective résumé and cover letter that will introduce you to a prospective employer.

- When you have been granted an interview, keep in mind that the first four seconds are the most critical, followed by the next five minutes. However, the body of the interview and the closing are also important in determining whether you get a second interview or a job offer.

- When it comes to salary, your pay is based on your worth to the marketplace. The higher the demand for your skills, the more value will be placed on them and the higher salary you will be paid. Salary is not determined by your worth as a person, your needs, your length of employment, or the company's profits.

## Assignments

Complete the Questions for Review.
Complete Exercises 16–1 through 16–7.
Practice gaining speed and accuracy by repeating Exercises 16–2 and 16–3 until you have mastered the feel of the keys.

## Questions for Review

**Directions:**   Answer the following questions without looking back at the material just covered. Write your answers in the space provided.

1. The _____ key completes multiplication and division operations and shows the results as a decimal.

2. What function does the divide key perform? _____

_____

**3.** The _____ key completes any pending operations.

**4.** What is the function of the total key? _____

_____

**5.** The memory total key displays and prints the value currently in _____, then clears the _____.

**6.** The numeric keypad is used for _____ when the Num Lock is on.

**7.** The space bar performs two functions. What are they?

   **1.** _____

   **2.** _____

**8.** What two functions does the Enter key perform?

   **1.** _____

   **2.** _____

**9.** Function keys perform what function? _____

_____

**10.** The cursor is _____

_____

**11.** What three points should your written marketing plan cover?

   **1.** _____

   **2.** _____

   **3.** _____

**12.** To determine your _____, consider the responsibilities you want on your next job, the industry in which you want to work, and what you can reasonably expect in the way of title and salary.

**13.** Your _____ lets the employer know what your goals are.

**14.** What is your résumé? _____

**15.** (True or False?) Never use an active voice or concise phrasing in your résumé. _____

**16.** A _____ is a way to toot your own horn.

**17.** (True or False?) Do not put anything in your cover letter that you cannot substantiate in an interview. _____

**18.** You should not job-hunt but instead _____ yourself.

**19.** Working adults normally make how many career changes in a lifetime? _____

**20.** (True or False?) The only way to achieve a significant increase in pay is to change jobs. _____

   If you were unable to answer any of these questions, refer back to that section and then fill in the answers.

# Exercise 16–1

**Directions:** Add each of the following columns of numbers and then subtract the numbers from your total to arrive at zero. Clear the entries from your calculator and subtract the following columns of numbers and total, then add the numbers to your total to arrive at zero. Use the printer tape to check accuracy.

| | | | |
|---|---|---|---|
| 71459 | 12181 | 128.49 | 12.89 |
| 28695 | 57926 | 321.67 | .92 |
| 13579 | 71349 | 014.89 | 7.16 |
| 58246 | 02763 | 906.76 | 18.21` |
| 69021 | 75396 | 741.08 | 267.93 |
| 54321 | 74185 | 529.63 | 1234.56 |
| 67891 | 29630 | 369.25 | 892.10 |
| 83214 | 36925 | 801.47 | 809.13 |
| 47986 | 80147 | 753.85 | 693.21 |
| 32694 | 42569 | 102.36 | 5679.32 |
| 15723 | 00147 | 564.12 | 137.14 |
| 38014 | 73528 | 321.65 | 432.78 |
| 98752 | 60413 | 498.70 | 6789.50 |
| 20361 | 13311 | 321.65 | 1090.17 |
| 13979 | 21769 | 789.93 | 578.15 |
| 02031 | 24989 | 456.89 | 692.00 |
| 11484 | 67400 | 999.01 | 780.29 |
| 25763 | 09121 | 847.03 | 566.17 |

# Exercise 16-2

**Directions:** Perform the function indicated for each list of numbers. Try not to watch your hands. Speed is not important at the beginning of performing these exercises. It will come later as you become more familiar with the keys.

1. Add the following numbers.

| A. | 12 | B. | 65 | C. | 44 | D. | 334 |
|---|---|---|---|---|---|---|---|
| | 24 | | 70 | | 69 | | 781 |
| | 67 | | 49 | | 26 | | 456 |
| | 41 | | 52 | | 73 | | 241 |
| | 92 | | 100 | | 84 | | 908 |
| | 34 | | 99 | | 35 | | 528 |
| | 72 | | 34 | | 21 | | 803 |

| E. | 295 | F. | 4576 | G. | 54 | H. | 32.514 |
|---|---|---|---|---|---|---|---|
| | 630 | | 8493 | | 835 | | 8.123 |
| | 816 | | 90.56 | | 046 | | 61.54 |
| | 902 | | 3809 | | 516 | | 123.64 |
| | 517 | | 9238 | | 943 | | 543.55 |
| | 703 | | 12.98 | | .0015 | | 999.83 |
| | 491 | | 540.5 | | | | |

2. Enter the first number, then subtract the following numbers.

| A. | 9999 | B. | 7654 | C. | 4329 |
|---|---|---|---|---|---|
| | 45 | | 11 | | 649 |
| | 66 | | 92 | | 42 |
| | 90 | | 561 | | 631 |
| | 1504 | | 341 | | 42 |
| | 3535 | | 940 | | 792 |
| | 901 | | 52 | | 406 |

| D. | 1000.00 | E. | 564.000 | F. | 410014 |
|---|---|---|---|---|---|
| | 10.00 | | .630 | | .123 |
| | .20 | | .920 | | 654.456 |
| | 341.00 | | 162.000 | | 84.25 |
| | 1.78 | | .789 | | 67.48 |
| | .78 | | 231.000 | | 138.03 |
| | 592.00 | | 501.000 | | 486.381 |

# Exercise 16-3

**Directions:** Perform the function indicated for each list of numbers. Try not to watch your hands. Speed is not important at the beginning. It will come later as you become more familiar with the keys.

**1.** Multiply the following.

| | | | |
|---|---|---|---|
| A.  231 | B.  5482 | C.  7602 | D.    891 |
| $\times 42$ | $\times 61$ | $\times 201$ | $\times 23.61$ |

| | | | |
|---|---|---|---|
| E. 43.92 | F. 24.51 | G. 903.45 | H. 2503.99 |
| $\times .639$ | $\times 70\%$ | $\times 85\%$ | $\times 90\%$ |

| | | | |
|---|---|---|---|
| I. 492.67 | J. 29.16 | K. 564465 | L. 654.21 |
| $\times 75\%$ | $\times 55\%$ | $\times 21\%$ | $\times 75\%$ |

**2.** Divide the first number by the second number in the following equations.

| | | | |
|---|---|---|---|
| A. 5634 | B. 56348 | C. 999999 | D.  3541 |
| 51 | 543 | .99 | 66 |

| | | | |
|---|---|---|---|
| E. 1000 | F. 65430 | G. 514623 | H.  5100 |
| .01 | 125 | 1523 | 45 |

# Exercise 16-4

**Directions:** Complete the following items.

**1.** Fill out the Résumé Questionnaire on the following pages (**Figure 16–1**).

**2.** Using the résumés on the following pages as examples (**Figures 16–2 through 16–4**), create your own résumé.

**3.** Using the following cover letter as an example (**Figure 16–5**), create your own cover letter.

# Résumé Questionnaire

First Name _____ M.I. _____ Last Name _____

Street _____

City _____ State _____ Zip _____

Day Phone _____ Eve. Phone _____ Soc. Sec. # _____

**Position Objective:** In the spaces below, enter the Occupational Titles of those positions which you feel you would be best qualified to fill. Opposite each position, enter the total years experience you have. Then indicate your minimum acceptable annual salary. "OPEN" is unacceptable. (Salary information is for your use and should not be included on an application.)

| | Years Experience | Desired Annual Salary |
|---|---|---|
| Occupational or Professional Title(s) | | |
| _____ | _____ | $_____ |
| _____ | _____ | $_____ |
| _____ | _____ | $_____ |
| | _____ | $_____ |

**Experience Summary:** Please summarize briefly your overall experience and accomplishments.

_____

_____

_____

**Education:**   Type of Degree, Diploma, Certificate, or Years completed: (i.e., HS Diploma, # year(s) College, AA/BA) Highest Level: Type: _____ Major _____

Name of School, College or University _____

Additional Courses/Seminars Taken, and/or Awards: _____

_____

_____

**U.S. Citizenship:** Yes _____ No _____

Type of Employment: _____ Full Time _____ Part Time _____ Temp _____ Contract _____

Geographic Area: _____ Open to Any Area   Area Desired _____

**Skills/Abilities:** Include any skills and abilities that may be of benefit to an employer. _____

_____

_____

_____

_____

■ **Figure 16–1** Résumé Questionnaire

*(continued on next page)*

**Work History**: Under each position title, describe your duties, responsibilities, and accomplishments. Be sure to list your present or last employer first.

From/To (Mo/Yr) _____ Company Name _____

Location (City & State) _____

Position Title _____ Salary $ _____

Type of Firm or Industry _____

Responsibilities/Accomplishments: _____

_____

From/To (Mo/Yr) _____ Company Name _____

Location (City & State) _____

Position Title _____ Salary $ _____

Type of Firm or Industry _____

Responsibilities/Accomplishments: _____

_____

From/To (Mo/Yr) _____ Company Name _____

Location (City & State) _____

Position Title _____ Salary $ _____

Type of Firm or Industry _____

Responsibilities/Accomplishments: _____

_____

**Other Experience/Accomplishments:** List briefly any additional experience or accomplishments that you would consider significant. _____

_____

_____

**Industry Experience:** Please indicate the industries in which you have experience and specify type(s) (i.e., agriculture, construction). _____

_____

_____

_____

**Foreign Language(s):** _____

I hereby certify that all of the information contained herein is complete and accurate and I agree to report any changes promptly.

Signature: _____ Date: _____

■ **Figure 16–1** Résumé Questionnaire *(continued)*

**SALLY STUDENT**
**12345 SUMMER STREET**
**SANDY, SC 20000**
**(803) 555-1234**

**Sample Résumé #1**

**OBJECTIVE:**
To obtain a position in the medical industry which will enable me to use my billing and communications background, supervisory experience, administrative skills, and creative talents.

**QUALIFYING STATEMENT:**
I am hard working and have excellent verbal and communication skills in both English and Spanish. I also have the ability to handle a variety of tasks and have good organizational skills.

**EXPERIENCE:**
Medical Biller/Receptionist—Spring Street Medical Offices, 1234 Spring Street, Sandy, SC, 20001. Duties included: Billing for services using HCFA-1500 and UB-92 billing forms, billing Medicare and Medicaid patients, maintaining medical records, setting appointments, answering phones, typing correspondence, greeting clients, ordering supplies. Job was an internship for completion of requirements for Medical Billing Certificate from The Suburban School. 2/02 - present

Waitress—The Scrumptious Supper, 4567 Sister Street, Sandy, SC 20030. Duties included: Taking orders, serving customers, cashiering, assisting with making of desserts and other items, bussing tables, acting as hostess. 9/00 - 2/02

Cook/Server—McStephens Fast Hamburgers, 98765 Stale Street, Sandy, SC 20002. Duties included: Taking orders, serving customers, receiving moneys, keeping an accurate cash drawer, cooking foods (including hamburgers and fries), preparing and maintaining salad bar and condiments bar. 4/98 - 9/00

**EDUCATION:**
Medical Billing Certificate, The Suburban School, 8765 Sullen Street, Sandy, SC 20022. Maintained a 3.95 GPA and graduated among the top in the class.

Sandy Adult Community School, 84756 Seashore Street, Sandy, SC 20007. Took classes and seminars in Computer Basics, Creative Writing, Working with DOS, Windows, and Word.

Diploma. Sandy High School, 3456 Sunset Street, Sandy, SC 20012. GPA 3.75 Perfect attendance certificate, 1995, 1994. Also took two business courses.

**SKILLS:**
Computer literate in PowerPoint, Word, Quicken, type (50 wpm), 10 key (6,000 kph), understand medical terminology, knowledgeable in proper business correspondence. Speak and write in both English and Spanish. Hobbies include writing and learning computer programs.

■ **Figure 16–2** Sample Résumé #1

*(continued on next page)*

---

# RÉSUMÉ                                    **Sample Résumé #2**

**NAME:**        Holly Hopeful

**ADDRESS:**     4536 Hammer Way
                 Hollywood, CA 90611

**PHONE:**       (818) 555-1772

**EDUCATION:**   Certificate—Administrative Assisting 2004, Success School

**EXPERIENCE:**  2003–present—Program Assistant. In charge of data entry, answering telephones, typing, and creating files, flyers and circulars. I also took care of sign-in logs and scheduling appointments.

                 2002–2003—Office Manager for Sam's Shoe Store. Assisted with running the office, hiring and firing duties and maintained and ordered the stock/inventory. I also scheduled employees and handled financial records.

                 2000–2002—Sales Clerk for Sarah's Sweet Shoppe. I assisted customers, maintained the cash drawer, and maintained and ordered stock. I also handled customer service and dealt with returns and dissatisfied customers.

■ **Figure 16–3** Sample Résumé #2

| | |
|---|---|
| **Ivana Job** | **Sample Résumé #3** |
| 4646 Jessup Court | |
| Jacobs, IL 60911 | |
| (815) 555-0101 | |

**OBJECTIVE:**   A challenging position utilizing my administrative assisting skills and experience.

**QUALITIES:**   Excellent organizational and problem solving abilities. Effectively handle multiple priorities and working under pressure. Skilled with people. Computer literate. Intelligent, accurate, goal-oriented and self-motivated. Superior work ethics.

**SUMMARY OF EXPERIENCE:**   Over 15 years experience in accounting and office work with an emphasis in managing personnel for a large drug store and pharmacy.

**WORK HISTORY:**
**2003–Present**   <u>STORE MANAGER</u>: Responsible to CEO for overall operation of drug store. Administered all human resource functions including hiring, employee relations, payroll and work scheduling. Supervised and set operating procedures for numerous departments. Assisted accounting department with accounts payable, accounts receivable, general ledger and collections. Responsible for multi-account bank reconciliations, tax returns and monthly financial statements. Wrote employee policy and training manual.

**2002–2003**   <u>BUYER</u>: Extensive purchasing and merchandising responsibilities including vendor negotiations, inventory controls and setting displays. Handled advertising, sales, and promotions. Improved level of customer service.

**1998–2002**   <u>PHARMACY TECHNICIAN</u>:  Assisted pharmacists in fulfilling prescriptions. Coordinated activities of pharmacy personnel. Obtained broad technical knowledge of drugs and medical terminology. Voted employee of the month three times.

**EDUCATION, LICENSES:**   Certificate, Administrative Assisting.
Savemore School, Sandy, SC
State of SC Pharmacy Technician License #TCH 000000

■ **Figure 16–4** Sample Résumé #3

**Holly Hopeful**          **Sample Cover Letter #1**
**4536 Hammer Way**
**Hollywood, CA 90611**
**(818) 555-1772**

January 2, CCYY

Steve Springer
Personnel Supervisor
Stupendous Supports
102938 Sports Street
Sandy, SC  20020

Dear Mr. Springer:

Please consider me for an administrative assistant position with your firm.

I recently completed my education at The Suburban School, where I received a certificate in administrative assisting. I completed the course with a 3.95 grade point average and was among the top students in my class. The course covered everything an administrative assistant should know, including using reference books, time management skills, legal issues, general office procedures, computer basics, calculator basics, typing, speedwriting, proofreading, correspondence writing, Word, PowerPoint, basic office accounting, customer service, event planning and travel arrangements. I am familiar with the use of Quicken Accounting and Billing, type 50 words per minute and can enter 6,000 keystrokes per hour on the ten key.

I also completed a three-month internship at Spring Street Offices in conjunction with this course, which utilized the knowledge that I had learned. During this internship I completed administrative assistant, billing and receptionist duties for an office that staffed eight professionals and had over 7,500 customers.

I am a conscientious, enterprising person who works very hard to turn in a good performance. I enjoy being creative and industrious. I learn quickly and am more than willing to take on the challenge of learning new things. I am dependable and loyal, and have had perfect attendance at my jobs for the past three years. I also get along well with co-workers and supervisors.

Thank you for taking the time to consider my résumé. I would be happy to interview with you at your convenience.

Sincerely,

*Holly Hopeful*
Holly Hopeful

■ **Figure 16–5**   Sample Cover Letter #1

# Exercise 16-5

**Directions:**  Find and circle the words listed below. Words can appear horizontally, vertically, diagonally, forward, or backward.

```
B I D T C R S J U L X W R A W E F
C N I E O K E R J J E J H X X V K
Q N F H M V Q C B Q J R L J J I D
V C C K P Q B J O T N W S Q C R U
E J B O U C P V D W U W O O D D L
P L S M T R M E V M U O V Q I D X
P U F I E J O P Q N K E B A O R D
J Z K S R P O T Z A R R H Z Y A R
K M U B D T I E A L O K B A C H B
W S W F I E V Z E L Y T P B V G F
D V M Y S B B T J S U P D E T P D
N T N V K H T B X Z G C G R A D T
Z Y B A D E A K D T I E L C K E S
O W G D R J Q U H Z Y N D A M L I
M Q R T I U C L F I C W Y O C H V
Q V S A V A G F Q W R A X F L O K
V P L Y E U H C T I W S R E W O P
```

1. Calculator
2. Computer Disk Drive
3. Cover Letter
4. Hard Drive
5. Power Switch

# Exercise 16–6

**Directions:** Complete the crossword puzzle by filling in a word from the keywords that fits each clue.

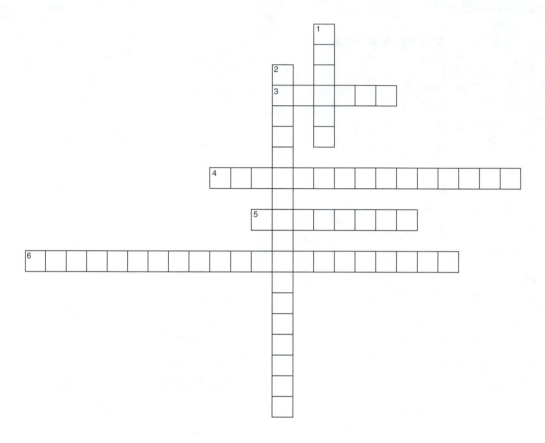

**Across**

3. A summary of employment experience and qualifications.

4. A knob that turns the contrast up and down between varying fields.

5. The primary means of communicating with your computer.

6. The rectangular box that houses the memory and functional components of the computer.

**Down**

1. The small-lighted symbol on the monitor screen that indicates where you are in the program or document.

2. A knob that changes the brightness of the image on the screen.

# Exercise 16-7

**Directions:** Match the following terms with the proper definition by writing the letter of the correct definition in the space next to the term.

**1.** _____ Central Processing Unit

**2.** _____ Computer Disk Drive

**3.** _____ Power Switch

**4.** _____ Computer Monitor

**5.** _____ Cover Letter

a. Turns the monitor on and off.

b. The screen that is connected to the computer.

c. The rectangular box that houses the memory and functional components of the computer.

d. An introduction to your résumé.

e. A place for the storage of information.

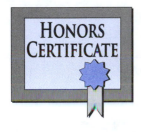

## Honors Certification™

The Honors Certification™ for this section is a timed test. You will be given several tests with problems similar to those found in Exercises 16–1 through 16–3 and will be asked to complete the problems and write in your answers. Each incorrect keystroke will result in a 2% deduction from your grade. You must achieve a score of 85% or higher to pass this test. If you fail the test on your first attempt, you may take the test one additional time. The items included in the second test may be different from those included in the first test.

There will also be a five-minute timed test to determine your average keystrokes per minute. You must achieve a speed of 200 keystrokes per minute in order to pass this test. If you fail the test on your first attempt, you may take the test one additional time. The items included in the second test may be different from those included in the first test.

## Résumé and Cover Letter

Create a perfect résumé and cover letter. This is a pass/fail item. You must be sure that there are no errors in either the cover letter or the résumé. If any errors are found, you must correct them before this item will be considered complete. When finished, your résumé and cover letter should be printed on nice paper. You may take as long as necessary to complete this challenge.

## Interview

You will be interviewed by your teacher or one of your classmates. The interview will take place in front of your class. You must dress appropriately for the interview and conduct yourself as you would in a real interview situation. This is a pass/fail situation. Whether you pass or fail will be determined by whether a majority of your classmates would give you a job based on your interview. If 85% of the class would hire you, you pass. If you fail the test on your first attempt, you may retake the test one additional time. However, 90% of the students must give you a passing score on the second interview.

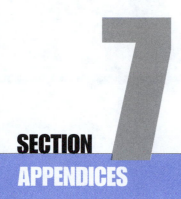

# SECTION 7
## APPENDICES

# Appendix A
# Contracts

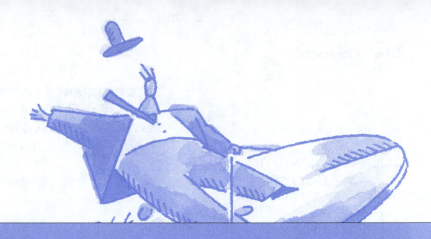

**BALL INSURANCE CARRIERS**
**(800) 555-5432**

*3895 BUBBLE BLVD. STE. 283,*
*BOXWOOD, CO 85926 (970) 555-5432*

INSURANCE CONTACT:___Betty Bell____
Policy: **XYZ Corporation**
**Basic/Major Medical Plan**

PHONE NUMBER:___(970) 555-5433____
Insurance Group # and Suffix: **62958/XYZ**
**Effective 09/1/2003**

**ELIGIBILITY** EMPLOYEE: Must work a minimum of 30 hours per week. Is eligible for coverage the first of the month following three consecutive months of continuous employment.

DEPENDENTS: Are eligible for coverage from birth to age 19 or to age 23 if a full-time student or handicapped prior to age 19/23 (proof of disability must be furnished within 31 days after dependent reaches limiting age). Not eligible as a dependent if eligible as an employee. Unmarried natural children, legally adopted and foster children are included (includes legal guardianship). If both parents are covered by the plan, children may be covered by one employee only.

**EFFECTIVE DATE** EMPLOYEE: If written application is made prior to eligibility date, coverage becomes effective the first of the month following three months of continuous employment.

DEPENDENTS: The date acquired by the covered employee becomes the effective date if written application is made within 31 days of eligibility date. If confined in a hospital on date of eligibility, coverage will not start until the first of the month following the date the confinement ends. Newborns are automatically covered for the first 30 days following birth. Coverage will be terminated after 30 days unless written application for coverage is submitted by the employee within 31 days of birth.

**TERMINATION OF COVERAGE** EMPLOYEE: Coverage terminates the last day of the month following termination of employment, or when the employee ceases to qualify as an eligible employee, or following request for termination of coverage.

DEPENDENTS: Coverage terminates the date the employee's coverage terminates or the last day of the month during which the dependent no longer qualifies as an eligible dependent.

### BASIC BENEFITS

**PREADMISSION TESTING**—Outpatient diagnostic tests performed prior to inpatient admissions; paid at 100% of UCR.

**SUPPLEMENTAL ACCIDENT EXPENSE**—100% of the first $300 for services incurred within 90 days of accident.

**INPATIENT HOSPITAL EXPENSE**
DEDUCTIBLE: $50.
ROOM AND BOARD: 100% Up to semi-private room charge. ICU up to $600 per day.
MISCELLANEOUS FEES: 100% Unlimited.
MAXIMUM PERIOD: Ten days per period of disability.
**SURGERY** CONVERSION FACTOR: $8.50.
CALENDAR YEAR MAXIMUM: $1,600 per person.
REMARKS: Voluntary sterilizations covered.
**ASSISTANT SURGERY**
CONVERSION FACTOR: $8.50.
CALENDAR YEAR MAXIMUM ALLOWANCE: $320 per person. Maximum of 20% of surgeon's allowance or billed charge, whichever is less.
REMARKS: Voluntary sterilizations covered for women only.
**IN-HOSPITAL PHYSICIANS**
DAILY MAXIMUM: $21 for the first day; $8 per day thereafter.
MAXIMUM PERIOD: Ten days per period of disability.
REMARKS: Only one doctor can be paid per day.
**ANESTHESIA**
CONVERSION FACTOR: $7.50.
CALENDAR YEAR MAXIMUM: $300 per person.
REMARKS: Voluntary sterilizations covered.
**OUTPATIENT PHYSICIANS VISITS**
CONVERSION FACTOR: $7.50.
CALENDAR YEAR MAXIMUM: $300 per person.
REMARKS: Chiropractors, M.D.s, D.O.s and acupuncturists allowed.
**X-RAY AND LABORATORY**
CONVERSION FACTOR: $7.
CALENDAR YEAR MAXIMUM: $200 per person.
REMARKS: Professional component charges covered at 40% of UCR allowance for procedure. Routine procedures are not covered.

### MAJOR MEDICAL EXPENSES

**INDIVIDUAL CALENDAR YEAR DEDUCTIBLE:** $125; three month carryover provision.
**FAMILY MAXIMUM DEDUCTIBLE:** Two family members must satisfy their individual calendar year deductible in order to satisfy the family deductible.
**STANDARD COINSURANCE:** 80%.
COINSURANCE LIMIT: $400 out-of-pocket per individual; $800 out-of-pocket per family (not to include deductible); aggregate.

**APPLICATION OF COINSURANCE LIMIT:** Coinsurance limit applies in the calendar year in which the limit is met and the following calendar year.

**OUTPATIENT MENTAL/NERVOUS EXPENSE:** 50% coinsurance while not a hospital inpatient.

**LIFETIME MAXIMUM:** $1,000,000 per person.

**ROOM LIMIT:** Semi-private room rate.

**HOSPITAL DEDUCTIBLE:** Not covered.

**HOME HEALTH CARE:** 120 visits per calendar year. Prior hospital confinement required.

**PREEXISTING LIMITATION:** If treatment received within six months prior to effective date, $2,000 maximum payment until patient has been covered continuously under the plan for 12 months.

**ANESTHESIA:** Calculated using actual time.

## MEDICARE

TYPE: Coordination of Benefits.

REMARKS: Assume all Medicare benefits whether or not individual actually enrolled. Subject to all other plan provisions.

## EXCLUSIONS

1. Expenses resulting from self-inflicted injuries.
2. Work-related injuries or illnesses.
3. Services for which there is no charge in the absence of insurance.
4. Charges or services in excess of UCR or not medically necessary.
5. Charges for completion of claim forms and failure to keep appointments.
6. Routine or preventative or experimental services.
7. Eye refractions, contacts or glasses, orthotics (eye exercises); radial keratotomy, or other procedures for surgical correction of refractive errors.
8. Custodial care.
9. Cosmetic surgery unless for repair of an injury or surgery incurred while covered or result of mastectomy.
10. Dental care of teeth, gums or alveolar process (TMJ) except: a) reduction of fractures of the jaw or facial bones; b) surgical correction of harelip, cleft palate or prognathism; c) removal of salivary duct stones; d) removal of bony cysts of jaw, torus palatinus, leukoplakia, or malignant tissues.
11. Reversal of voluntary sterilization.
12. Diagnosis or treatment of infertility including artificial insemination, in vitro fertilization, etc.
13. Contraceptive materials or devices.
14. Non-therapeutic abortions except where the life of the mother is endangered.
15. Expenses for obesity, weight reduction, or diet control unless at least 100 lbs. overweight.
16. Vitamins, food supplements and/or protein supplements.
17. Sex-altering treatments or surgeries or related studies.
18. Orthopedic shoes or other devices for support or treatment of feet except as medically necessary following foot surgery.
19. Bio-feedback related services or treatment.
20. Experimental transplants.
21. EDTA Chelation therapy.

## COMPREHENSIVE DENTAL BENEFITS

**DEDUCTIBLE:** $50.

**FAMILY DEDUCTIBLE LIMIT:** $150; nonaggregate.

**COINSURANCE:** 80%.

**MAXIMUM:** No lifetime maximum. $1,000 per calendar year maximum.

**SPACE MAINTAINER ELIGIBILITY:** Employees and dependents.

**FLUORIDE ELIGIBILITY:** Dependents up to age 18 only.

**ORTHODONTIA:** No coverage.

**CLAIM COST CONTROL:** Predetermination of benefits and alternate course of treatment based on customarily employed methods.

**PROSTHETIC REPLACEMENTS:** Five-year replacement rule applies to replacements of any previously installed prosthetics.

**ORDERED AND UNDELIVERED:** Excludes expenses for any devices installed or delivered after 30 days following termination of insurance.

**ORAL SURGERY:** Covered at regular coinsurance rate, subject to calendar year maximum.

**EXTENSION OF BENEFITS:** 12 months.

**MISSING AND UNREPLACED:** Applies.

**ROVER INSURERS INC**
**5931 ROLLING ROAD**
**RONSON, CO 81369**
**(970) 555-1369**

INSURANCE CONTACT: __Ravyn Ranger__                    PHONE NUMBER: __(970) 555-1360__

POLICY: **NINJA ENTERPRISES**, 1234 Nockout Road, Newton, NM 88012          Effective 01/01/2001
INSURANCE GROUP # AND SUFFIX:     **21088/NIN**

## ELIGIBILITY

EMPLOYEES must work a minimum of 30 hours per week. They are eligible for coverage the first of the month following one consecutive month of continuous employment. DEPENDENTS are eligible for coverage from birth to age 19, or to age 25 if a full-time student or handicapped prior to age 19/25. Is not eligible as a dependent if eligible as an employee. Unmarried natural children, legally adopted children, foster children, and legal guardianship children are included. If both parents are covered by the plan, children may be covered by one parent only.

**EFFECTIVE DATE** - EMPLOYEE becomes effective, if written application is made prior to eligibility date, on the first of the month following 30 days of continuous employment. If employee is absent from work due to disability on the date of eligibility, coverage will not start until the first of the month following the date of return to active work.
DEPENDENTS become effective on the date the covered employee becomes effective, if written application is made within 31 days of eligibility date. If confined in a hospital on the date of eligibility, coverage will not start until the first of the month following the date the confinement ends. Newborns are automatically covered for the first 14 days following birth. Coverage terminates after 14 days unless written application for coverage is submitted by the employee within 31 days of birth.

**TERMINATION OF COVERAGE** - EMPLOYEE'S coverage terminates the last day of the month following termination of employment or when the employee ceases to qualify as an eligible employee, or following request for termination of coverage. DEPENDENTS' coverage terminates the date the employee's coverage terminates, or the last day of the month during which the dependent no longer qualifies as an eligible dependent.

**EXTENSION OF BENEFITS** - If covered under the plan when disabled, may continue coverage in accordance with COBRA. No other extension available.

## COMPREHENSIVE MEDICAL BENEFITS

**PREADMISSION TESTING** - Outpatient diagnostic tests performed prior to inpatient admissions are paid at 100% whether through a network provider or not.

**PRECERTIFICATION** - Voluntary, nonemergency inpatient admissions must be approved at least five days prior to admission. Emergency admissions must be precertified within 48 hrs. of admission. Benefits are reduced to 50% if not performed as required.

**SECOND SURGICAL OPINION** - The SSO is paid at 100% of UCR. It is required for the following: bunionectomy, cataract extraction, chemonucleolysis, cholecystectomy, coronary bypass, hemorrhoidectomy, hysterectomy, inguinal herniorrhaphy, laparotomy, laminectomy, mastectomy, meniscectomy, oophorectomy, prostatectomy, salpingectomy, submucous resection, total joint replacement (hip or knee), tenotomy, varicose veins (all procedures). **IF SSO NOT PERFORMED, ALL RELATED EXPENSES PAYABLE AT 50%.**

**SUPPLEMENTAL ACCIDENT EXPENSE** - 100% is paid on the first $500 for services incurred within 90 days of the date of accident. Subject to $20 copayment. After $500, payments are subject to calendar year deductible. Provider does not have to be a network member to receive 100% benefit. Common accident provision applies.

**OUTPATIENT FACILITY CHARGES PAYABLE AT 100%** - Network outpatient facility expenses for following procedures paid 100%. Does not include professional charges: arthroscopy, breast biopsy, cataract removal, bronchoscopy, deviated nasal septum, pilonidal cyst, myringotomy w/tubes, esophagoscopy, colonoscopy, herniorrhaphy (umbilical, to five years old), skin and subsequent lesions, benign and malignant (2cms+).

**INDIVIDUAL CALENDAR YEAR DEDUCTIBLE** - $150; three month carryover provision. All plan services subject to deductible unless otherwise indicated.

**FAMILY MAXIMUM DEDUCTIBLE** - $300, nonaggregate. Two family members must meet individual deductible limit.

**STANDARD COINSURANCE** - 80% for Network providers; 60% for Non-network providers.
**COINSURANCE LIMIT** - $1,250 out-of-pocket per individual; $2,500 out-of-pocket per family. Two individuals must meet their individual out-of-pocket limit to satisfy the family limit. Limits not to include deductible, surgery expenses reduced because SSO not performed, or hospital benefits reduced because precertification not performed. 100% of allowed amount paid thereafter for network providers; 80% for non-network providers.

**LIFETIME MAXIMUM** - $1,000,000 per person.

**PREEXISTING LIMITATION** - If treatment is received within 90 days prior to effective date, no coverage on that condition for six months from the effective date (continuously covered for six consecutive months) unless treatment free for three consecutive months which ends after the effective date of coverage.

**INPATIENT HOSPITAL EXPENSE**               **IF NO PRECERTIFICATION, ADMISSION PAID AT 50%**
**DEDUCTIBLE - $200,** waived for network facilities, applies to non-network. Inpatient hospital expenses not subject to regular Major Medical deductible.
ROOM AND BOARD - Network providers: 80% of semi-private/ICU; Non-network providers: 60% of semi-private/ICU.
MISCELLANEOUS FEES - Network: 80%; Non-network: 60%.
EXCLUSIONS - Well baby care. Automatic coverage for first seven days if baby is ill. Otherwise, no coverage.

**MENTAL/NERVOUS/PSYCHONEUROTIC** - Includes substance abuse and alcoholism.
    <u>OUTPATIENT MENTAL AND NERVOUS TREATMENT</u>
    PAYABLE - $60 per visit for first 5 visits; $30 per visit for next 21 visits.
    COINSURANCE - 80% for first five visits (maximum payable: $60 per visit), 50% per visit for next 21 visits      (maximum payable: $30 per visit).
    CALENDAR YEAR MAXIMUM - 26 visits.
    <u>INPATIENT MENTAL AND NERVOUS TREATMENT</u>
    PHYSICIAN SERVICES - 70% applies to network and non-network providers.
    HOSPITAL SERVICES - 70% network and non-network providers.

**MAMMOGRAMS**
COINSURANCE - 80% Network providers; 60% Non-network providers.
REQUIREMENTS - Baseline mammogram for women age 35–39; for ages 40–49, one allowed every two years; for ages 50+, one allowed every year.

**X-RAY AND LABORATORY** - PROFESSIONAL COMPONENTS - Professional charges paid at 25% of UCR.

**DURABLE MEDICAL EQUIPMENT**
COINSURANCE - 50%.
REQUIREMENTS - Prescribed by M.D.; must not be primarily necessary for exercise, environmental control, convenience, comfort or hygiene. Must be an article only useful for the prescribed patient. Covered up to purchase price only.

**ANESTHESIA:** Use actual time.

**MEDICARE**
TYPE - Maintenance of benefits.
REMARKS - Assume all Medicare benefits whether or not individual actually enrolled. Subject to all other plan provisions.

**EXCLUSIONS**
1. Expenses resulting from self-inflicted injuries.
2. Work-related injuries or illnesses.

3. Services for which there is no charge in the absence of insurance.
4. Charges or services in excess of UCR or not medically necessary.
5. Pre-existing conditions.
6. Charges for completion of claim forms and failure to keep appointments.
7. Routine or preventative or experimental services.
8. Eye refractions; contacts or glasses; orthotics (eye exercises); radial keratotomy, or other procedures for surgical correction of refractive errors.
9. Custodial care.
10. Cosmetic surgery unless for repair of an injury or surgery incurred while covered or result of mastectomy.
11. Biofeedback related services or treatment.
12. Dental care of teeth, gums or alveolar process (TMJ) except: a) reduction of fractures of the jaw or facial bones; b) surgical correction of harelip, cleft palate or prognathism; c) removal of salivary duct stones; d) removal of bony cysts of jaw, torus palatinus, leukoplakia, or malignant tissues.
13. Reversal of voluntary sterilization.
14. Diagnosis or treatment of infertility including artificial insemination, in vitro fertilization, etc.
15. Contraceptive materials or devices.
16. Pregnancy; pregnancy-related expenses of dependent children for the delivery including Caesarian section. Related illnesses may be covered such as pre-eclampsia, vaginal bleeding, etc.
17. Non-therapeutic abortions except where the life of the mother is endangered.
18. Vitamins.

**WINTER INSURANCE COMPANY**
**9763 WESTERN WAY, WHITTIER,**
**CO 82963, (970) 555-2963**

POLICY: ABC CORPORATION, POLICY NAME: ABC, EFFECTIVE DATE: 06/01/02
INSURANCE GROUP # and SUFFIX: 36928/ABC
INSURANCE CONTACT:   Wilma Williams

PHONE NUMBER:   (970) 555-2964

**ELIGIBILITY** EMPLOYEE: Must work a minimum of 35 hours per week. Is eligible for coverage the first of the month following 60 consecutive days of continuous employment.

DEPENDENTS: Are eligible for coverage from birth to age 19, or to age 24 if a full-time student or handicapped prior to age 19/24 (proof of disability must be furnished within 31 days after dependent reaches limiting age). Dependent is not eligible as a dependent if eligible as an employee. Unmarried natural children, legally adopted and foster children are included (also includes legal guardianship). If both parents are covered by the plan, children may be covered by one employee only.

**EFFECTIVE DATE** EMPLOYEE: If written application is made prior to the eligibility date, coverage becomes effective the first of the month following 60 days of employment.

DEPENDENTS: The date acquired by the covered employee becomes the effective date if written application is made within 31 days of the eligibility date. Newborns are automatically covered for the first seven days following birth; well-baby charges excluded. Coverage will terminate after seven days unless written application for coverage is submitted by the employee within 31 days of birth.

**TERMINATION OF COVERAGE** EMPLOYEE: Coverage terminates the last day of the month following termination of employment or when the employee ceases to qualify as an eligible employee, or following request for termination of coverage.

DEPENDENTS: Coverage terminates the date the employee's coverage terminates, or the last day of the month during which the dependent no longer qualifies as an eligible dependent.

**EXTENSION OF BENEFITS** If covered under the plan when disabled, employee may continue coverage for 12 months following the date of termination or until no longer disabled, whichever is less.

### COMPREHENSIVE MEDICAL BENEFITS

**SUPPLEMENTAL ACCIDENT EXPENSE** 100% of first $300 for services incurred within 120 days of date of accident. Not subject to deductible.

**PLAN BENEFITS**
INDIVIDUAL CALENDAR YEAR DEDUCTIBLE: $100; three month carryover provision.
FAMILY MAXIMUM DEDUCTIBLE: $200, aggregate.
STANDARD COINSURANCE: 90% except 100% of hospital room and board expenses for 365 days per lifetime.
COINSURANCE LIMIT: $750 out-of-pocket per individual; $1,500 out-of-pocket per family. Two separate members must satisfy the individual limit, not to include deductible. Applies only in the calendar year in which the limit is met.
LIFETIME MAXIMUM: $300,000 per person.
PREEXISTING LIMITATION: On 6/1/99 no restriction. After 6/1/99, if treatment received within 90 days prior to effective date, no coverage for that condition for 12 months from the effective date (continuously covered for 12 months) unless treatment free for three consecutive months ending after the effective date of coverage.

**X-RAY AND LABORATORY**
REMARKS: Professional component charges covered at 40% of UCR allowance for procedure. Routine procedures are not covered.

**INPATIENT HOSPITAL EXPENSE**
Room and board payable at 100% of semi-private room rate. Miscellaneous expenses covered at 90%. Nonmedically necessary, well baby care and cosmetic services excluded. Personal comfort items not covered.

**MENTAL/NERVOUS/PSYCHONEUROTIC**
INCLUDES SUBSTANCE ABUSE AND ALCOHOLISM.
OUTPATIENT MENTAL/NERVOUS TREATMENT
COINSURANCE: 50% while not hospital confined.
CALENDAR YEAR MAXIMUM: None.
INPATIENT MENTAL/NERVOUS TREATMENT
PHYSICIAN SERVICES: Covered at 90%.
HOSPITAL SERVICES: Covered at 90%.
ALLOWED PROVIDERS: Psychiatrists and clinical psychologists. Marriage and Family Child Counselor and Licensed Clinical Social Worker allowed with referral from M.D.

**EXTENDED CARE FACILITY**
LIFETIME MAXIMUM: 60 days.

HOSPITAL SERVICES: 80% of billed room and board charge.

REQUIREMENTS: Stay must begin within 14 days of acute hospital stay of at least three days. Extended care must be due to same disability that caused hospitalization and continued hospital care would otherwise be required.

## DURABLE MEDICAL EQUIPMENT

COINSURANCE: Covered at 90%.

REQUIREMENTS: Must be prescribed by M.D. Must not be primarily necessary for exercise, environmental control, convenience, comfort, or hygiene. Must only be useful for the prescribed patient. Covered up to purchase price only.

## ANESTHESIA

Computed using block time.

## REMARKS

Covered expenses include charges for the initial set of contact lenses which are necessary due to cataract surgery. Handicapped children are limited to a $15,000 lifetime maximum after attainment of age 19. Coordination of Benefits according to National Association of Insurance Carriers (NAIC) guidelines. Subject to Third Party Liability and subrogation.

## MEDICARE INTEGRATION

TYPE: Nonduplication of benefits applies.

REMARKS: Assume all Medicare benefits whether or not individual actually enrolled.

## EXCLUSIONS

1. Expenses resulting from self-inflicted injuries, work related injuries, or illnesses.
2. Charges or services: in excess of UCR, not medically necessary, for completion of claim forms, for failure to keep appointments; for routine, preventative, or experimental services.
3. Eye refractions; contacts or glasses; orthotics (eye exercises); radial keratotomy, or other procedures for surgical correction of refractive errors.
4. Custodial care and/or convalescent facility coverage.
5. Cosmetic surgery unless for repair of an injury or surgery incurred while covered or result of mastectomy.
6. Diagnosis or treatment of infertility including artificial insemination, in vitro fertilization, etc., contraceptive materials or devices, non-therapeutic abortions except where the life of the mother is endangered, reversal of voluntary sterilization.
7. Pregnancy-related expenses for dependent children.
8. Expenses for obesity, weight reduction, or diet control unless at least 100 lbs. overweight.
9. Vitamins, food supplements, and/or protein supplements.
10. Sex altering treatments or surgeries or related studies.
11. Orthopedic shoes or other devices for support or treatment of feet except as medically necessary following foot surgery.
12. Bio-feedback related services or treatment, EDTA chelation therapy.

## COMPREHENSIVE DENTAL BENEFITS

INTEGRATED: Deductible provisions, lifetime maximum and coinsurance limit combined with comprehensive Major Medical.

CALENDAR YEAR DEDUCTIBLE: $100.

DEDUCTIBLE CARRYOVER: No carryover.

FAMILY DEDUCTIBLE LIMIT: $200, aggregate.

COINSURANCE: 90%.

COINSURANCE LIMIT: $500 (Patient responsibility, not to include disallowed amounts or the deductible.)

APPLICATION OF COINSURANCE LIMIT: Applies only in the calendar year in which the limit is met.

FAMILY COINSURANCE LIMIT: $1,000.

MAXIMUM: $300,000 lifetime.

MAXIMUM PER CALENDAR YEAR: $1,500.

ORTHODONTIA ELIGIBILITY: Dependents only.

SPACE MAINTAINER ELIGIBILITY: Dependents only.

FLUORIDE ELIGIBILITY: Employees and dependents.

ORTHODONTIC: 90% coinsurance.

ORTHODONTIC MAXIMUM: $800 lifetime; not subject to the $1,500 calendar year maximum.

CLAIM COST CONTROL OPTIONS: Predetermination of benefits required on claims over $500; alternate course of treatment based on customarily employed method. Benefits cut to 50% if no predetermination done.

PROSTHETIC REPLACEMENTS: Five-year rule applies to replacement of any previously installed prosthetics.

ORDERED AND UNDELIVERED: Excludes expenses for any devices installed or delivered after 30 days following termination date of insurance.

MISSING AND UNREPLACED EXCLUSION: Applies.

REMARKS: Orthodontic benefits are payable as incurred, rather than amortized over the period of time during which work is performed.

## *SMALL GROUP HMO CONTRACT*

[Carrier] **Summer Insurance Company**
18932 Spring Road, Autumn, CO 82974
(970) 555-9631

INSURANCE CONTACT:___Sammy Rock

**CONTRACT HOLDER:** Rocky Company
1234 Ribbon Road, Rudolph, CO 81208
**Effective Date of Contract:** January 1, 1998
**Insurance Group # and Suffix:** 67980/ROC
PHONE NUMBER:___(970) 555-9632

**ELIGIBILITY** EMPLOYEES: Actively at work for a minimum of 35 hours per week. Is eligible after 30 continuous work days.

Employees who enroll more than 30 days after their employment date are considered Late Enrollees. Late Enrollees are subject to this Contract's Preexisting Conditions limitation.

Coverage terminates the date an Employee ceases to be an Actively-at-Work, Full-time Employee for any reason.
DEPENDENTS: Dependents include the Employee's legal spouse, the Employee's unmarried Dependent children who are under age 19, and the Employee's unmarried Dependent children, from age 19 until their 23rd birthday, who are enrolled as full-time students at accredited schools.
EXCEPTION: Any dependent who does not reside in the Service Area is not an eligible Dependent. Eligible Dependents will not include any Dependent who is covered by this Contract as an Employee or on active duty in the armed forces of any country.

"Unmarried Dependent children" include legally adopted children, step-children if they depend on the Employee for most of their support and maintenance, and children under a court appointed guardianship.

### THE ROLE OF A MEMBER'S PRIMARY CARE PHYSICIAN (PCP)

A Member's PCP provides basic health maintenance services and coordinates a Member's overall health care. Anytime a Member needs medical care, the Member should contact his or her Primary Care Physician. In a Medical Emergency, a Member may go directly to the emergency room. If a Member does, then the Member must call his or her Primary Care Physician or the Care Manager and Member Services within 48 hours, or We will provide services under this HMO Plan only if We determine that notice was given as soon as was reasonably possible.

### REFERRAL FORMS

A Member can be referred for Specialist Services by a Member's PCP. Except in the case of a Medical Emergency, a Member will not be eligible for any services provided by anyone other than a Member's PCP (including but not limited to Specialist Services) if a Member has not been referred by his or her PCP. Referrals must be obtained prior to receiving services and supplies from any Practitioner other than the Member's PCP.

### MEDICAL NECESSITY

Members will receive designated benefits only when Medically Necessary and Appropriate. We or the Care Manager may determine whether any benefit was Medically Necessary and Appropriate, and We have the option to select the appropriate Participating Hospital to render services if hospitalization is necessary. Decisions as to what is Medically Necessary and Appropriate are subject to review by our quality assessment committee or its physician designee.

### LIMITATION ON SERVICES

Except in cases of Medical Emergency, services are available only from Participating Providers. We shall have no liability or obligation to cover any service or benefit sought or received by a Member from any Physician, Hospital, other Provider unless prior arrangements are made by Us.

### SCHEDULE OF SERVICES AND SUPPLIES

The services or supplies covered under the contract are subject to all copayments and are determined per calendar year per Member, unless otherwise stated. Maximums apply only to the specific services provided.

### SERVICES COPAYMENTS:

Copayment $15, unless otherwise stated.
Emergency Room Copayment $50, credited toward Inpatient admission if admitted within 24 hours.
Coinsurance 0% except as stated on the Schedule of Services and Supplies for Prescription Drugs.
### MAXIMUM LIFETIME BENEFITS
Unlimited, **except** as otherwise stated.

### HOSPITAL SERVICES:

**INPATIENT** $150 Copayment/day for a maximum of five days/admission. Maximum Copayment $1,500 per Calendar Year. Unlimited days.
**OUTPATIENT** $15 Copayment/visit.

### PRACTITIONER SERVICES RECEIVED AT A HOSPITAL:

**INPATIENT VISIT** $0 Copayment.
**OUTPATIENT VISIT** $15 Copayment/visit; no Copayment if any other Copayment applies.
EMERGENCY ROOM $50 Copayment/visit/Member (credited toward Inpatient Admission if Admission occurs within 24 hours).

**SURGERY:**
**INPATIENT** $0 Copayment.
**OUTPATIENT** $15 Copayment/visit.
**HOME HEALTH CARE** Unlimited days, if preapproved; $0 Copayment.
**HOSPICE SERVICES** Unlimited days, if preapproved; $0 Copayment.
**MATERNITY/PRENATAL CARE** $25 Copayment for initial visit only; $0 Copayment thereafter.

**MENTAL NERVOUS CONDITIONS AND SUBSTANCE ABUSE:**
**OUTPATIENT** $15 Copayment/visit maximum 20 visits/Calendar Year.
**INPATIENT** $150 Copayment/day for a maximum of five days per admission. Maximum Copayment: $1,500/ Calendar Year. Maximum of 30 days inpatient care/ Calendar Year. One Inpatient day may be exchanged for two Outpatient visits.

**THERAPEUTIC MANIPULATION** $15 Copayment/visit; maximum 30 visits/Calendar Year.
**PODIATRIC** $15 Copayment/visit (excludes Routine Foot Care).
**PREADMISSION TESTING** $15 Copayment/visit.
**PRESCRIPTION DRUG** 50% Coinsurance (May be substituted by Carrier with $15 Copayment.)
**PRIMARY CARE PHYSICIAN** $15 Copayment/visit.
**OR CARE MANAGER SERVICES (OUTSIDE HOSPITAL)**
**PRIMARY CARE SERVICES** $15 Copayment/visit.
**REHABILITATION SERVICES** Subject to the Inpatient Hospital Services Copayment above. The Copayment does not apply if Admission is immediately preceded by a Hospital Inpatient Stay.
**SECOND SURGICAL OPINION** $15 Copayment/visit.
**SPECIALIST SERVICES** $15 Copayment/visit.
**SKILLED NURSING CENTER** Unlimited days, if preapproved; $0 Copayment.
**THERAPY SERVICES** $15 Copayment/visit.
**DIAGNOSTIC SERVICES.**
**INPATIENT** $0 Copayment.
**OUTPATIENT** $15 Copayment/visit.

**NOTE:** No services or supplies will be provided if a Member fails to obtain preauthorization of care through his or her primary care physician or health center or care manager. Read the Member provisions carefully before obtaining medical care, services, or supplies. Refer to the section of this contract called "Noncovered Services and Supplies" for a list of the services and supplies for which a Member is not eligible for coverage under this contract.

**COVERED SERVICES & SUPPLIES**
Under this HMO Plan, Members are entitled to receive the benefits in the following sections when Medically Necessary and Appropriate, subject to the payment by Members of applicable copayments as stated in the applicable Schedule of Services and Supplies.

**(a) OUTPATIENT SERVICES.** The following services are covered only at the PCP's office, or elsewhere upon prior written Referral by a Member's PCP:

1. **Office visits** during office hours, and during non-office hours when Medically Necessary.
2. **Home visits** by a Member's PCP.
3. **Periodic health examinations** to include:
    a. Well child care from birth including immunizations.
    b. Routine physical examinations, including eye examinations.
    c. Routine gynecologic exams and related services.
    d. Routine ear and hearing examination.
    e. Routine allergy injections and immunizations (but not if solely for the purpose of travel or as a requirement of a Member's employment).
4. **Diagnostic Services.**
5. **Casts and dressings.**
6. **Ambulance Service** when certified in writing as Medically Necessary by a Member's PCP and approved in advance by Us.
7. **Procedures and prescription drugs to enhance fertility,** except where specifically excluded in this Contract.
8. **Prosthetic Devices** when We arrange for them. We cover only the initial fitting and purchase of artificial limbs and eyes, and other prosthetic devices. We do not cover replacements, repairs, or wigs.
9. **Durable Medical Equipment** when ordered by a Member's PCP and arranged through Us.
10. **Prescription Drugs and contraceptives which require a Practitioner's prescription,** insulin syringes and needles, glucose test strips and lancets, colostomy bags, belts, and irrigators when obtained through a Participating Provider. A prescription or refill will not include more than:
    a. the greater of a 30 day supply or 100 unit doses for each prescription or refill; or
    b. the amount usually prescribed by the Member's Participating Provider.
11. **Nutritional Counseling** for the management of disease.
12. **Dental x-rays** when related to Covered Services.
13. **Oral surgery** in connection with bone fractures, removal of tumors and orthodontogenic cysts, and other surgical procedures, as We approve.
14. **Food and Food Products for Inherited Metabolic Diseases**: We cover charges incurred for the therapeutic treatment of inherited metabolic diseases, including the purchase of medical foods

(enteral formula) and low protein modified food products. For the purpose of this benefit: "inherited metabolic disease" means a disease caused by an inherited abnormality of body chemistry for which testing is mandated by law.

**(b) INPATIENT HOSPICE, HOSPITAL, REHABILITATION CENTER, AND SKILLED NURSING CENTER BENEFITS.** The following services are covered when hospitalized by a Participating Provider at Participating Hospitals (or at Nonparticipating facilities upon prior written authorization by Us):

1. Semi-private room and board accommodations Except as stated below, We provide coverage for Inpatient care for:
   a. a minimum of 72 hours following a modified radical mastectomy.
   b. a minimum of 48 hours following a simple mastectomy.

   We also provide coverage for the mother and newly born child for:
   a. up to 48 hours of inpatient care following a vaginal delivery.
   b. a minimum of 96 hours of inpatient care following a cesarean section.

   We provide such coverage subject to the following:
   a. the attending Practitioner must determine that inpatient care is medically necessary; or
   b. the mother must request the inpatient care.

2. Private accommodations will be provided only when approved in advance by Us. If a Member occupies a private room without such certification, Member shall be liable for the difference between payment by Us to the Provider and the private room rate.
3. General nursing care.
4. Use of intensive or special care facilities.
5. X-ray examinations including CAT scans but not dental x-rays.
6. Use of operating room and related facilities.
7. Magnetic resonance imaging "MRI".
8. Drugs, medications, biologicals.
9. Cardiography/Encephalography.
10. Laboratory testing and services.
11. Pre- and postoperative care.
12. Special tests.
13. Nuclear medicine.
14. Therapy Services.
15. Oxygen and oxygen therapy.
16. Anesthesia and anesthesia services.
17. Blood, blood products, and blood processing.
18. Intravenous injections and solutions.
19. Surgical, medical, and obstetrical services; We also cover reconstructive breast Surgery, Surgery to restore and achieve symmetry between the two breasts, and the cost of prostheses following a mastectomy on one breast or both breasts.
20. Private duty nursing only when approved in advance by Us.
21. The following transplants: Cornea, Kidney, Lung, Liver, Heart, and Pancreas.
22. Allogeneic bone marrow transplants.
23. Autologous bone marrow transplants and associated dose intensive chemotherapy: only for treatment of Leukemia, Lymphoma, Neuroblastoma, Aplastic Anemia, Genetic Disorders (SCID and WISCOT Alldrich) and Breast Cancer, when approved in advance by Us, if the Member is participating in a clinical trial.
24. Peripheral Blood Stem Cell Transplants.

**(c) BENEFITS FOR SUBSTANCE ABUSE AND NON-BIOLOGICALLY-BASED MENTAL ILLNESSES.** The following services are covered when rendered by a Participating Provider at Provider's office or at a Participating Substance Abuse Center or Health Center upon prior written referral by a Member's PCP. This section does not address coverage for a Biologically-based Mental Illness.

1. **Outpatient.** Members are entitled to receive up to twenty (20) outpatient visits per Calendar Year. Benefits include diagnosis, medical, psychiatric and psychological treatment and medical referral services by a Member's PCP or the Care Manager for the abuse of or addiction to drugs and Non-Biologically-based Mental Illnesses. Payment for non-medical ancillary services (such as vocational rehabilitation or employment counseling) is not provided. Members are additionally eligible, upon referral by a Member's PCP or the Care Manager, for up to sixty (60) more outpatient visits by exchanging one or more of the inpatient hospital days described below where each exchanged inpatient day provides two outpatient visits.
2. **Inpatient Hospital Care.** Members are entitled to receive up to thirty (30) days of inpatient care benefits for detoxification, medical treatment for medical conditions resulting from the substance abuse, referral services for substance abuse or addiction, and Non-Biologically-based Mental Illnesses.

**(d) BENEFITS FOR BIOLOGICALLY-BASED MENTAL ILLNESS OR ALCOHOL ABUSE.** We cover treatment of a Biologically-based Mental Illness or Alcohol Abuse the same way We would for any other illness. We do not pay for Custodial care, education, or training.

**(e) EMERGENCY CARE BENEFITS - WITHIN AND OUTSIDE OUR SERVICE AREA.** The following Services are covered under this HMO Plan without prior written referral by a Member's PCP in the event of a Medical Emergency as Determined by Us.

1. A Member's PCP is required to provide or arrange

for on-call coverage twenty-four (24) hours a day, seven (7) days a week. Unless a delay would be detrimental to a Member's health, Member shall call a Member's PCP or Health Center or Us or the Care Manager prior to seeking emergency treatment.

2. In the event Members are hospitalized in a Nonparticipating Facility, coverage will only be provided until Members are medically able to travel or be transported to a Participating Facility. If Members elect to continue treatment with Nonparticipating Providers, We shall have no responsibility for payment beyond the date Members are Determined to be medically able to be transported. If transportation is Medically Necessary, We will cover the reasonable and customary cost. Members will be subject to all Copayments which would have been required had similar benefits been provided upon prior written referral to a Participating Provider.

3. The Copayment for an emergency room visit will be credited toward the Hospital Inpatient Copayment if Members are admitted as an Inpatient to the Hospital as a result of the Medical Emergency.

**(f) THERAPY SERVICES.** The following Services are covered.

1. Speech, Physical, Occupational, and Cognitive Therapies are covered for non-chronic conditions and acute Illnesses and Injuries. This benefit consists of treatment for a 60 day period per incident of Illness or Injury, beginning with the first day of treatment, provided that a Member's PCP certifies in writing that the treatment will result in a significant improvement of a Member's condition within this time period and treatment is approved in writing by Us.

2. Chelation Therapy, Chemotherapy treatment, Dialysis Treatment, Infusion Therapy, Radiation Therapy, and Respiration Therapy.

**(g) HOME HEALTH SERVICES.** The following Services are covered.

1. **Skilled nursing services,** provided by or under the supervision of a registered professional nurse.

2. Services of a **home health aide**, under the supervision of a registered professional nurse, or if appropriate, a qualified speech or physical therapist.

3. **Medical Social Services** by or under the supervision of a qualified medical or psychiatric social worker, in conjunction with other Home Health Services, if the PCP certifies that such services are essential for the effective treatment of a Member's medical condition.

4. **Therapy Services** as set forth above.

5. **Hospice Care** if Members are terminally Ill or terminally Injured with life expectancy of six months or less, as certified by the Member's PCP. Services may include home and hospital visits by nurses and social workers; pain management and symptom control; instruction and supervision of family Members, inpatient care; counseling and emotional support; and other Home Health benefits listed above. Nothing in this section shall require Us to provide Home Health Benefits when in Our Determination the treatment setting is not appropriate, or when there is a more cost effective setting in which to provide Medically Necessary and Appropriate care.

**(h) DENTAL CARE AND TREATMENT.** The following services are covered when rendered by a Participating Practitioner upon prior Referral by a Member's PCP. We cover:

   a. the diagnosis and treatment of oral tumors and cysts

   b. the surgical removal of bony impacted teeth.

1. We also cover treatment of an Injury to natural teeth or the jaw, but only if:

   a. the Injury occurs while the Member is covered under any health benefit plan;

   b. the Injury was not caused, directly or indirectly by biting or chewing; and

   c. all treatment is finished within six months of the date of the Injury.

2. Treatment includes replacing natural teeth lost due to such Injury. But in no event do we cover orthodontic treatment.

3. For a Member who is severely disabled or who is a child under age six, we cover:

   a. general anesthesia and Hospitalization for dental services; and

   b. dental services rendered by a dentist regardless of where the dental services are provided for a medical condition covered by this Contract which requires Hospitalization or general anesthesia.

**(i) TREATMENT FOR TEMPOROMANDIBULAR JOINT DISORDER (TMJ)** Not covered. We do not cover any services or supplies for orthodontia, crowns, or bridgework.

**(j) THERAPEUTIC MANIPULATION** Limited to 30 visits per Calendar Year, and no more than two modalities per visit.

**(k) NONCOVERED SERVICES AND SUPPLIES:**
**THE FOLLOWING ARE NOT COVERED SERVICES UNDER THIS CONTRACT.**
**Acupuncture** except when used as a substitute for other forms of anesthesia.
**Ambulance services** for transportation from a Hospital or other health care Facility, unless Member is being transferred to another Inpatient health care Facility.
**Broken Appointments** (Charges for)
**Blood or blood plasma** which is replaced by or for a Member.

Care and/or treatment by a **Christian Science Practitioner**.

**Completion of claim forms.**

**Cosmetic Surgery**, except as otherwise stated in this Contract; complications of Cosmetic Surgery; drugs prescribed for cosmetic purposes.

**Custodial** or **domiciliary** care.

**Dental care** or treatment, including appliances, except as otherwise stated in this Contract.

**Dose intensive chemotherapy**, except as otherwise stated in this Contract.

**Educational services and supplies** providing: training in the activities of daily living; instruction in scholastic skills such as reading and writing; preparation for an occupation; or treatment for learning disabilities.

**Experimental or Investigational** treatments, procedures, hospitalizations, drugs, biological products or medical devices, except as otherwise stated in this Contract.

**Extraction of teeth**, except for bony impacted teeth. Services or supplies for or in connection with:

a. except as otherwise stated in this Contract, exams to determine the need for (or changes of) **eyeglasses** or lenses of any type.

b. eyeglasses or lenses of any type except initial replacements for loss of the natural lens.

c. eye surgery such as radial keratotomy, when the primary purpose is to correct myopia (nearsightedness), hyperopia (farsightedness) or astigmatism (blurring).

Services or supplies provided by Members of the Employee's **family**.

**Fertility treatments** including harvesting, storage and / or manipulation of eggs and sperm. This includes, but is not limited to: in vitro fertilization; embryo transfer; embryo freezing; and Gamete intra-fallopian Transfer (GIFT) and Zygote Intrafallopian Transfer (ZIFT), drugs and drug therapy.

**Hearing aids and hearing examinations** to determine the need for hearing aids or the need to adjust them.

**Herbal medicine.**

**Hypnotism.**

**Illegal occupations or activities.**

**Work-related Illness or Injury**, including a condition which is the result of disease or bodily infirmity, which occurred on the job and which is covered or could have been covered for benefits provided under workers' compensation.

**Local anesthesia charges.**

**Membership costs** for health clubs, weight loss clinics, and similar programs.

**Marriage, career or financial counseling, sex therapy or family therapy, and related services.**

**Methadone** maintenance.

**Nonprescription drugs** or supplies, except;

a. insulin needles, syringes, glucose test strips, and lancets.

b. colostomy bags, belts, and irrigators.

c. as stated in this Contract for food and food products for inherited metabolic diseases.

**Pastoral counseling services.**

**Personal convenience** or comfort items.

Any service provided without prior written Referral by the Member's **PCP**, except as specified in this Contract. In the event of a Medical Emergency, any amount which is greater than the amount We Determine to be the **reasonable and customary charge**.

**Rest or convalescent cures.**

**Room and board charges** for any period of time during which the member was not physically present overnight in the Facility.

**Routine Foot Care, except:**

a. an open cutting operation to treat weak, strained, flat, unstable or unbalanced feet, metatarsalgia, or bunions.

b. the removal of nail roots.

c. treatment or removal of corns, calluses, or toenails in conjunction with the treatment of metabolic or peripheral vascular disease.

**Self-administered services** such as: biofeedback, patient-controlled analgesia on an Outpatient basis, related diagnostic testing, self-care and self-help training.

**Services or supplies:**

a. eligible for payment under either federal or state programs (except Medicaid and Medicare).

b. for which a charge is not usually made.

c. for which a Member would not have been charged if he or she did not have healthcare coverage.

d. provided by or in a Government Hospital unless the services are for treatment:
  • of a nonservice Medical Emergency; or
  • by a Veterans' Administration Hospital of a nonservice related Illness or Injury.

**Sterilization reversal.**

**Sex-alteration treatment**, including surgery, sex hormones, and related medical, psychological, and psychiatric services; services and supplies arising from complications of sex transformation.

**Telephone consultations.**

**Transplants**, except as otherwise listed in the Contract.

**Transportation.**

**Vision therapy.**

**Vitamins and dietary supplements.**

Services or supplies received as a result of a **war**, declared or undeclared; police actions; services in the armed forces; or riots or insurrection.

**Weight reduction or control**, unless there is a diagnosis of morbid obesity; special foods, food supplements, liquid diets, diet plans, or any related products.

**Wigs, toupees, hair transplants, hair weaving, or any drug** if such drug is used in connection with baldness.

**COORDINATION OF BENEFITS AND SERVICES:**
OBD rules apply for coordination of benefits.

| Covered Services | MEDICARE | | COMMERCIAL | | | | | | |
| --- | --- | --- | --- | --- | --- | --- | --- | --- | --- |
| | Standard | Medi-Medi | AMG | Rocky | CAT | MIPC | CAIT | SBA | RICE |
| Anesthesia for opening upper femur (01230) | P | P | P | P | P | P | P | P | P |
| Crutches (E0114) | - | G | G | G | G | G | G | G | G |
| Emergency department visit, emergency medicine given. (99284) | P | P | P | P | P | P | P | P | G |
| Emergency Transport, BLS (A0429) | P | P | P | P | P | P | P | P | P |
| Magnetic resonance lower extremity, without contrast (73718) | P | P | P | P | P | P | P | P | P |
| New patient, counseling, regular visits (99203) | G | G | G | G | G | G | G | G | G |
| Outpatient surgery | | | | | | | | | |
|   Facility charges | P | P | P | P | P | P | P | P | P |
|   Physician visits | G | G | G | G | G | G | G | G | G |
|   Surgeon | P | P | G | G | P | G | G | G | G |
|   Assistant surgeon | P | P | G | G | P | G | G | G | G |
|   Anesthesiologist | P | P | P | P | P | P | P | P | P |
|   X-ray technician | P | P | P | P | P | P | P | P | P |
| Plaster or casting, knee ankle and foot (L2122) | G | G | G | G | G | G | G | G | G |
| Radiologic examination of femur (73550) | G | G | G | G | G | G | G | G | G |
| Removal of, foreign body thigh or knee area (27372) | G/P¹ | G/P¹ | G/P¹ | G/P¹ | G/P¹ | G/P¹ | G/P¹ | G/P¹ | G/P¹ |

¹See Outpatient surgery for surgery done on an outpatient basis; see Inpatient Surgery for charges done on an inpatient basis.

Legend: G = Medical Group Responsibility; P = Plan/HMO Responsibility; G/P = Shared Responsibility; - = Not Covered
This chart shows a sampling of CPT codes and the party that bears responsibility for covering costs for each procedure under numerous different plans. It is important to check the correct column for the plan being processed to determine if services are covered or not.

**Figure AA–1** Distribution of Responsibility

## Rocky Fee Schedule

| CPT®/ HCPCS* | Description | Allowed Amount | Follow-up Days |
|---|---|---|---|
| 00400 | ANESTHESIA, INTEGUMENTARY SYSTEM, EXTREMITIES | 94.23 | -- |
| 00520 | ANESTHESIA FOR CLOSED CHEST PROCEDURES | 188.46 | -- |
| 00534 | ANESTHESIA FOR TRANSVENOUS INSERTION | 219.87 | -- |
| 00868 | ANESTHESIA FOR RENAL TRANSPLANT | 314.10 | -- |
| 01230 | ANESTHESIA FOR UPPER 2/3 OF FEMUR, OPEN | 188.46 | -- |
| 01480 | ANESTHESIA, ON BONES OF LOWER LEG, OPEN | 94.23 | -- |
| 15952 | EXCISION TROCHANTERIC PRESS ULCER | 293.04 | 90 |
| 19125 | EXCISION OF BREAST LESION | 256.41 | 30 |
| 20205 | BIOPSY, MUSCLE DEEP | 87.92 | 15 |
| 27372 | REMOVAL OF FOREIGN BODY, DEEP, THIGH REGION | 190.48 | 30 |
| 27758 | OPEN TREATMENT OF TIBIAL SHAFT FRACTURE | 36.63 | 30 |
| 27784 | OPEN TREATMENT OF PROXIMAL FIBULA | 465.21 | 90 |
| 31200 | ETHMOIDECTOMY | 256.41 | 90 |
| 33217 | INSERTION OF A TRANSVENOUS ELECTRODE | 347.99 | 15 |
| 36430 | TRANSFUSION, BLOOD | 14.66 | 00 |
| 39545 | IMBRICATION OF DIAPHRAGM FOR EVENTRATION | 439.56 | 90 |
| 40808 | BIOPSY, VESTIBULE OF MOUTH | 25.65 | 00 |
| 47630 | BILIARY DUCT STONE EXTRACTION | 256.41 | 45 |
| 49560 | REPAIR INITIAL INCISIONAL OR VENTRAL HERNIA | 421.25 | 45 |
| 61703 | SURGERY OF INTRACRANIAL ANEURYSM | 476.19 | 90 |
| 62000 | ELEVATION OF DEPRESSED SKULL FRACTURE | 304.03 | 90 |
| 65800 | PARACENTESIS OF ANTERIOR CHAMBER OF EYE | 109.89 | 00 |
| 69400 | EUSTACHIAN TUBE INFLATION | 10.99 | 00 |
| 70250 | RADIOLOGIC EXAM, SKULL | 85.16 | -- |
| 73130 | RADIOLOGIC EXAM, HAND, MINIMUM 3 VIEWS | 76.92 | -- |
| 73550 | RADIOLOGIC EXAM, UPPER LEG | 76.92 | -- |
| 73590 | RADIOLOGIC EXAM, LOWER LEG | 68.68 | -- |
| 73718 | MRI LEG | 1,510.85 | -- |
| 74250 | RADIOLOGIC EXAM, SMALL BOWEL | 181.31 | -- |
| 76092 | SCREENING MAMMOGRAPHY, BILATERAL | 123.62 | -- |
| 80048 | BASIC METABOLIC PANEL | 35.72 | -- |
| 80053 | COMPREHENSIVE METABOLIC PANEL | 43.96 | -- |
| 81000 | URINALYSIS | 19.23 | -- |
| 82310 | CALCIUM, TOTAL | 27.47 | -- |
| 83540 | IRON | 43.96 | -- |
| 85025 | BLOOD COUNT, COMPLETE, AUTOMATED | 21.98 | -- |
| 85610 | PROTHROMBIN TIME | 16.49 | -- |
| 86901 | BLOODTYPING, RH (D) | 30.22 | -- |
| 87040 | CULTURE, BACTERIAL; BLOOD | 32.97 | -- |
| 87070 | CULTURE, BACTERIAL | 35.72 | -- |
| 88150 | CYTOPATHOLOGY, SLIDES, CERVICAL OR VAGINAL | 24.73 | -- |
| 90782 | THERAPEUTIC, INJECTION | 80.13 | -- |
| 97116 | GAIT TRAINING | 224.35 | -- |
| 99201 | OFFICE OR OTHER OUTPATIENT VISIT, NEW | 208.33 | -- |
| 99213 | ESTABLISHED PATIENT, EXPANDED | 288.45 | -- |
| 99284 | EMERGENCY VISIT, DETAILED | 801.25 | -- |
| 99285 | EMERGENCY VISIT, COMPREHENSIVE | 1,185.85 | -- |
| A0429 | EMERGENCY TRANSPORT | 175.00 | -- |
| E0114 | CRUTCHES | 65.00 | -- |
| L2126 | PLASTER OR CASTING,KNEE, ANKLE AND FOOT | 116.55 | -- |

■ **Figure AA–2** Rocky Fee Schedule

# Appendix B
# Conversion Factors
## and Relative Value Studies

## Table of Contents

# Medical UCR Conversion Factor Report

The following list of medical conversion factors is to be used for training purposes only.

| Zip | Area | Including Zip Codes | Surgery | Medicine | X-Ray & Lab (DXL) | Anesthesia |
|-----|------|--------------------|---------|----------|-------------------|------------|
| 006 | Puerto Rico | 006-009 | 35.58 | 31.13 | 26.68 | 22.14 |
| 039 | Maine | 039-049 | 31.01 | 27.13 | 23.26 | 31.34 |
| 100 | New York City | 100-102 | 66.02 | 57.77 | 49.51 | 30.30 |
| 125 | Poughkeepsie, Monticello, NE NY | 125, 127-129, 136 | 40.71 | 35.62 | 30.53 | 32.71 |
| 153 | Southwestern PA | 153-158 | 36.76 | 32.16 | 27.57 | 25.25 |
| 210 | Baltimore Area | 210, 211, 214 | 48.00 | 42.00 | 36.00 | 35.35 |
| 255 | Huntington, Wheeling, Parkesburg, Morgantown | 255, 257, 260, 261, 265 | 32.94 | 28.82 | 24.70 | 31.14 |
| 302 | Atlanta | 302, 303 | 38.86 | 34.00 | 29.14 | 47.43 |
| 354 | Alabama-miscellaneous | 354-357, 359-360, 363-365, 368, 324 | 30.90 | 27.04 | 23.18 | 32.06 |
| 441 | Cleveland, Youngstown Area | 441, 444 | 37.10 | 32.46 | 27.83 | 38.69 |
| 480 | Detroit | 480-482, 485 | 36.63 | 32.05 | 27.47 | 31.41 |
| 550 | Minneapolis-St Paul Area | 550, 551, 553 | 26.42 | 23.12 | 19.81 | 29.46 |
| 580 | North Dakota | 580-588 | 28.00 | 24.50 | 21.00 | 23.12 |
| 606 | Chicago | 606 | 45.64 | 39.94 | 34.23 | 49.57 |
| 640 | Kansas City Area | 640-641, 661-662 | 33.48 | 29.29 | 25.11 | 40.30 |
| 770 | Houston | 770, 772, 775 | 40.60 | 35.52 | 30.45 | 42.66 |
| 777 | Austin & Beaumont | 777, 779, 787, 788 | 33.10 | 28.96 | 24.82 | 50.31 |
| 801 | Denver, CO Springs, Alamosa, Glenwood Springs Area | 801-803, 806, 808, 811, 816 | 32.32 | 28.28 | 24.24 | 41.69 |
| 890 | Reno & Area | 890, 895, 897 | 34.38 | 30.08 | 25.78 | 49.11 |
| 904 | Santa Monica, Long Beach, Glendale | 904, 908, 912 | 45.18 | 39.53 | 33.89 | 47.94 |
| 970 | Portland & Western OR | 970, 971, 974, 975 | 30.87 | 27.01 | 23.15 | 34.20 |

■ **Table AB–1** Medical UCR Conversion Factor Report

# Medical Relative Value Study

The following list of CPT® code unit values is to be used for training and reference purposes only.

| CPT ®/HCPCS * | Description | Total RVUs | Follow-up Days |
|---|---|---|---|
| 00215 | ANESTHESIA FOR CRANIOPLASTY | 9.0 | -- |
| 00400 | ANESTHESIA, INTEGUMENTARY SYSTEM, EXTREMITIES | 3.0 | -- |
| 00520 | ANESTHESIA FOR CLOSED CHEST PROCEDURES | 6.0 | -- |
| 00534 | ANESTHESIA FOR TRANSVENOUS INSERTION | 7.0 | -- |
| 00868 | ANESTHESIA FOR RENAL TRANSPLANT | 10.0 | -- |
| 01230 | ANESTHESIA FOR UPPER 2/3 OF FEMUR, OPEN | 6.0 | -- |
| 01480 | ANESTHESIA, ON BONES OF LOWER LEG, OPEN | 30 | -- |
| 01990 | PHYSIOLOGICAL SUPPORT, BRAIN-DEAD PATIENT | 7.0 | -- |
| 15570 | FORMATION OF DIRECT OR TUBED PEDICLE | 10.0 | 90 |
| 15952 | EXCISION TROCHANTERIC PRESSURE ULCER | 8.0 | 90 |
| 19125 | EXCISION OF BREAST LESION | 7.0 | 30 |
| 19126 | EXCISION OF BREAST LESION, EACH ADDITIONAL | 3.5 | 30 |
| 20205 | BIOPSY, MUSCLE, DEEP | 2.4 | 15 |
| 21800 | CLOSED TREATMENT OF RIB FRACTURE, EACH | 18.0 | 90 |
| 24102 | ARTHROTOMY, ELBOW WITH SYNOVECTOMY | 14.5 | 90 |
| 25622 | CLOSED TREAT OF CARPAL SCAPHOID FRACTURE | 3.5 | 60 |
| 27350 | PATELLECTOMY OR HEMIPATELLECTOMY | 12.0 | 60 |
| 27372 | REMOVAL OF FOREIGN BODY, DEEP, THIGH REGION | 5.2 | 30 |
| 27758 | OPEN TREATMENT OF TIBIAL SHAFT FRACTURE | 12.7 | 30 |
| 27784 | OPEN TREATMENT OF PROXIMAL FIBULA SHAFT FX | 12.7 | 90 |
| 28456 | PERCUTANEOUS SKELETAL FIXATION OF TARSAL BONE FX | 3.9 | 90 |
| 30125 | EXCISION DERMOID CYST NOSE, UNDER BONE | 8.5 | 30 |
| 31200 | ETHMOIDECTOMY | 7.0 | 90 |
| 31225 | MAXILLECTOMY WITHOUT ORBITAL EXENTERATION | 22.5 | 120 |
| 32800 | REPAIR LUNG HERNIA THROUGH CHEST WALL | 12.0 | 30 |
| 33217 | INSERTION OF A TRANSVENOUS ELECTRODE, DUAL CHAMBER | 9.5 | 15 |
| 33225 | INSERTION OF PACING ELECTRODE | BR | -- |
| 33240 | INSERTION OF SINGLE OR DUAL CHAMBER PACING | 0.7 | 15 |
| 36430 | TRANSFUSION, BLOOD | 0.4 | 00 |
| 38100 | SPLENECTOMY, TOTAL | 16.0 | 45 |
| 39520 | REPAIR, DIAPHRAGMATIC HERNIA | 17.0 | 90 |
| 39545 | IMBRICATION OF DIAPHRAGM FOR EVENTRATION | 12.0 | 90 |
| 40808 | BIOPSY, VESTIBULE OF MOUTH | 0.7 | 00 |
| 43840 | GASTRORRHAPHY, SUTURE PERFORATED ULCER | 14.0 | 45 |
| 47630 | BILIARY DUCT STONE EXTRACTION | 7.0 | 45 |

■ **Table AB–2** Medical RVS Schedule

*(continued on next page)*

| 49560 | REPAIR INITIAL INCISIONAL OR VENTRAL HERNIA | 11.5 | 45 |
|---|---|---|---|
| 52500 | TRANSURETHRAL RESECTION OF BLADDER NECK | 10.0 | 90 |
| 58700 | SALPINGECTOMY, COMPLETE OR PARTIAL | 11.4 | 90 |
| 59400 | ROUTINE OBSTETRIC CARE | 20.0 | 45 |
| 59820 | TREATMENT OF MISSED ABORTION | 4.5 | 30 |
| 61703 | SURGERY OF INTRACRANIAL ANEURYSM | 13.0 | 90 |
| 62000 | ELEVATION OF DEPRESSED SKULL FRACTURE | 8.3 | 90 |
| 65800 | PARACENTESIS OF ANTERIOR CHAMBER OF EYE | 3.0 | 00 |
| 69400 | EUSTACHIAN TUBE INFLATION | 0.3 | 00 |
| 70250 | RADIOLOGIC EXAM, SKULL | 3.1 | -- |
| 70260 | RADIOLOGIC EXAM, SKULL, COMPLETE | 5.0 | -- |
| 70450 | CAT SCAN, SKULL | 21.7 | -- |
| 71020 | RADIOLOGIC EXAM, CHEST | 3.2 | -- |
| 73100 | RADIOLOGIC EXAM, WRIST | 2.5 | -- |
| 73130 | RADIOLOGIC EXAM, HAND, MINIMUM 3 VIEWS | 2.8 | -- |
| 73550 | RADIOLOGIC EXAM, FEMUR | 2.8 | -- |
| 73590 | RADIOLOGIC EXAM, TIBIA AND FIBULA | 2.5 | -- |
| 73718 | MRI LEG | 55.0 | -- |
| 74250 | RADIOLOGIC EXAM, SMALL INTESTINE | 6.6 | -- |
| 76090 | MAMMOGRAPHY, UNILATERAL | 4.5 | -- |
| 76092 | SCREENING MAMMOGRAPHY, BILATERAL | 4.5 | -- |
| 76870 | ULTRASOUND, SCROTUM AND CONTENTS | 8.0 | -- |
| 76872 | ULTRASOUND, TRANSRECTAL | 13.8 | -- |
| 78811 | TUMOR IMAGING | 100.0 | -- |
| 80048 | BASIC METABOLIC PANEL | 1.3 | -- |
| 80053 | COMPREHENSIVE METABOLIC PANEL | 1.6 | -- |
| 81000 | URINALYSIS | 0.7 | -- |
| 82310 | CALCIUM, TOTAL | 1.0 | -- |
| 83540 | IRON | 1.6 | -- |
| 85025 | BLOOD COUNT, COMPLETE, AUTOMATED | 0.8 | -- |
| 85610 | PROTHROMBIN TIME | 0.6 | -- |
| 86901 | BLOODTYPING, RH (D) | 1.1 | -- |
| 87040 | CULTURE, BACTERIAL; BLOOD | 1.2 | -- |
| 87070 | CULTURE, BACTERIAL OTHER SOURCE | 1.3 | -- |
| 88150 | CYTOPATHOLOGY, SLIDES, CERVICAL OR VAGINAL | 0.9 | -- |
| 90772 | THERAPEUTIC, INJECTION | 2.5 | -- |
| 93000 | EKG | 7.8 | -- |
| 93545 | INJECTION DURING ANGIOGRAPHY | 22.0 | -- |
| 94060 | BRONCHOSPASM EVALUATION | 20.0 | -- |
| 97116 | GAIT TRAINING | 7.0 | -- |

*(continued)*

| 99201 | OFFICE OR OTHER OUTPATIENT VISIT, NEW, STRAIGHTFORWARD | 6.5 | -- |
|-------|--------------------------------------------------------|------|----|
| 99203 | OFFICE OR OTHER OUTPATIENT VISIT, NEW, DETAILED | 8.0 | -- |
| 99213 | OV ESTABLISHED PATIENT, EXPANDED | 9.0 | -- |
| 99284 | EMERGENCY VISIT, DETAILED | 25.0 | -- |
| 99285 | EMERGENCY VISIT, COMPREHENSIVE | 37.0 | -- |
| A0427 | ALS1–EMERGENCY | 41.0 | -- |
| A0429 | BLS–EMERGENCY | 40.0 | -- |
| A0433 | ADVANCED LIFE SUPPORT, LEVEL 2 | 41.0 | -- |
| E0114 | CRUTCHES, UNDERARM | 3.5 | -- |
| E0144 | WALKER, ENCLOSED, FOUR-SIDED FRAME | 4.5 | -- |
| E0617 | EXTERNAL DEFIBRILLATOR | 7.5 | -- |
| L2126 | KNEE-ANKLE-FOOT-ORTHOSIS | 3.0 | -- |

*(continued)*

# Hospital Services Payment Worksheet
## Type of Service Codes

| Description of Service | Code |
|---|---|
| Room and Board Charges | R/B |
| Specialized Unit (ICU, CCU, etc.) | R/B–ICU |
| Private | PVT |
| Ancillary Expenses | MISC |
| Personal Items | PTCON |
| Professional Fees | PROF |
| Outpatient Surgery | OP/SURG |
| Outpatient Ancillary | OP/MISC |
| Preadmission Testing | PAT |
| Outpatient Facility Payable at 100% | OP/FAC |
| Not Covered | N/C |

■ **Table AB–3** Hospital Services Payment Worksheet Type of Service Codes

## Remarks List

| |
|---|
| No Deductible Taken Due To Common Accident Provision. |
| Accident Benefit, First $500 Payable At 100%. |
| Accident Benefit Has Already Been Applied For On This Accident. |
| Lifetime Maximum Has Been Reached. $"amount" Exceeds Your Lifetime Maximum. |
| Charges Have Been Applied To Your CCYY Deductible. |
| 20YY Individual Deductible Limit Has Previously Been Met. |
| 20YY Individual Deductible Has Been Met On This Claim. |
| CCPY Carryover Deductible Does Not Apply To CCYY Family Deductible Limit. |
| CCYY Family Deductible Limit Has Previously Been Met. |
| CCYY Family Deductible Has Been Met On This Claim. |
| CCYY Individual and Family Deductibles Have Been Met On This Claim. |
| CCYY Individual and Family Deductible Limits Have Previously Been Met. |
| CCYY Individual Out Of Pocket Limit Has Previously Been Met. |
| CCYY Individual Out Of Pocket Limit Has Been Met On This Claim. |
| CCYY Family Aggregate Out Of Pocket Limit Has Been Met On This Claim. |
| CCYY Family Aggregate Out Of Pocket Limit Has Previously Been Met. |
| CCYY Family Coinsurance Limit Has Been Met On This Claim. |
| CCYY Family Coinsurance Limit Has Previously Been Met. |
| CCYY Individual And Family Coinsurance Limits Have Previously Been Met. |
| CCYY Individual And Family Coinsurance Limits Have Been Met On This Claim. |
| CCYY Individual Coinsurance Limit Has Previously Been Met. |
| CCYY Individual Coinsurance Limit Has Been Met On This Claim. |
| Benefits Reduced To #%. |
| Benefits Payable At #%. |
| Non-Network Provider Benefits Payable At #%. |
| Benefits Have Been Adjusted Due To Medicare's Payment. |
| Credit Reserve = $"amount" |
| Medicare's Payment Exceeds Your Plan Normal Liability Therefore No Benefit Is Payable. |
| Provider Does Not Accept Medicare Assignment. |
| Provider Accepts Medicare Assignment. |
| Lab Professional Charges Paid at #% of UCR. |

■ **Table AB–4** Remarks List

*(continued on next page)*

| |
|---|
| Deductible Waived For Network Facilities. |
| Network Provider. Benefits paid at #%. |
| Network Facility. Benefits paid at #%. |
| Maximum dental benefit payable is $1,000.00 per calendar year. |
| Maximum Payable For Ambulance Is $150.00 Each Way. |
| Hospital Inpatient Deductible $200.00 |
| Benefits Have Been Adjusted Due To COB With Primary Carrier. |
| Benefits are adjusted due to payment by primary payer. |

*(continued)*

# Denial Reasons

| |
|---|
| Charge exceeds amount covered under your plan. |
| This procedure does not require the attendance of an assistant surgeon. |
| Personal convenience items are not covered under your plan. |
| "item" – Duplicate Charge. |
| "item(s)" is/are not covered under your plan. |
| Services not covered. Patient is over the age limit. |
| Services were denied as not medically necessary. |
| Non-prescription medication not covered under your plan. |
| "patient" is not covered under this plan. |
| Test performed is not related to the diagnosis indicated. |
| Pended. Additional Information Needed. |
| Pended. Please verify if charges are for professional services or facility fees. |
| Pended. Need anesthesia time. |
| Pended. Please submit narrative explaining use of Polaroid camera. |
| Charge exceeds Medicare's approved amount. |
| Group responsibility, covered under capitation. |
| Charges included in global maternity fee. |
| Charges incidental to above procedure. |
| "procedure" is not covered under your plan. |
| Charge exceeds amount covered under your plan. All x-rays combined under full mouth x-ray w/ bitewings. |
| Fluoride treatment only covered for children under 14. |
| No additional base units allowed for secondary procedures. |
| Monitoring blood gasses is an integral part of anesthesia. No extra units allowed. |
| Room and Board covered up to $"amount" per day. |
| Charge exceeds average semiprivate room rate. |
| Charges due to preexisting conditions which are excluded under your plan. |
| Exceeds purchase price of rental item. |
| Not covered, exceeds maximum amount covered for this service. |

■ **Table AB–5** Denial Reasons

# Dental Conversion Factor Report

The following list of dental conversion factors is intended to be used for training and reference purposes only. Because claim exercises are within the state of California and Pennsylvania, only California and Pennsylvania conversion factor codes are listed.

| State: | California | | | |
|---|---|---|---|---|
| Area | Zip Codes | A. Diagnostic And Preventive | B. All Other Excl. Gold Restorations Crowns, Prosthetics | C. Gold Rest. Crowns, Prosthetics |
| Los Angeles, Long Beach, Code 900 | 900-918 | 40.00 | 41.75 | 37.35 |
| San Diego, Code 920 | 920-921 | 34.00 | 36.50 | 33.00 |
| San Bernardino, Riverside, Palm Springs, Code 922 | 922-925 | 35.00 | 36.50 | 31.75 |
| Orange County, Code 926 | 926-928 | 40.00 | 41.00 | 35.00 |
| Ventura, Santa Barbara, Code 930 | 930-931 | 35.75 | 38.25 | 33.50 |
| San Francisco, Oakland, San Jose, Code 940 | 940-951 | 40.00 | 41.25 | 36.00 |
| Sacramento, Stockton, Code 952 | 952-953, 956-958 | 35.75 | 35.00 | 30.75 |
| Other California | 932-937, 939, 954, 955, 959-966 | 35.75 | 35.25 | 31.00 |

| State: | Pennsylvania | | | |
|---|---|---|---|---|
| Area | Zip Codes | A. Diagnostic And Preventive | B. All Other Excl. Gold Restorations Crowns, Prosthetics | C. Gold Rest. Crowns, Prosthetics |
| Oliver Code 155 | 155-159 | 35.00 | 36.50 | 32.00 |

■ **Table AB–6** Dental Conversion Factor Report

# Dental Relative Value Study

The following list of CDT® code unit values is intended to be used for training and reference purposes only.

## I. Diagnostic  (D0100—D0999)

| ADA Code | Unit Value | Description of Service | ADA Code | Unit Value | Description of Service |
|---|---|---|---|---|---|
| D0120 | 0.5 A | Periodic oral evaluation | D0140 | 0.3 A | Limited oral evaluation |
| D0150 | 1.5 A | Comprehensive oral evaluation | D0210 | 1.4 A | Intraoral – complete series (w/bitewings) |
| D0220 | 0.3 A | Intraoral – periapical first film | D0230 | 0.2 A | Intraoral – peripical each additional film |
| D0240 | 0.5 A | Intraoral – occlusal film | D0250 | 0.4 A | Extraoral – first film |
| D0260 | 0.3 A | Extraoral – each additional film | D0270 | 0.4 A | Bitewing – first film |
| D0272 | 0.5 A | Bitewings – two films | D0274 | 0.7 A | Bitewings – four films |
| D0460 | 0.5 A | Pulp vitality tests | | | |

## II. Preventive  (D1000—D1999)

| ADA Code | Unit Value | Description of Service | ADA Code | Unit Value | Description of Service |
|---|---|---|---|---|---|
| D1110 | 1.0 A | Prophylaxis – adult | D1120 | 0.8 A | Prophylaxis – child |
| D1201 | 1.1 A | Fluoride (incl. prophylaxis) – child | D1203 | 0.3 A | Fluoride (prophylaxis not incl.) – child |
| D1204 | 0.4 A | Fluoride (incl. prophylaxis) – adult | D1205 | 1.4 A | Fluoride (prophylaxis not incl.) – adult |

## III. Restorative (D2000—D2999)

| ADA Code | Unit Value | Description of Service | ADA Code | Unit Value | Description of Service |
|---|---|---|---|---|---|
| D2140 | 1.1 B | Amalgam – one surface, prim. or perm. | D2150 | 1.4 B | Amalgam – two surfaces, prim. or perm. |

■ **Table AB–7** Dental Relative Value Study

*(continued on next page)*

| D2160 | 1.7 B | Amalgam – three surfaces, prim. or perm. | D2161 | 2.0 B | Amalgam – 4+ surfaces, prim. or perm. |
|---|---|---|---|---|---|
| D2330 | 1.3 B | Resin-based composite – 1 surf., anterior | D2331 | 1.8 B | Resin-based composite – 2 surf., anterior |
| D2332 | 2.3 B | Resin-based composite – 3 surf., anterior | D2391 | 1.5 B | Resin-based composite – 1 surf., posterior |
| D2392 | 2.0 B | Resin-based composite – 2 surf., posterior | D2393 | 2.5 B | Resin-based composite – 3 surf., posterior |
| D2394 | 2.8 B | Resin-based composite – 4+ surf., posterior | D2520 | 9.4 C | Inlay – metallic – 2 surfaces |
| D2542 | 9.5 C | Onlay – metallic 2 surfaces | D2721 | 10.5 C | Crown – resin w/base metal |
| D2751 | 11.4 C | Crown – porcelain fused to base metal | | | |

## IV. Endodontic (D3000—D3999)

| ADA Code | Unit Value | Description of Service | ADA Code | Unit Value | Description of Service |
|---|---|---|---|---|---|
| D3310 | 7.0 B | Anterior (excl. final restoration) | D3330 | 11.0 B | Molar (excl. final restoration) |
| D3410 | 8.0 B | Apicoectomy/ periradicular surgery – anterior | D3425 | 8.4 B | Apicoectomy/ periradicular surgery – molar |

## V. Periodontic  (D4000—D4999)

| ADA Code | Unit Value | Description of Service | ADA Code | Unit Value | Description of Service |
|---|---|---|---|---|---|
| D4210 | 6.0 B | Gingivectomy or gingivoplasty – four or more contiguous teeth or bounded teeth spaces per quadrant | D4211 | 5.0 B | Gingivectomy or gingivoplasty – one to three teeth, per quadrant |
| D4341 | 2.5 B | Periodontal scaling and root planning – four or more contiguous teeth or bounded teeth spaces per quadrant | D4342 | 1.9 B | Periodontal scaling and root planning – one to three teeth, per quadrant |

*(continued)*

## VI. Prosthodontic (D5000—D5999)

| ADA Code | Unit Value | Description of Service | ADA Code | Unit Value | Description of Service |
|---|---|---|---|---|---|
| D5110 | 16.5 C | Complete denture – maxillary | D5120 | 16.5 C | Complete denture – mandibular |
| D5211 | 14.0 C | Maxillary partial denture – resin base (incl. clasps, rests and teeth) | D5121 | 14.0 C | Mandibular partial denture – resin base (incl. clasps, rests and teeth) |
| D5213 | 18.0 C | Mandibular partial denture – cast metal framework w/resin bases (incl. clasps, rests and teeth) | D5214 | 18.0 C | Mandibular partial denture – cast metal framework w/resin bases (incl. clasps, rests and teeth) |

## X. Oral Surgery(D7000—D7999)

| ADA Code | Unit Value | Description of Service | ADA Code | Unit Value | Description of Service |
|---|---|---|---|---|---|
| D7111 | | Coronal remnants – deciduous tooth | D7140 | 1.4 B | Extraction, erupted tooth or exposed root (elevation and/ or forceps removal) |
| D7210 | 2.0 B | Surgical removal of erupted tooth requiring elevation of mucoperiosteal flap and removal of bone or section of tooth | D7220 | 2.5 B | Removal of impacted tooth – soft tissue |
| D7230 | 3.6 B | Removal of impacted tooth – partially bony | D7240 | 4.2 B | Removal of impacted tooth – completely bony |
| D7441 | 7.2 B | Excision of malignant tumor – over 1.25 cm | D7450 | 3.0 B | Removal of benign odontogenic cyst or tumor – up to 1.25 cm |
| D7451 | 6.0 B | Removal of benign odontogenic cyst or tumor – greater than 125 cm | D7460 | 3.0 B | Removal of benign nonodontogenic cyst or tumor – up to 1.25 cm |
| D7461 | 6.0 B | Removal of benign nonodontogenic cyst or tumor – greater than 1.25 cm | | | |

*(continued)*

# Appendix C
# Tables

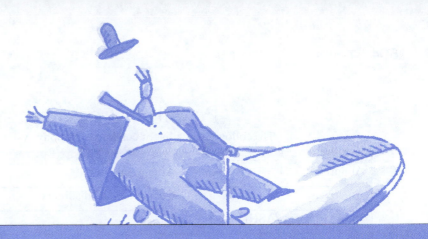

## Table of Contents

# Possible Preexisting Conditions

The following is a list of conditions by body system that are potentially preexisting.

| Cardiovascular System | Genitourinary System | Miscellaneous Conditions |
|---|---|---|
| Abnormal ECG | Albuminuria | Arthritis |
| Aneurysm | Congenital GU disorders | Back disorders, disc, sacro |
| Arteriosclerosis/ASHD | GU stone | Bone/joint disorders |
| Coronary disease | Hematuria | Cancer |
| Dyspnea | Hydronephrosis | Cataracts |
| Edema | Hysterectomy | Eye disorder |
| Enlarged heart | Kidney disorders | Glaucoma |
| Fibrillation | Nephrectomy | Gout |
| Heart disease/ASHD | Nephritis | Hodgkin's lymphoma |
| Heart failure | PID | Impaired vision |
| Heart murmurs | Prostatic disorder | Lupus erythematosus |
| Hemophilia | Pyelitis | Lymph node disorders |
| High blood pressure | Pyelonephrosis | Mastoiditis |
| Irregular pulse | Pyonephrosis | Meniere's disease, labyrinthitis |
| Leukemia | Sexually transmitted diseases | Muscular dystrophy |
| Pacemaker | Toxemia/eclampsia | Osteomyelitis |
| Rapid pulse | Unlisted or undiagnosed | Otitis media |
| Stroke/CVA | | Regional disorders |
| | | Skin cancer |
| | | Spinal curvature |
| | | TB |
| | | Tumors, malignant |
| | | Tumors, benign |

| Nervous System | Gastrointestinal System | Endocrine System |
|---|---|---|
| Autism | Colostomy/ileostomy | Adrenal disorders |
| Cerebral palsy | Duodenal ulcer | Diabetes |
| Headaches | Esophageal disorders | Elevated blood sugar |
| Mental retardation | Gastric ulcers | Hyperglycemia |
| Down's syndrome | GI hemorrhage | Pituitary disorders |
| Multiple sclerosis | Liver disorders | Thyroid disorders (except hypothyroidism) |
| Parkinson's disease | Pancreas disorders | |
| Psychoses | Peptic ulcer | |

■ **Table AC–1** Possible Preexisting Conditions

*(continued on next page)*

| Seizure disorders | Regional enteritis | |
| --- | --- | --- |
| Severe neuroses | Regional ileitis | |
| Suicide (attempted) | Ulcerative colitis | |
| Syncopy/vertigo | | |
| Tremors | | |

| Non-Physical Conditions | Respiratory System |
| --- | --- |
| Drug addiction | Asthma |
| Alcoholism | Bronchiectasis |
| | Chronic bronchitis |
| | Constructive pulmonary disease |
| | Emphysema |
| | TB/TBC |
| | Obstructive pulmonary disease |

*(continued)*

# Potential Medical Case Management Claims

The following list consists of diagnoses that are potentially medical case management claims. This list is intended to be used for training and reference purposes only, since the particular company or plan guidelines may differ from those stated.

**Section 1:** Potential medical case management claims listing by condition are as follows:

| Neurologic Patients | Neonatal Patients | Malignancy Patients |
| --- | --- | --- |
| Brain tumors | Premature birth | Multiple surgeries |
| TIA (transient ischemic attack) | Hydrocephalus | Radiation treatments |
| Closed head injury | Respiratory distress and in ICU over one week | Cancer in children |
| Unconsciousness (any cause) | Meningomyelocele | Chemotherapy |
| Cerebral aneurysm or AV malformation | Bronchopulmonary dysplasia | Acute leukemia |
| Meningitis or encephalitis | Major or multiple congenital anomaly | Aplastic anemia |
| Reye's syndrome | | Kaposi's sarcoma |
| Anoxic encephalopathy | TRANSPLANT/DIALYSIS PATIENTS | OBSTETRIC PATIENTS |
| Guillain-Barre | Heart, liver, or bone marrow transplant | Expected multiple birth of three or more infants |
| Quadriplegia | Organ rejection | Previous history of neonatal ICU confined infant |
| Paraplegia | Cardiomyopathy | Bleeding during pregnancy |
| Chronic stroke | Biliary atresia | |
| Multiple sclerosis (MS) | Renal failure | |
| Amyotrophic lateral sclerosis (ALS) | | |
| Alzheimer's disease | | |

| Psychiatric Conditions | Traumatically Injured Patients | Cardiovascular Conditions |
| --- | --- | --- |
| Anorexia nervosa | Thermal burns or frostbite | Ruptured abdominal aortic aneurysm |
| Adolescent adjustment reaction | Child over 10% or adult over 20% | Myocardial Interaction (heart attack) |
| Manic depression; bipolar disorder | Crash injuries | Intractable angina |
| Schizophrenia | Amputations | Peripheral vascular disease, w/ pending amputation |
| Sexual abuse | Multiple trauma or fractures | |
| Chemical dependency | Spinal cord injury | |
| Depression with or without suicide attempt | | |

| Respiratory Conditions | Other Diagnoses |
| --- | --- |
| Respirator dependency (any cause) | AIDS |
| Emphysema | Lupus |
| Chronic bronchitis or asthma | Any condition causing paralysis |

■ **Table AC–2** Potential Medical Case Management Claims

*(continued on next page)*

| Section II: Potential medical case management claims by ICD-9-CM® codes are as follows: | | | | |
|---|---|---|---|---|
| Cases ICD-9-CM | Description | | Cases ICD-9-CM | Description |
| **High-risk mothers** | | | **Other** | |
| 640.x – 644.0 | Complications of pregnancy | | 344.x | Other paralytic syndromes |
| 646.x – 648.x | | | 045.x | Poliomyelitis |
| 760 – 779 | Perinatal conditions | | | |
| **Highly suggestive of AIDS** | | | **Traumatic brain injury** | |
| 031.0 | Pulmonary infection by *Mycobacterium* | | 850.x—854.x | Various types of head injury |
| 112.0* | Candidiasis of mouth (thrush) | | 800.x—804.x | Skull fracture |
| 112.4 | Candidiasis pneumonia | | 780.0x | Coma and stupor |
| 112.5 | Systematic candidiasis | | **Non-traumatic brain injury** | |
| 112.81 – 112.89* | Candidiasis of other sites | | 191.x | Brain tumors |
| 114 | Coccidioidal meningitis | | 293.x | Transient organic psychotic conditions |
| 114.0 | Pulmonary coccidioidomycocis | | 294.x | Other organic psychotic conditions |
| 114.9 | Coccidioidomycocis, unspecified | | | |
| 115.0 – 115.9 | Histoplasmosis | | 310.x | Mental disorders due to organic brain damage |
| 130.0 | Toxoplasmosis encephalitis | | 348.x | Brain conditions |
| 130.3 – 130.9 | Toxoplasmosis of other sites | | 349.x | Other and unspecified diseases of CNS |
| 136.3 | *Pneumocystis carinii* pneumonia | | | |
| 176.x | Kaposi's sarcoma | | **Stroke** | |
| 279.3 | Deficiency of cell-mediated immunity | | 342.x | Hemiplegia |
| 279.3 | Unspecified immunity deficiency | | 430 | Subarachnoid hemorrhage |
| 279.9 | Unspecified disorder of immune system | | 431 | Intercerebral hemorrhage |
| | | | 432 | Other unspecified intracranial hemorrhage |
| 279.10 | Immunodeficiency with predominant T-cell defect, unspecified | | 433.x | Occlusion and stenosis of cerebral arteries |
| 279.19 | Other immune disorders | | | |
| 780.6* | Fever of unknown origin | | | |
| 785.6* | Lymphadenopathy | | | |
| 790.8* | Viremia, unspecified | | | |
| **Spinal cord injury** | | | **High-risk infants** | |
| 952.x | Spinal cord injury without evidence of spinal bone injury | | 343.x | Infantile cerebral palsy |
| | | | 741.x | Spina bifida |
| 805.x – 806.x | Fracture of neck and trunk | | 742.x | Other congenital anomalies of the nervous system |
| 336.x | Diseases of spinal cord | | 644.2 | Early onset of delivery |
| **Multiple fractures** | | | **Burns** | |
| 733.81 | Malunion (fx) | | 940.x—949.x | Burns |
| 733.82 | Nonunion (fx) | | | |

*(continued)*

# Durable Medical Equipment Coverage Guidelines

The following is a list of commonly billed DME items and coverage guidelines. This list is intended to be used for training and reference purposes only, since the particular company or plan guidelines may differ from the guidelines stated.

| Item | Description | Coverage Guidelines |
|---|---|---|
| **Action bath hydro massage** | (See Whirlpool.) | Rx required. Refer for medical review. |
| **Adjust-a-bed** | (Lounger.) | Not covered. Comfort item. |
| **Aero-massage** | (See Whirlpool.) | See Whirlpool. |
| **Aero-pulse Surgical Leggings** | (Non-reusable support leggings.) | Rx required following surgery. |
| **Air Conditioner** | (Circulates and cools the air in a home.) | Not covered. Environmental control equipment. |
| **Air-fluidized Bed** | (Institutional equipment.) | Not covered. Not for home use. |
| **Air Purifier** | (Electronically cleans house environment.) | Not covered. Environmental control equipment. |
| **Allergy-free Items** | (Not primarily medical.) | Not covered. Preventive in nature, nondurable |
| **Alternating Pressure Pads** | (Prevents pressure sores in bed or wheelchair confined person.) | Rx required when ordered for treatment of decubitus ulcers or when a person is susceptible to ulcers. |
| **Ankle Weights** | (As exercise equipment for postoperative care.) | Not a covered medical expense. Covered only when prescribed in a post-op situation to return function (i.e., knee surgery). |
| **Apnea Monitor** | (Monitors apnea, cessation of breathing, episodes in infants.) | Medical documentation of condition necessary. Rx required. |
| **Aqua-matic K-pad** | (Heating pad.) | Not covered. Comfort item, nondurable medical equipment. |
| **Aqua-matic K-thermia** | (Warm water system.) | Used only in institutions or acute care facility. Not covered. |
| **Aqua Massage Pump** | (See Whirlpool.) | See Whirlpool. |
| **Aqua-whirl** | (See Whirlpool.) | See Whirlpool. |
| **Arch Supports** | (Removable in-shoe support. See Orthotics.) | Not covered. Nondurable medical equipment. |
| **Arterio Sonde** | (Automatic blood pressure monitor.) | Covered as home blood pressure monitoring device. |
| **Artificial Kidney** | (Home hemodialysis unit.) | Covered for chronic renal disease; ancillary supplies essential to medical use may also be covered. Refer to medical review. |
| **Astromatic Bed, Astropedic Bed, Comfort-a-bed** | (Comfort bed. Not medical equipment.) | Not covered. Comfort item. |
| **Autolift, Bathtub** | (Bathtub lift.) | Possible convenience item. Rx required, patient's weight and statement of medical necessity; refer for medical review. |
| **Backtrak, Cotrell** | (Home back traction unit.) | Not covered. |
| **Barbells** | (As exercise equipment. For post-op rehabilitation.) | Not a covered medical expense. Covered only if prescribed in a post-op situation to return function. |
| **Bathtub Rail and Seat** | (Attached to bathtub for patient assistance.) | Rx required or statement of medical necessity. Covered for |

■ **Table AC–3** Durable Medical Equipment Coverage Guidelines

*(continued on next page)*

| | | paraplegics, quads, or stroke patients. |
|---|---|---|
| **Beautyrest Adjustable Bed** | (Not a hospital bed, not primary medical.) | Not covered. Convenience item. See Hospital bed (standard). |
| **Bed Bath** | (Hygienic equipment.) | Convenience item. Not for treating disease or injury. |
| **Bedboard** | (Provides firm support under mattress.) | Not covered. Not for treatment of disease or injury. |
| **Bed Lift** | (Sling, either manual or electronic; lifts person to and from bed.) | See Bathtub rail and seat. Rx required, patient's weight and statement of medical necessity. |
| **Bed Lounge, Power or Manual** | (Not a hospital bed.) | Convenience item (power or manual). Not covered. See Hospital bed, standard. |
| **Bed Mattress** | (Standard mattress for adjustable hospital bed.) | Covered when hospital bed is allowed. |
| **Bedpan** | (Hospital type.) | Covered for bed-confined or immobilized patients. |
| **Bed Siderail** | (Attached to hospital bed, protective device, often standard bed equipment.) | Covered if person is bed confined, or if condition of vertigo, seizure, or neurologic disorder is present; also covered for small children. |
| **Bed, Oscillating Type** | (Swings back and forth.) | Not covered for home use. Institutional equipment. |
| **Bell & Howell Master** | (Speech teaching machine, training aid.) | Not covered. |
| **Bendix-type Oxygen Concentrator** | (Concentrates room air oxygen to a therapeutic level.) | Rx required. Covered for person with severe breathing impairment. |
| **Bennett IPPB Machine** | (Intermittent positive-pressure breathing.) | Rx required. Covered for person with severe breathing impairment. |
| **Bicycle, Standard** | Not covered. | |
| **Bicycle, Stationary** | (For cardiac medical exercise program only.) | Refer for medical review. |
| **Bidet** | (Hygienic toilet item.) | Not primarily for treatment of disease or medical condition. Not covered. |
| **Bimler Appliance** | (Orthodontic dental appliance, corrects tongue thrust.) | Not covered. |
| **Bi-osteogenic Electromagnetic Treatment System** | (Electrical currents used to treat nonunion fracture.) | Covered to treat fractures. Medical documentation required. |
| **Bird Respirator** | (IPPB Machine for respiratory therapy.) | Rx required. Covered for person with severe breathing problem. |
| **Blood Pressure Cuff** | (Measures blood pressure; necessary for home management.) | Covered with documented diagnosis of hypertension; also used with home hemodialysis units. |
| **Body Braces, Back, Foot, Leg, Arm** | (Supportive devices.) | Rx required. Covered if durable and necessary. |
| **Bra, Jobst Surgical** | (Support item following surgery.) | Initial bra only following post-surgical reconstruction and mastectomy. |
| **Braille Teaching Aid** | (Training and vocational equipment.) | Not covered. |
| **Breast Pump** | (Assists mother in breastfeeding; may be either manual or electric.) | Not covered. Elective device for patient comfort. |

*(continued)*

| Canes | (Straight, quad, ambulatory aids.) | Covered for ambulatory impairments. |
|---|---|---|
| **Cardiac Phone Monitor** | (Telephone-relayed EKG reporting devices.) | Charges covered within physician's office fee. |
| **Cast Guards** | (A waterproof [usually plastic] coverlet for casts.) | Covered for all covered casting procedures. |
| **Cast Shoes (fracture boot)** | (A wood or rubber-based shoe with canvas sides to support casts in ambulation.) | Covered with documentation by diagnosis. |
| **Catheter** | (Medical supply item, not reusable.) | For bed-confined or similarly disabled persons; for urinary retention problems. |
| **Centrifuge Readocrit** | (Blood testing equipment.) | Rx required. Covered for person on home dialysis. |
| **Cervical Collar** | (Neck support item.) | Covered for appropriate diagnosis, such as cervical sprain. |
| **Cervical Pillow** | (Neck support item.) | Covered for appropriate diagnosis, such as cervical sprain. |
| **Colostomy Supplies, Bags and Accessories** | (Used after ostomy procedures.) | Covered for colostomy patients, post-rectal surgery. |
| **Commode** | (Bedside toilet chair.) | Covered for bed or wheelchair-confined person. |
| **Computerized Equipment for Mobility and Speech** | (For paraplegics.) | Not covered. |
| **Contact Lens, Bandage** | (Protects cornea following surgery or injury.) | Rx required. |
| **Contact Lens, Orthokeratology** | (Myopia or refractive.) | Refer for medical review. |
| **Corset** | (Supportive item.) | Covered with appropriate diagnosis, such as thoracic sprain. |
| **Crutches** | (Ambulatory aids.) | Covered for ambulatory impairments. |
| **Cushion-lift Power Seat** | (Assist person in/out of seat.) | Covered for person with hip, knee arthritis, or other neuromuscular conditions. |
| **Dehumidifier** | (Room or central system type.) | Not covered. Environmental control equipment. |
| **Deluxe Padding** | (Comfort item, special order for wheelchairs, other seating.) | Not covered. |
| **Denis Browne Splint or Bar** | (Metal support to maintain and correct adduction.) | Covered for child with clubfoot or metatarsus deformity, (includes one pair of shoes). |
| **Dextrometer/Glucometer/Diabetic Supplies** | (Measures blood sugar levels.) | Rx required. For diabetic treatment. |
| **Dialysis Equipment and Supplies** | (Artificial kidney.) | Covered for chronic renal disease. See hemodialysis. |
| **Diapulse Machine** | (Diathermy machine.) | Not covered for home use. |
| **Diathermy Equipment** | (Heat treatment.) | Not covered for home use. |
| **Disposable Sheets and Bags** | (Supplies.) | Not covered. Nondurable medical equipment. |
| **Ear Molds** | (Prevents water from entering inner ear canal.) | Refer for medical review. |
| **Ease-o-matic Bed Spring** | (Comfort item, not adaptable to hospital bed.) | Not covered. See Hospital bed (standard). |
| **Eaton E-Z Bath** | (Bathtub seat.) | See Bathtub rail and seat. |
| **Egg-crate Pad, Mattress** | (Portable pad for preventing | Rx required. For treatment of |

*(continued)*

| | bedsores.) | decubitus ulcers. |
|---|---|---|
| **Elastic stocking, Jobst type** | (Supportive, medical item following surgery.) | Rx required. Covered post-surgical expense or for diagnosis of circulatory problems. |
| **Electra-Rest Bed** | (Not a hospital bed) | Not covered. |
| **Electrocardiocorder** | (Diagnostic equipment.) | Covered only as part of a physician's diagnostic charge. |
| **Electrostatic Air Purifier Machines** | (Air cleanser, environment control apparatus.) | Not covered. Environmental control equipment. |
| **Elevators** | (Convenience item.) | Not covered. |
| **Emesis Basin** | (Basin for vomitus fluids.) | Covered expense for home bed-confined patients. |
| **Enema Supplies** | (For stimulating lower colon activity.) | Rx required. |
| **Enuresis Equipment** | (Monitoring and training devices for involuntary urination.) | Not covered. |
| **Enurtone** | (Training device for enuresis.) | Not covered. |
| **Ergometer** | (Tension measuring device for stationary bicycle.) | See bicycle (stationary). |
| **Esophageal Dilator** | (To open esophagus.) | Used only by physician. Not covered for home use. |
| **Exercise Equipment** | (Not primarily medical.) | Not covered. |
| **Exercise Pad** | (Flat soft surface.) | Not covered. |
| **Exercycle** | (Stationary bicycle.) | Rx required. For cardiac patients in active program. See Bicycle (stationary). |
| **Face mask, Oxygen** | (Necessity for oxygen therapy.) | Covered when oxygen therapy is required. |
| **Face mask, Surgical** | (For contagious diseases, isolation care.) | Rx required. |
| **Flowmeter, Oxygen** | (Oxygen regulator.) | Covered when oxygen therapy is required. |
| **Fluidic Breathing Assistor** | (Positive-pressure machine.) | Covered when IPPB care is necessary. |
| **Foundation Garment** | (Padding, bras, etc.) | Not covered. Check under specific items such as Corset. |
| **Freika Pillow Splint** | (Maintains adduction.) | Covered for small child with hip disorder. |
| **Gatchboard** | (Bedboard.) | Not covered. |
| **Gel Flotation Pad and Mattress** | (Treats and prevents pressure sores.) | Covered for treatment of decubitus ulcers. |
| **Glideabout Chair** | (Chair with small wheels.) | Rx required. Covered in lieu of wheelchair. |
| **Glucometers** | (Measures blood sugar levels.) | Rx required. For medical management of covered conditions. |
| **Gravitronics Gravity Device** | (Antigravity treatment for back condition.) | Not generally accepted medical practice. |
| **Hand-E-Jet** | (Portable whirlpool machine.) | See Whirlpool. |
| **Hand-D-Vent** | (Similar to IPPB machine; manual respiratory therapy.) | Rx required. Covered for severe respiratory impairment. |
| **Hearing Aid** | (To assist hearing.) | No coverage when specifically excluded by policy. |
| **Heating Lamp** | (External thermal applicator.) | Not covered outside hospital setting. |

*(continued)*

| Heating Pad | (Applies external heat.) | Not covered. Nondurable medical equipment. |
|---|---|---|
| Hemodialysis Equipment | (Artificial kidney device for blood filtering.) | Rx required. For chronic renal disease. |
| Holter Monitor | (24-hour cardiac measurement.) | Used only in physician's office. Charges payable within office fee as billed by physician. |
| Hospital bed, Electric | (Power multipurpose bed.) | Rx required. May be necessary when person is required to self-change bed position. Refer for medical review. |
| Hospital bed, Standard | (Multilevel positioning bed.) | Rx required. For bed-confined person who requires frequent position changes. |
| Hot Tub | (Thermal home spa system.) | Not covered. |
| Hoyer lift, Hydraulic | (Hydraulic patient lift.) | Rx required. Generally a convenience for lifting person from bed to wheelchair, etc. Patient's weight and statement of medical condition necessary. Refer for medical review. |
| Humidifier, Component of Oxygen Equipment | (Adds moisture to oxygen.) | Covered when oxygen therapy unit is covered. |
| Humidifier, Room or Central | (Environmental control.) | Not covered. Environmental control equipment. |
| Hydrocollator Heating Unit | (Applies local external heat.) | Rx required. Expense should be incurred through physician's office. |
| Hydro-jet Whirlpool Bath | (Comfort whirlpool.) | See Whirlpool. |
| Hypodermic Needles and Supplies, Hypospray | (Administration of intramuscular, intradermal injections.) | Rx required. For medical management of covered condition. |
| Incontinence Pads | (Nondurable, disposable supply.) | Covered only for post-surgical urinary conditions for one month. |
| Infusion Pump | (Stimulates constant infusions of medication subcutaneously or intra-arterially.) | Rx required. Refer for medical review. |
| Insulin Pump | (Artificial pancreas function surgically implanted.) | Procedures still investigational. Submit records for medical review. |
| Inhalator | (Respiratory assistance.) | Rx required. |
| IPPB Machines | (For respiratory therapy.) | Rx required. |
| Irrigation Kit | (For hygienic use.) | Covered for respiratory paralysis, wound drainage, etc. 60 days rental. |
| Jacuzzi Portable Pump | (For use in bathtubs.) | Rx required. Refer for whirlpool medical review. |
| Jobst Hydro Float | (Special floatation cushion.) | Covered for prevention or treatment of decubitus ulcers. |
| Jobst Pneumatic Appliance and Compressor, Pump | (Pneumatic full-limb appliance that maintains surface pressure.) | Rx required. Covered for intractable edema, post-radical mastectomy, etc. Refer for medical review. |
| Jobst Fabric Support, Houses, Sleeves, Stockings | (Non-reusable items, anti-embolism hose.) | Rx required. For circulatory conditions, pre- and post-op situations. |
| Lambs Wool Pad | (Soft padding, deluxe item, | Covered for bed sores, etc. |

*(continued)*

| | nondurable.) | |
|---|---|---|
| **Laser Equipment, any kind** | (High-intensity light source.) | Covered service only in physician's office. |
| **Lattoflex Spring Base** | (Not a hospital-type bed.) | Not covered. Comfort item. |
| **Lenox Hill Knee Brace** | (Supportive orthopedic device.) | Rx required. Charges based on individual custom-ordered appliance. |
| **Leotards** | (Tight body apparel.) | Not covered. |
| **Life-O-Gen Tank** | (Portable oxygen.) | Rx required. Covered for persons with respiratory impairment. |
| **Limb-O-Cycle** | (Exercise equipment.) | Not covered. |
| **Linde Oxygen Walker** | (Portable oxygen system.) | Rx required. Covered for persons with respiratory impairment. |
| **Lumex Chair Table** | (Like a rollabout chair.) | Covered in lieu of regular wheelchair. |
| **Lymphedema Pump** | (Appliance that maintains surface pressure.) | Rx required. Covered for intractable edema of extremity. |
| **Mask Devices** | (To mask out ringing in ears.) | Refer for medical review. |
| **Mask, Oxygen** | (Used to deliver oxygen.) | Covered for persons who require oxygen. |
| **Massage Devices** | (Comfort item.) | Not covered. |
| **Massage Pillow** | (Comfort item.) | Not covered. |
| **Mattress, Medical** | (For use with hospital bed.) | Covered when hospital bed is allowed. |
| **Maxi-Mist Machine** | (Delivers medicines as mist to be inhaled.) | Rx required. |
| **Medasphere Portable Oxygen Unit** | (Portable oxygen system.) | Covered when oxygen is necessary with exercise or walking. |
| **Medcolator** | (Physical therapy equipment.) | Not covered. |
| **Medi-Cool Refrigerator** | (For cooling medication.) | Not covered. |
| **Medi-Jector, Injection Gun** | (Delivers insulin without use of needles, Convenience item.) | Not covered. |
| **Micronaire Environmental Control** | (Equipment to control environment; air purifier.) | Not covered. Environmental control equipment. |
| **Milwaukee Back Brace** | (Supportive orthopedic brace.) | Rx required. |
| **Mobile Geriatric Chair** | (Wheelchair with smaller than normal wheels.) | Covered in lieu of regular wheelchair. |
| **Nebulizer** | (Delivers medicine in mist form for inhalation.) | Covered for respiratory impairment. |
| **Neck Halter** | (Supportive device.) | Rx not required. |
| **Nolan Bath Chair** | (For assistance in bathtub.) | Rx required. Possible convenience item. Statement of medical necessity. See Bathtub rail and seat. |
| **Non-vocal Communication System** | (Daily living assistance system, electronic.) | Not covered. |
| **Obturator** | (Oral prosthesis.) | Rx required. Cleft palate prosthesis. |
| **Orthopedic Shoes** | (Custom shoes.) | Not covered. |
| **Orthosis** | (Adjustable back brace.) | Rx required. |
| **Orthotics, Foot Stabilizers** | (Acrylic arch supports.) | Covered only when dispensed by physician and when not excluded by policy provisions. |
| **Osci Lite** | (Heat lamp.) | Not covered. |

*(continued)*

| | | |
|---|---|---|
| **Oscillating Bed** | (Alternating motion bed.) | Not covered for home use. |
| **Ostomy Bags** | (Used after ostomy procedures.) | Covered post-surgically. |
| **Ottobock Cosmetic Stockings** | (Covers existing prosthesis.) | Not covered. Nondurable medical equipment. |
| **Overbed Tables** | (For use with hospital bed, comfort item.) | Not covered. |
| **Oxygen** | (Compressed gas or liquid in tank.) | Rx required. |
| **Oxygen Concentrator** | (Condenses oxygen from room air.) | Rx required. Covered for persons with severe respiratory impairment. |
| **Oxygen Humidifier** | (Adds moisture to oxygen before inhalation.) | Rx required. Used in conjunction with oxygen tank system. |
| **Oxygen Regulator** | (Measures oxygen flow.) | Covered when oxygen unit is allowable. |
| **Oxygen Tent** | (Plastic overbed cover.) | Rx required. |
| **Oxygen Tank, Spare** | (Precautionary supply.) | Not covered. |
| **Pace Trac** | (Pacemaker monitor.) | Rx required. Refer for medical review. |
| **Poli-Axial Knee Cage Brace System** | (Lightweight supportive athletic knee cage and brace; very costly.) | Not covered. Athletic support device. |
| **Paraffin bath Unit, Portable and Standard** | (Wax immersion of affected joints.) | Covered for home use for arthritis patients. |
| **Parallel Bars** | (Exercise equipment.) | Not covered. |
| **Penile Implant** | (Inflatable penile prosthesis.) | Covered for those with diabetes, spinal cord injury, vascular disease, hypertension, post-surgical impotence. |
| **Penile Monitor** | (Electronic measuring device.) | Covered only in hospital under medical supervision. |
| **Percusser** | (Striking instrument used to perform percussion.) | Refer for medical review. |
| **Phonic Mirror, Handi-Voice** | (Electronic device that produces words by pressing buttons.) | Not covered. |
| **Pogon Buggy, Stroller Type** | (Adaptive wheelchair for child.) | Covered for non-ambulatory child who requires more support than standard wheelchair provides. |
| **Pollen Extractor** | (For home environment use air purifier.) | Not covered. Environmental control equipment. |
| **Portable Oxygen System** | (Transportable.) | Regulated, adj. flow. Rate – Rx required. – Preset, one flow rate – (For general use.) – Not covered. |
| **Portable Room Heater** | (Environmental control.) | Not covered. |
| **Posture Support Chairs** | (Comfort item.) | Not covered. |
| **Posturpedic Mattress** | (Special mattress.) | Covered only when a hospital bed is allowable. |
| **Pressure-Eze Pad** | (Alternating pressure pad.) | Covered for treatment of decubitus ulcer. |
| **Pressure Leotard** | (Form-fitting apparel.) | Not covered. |
| **Pulmo-Aide** | (Medicated nebulizer system.) | Covered for upper respiratory disease. |
| **Pulse Tachometer** | (Electronic pulse reader.) | Not covered. |
| **Reading Lamp** | (For home use.) | Not covered. |
| **Rib Belt** | (Supportive elastic item.) | Rx not required. Covered for appropriate diagnosis such as rib injury. |

*(continued)*

| | | |
|---|---|---|
| **Sacro-Ease Car Seat** | (For auto use.) | Not covered. |
| **Sanitation Equipment** | (For environmental use.) | Not covered. |
| **Sauna Bath** | (Comfort item.) | Not covered. |
| **Scolitron Stimulator** | (For curvature of the back, similar to TENS unit.) | Refer for medical review. |
| **Seat Lift** | (Seat that raises and lowers person in and out of chair.) | Rx required. For arthritis or other degenerative type diseases when the person is ambulatory. |
| **Selectron Air Purifier** | (Air cleaner for environmental control.) | Not covered. Environmental control equipment. |
| **Shoe Wedging** | (Sole modification.) | Rx required. |
| **Shoes** | (Wearing apparel item.) | Not covered. See Orthopedic shoes. |
| **Sitz Bath** | (Moist heat application.) | Not covered for home use. |
| **Sleek Seat.** | (Supportive chair for atonic child.) | Rx required. For children with atonic muscle condition. |
| **Spectrowave Machine** | (Diathermy machine.) | Not covered for home use. |
| **Speech Teaching Aids** | (Education devices.) | Not covered. |
| **Sphygmomanometer** | (Blood pressure equipment.) | Covered with documented diagnosis of hypertension; also used with home hemodialysis units. |
| **Spircare Incentive Breathing Device** | (Usually shows pulmonary function.) | Not covered. |
| **Stairglide** | (Home elevator system.) | Not covered. |
| **Stand Alone** | (Device that allows a paraplegic to stand without assistance. Comfort item.) | Not covered. |
| **Standing Table** | (Special table for use in standing position.) | Not covered. |
| **Stethoscope** | (Blood pressure monitoring equipment.) | Covered only with home blood pressure monitoring system. |
| **Stimulators, TENS** | (Electronic pulse.) | Rx required. Refer for medical review. |
| **Stryker Flotation Pad and Mattress** | (Gel flotation pad treats and prevents pressure sores.) | Rx required. |
| **Suction Machine** | (Removes secretions from airway, etc.) | Rx required. Must have qualified person in home to handle machine. |
| **Sun Lamp** | (Thermal application to skin.) | Not covered. |
| **Superpulse Machine** | (Diathermy machine.) | Not covered for home use. |
| **Surgical Stockings and Leggings** | (Support apparel, anti-embolism hose.) | Rx required. See Jobst fabric. |
| **Telemedic II** | (Telephone cardiac monitor.) | Covered only when done in physician's office. |
| **Telephone Arm** | (Attaches to receiver, comfort item.) | Not covered. |
| **Thermo-Jet** | (Whirlpool pump.) | See Whirlpool. |
| **Thermometer, Clinical** | (Measures temperature.) | Not covered. |
| **Thermophore Fomentation Device** | (Heat applicator, external heat source moist heating pad.) | Not covered. Nondurable medical equipment. |
| **Tilt Table** | (Adjustable exercise table.) | Not covered. |
| **Toilet Seat, Raised** | ------------------------ | Rx required. Hip replacement surgeries. See seat lift for other conditions. |

*(continued)*

| Traction Device | (Weighted device for physical therapy.) | Rx required. |
|---|---|---|
| Trapeze Bar | (Supportive device used for lifting self in hospital bed.) | Rx required. For use with a standard hospital bed only. |
| Treadmill Devices | (Home walking exercise unit.) | Rental covered with Rx and appropriate cardiac diagnosis. |
| Truss | (Hernia support.) | Rx not required. Covered with appropriate diagnosis. |
| Tub Chair | (Bathtub use. Comfort item.) | Not covered. |
| Twister Cable Medical Device | (Pediatric orthopedic.) | Rx required. Refer for medical review. |
| Ultrasound Machine | (Sound waves applied to muscles, tendons, etc.) | Covered only in physician's office. Not for home use. |
| Ultraviolet Equipment | (Directs ultraviolet light to body areas.) | Covered for persons with psoriasis when medical necessity is documented and home use approved by physician. |
| Urinal, Autoclaveable Hospital Type | (Not a comfort item) | Rx not required. Covered for bed-confined able person. |
| Vaporizer | (Delivers water mist to limited area in home.) | Not covered. Does not dispense medication as a nebulizer does. |
| Vasculating Bed | (Special hospital bed providing movement.) | Not covered for home use. |
| Vision Therapy Training Aids | (For adjunctive home use with vision therapy program.) | Not covered. |
| Walker | (Ambulatory aid.) | Rx not required. |
| Water Bed | (Comfort item.) | Not covered. See standard adjustable hospital bed. |
| Water Pressure Pad and Mattress | (Treats and prevents pressure sores, hospital bed type.) | Rx required. |
| Weighted Quad Boot | (Physical fitness equipment.) | Not covered. See ankle weights. |
| Wheel-O-Vater | (Home elevator.) | Not covered. |
| Wheelchair | Regular manual standard model. | Rx not required if documented by diagnosis |
| Wheelchair | Electric type. | Rx required. Person must require independent mobility |
| Wheelchair | Accessories and repair to function. | |
| Wheelchair | (Rubber wheel linings, ball appropriate and bearings, batteries, seat pad.) | Rx required. Covered only when policy provisions do not exclude. Convenience items or modifications not functional in nature such as color coordination, deluxe padding, and trays are not covered expense. |
| Travel Type | Covered in lieu of regular wheelchair. | |
| Wheelchair Insert | (For small child, when chair seat does not fit.) | Rx not required |
| Whirlpool Pumps | (Portable units for home use in baths.) | Rx required. Refer for medical review. |
| Wigs and Toupees | (Cosmetic appliance for conditions of alopecia, hair loss.) | Refer for medical review. |

*(continued)*

# Assistant Surgeon Procedures

Following is a list of surgical procedures by CPT® code for which an assistant surgeon is considered NOT necessary. This list and is intended to be used for training and reference purposes only, as the particular company or plan guidelines may differ from those guidelines stated.

| | | | | |
|---|---|---|---|---|
| 17108 | 19125 | 19126 | 19328 | 21616 |
| 23020 | 24101 | 24105 | 24110 | 24351 |
| 25295 | 25909 | 26037 | 26358 | 26516 |
| 27358 | 27619 | 27831 | 28290 | 30130 |
| 30140 | 30520 | 30620 | 31502 | 33470 |
| 36469 | 37700 | 42220 | 46700 | 52510 |
| 54110 | 54430 | 55040 | 55680 | 56304 |
| 58660 | 59821 | 61556 | 62142 | 63308 |
| 63746 | 64862 | 65155 | 66605 | 67101 |
| 67311 | 67875 | 68505 | 69631 | 69670 |

■ **Table AC–4** Assistant Surgeon Procedures

# State Abbreviations

| Name of State | Abbreviation |
|---|---|
| Alabama | AL |
| Alaska | AK |
| American Samoa | AS |
| Arizona | AZ |
| Arkansas | AR |
| California | CA |
| Colorado | CO |
| Connecticut | CT |
| Delaware | DE |
| District of Columbia | DC |
| Florida | FL |
| Georgia | GA |
| Guam | GU |
| Hawaii | HI |
| Idaho | ID |
| Illinois | IL |
| Indiana | IN |
| Iowa | IA |
| Kansas | KS |
| Kentucky | KY |
| Louisiana | LA |
| Maine | ME |
| Maryland | MD |
| Massachusetts | MA |
| Michigan | MI |
| Minnesota | MN |
| Mississippi | MS |
| Missouri | MO |
| Montana | MT |
| Nebraska | NE |
| Nevada | NV |
| New Hampshire | NH |
| New Jersey | NJ |
| New Mexico | NM |
| New York | NY |
| North Carolina | NC |
| North Dakota | ND |
| Ohio | OH |
| Oklahoma | OK |
| Oregon | OR |
| Pennsylvania | PA |
| Puerto Rico | PR |
| Rhode Island | RI |
| South Carolina | SC |
| South Dakota | SD |
| Tennessee | TN |
| Texas | TX |
| Utah | UT |
| Vermont | VT |

■ **Table AC–5** State Abbreviations          *(continued on next page)*

| Virginia | VA |
|---|---|
| Virgin Islands | VI |
| Washington | WA |
| West Virginia | WV |
| Wisconsin | WI |
| Wyoming | WY |

*(continued)*

# Other Address Abbreviations

| Other Address | Abbreviation |
|---|---|
| Alley | Aly |
| Avenue | Ave |
| Boulevard | Blvd |
| Branch | Br |
| Bypass | Byp |
| Causeway | Cswy |
| Center | Ctr |
| Circle | Cir |
| Court | Ct |
| Courts | Cts |
| Crescent | Cres |
| Drive | Dr |
| Expressway | Expy |
| Extension | Ext |
| Freeway | Fwy |
| Gardens | Gdns |
| Grove | Grv |
| Heights | Hts |
| Highway | Hwy |
| Lane | Ln |
| Manor | Mnr |
| Place | Pl |
| Plaza | Plz |
| Point | Pt |
| Post Office | PO |
| Road | Rd |
| Rural | R |
| Rural Route | RR |
| Square | Sq |
| Street | St |
| Terrace | Ter |
| Trail | Trl |
| Turnpike | Tpke |
| Viaduct | Via |
| Vista | Vis |

■ **Table AC–6** Other Address Abbreviations

# Appendix D
# Forms

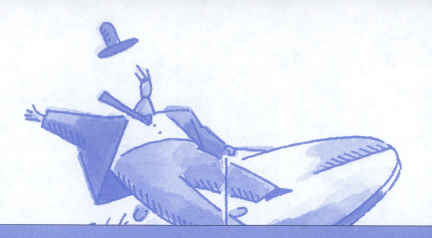

## Table of Contents

# Payment Worksheet

| Eligible Employee: | | Accident Benefit: | $ | (CCYY) |
|---|---|---|---|---|
| Company: | | Lifetime Max: | $ | |
| Insured's ID Number: | | Deductible: | $ | (CCYY) |
| Patient: | | Carryover Ded: | $ | (CCNY) |
| Relationship: | | Coinsurance: | $ | (CCYY) |
| Provider's Zip Code: | | Date of Injury: | | |

| Procedure Type of Service | Dates of Service | Billed Amount | Excluded Amounts* | Allowed | Basic/ Accident 100% | Maj. Med. ___% | ___% | UCR Calcula- tions |
|---|---|---|---|---|---|---|---|---|
| 1. | | $ | $ | $ | $ | | | |
| 2. | | | | | | | | |
| 3. | | | | | | | | |
| 4. | | | | | | | | |
| 5. | | | | | | | | |
| 6. | | | | | | | | |
| **Remarks:** | **Totals:** | $ | $ | $ | $ | | | |
| | Deductible: | | | | $ | | | |
| | Amount Subject to Coinsurance: | | | | $ | | | |
| | Coinsurance: | | | | $ | | | |
| | Amount Subject to Adjustment: | | | | $ | | | |
| | Adjustment (See Remarks): | | | | $ | | | |
| | Payment Amount: | | | $ | $ | | | |

| *Denial Reasons |
|---|
| 1. |
| 2. |
| 3. |
| 4. |
| 5. |
| 6. |

| Payees |
|---|
| 1. |
| 2. |
| 3. |
| 4. |
| 5. |
| 6. |

If you disagree with our decision on your claim, you have the right by law to request that your claim be reviewed by your plan administrator. This request must be made in writing within 60 days of receipt of this notice. If you wish, you may submit your written comments and views. Please consult your plan's claim review procedures. See your employer regarding any other ERISA questions.

■ **Figure AD–1**  Payment Worksheet

# Coordination of Benefits Calculation Worksheet

Patient's Name: _____  Year: _____

**Payment Calculation:**

1. Total allowable amount for this claim is the higher of either the primary plan's allowable amount or the secondary plan's allowable amount.  _____

2. Total primary insurance carrier payment for this claim.  _____

3. Difference between Line 1 and Line 2.  _____

4. Secondary insurance carrier's normal liability for this claim.  _____

5. The lesser of Line 3 or Line 4.
   This is the amount of the secondary insurance carrier actual payment on this claim.  _____

**Credit Reserve:**

6. Normal liability for this claim (Line 4 above).  _____

7. Actual payment for this claim (line 5 above).  _____

8. Subtract Line 7 from Line 6.  _____

9. Credit reserve on all previous claims for this patient.  _____

10. Total credit reserve (add Line 8 and Line 9).  _____

**Instructions:**
Place the patient's name and the year that services were rendered in the box on the top of the COB calculation sheet.
1. Enter the total allowable amount on this claim. The total allowable amount is the greater of either the primary plan's allowable amount or the secondary plan's allowable amount.
2. Enter the total amount that other insurance companies have paid on this claim.
3. Subtract line 2 from line 1.
4. Enter the normal liability amount for this insurance company for this claim.
5. Enter the lesser of either Line 3 or Line 4. This is the actual amount of the secondary insurance payor on this claim.

**To Calculate Credit Reserve:**
6. Enter the normal liability amount for the secondary insurance carrier for this claim.
7. Enter the actual payment for the secondary insurance carrier for this claim.
8. Subtract Line 7 from Line 6. This is the amount of money the secondary carrier has saved by paying secondary on this claim. This amount becomes part of the credit reserve.
9. Enter the credit reserve amount for all previous claims for this patient.
10. Add Line 8 and Line 9. This is the total credit reserve for this patient.

■ **Figure AD–2** Coordination of Benefits Calculation Worksheet

PLACE STICKER AT THE BOTTOM OF THE PACKAGE
FOLD AT DOTTED LINE

## Certified Mail

1000 0555 0001 2222 5555

0001 0222 1000 5555 2222

| | |
|---|---|
| **Provider Postal Services-Certified Mail** | |
| Sender's Name | |
| Street, Apt. No.; or PO Box No. | |
| City, State, ZIP + 4 | |
| Postage $ | |
| Certified Fee $ | |
| Total Postage $ | |
| Recipient's Name (To be completed by mailer) | |
| Street, Apt. No.; | |
| City, State, ZIP + 4 | |

■ **Figure AD–3** Certified Mail Form

PROVIDER POSTAL SERVICES

First-Class Mail
Postage & Fees Paid
PPS
Permit No. P-18

●Sender: Please print your name, address, and ZIP+4 in this box●

---

**SENDER:** *COMPLETE THIS SECTION*

- Complete items 1, 2, and 3. Also complete item 4 if Restricted Delivery is desired.
- Print your name and address on the reverse so that we can return the card to you.
- Attach this card to the back of the maiilpiece, or on the front if space permits.

1. Article Addressed to:

2. Article Number
   *(Transfer from service label)*

**COMPLETE THIS SECTION ON DELIVERY**

A. Signature

X
☐ Agent
☐ Addressee

B. Received by (Printed Name) | C. Date of Delivery

D. Is delivery address different from item 1? ☐ Yes
   If YES, enter delivery address below: ☐ No

3. Service Type
   ☐ Certified Mail     ☐ Express Mail
   ☐ Registered         ☐ Return Receipt for Merchandise
   ☐ Insured Mail       ☐ C.O.D

4. Restricted Delivery? *(Extra Fee)*     ☐ Yes

PPS Form 2894          Domestic Return Receipt          105535-06-P-6211

■ **Figure AD–4** Domestic Return Receipt (Front and Back)

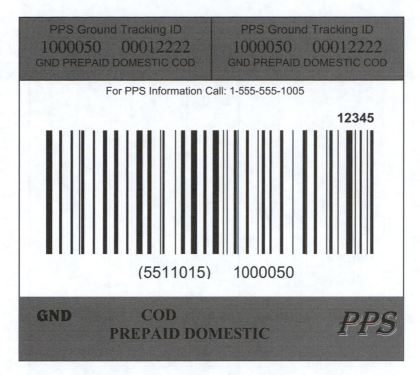

**■ Figure AD–5** Ground Tracking COD Form

## PPS EXPRESS *C.O.D Airbill*

*PPS Tracking Number 1005 1222*

5005

### 1 From *Please print and press hard.*

Date

Sender's PPS
Account Number 1005-5505-5

Sender's
Name _____ Phone ( )

Company _____

Address _____

Dept./Floor/Suite/Room

City _____ State _____ ZIP _____

### 2 Your Internal Billing Reference
First 4 characters will appear on invoice.

### 3 To

Recipient's
Name _____ Phone ( )

Company _____

Address _____

To "HOLD" at PPS location, print PPS address. We cannot deliver to P.O. boxes or P.O. ZIP codes.

Address _____

Dept./Floor/Suite/Room

City _____ State _____ ZIP _____

**Questions? Call 1-555-555-1005**

---

Form
I.D. No.         **1055**          Sender's Copy

### 4a Express Package Service          *Packages up to 150lbs.*

□ **PPS Priority Overnight**       □ **PPS Standard Overnight**   □ **PPS First Overnight**
Next business morning           Next business afternoon      Earliest next business morning
                                delivery to select locations

□ **PPS 2Day**                    □ **PPS Express Saver**
Second business day             Third business day
                                PPS Envelope rate not available. Minimum charge: One-pound rate
Delivery commitment may be later in some areas.

### 4b Express Freight Service          *Packages over 150 lbs.*

□ **PPS 1Day Freight***          □ **PPS 2Day Freight**          □ **PPS 3Day Freight**
Next business day               Second business day            Third business day
*Call for confirmation:_____
Delivery commitment may be later in some areas.

### 5 Packaging

□ **PPS Envelope***   □ **PPS Pak***   □ **Other**
                      Includes Small,        Declared value limit $500
                      Large and Sturdy Pak

### 6 Special Handling          [Include PPS address in Section 3]

□ **SATURDAY Delivery**   □ **HOLD Weekday**       □ **HOLD Saturday**
at PPS Location            at PPS Location

### 7 Payment    *Bill to:*   [Enter PPS Acct. No. or Credit Card No. below.]

□ Sender        □ Recipient     □ Third Party     □ Credit Card     □ Cash/Check
Acct. No. in
Section 1 will be billed.

PPS Acct. No.
Credit Card No. _____              Exp.
                                             Date

Total Packages   Total Weight   Total Declared Value†

$ _____ .00
                PPS Use Only

†Our Liability is limited to $100 unless you declare a higher value.

### 8 Release Signature

*Sign to authorize delivery without obtaining signature.*

_____

By signing you authorize us to deliver this shipment without obtaining a signature
and agree to indemnify and hold us harmless from any resulting claims.

**■ Figure AD–6** PPS Express COD Airbill

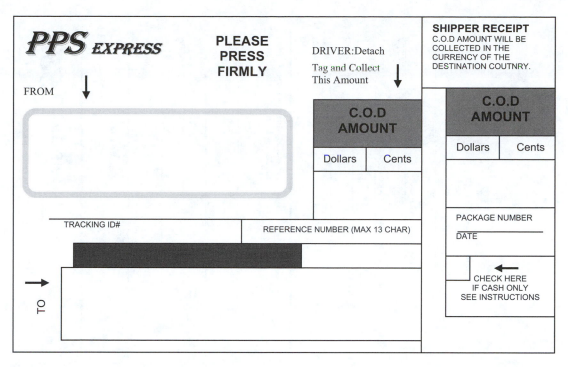

■ **Figure AD–7**  COD Shipper Receipt

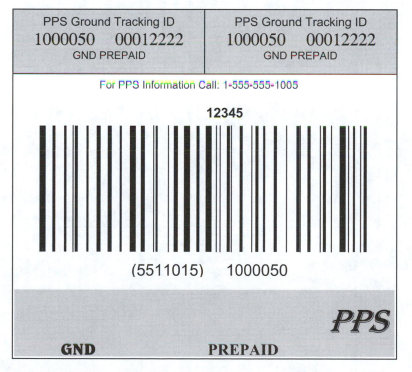

■ **Figure AD–8**  Ground Tracking ID Prepaid Form

## PPS EXPRESS  *Airbill*

PPS Tracking Number   1005  1222

5005

### 1 From *Please print and press hard.*

Sender's PPS
Account Number 1005-5505-5

Date

Sender's
Name _____   Phone ( )

Company _____

Address _____

City _____ State _____ ZIP _____

Dept./Floor/Suite/Room

### 2 Your Internal Billing Reference

First 4 characters will appear on invoice.

_____

### 3 To

Recipient's
Name _____   Phone ( )

Company _____

Address _____
To "HOLD" at PPS location, print PPS address.   We cannot deliver to P.O. boxes or P.O. ZIP codes.

Address _____

City _____ State _____ ZIP _____

Dept./Floor/Suite/Room

**Questions? Call 1-555-555-1005**

---

Form
I.D. No.                          **1055**

### Sender's Copy

### 4a Express Package Service
*Packages up to 150lbs.*

☐ **PPS Priority Overnight**
Next business morning

☐ **PPS Standard Overnight**
Next business afternoon
delivery to select locations

☐ **PPS First Overnight**
Earliest next business morning
Delivery commitment may be later in some areas.

☐ **PPS 2Day**
Second business day

☐ **PPS Express Saver**
Third business day
**PPS Envelope rate not available. Minimum charge: One-pound rate**

### 4b Express Freight Service
*Packages over 150 lbs.*

☐ **PPS 1Day Freight***
Next business day
*Call for confirmation:

☐ **PPS 2Day Freight**
Second business day

☐ **PPS 3Day Freight**
Third business day
Delivery commitment may be later in some areas.

### 5 Packaging

☐ PPS Envelope*    ☐ PPS Pak*    ☐ Other
Includes Small,
Large and Sturdy Pak
Declared value limit $500

### 6 Special Handling

☐ **SATURDAY Delivery**
at PPS Location

☐ **HOLD Weekday**
at PPS Location

[Include PPS address in Section 3]

☐ **HOLD Saturday**

### 7 Payment    *Bill to:*

☐ **Sender**
Acct. No. in
Section 1 will be billed.

☐ **Recipient**    ☐ **Third Party**    ☐ **Credit Card**    ☐ **Cash/Check**

[Enter PPS Acct. No. or Credit Card No. below.]

PPS Acct. No.
Credit Card No. _____   Exp.
Date _____

Total Packages | Total Weight | Total Declared Value†

$ _____ .00

PPS Use Only

†Our Liability is limited to $100 unless you declare a higher value.

### 8 Release Signature

*Sign to authorize delivery without obtaining signature.*

By signing you authorize us to deliver this shipment without obtaining a signature
and agree to indemnify and hold us harmless from any resulting claims.

---

# Glossary

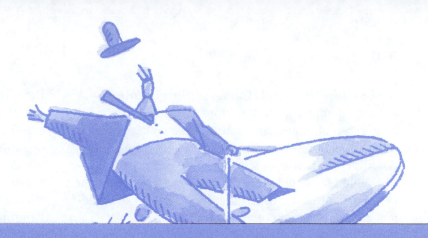

**Abortion**—A premature expulsion of an embryo or nonviable fetus.

**Abscess**—A collection of pus that results in disintegration or displacement of tissues.

**Abutment**—A tooth that is used to support or stabilize one end of a prosthetic appliance.

**Accident**—Defined as an unintentional injury which has a specific time, date, and place.

**Accidental Injury**—A sudden and unforeseen event, definite as to time and place. This includes trauma happening involuntarily or as a result of a voluntary act entailing unforeseen consequences.

**Accumulation Period**—The period of time in which to satisfy the deductible, accumulate COB credit reserves, reach maximums, and so on.

**Active Work (Actively at Work)**—Usually means performing the regular duties for a full workday for the employer.

**Actively-at-work**—A stipulation included in many contracts that states that a person must be at work (or actively engaged in their normal activities if a dependent) on the date coverage becomes effective.

**Acts of Third Parties (ATP)**—A provision that allows the insurance carrier to recoup medical expenses paid if it is found that a third party is liable for damages.

**Actuarial Statistics**—Studies that an insurance company uses. For a carrier which covers health insurance, these can include statistics covering average life span, number of days in hospital per year for each age group, number of doctor visits, costs of all medical services, etc.

**Acupuncture**—The ancient Chinese practice of inserting fine needles into various points in the body to relieve pain, induce anesthesia, and to regulate and improve body functions.

**Adjunctive General Services**—Miscellaneous services, treatments not listed elsewhere on a dental code listing.

**Adjustment**—The reprocessing of a claim to correct prior errors.

**Aggregate**—Any amounts paid toward the deductible by any member of the family will be added up to reach the deductible.

**Air Ambulance**—A helicopter or other flight vehicle used to transport a severely injured or ill person to a hospital.

**Allowable Expense**—Any necessary, reasonable, and customary item of a medical or dental expense, at least partly covered under at least one of the plans.

**Allowed Amount**—Same as UCR amount.

**Alternative Benefit Provision (ABP)**—This provision determines the level of care/treatment that can be provided under the plan.

**Alternative Birthing Centers (ABC)**—Outpatient care centers that provide special rooms for routine deliveries.

**Alveolar Process**—The portion of the mandible or maxilla that contains the tooth socket.

**Alveoloplasty**—Surgical preparation of a ridge for dentures.

**Ambulance Expenses**—Charges billed for transporting an injured or ill person to a medical facility.

**Ambulatory Surgical Centers (Surgi-centers)**—A center equipped to allow for the performance of surgery on an outpatient basis. These centers may be freestanding or attached to a major acute care facility.

**Ancillary Expenses**—Miscellaneous services or supplies that are provided by the hospital on an inpatient or outpatient basis, which are necessary for the medical care or treatment of an individual.

**Anesthesia**—The artificially induced loss of feeling and sensation with or without loss of consciousness.

**Ankyloglossia**—A shortened frenulum of the tongue, preventing proper movement of the tongue.

**Apex**—The terminus or end of the root.

**Apexification**—Performed on the permanent tooth of a young person when the apex of the tooth is incompletely formed.

**Appliance**—Any device or brace that includes banding or wiring used to reposition teeth, jaw joint, or lower jaw to restore normal occlusion.

**Arthroplasty**—A procedure in which a portion of the joint is surgically removed and the toe is straightened.

**Assignment of Benefits**—A statement, usually included on the claim form, which permits the member to authorize the administrator to pay benefits directly to the person or institution that provided the service.

**Assistant Surgeon**—A surgeon who assists a primary surgeon. An assistant surgeon may perform the closing of the operative wound, hemostasis of the wound edges, and suturing of vessels.

**Automatic Annual Reinstatement (AAR)**—A contractually specified amount of money that may be added to the balance of available lifetime benefits.

**Balance Billing**—In Medicare, charging patients for more than the Medicare allowance.

**Banding Fee**—Portion of the total case fee.

**Basic Benefit**—Benefits which are paid before major medical benefits, and which provide a specified allowance for a certain type of service. Usually, the allowance is 100% of either UCR (as defined by the plan) or some other amount based on the relative value study (RVS) and conversion factors.

**Basic Dental Plan**—Pays dental benefits at 100% of either the UCR or a scheduled amount.

**Batch Files**—Files which are kept in batches or groups based on the date they were processed and the person who processed them.

**Beneficiary**—The person who receives payment on a claim, often the person who receives the benefit in the case of a deceased member.

**Benefit**—An item covered by an insurance policy, or something paid to or on behalf of a recipient.

**Benefit Period**—A period that begins with the first day of admission to the hospital. A benefit period ends after the patient has been discharged from the hospital or skilled nursing facility for a period of 60 consecutive days (including the day of discharge).

**Bilateral Procedures**—Surgeries that involve a pair of similar body parts (i.e., breasts, eyes).

**Binding Machines**—Machines that bind several pages of a document together, often with a strip down the left-hand side of the document.

**Biofeedback**—Training an individual to consciously control automatic, internal bodily functions.

**Bitewing X-rays**—X-rays that show the relationship of the teeth in two opposing dental arches.

**Block Procedures**—Multiple surgical procedures performed during the same operative session in the same operative area.

**Body**—Part of the correspondence that contains the main text or message.

**Bone Spur**—A bony overgrowth on the bone.

**Brightness Control**—Changes the brightness of the image on the screen.

**Bruxism**—Grinding of the teeth.

**Buccal (B)**—The surface nearest the cheek.

**Bunion**—An enlargement of a bone in a joint at the base of the big toe.

**By Report (BR)**—Procedures that are so unusual or variable that it is impossible to determine a standard UCR or unit value allowance. The RVS may refer to these procedures as Relative Value Not Established (RNE).

**Calculator**—A machine that computes numbers.

**Calculus**—Calcified dental plaque.

**Capillaries**—Supply blood nourishment to the tooth.

**Capitation**—A monthly fee paid to a provider in exchange for handling the healthcare needs of a patient.

**Capsulotomy**—A procedure performed to release the buckling and the top and bottom tendons.

**Carryover Deductible**—Means that any amounts which the patient pays toward their deductible in the last three months of the year will carry over and will be applied toward the next year's deductible.

**Cementum**—A bone-like material that although hard, is not the same category as the enamel or the dentin.

**Central Processing Unit (CPU)**—The rectangular box that houses the memory and functional components of the computer.

**Certified Mail**—A package or envelope that must be signed for upon delivery.

**Cheilitis**—Inflammation of the lips.

**Cheiloschisis**—A deep groove in the lip. It is also known as a harelip or cleft lip.

**Chromosomal Analysis**—A diagnostic study performed on the fluid to study the number and structure of the chromosomes to determine whether any abnormalities are present.

**Claim**—A written request by the insured individual for payment by the insurance company of covered expenses under the insurance policy.

**Claim Determination Period**—A period in which COB is determined, usually a calendar year.

**Claim Files**—Files for holding claims and other processing information.

**Claim Investigation**—Making a detailed inquiry to verify facts pertaining to a claim submitted.

**Claim Payment Worksheet**—A form that is equivalent to an explanation of benefits. A copy of this form will be sent to the insured to explain the benefit payment for the claim.

**Claim Processing**—To determine benefit amounts and pay a claim.

**Clarity in Writing**—Exactness of language.

**Cleft Palate**—A deep fissure of the palate. It may involve the soft palate, the hard palate, the lip, or all three.

**CMS-1500**—The claim form most commonly used to bill for provider's services.

**Coherence in Writing**—Information that follows logically flow from one idea to the next.

**Coinsurance**—The arrangement by which both the member and the plan share, in a specific ratio, the covered losses under the policy.

**Coinsurance Limit**—This limit stipulates that if the coinsurance amount reaches a certain level, all subsequent claims will be paid at 100% of the allowed amount.

**Collate**—To put copies in the original order of the pages.

**Common Accident Provision**—A provision whereby only one deductible is taken for all members of a family involved in the same accident.

**Company Activities**—An injury sustained while attending an activity sponsored by an employer for the purpose of obtaining some business gain or an activity which the company provides remuneration and an injury sustained while in the course of a person's occupation.

**Compensatory Damages**—Damages designed to compensate an insured for all of the actual losses or damages to make that person whole again.

**Complex Cavities**—Involve three or more surfaces of a tooth.

**Complimentary Close**—Where you bring your letter to an end in a short polite manner.

**Compound Cavities**—Involve two surfaces of a tooth.

**Computer Disk Drive**—A place for the storage of information.

**Computer Monitor**—The screen that is connected to the computer.

**Concurrent Review**—Determines whether the estimated length of time and scope of the inpatient stay is justified by the diagnosis and symptoms. This review is conducted periodically during the projected length of stay.

**Consideration**—Anything that is given, done, promised, forbidden, or suffered by one party as an inducement for the agreement.

**Consolidated Omnibus Budget Reconciliation Act of 1985 (COBRA)**—Also referred to as Continuation of Coverage. The law requires employers to permit employees and their dependents to purchase transitional healthcare coverage at favorable group rates until replacement coverage could be obtained. The intended result was to reduce the number of people without healthcare coverage.

**Consultation**—An opinion provided by a specialist.

**Contract**—A legal and binding written document that exists between two or more parties.

**Contrast Control**—Turns the contrast up and down between varying fields.

**Contributory Plan**—The employees contribute to the cost of the coverage, usually through payroll deductions.

**Convalescent Facilities**—Usually considered to be midrange facilities that provide nonacute care for persons recovering from an acute illness or injury.

**Conversion**—Permits employees and dependents to continue their insurance protection on an individual basis when their coverage under a group plan ceases.

**Conversion Factor**—A dollar amount determined for a specific service type or a particular region. Each region may have a unique set of conversion factors, and each service type may be assigned a specific conversion factor.

**Coordination of Benefits (COB)**—A process that occurs when two or more group plans provide coverage on the same person so that the insured does not make money from an illness or injury.

**Copayment**—A provision requiring the member to pay a set or fixed dollar amount (i.e., $5, $10, or $25) each time a particular medical service is used. Copayment provisions are frequently found in PPO and HMO plans.

**Correspondence**—Written communication between two people.

**Cosmetic Procedure**—A surgical procedure performed solely to improve appearance.

**Cosmetic Surgery**—A surgical procedure performed solely to improve appearance and is usually not covered by benefit plans.

**Cosurgeons**—Under some circumstances, two surgeons, usually with similar skills, may operate simultaneously as primary surgeons performing distinct, separate parts of a total surgical service.

**Cover Letter**—An introductory letter to your resume.

**Covered Expense**—Any expense for which complete or partial payment is provided under the insurance policy.

**Credible Coverage**—Like or similar coverage. For example if the former coverage was medical only, and the new coverage is medical, dental, and vision, only the medical portion would be considered credible. Therefore, the employee would be given credit for prior medical coverage, but preexisting exclusions could be applied to dental and vision services.

**Credit Reserve (CR)**—A cumulative amount within a claim determination period that is derived from the amount of funds that a plan has saved by being the secondary carrier.

**Crown**—A covering that is placed on a tooth.

**CT (Computed Tomography) Scans**—Is a process that uses multiple x-ray images to create three-dimensional images of body structures.

**Cumulative Benefit**—One of the more common types of MWH benefit. To calculate benefits under this provision, the number of days hospitalized is multiplied by the benefit amount.

**Current Dental Terminology (CDT)**—A reference manual published by the American Dental Association that contains dental procedure codes.

**Cursor**—The small lighted symbol on the monitor screen that indicates where you are in the program.

**Cuspids (Canines)**—Are located behind the incisors. They are used for tearing and piercing. The normal adult has four, one behind each set of incisors.

**Custodial Care**—Care that is primarily for the purpose of meeting the personal daily needs of the patient and can be provided by personnel without medical care skills or training.

**Cyst**—An enclosed pouch that contains fluid, semifluid, or solid material.

**Day Care Centers**—Provide treatment during the daylight hours with the patient being released at night.

**Death Benefits**—Benefits which compensate the family of a deceased employee for the loss of income which the employee would have provided to the family.

**Deciduous Teeth (Primary Teeth)**—Numbered one to 20 and apply to children. These teeth are lettered rather than numbered to avoid confusion with the adult numbering system.

**Deductible**—The amount of covered expenses that must be paid by the insured/member before benefits become payable by the insurer/plan under the Major Medical portion of the contract.

**Deficit Reduction Act of 1984, (DEFRA)**—The Act that amended TEFRA so that spouses, aged 65 years and older, of active employees who are under age 65 can elect their primary coverage, as either Medicare or the private group plan.

**Dental Caries or Cavities**—Holes or decayed portions of the tooth. They are caused by the progressive decalcification of the tooth.

**Dental Claim Form**—A form that lists specific information regarding the patient and the services that have been or are going to be performed.

**Dental Plaque**—A mass of microorganisms that grows on the exposed portions of the teeth and may spread under the gum line.

**Dental Relative Value Study**—A scheme used to determine how much a provider should be paid by assessing a unit value to each CDT® code.

**Dentalgia**—A toothache or pain in the tooth.

**Dentin**—Sometimes called the ivory, which forms the bulk of the tooth.

**Dentistry**—The department of the healing arts that is concerned with the teeth, the oral cavity (mouth) and its associated structures.

**Dentists**—Doctors who have received a Doctor of Medical Dentistry (D.M.D.) degree.

**Department of Insurance**—The legal entity that oversees the operations of all insurance companies.

**Dependent**—The employee's legal spouse or domestic partner, and unmarried children within the age limitations specified by the plan who rely on the employee for daily maintenance and care.

**Diagnosis Related Group Billing (DRG)**—A flat rate payment is made based on the patient's diagnosis rather than the hospital's itemized billing.

**Diagnostic**—Routine services designed to assist in the diagnosis and planning of required treatment.

**Diagnostic Casts**—Models that duplicate the structure of the mouth.

**Diagnostic Charges**—For initial testing to confirm a diagnosis or to rule out other diagnoses.

**Diagnostic Photographs**—Colored photographs of the oral cavity that are used to show various conditions of the teeth and mouth structures.

**Diagnostic Procedures**—Procedures performed to determine the presence of disease or the cause of the patient's symptoms.

**Diagnostic X-rays**—Flat or two-dimensional pictures of a particular body part or organ.

**Dialysis**—A treatment given to patients who have suffered acute kidney failure and must have their kidney functions taken over artificially.

**Disclaimer**—A denial or renunciation, as of responsibility.

**Distal (D)**—The surface farthest away from the midline.

**Distoclusion**—Occurs when the maxillary arch protrudes out from the mandibular arch.

**Doctor's First Report of Occupational Injury or Illness (First Report)**—The report completed by a doctor at a Workers' Compensation patient's first visit.

**Documentation**—The orderly organization and communication of important facts that can be used to furnish decisive evidence of claim handling or processing.

**Dorsal Osteotomy**—A procedure performed by removing a small wedge of bone from the top (dorsal) side of the base of the fifth metatarsal bone.

**Durable Medical Equipment (DME)**—Items that can be used for an extended period of time without significant deterioration.

**Dwyer Procedure**—Treatment for a deformity of the calcaneus or large heel bone.

**Edentulous**—Without teeth.

**Effective Date**—The date a contract began to be in force.

**Effectiveness in Writing**—Being able to evoke the type of response you want your reader to have, whether you want the reader to subscribe to a magazine or to purchase a product or service.

**Electronic Claims**—Claims that are routinely submitted electronically.

**Electronic Claims Submission**—A process whereby insurance claims are submitted via computerized data (either by data diskette or modem) directly from the provider to the insurance company.

**Eligibility**—The qualifications that make the person eligible for coverage.

**Eligibility Roster**—A listing which shows the effective dates of the patient's coverage, what contract they are covered under, and their primary care provider.

**Embezzlement**—The act of an employee illegally taking funds from a company they work for.

**Emergency Medical Technician (EMT)**—A person trained in basic life support.

**Employee Benefit**—Anything other than wages offered to an employee. This can include insurance coverage, vacation time, pension or retirement plans, sick pay, etc.

**Enclosures**—Anything that you are sending along with the letter.

**Endodontics**—Treatment of dental pulp or other internal structures of the teeth.

**Endogenous Obesity**—Obesity caused by an internal malfunction, usually hormonal (i.e., thyroid disorder).

**End-Stage Renal Disease (ESRD)**—The condition in which a person's kidneys fail to function.

**Epidural Anesthesia**—Anesthesia which blocks the nerves in the epidural space.

**ERISA Right of Review Statement**—A statement which must be included on all denied claims.

**Etiquette**—The practices and forms prescribed by convention or by authority. In essence, etiquette is manners.

**Evidence of Insurability**—The employee will be required to submit proof of good health usually by filling out a health questionnaire.

**Exclusions**—Conditions or types of services that the policy does not cover.

**Exclusive Provider Organization (EPO)**—The patient selects a primary care giver and can use only physicians who are part of the network or who are referred by the primary care physician.

**Exogenous Obesity**—Obesity caused by overeating.

**Explanation of Benefits (EOB)**—A letter of explanation of benefits from a payer indicating how a member's benefits have been applied.

**Extended Benefits**—The continued entitlement of a member, under certain circumstances, to receive benefits after the coverage has terminated.

**Extraoral X-rays**—Rays taken with the film placed outside the mouth.

**Facility Services**—Services provided at a "place," for example, a hospital or clinic. Equipment usage and room fees (i.e., x-ray equipment, operating room) are considered facility expenses.

**Facsimile Machine**—More commonly known as a fax machine. It sends pictures over the phone lines by transmitting a series of dot messages.

**False Nail**—A tough skin that mimics a real nail.

**Family Files**—Folders of claims that are kept for each family of claimants.

**Fee Schedule**—Allowable amount for that particular procedure assigned according to the particular CPT® code.

**Filling Restorations**—Include a base, polishing, and local anesthetic.

**Flat Feet (Pes Planus)**—A hereditary condition that is caused by a muscle imbalance.

**Fluoride Treatments**—The application of a topical fluoride substance to the teeth.

**Follow-up Days**—Days immediately following a surgical procedure in which a doctor must monitor a patient's condition for that particular procedure.

**Fraud**—Deception to cause a person to give up property or something of lawful right.

**Full Credit Adjustment**—An adjustment that completely reverses a claim payment.

**Full Dentures**—Appliances that replace all of the patient's natural teeth.

**Full-mouth X-ray Limitation**—If the dollar amount payable for the total number of x-rays taken exceeds the dollar amount payable for a set of full-mouth x-rays, the allowable amount would be based on the full-mouth x-ray allowance because the dentist could have taken an entire x-ray series to see all tooth structures.

**Ganglion**—A fluid-filled sac that may grow on a joint capsule or tendon.

**Garnishment**—A method of collecting an unpaid debt, which may only be utilized after a lawsuit has been filed, and a judgment is obtained.

**Gatekeeper PPO**—The member chooses a family provider or physician and must see him or her before being referred to a specialist. The specialist may or may not be within the network.

**Gender rule**—States that the plan covering the male employee is primary, and the plan covering the female employee is secondary.

**General Anesthesia**—Anesthesia that produces a state of unconsciousness.

**Gingivitis**—Inflammation of the gums. It may include swelling, redness, pain, bleeding, or difficulty in chewing. Possible causes are improper dental hygiene, dentures or dental appliances that fit improperly, or improper occlusion (closure) of the teeth. Occasionally, gingivitis accompanies upper respiratory infections or diseases such as scurvy or metallic poisoning.

**Global Approach**—The total billed amount should be compared with the total UCR amount. In our example, the total UCR amount is $700; however, the total billed amount is $900. The amounts in excess of the global UCR should be denied.

**Global COB**—COB applied to both medical and dental charges combined. All savings are kept intermingled.

**Group Contract**—An instrument through which an insurance company can meet the financial security needs of a group of persons. It is an agreement between the insurance company and the policyholder to insure the lives and health of the members of a defined group of persons and to pay the insurance benefits to the insured person or their beneficiaries.

**Group Insurance**—Provides coverage for several people under one contract, called a master contract. It is available to all people who qualify on a class basis, regardless of individual considerations.

**Group Model**—An HMO that contracts with providers or provider groups to provide services. These practitioners agree to see only HMO members, but they do so at their own facilities.

**Group Policy Holder**—An employer or entity (i.e., union) who purchases a group policy.

**Gum (Gingiva)**—The firm but soft tissue that surrounds the alveolar process and the mandibular and maxillary bones.

**Hammertoes**—Inherited muscle imbalances or abnormal bone lengths that can make the toes buckle under, causing the joints to contract.

**Hard Drive**—Provides space (memory) for information to be stored within the computer itself.

**Hard Palate**—Along with the soft palate, forms the roof of the mouth. It is located toward the front and is so named because it is a hard, bony structure. It is formed by portions of the maxillary and palatine bones.

**Heading**—Contains the return address, date, and a reference line and other notations if applicable.

**Health Care Common Procedure Coding System (HCPCS)**—A coding book which came about because of the limitations in the CPT® and RVS for billing injections, medication, supplies, and durable medical equipment.

**Health Insurance Payment Demand (HIPD)**—A bill that lists the healthcare services paid by the Medicaid program on behalf of a person who has other healthcare coverage benefits available.

**Health Maintenance Organization (HMO)**—A policy where members pay a set amount every month and the HMO agrees to provide all their care, or to pay for the covered care they cannot provide.

**Heel Spur**—An overgrowth on the heel bone.

**High-arched Feet (Pes Cavus)**—An imbalance of muscles and nerves and is often inherited.

**Hospice Care**—A healthcare program providing coordinated services in a home setting.

**Hospital Services**—Services performed in a hospital setting.

**Hospital Staff Anesthesiologist**—An anesthesiologist employed by the hospital.

**Hypnosis**—A state where the subconscious mind is allowed to take over and the conscious mind is more or less inactive.

**Impacted Tooth**—A tooth that is positioned or wedged against another tooth, bone, or soft tissue and is prevented from erupting normally.

**Implant**—To transfer or to graft something additional onto or into an existing surface.

**In Vitro Fertilization**—The fertilization of the ovum within a test tube.

**Incentive plans**—Encourage regular dental care, thus decreasing the possibility that a minor problem will remain untreated until it becomes a major problem.

**Incidental Procedure**—Surgery that does not add significant time or complexity to the operative session. In such a case, the allowed amount will be that of the major procedure only.

**Incisal (I)**—The biting edge or surface of the tooth.

**Incisors**—Are located at the front of the mouth and have a sharp edge that is used for biting. The normal adult has eight incisors, four on the top and a matching set of four on the bottom.

**Independent Anesthesiologist**—An anesthesiologist who is self-employed or not employed by the hospital.

**Independent Physician Associations (IPAs)**—Groups of providers who have banded together for the sole purpose of signing a contract with an MCP.

**Individual Practice Organizations (IPOs)**—Legal entities, comprised of networks of private physicians who have organized to negotiate contracts with insurance companies and HMOs.

**Individual Deductible**—The amount of covered expense that must be paid by the individual family member before benefits become payable by the plan.

**Individual Insurance**—Issued to insure the life or health of a named person or persons, rather than the life or health of the members of a group.

**Infusion Pump**—A machine which contains medication and administers a small dose when a button is depressed.

**Ingrown Toenail**—A nail where one or both corners or sides of the nail grow into the skin of the toe.

**Inlay**—A gold alloy or porcelain casting that lies on the occlusal surface of the patient's cusps (the pronounced elevation or edge of the tooth).

**In-Network**—Those providers approved by a plan.

**Inpatient Care**—The patient is admitted into a hospital or a similar facility and stays for a period of time, usually a minimum of 24 hours. There must be a room and board charge.

**Inside Address**—The address to which the letter is being sent.

**Insular COB**—COB applied separately to medical and dental charges. All savings are kept separately.

**Insurance**—An agreement whereby an insurance carrier agrees to cover certain benefits in exchange for premium payments.

**Insurance Carrier**—The company which offers the health insurance policy; a corporation or association whose business is to make contracts of insurance.

**Insurance Company**—Often used to refer to companies that sell policies offered by insurance carriers.

**Insurance Policy**—A written contract defining the insurance plan, its coverage, exclusions, eligibility requirements, and all benefits and conditions that apply to individuals insured under the plan.

**Insurance Premium**—The amount of money required for coverage under a specific insurance policy for a given period of time. Depending on the policy agreement, the premium may be paid monthly, quarterly, semiannually, or annually.

**Insurance Speculation**—A person or entity buying insurance or maintaining coverage for the purpose of making a profit.

**Insured** (also called **Member**)—The person who obtains or is otherwise covered by insurance on his health, life, or property.

**Intermediaries**—Private insurance companies that process Part A claims.

**International Classification of Disease–9th Revision Clinical Modification (ICD-9-CM)**—An indexing of conditions.

**Intractable Pain**—A pain which is hard to manage and is often severe enough to limit a patient's movement or abilities.

**Intraoral X-rays**—X-rays taken with the film placed inside the mouth.

**Intravenous (IV) Sedation**—A medication composed of a sedative and a painkiller administered intravenously. A semiconscious state is produced.

**In-utero Fetal Surgery**—Surgery on a fetus while it is in the mother's womb; and also to remove the fetus from the womb, perform surgery, and return it back to the womb, with the pregnancy continuing to term.

**Investigation**—An organized effort to discover the facts or truth of the matter.

**Job Related Injuries**—Include any injuries which happen during the performance of work-related duties whether they are in or out of the office.

**Joint**—The place where two bones meet.

**Jump**—The replacement of the base of the denture because of deterioration or tissue changes.

**Keyboard**—Primary means of communicating with your computer.

**Labial (La, L)**—The surface on the anterior teeth nearest the lip, and the incisal (I).

**Labial Veneer**—A cosmetic procedure that coats the tooth.

**Laboratory Examinations**—The analyzing of body substances to determine their chemical or tissue makeup.

**Lapse in Coverage**—A break in continuous insurance coverage, usually resulting from nonpayment of premium.

**Legal Damages**—Monetary awards that a plan member may attempt to recover, which are above and beyond the benefits provided by the group plan.

**Lien**—A legal document that expresses claim on the property of another for payment of a debt.

**Lifetime Maximum**—The total dollar payments the insurance carrier will make toward the care of this member.

**Ligaments**—Flexible bands of fiber joining bone to bone.

**Limiting Charge**—The maximum amount that the Federal Government allows nonparticipating physicians to charge Medicare patients for a given service.

**Lingual (Li)**—The surface nearest to the tongue.

**Lingual Bar**—The support that runs along the bottom of the mouth.

**Local Anesthesia**—Anesthesia that affects only a localized area.

**Loss Date**—The date of an accident.

**Maintenance of Benefits**—A COB provision in many group health plans that allows the person who has Medicare to "maintain" the same group benefits as members who do not have Medicare.

**Maintenance Therapy**—Refers to the various kinds of treatment (usually medical) given to patients to enable them to maintain their health in a disease-free or limited disease state.

**Major Medical Benefits**—Those benefits paid after basic benefits and which are usually subject to a deductible and coinsurance.

**Malice**—Intentional conduct to cause injury, or conduct that is carried on with the conscious disregard of the rights of others.

**Managed Care**—A strategy for reducing or controlling healthcare costs by tightly monitoring and restricting the use and cost of services. With this type of system, the insurer manages the delivery of healthcare and often emphasizes primary and preventive care services.

**Management Service Organization (MSO)**—A corporation set up to provide management services to a medical group for a fee.

**Mandates**—Laws enacted by state legislatures that require insurance carriers to cover certain services or dependents, or services provided by certain providers.

**Mandatory Program**—Requires the patient to obtain an SSO for special procedures, or there is an automatic reduction or denial of benefits.

**Mandible**—The lower jaw that is nonfixed (movable), which allows for not only biting and chewing food, but for speech, vocalization (speech and sound), and opening and closing the mouth.

**Matrixectomy**—Removal of a nail margin.

**Maxilla**—The upper fixed (nonmovable) bone. It is actually made up of two maxillae which form the skeletal base of most of the upper face, the roof of the mouth, the sides of the nasal cavity, and the floor of the orbit (the portion of the skull that contains and protects the eyeball).

**Maxillofacial Prosthetics**—The prosthetic rehabilitation of regions of the head and neck that are missing or defective.

**Maximum**—The greatest amount payable by the plan.

**Medicaid**—A jointly funded federal-state entitlement program, designed to provide healthcare services to certain low-income and needy people.

**Medical Case Management (MCM)**—The process of evaluating the effectiveness and frequency of medical treatments by reviewing to determine whether the care that is being rendered or that is going to be rendered is appropriate.

**Medical Dictionary**—A book that lists medical terms and their definitions, synonyms, illustrations, and supplemental information.

**Medical Groups**—Groups of physicians who are signed under or work for the same company.

**Medical Management**—X-ray and laboratory charges that are incurred to control or manage a diagnosis (i.e., monitoring blood glucose levels on a patient with diabetes).

**Medically Oriented Equipment**—Items primarily and customarily used for medical purposes.

**Medicare**—The Federal Health Insurance Benefit Plan for the Aged and Disabled.

**Medicare Allowance**—The amount Medicare deems an appropriate fee for the particular service or procedure.

**Medicare Remittance Notice (MRN)**—An explanation of benefits issued to providers for claims submitted to Medicare for a certain period of time.

**Medicare Summary Notice (MSN)**—An explanation of benefits sent to the Medicare beneficiary, detailing the processing of claims submitted for payment.

**Medicare Supplements**—Separate plans written exclusively for Medicare participants that cover items Medicare does not cover.

**Medicated Filling**—Temporary fillings to help relieve pain. Also called sedative fillings.

**Member Files**—Files that contain only one member's claim documents per file, and include documents for all years.

**Memo**—Short for memorandum, it is a letter intended for distribution within a company.

**Mental/Nervous Expenses**—Expenses for psychiatric treatment, marriage and family counseling, and drug and alcohol treatment.

**Merck Manual**—A manual that assists in identifying the symptomatology, prognosis, treatment protocols, etiology, and other miscellaneous information regarding diagnoses.

**Mesial (M)**—The surface nearest the midline. It is an imaginary line drawn between the maxillary centrals and the mandibular centrals.

**Mesioclusion**—Occurs when the mandibular arch protrudes in front of the maxillary arch.

**Metatarsal Plantar Callus**—A condition that occurs when the metatarsal bone is longer or lower than the others so that it hits the ground first at every step with more force than it is equipped to handle.

**Miscellaneous Services**—All other types of services not included under professional or facility services. For example, prescriptions, medical equipment (i.e., wheelchairs, crutches), and ambulance charges are all considered miscellaneous services.

**Missing and Unreplaced Rule**—This rule limits coverage for the replacement of teeth that are lost before the patient was covered by the plan.

**Mobile Intensive Care Unit**—A life support vehicle equipped to provide care to critically ill patients during transportation to a hospital.

**Modifier Codes**—Two-digit numerical codes attached to a CPT® code to indicate special circumstances for that particular service. This may mean that the unit value or UCR amount should be increased or decreased because of those special circumstances.

**Molars (Tricuspids)**—Are located behind the premolars and have three cusps.

**Monitored Anesthesia Care (MAC)**—The monitoring of a patient's vital signs during an operation in anticipation of the need for a general anesthesia.

**Mouth**—The organ primarily responsible for the introduction of air, food, and other substances into the body.

**Mucus**—A liquid containing mucin, leukocytes, inorganic salts, epithelial cells, and water.

**Multiline Phones**—With multiline phones the caller needs only to dial the original number, and if that line is busy, the call will automatically roll over to the first available line.

**Multiple Procedures**—More than one surgical procedure performed during the same operative session.

**Necessity**—Equipment is necessary when it is expected to make a meaningful contribution to the treatment of the patient's illness or injury or to the improvement of the functioning of a malformed body part.

**Neck**—The portion of the tooth covered by the gum which links the crown to the root.

**Neoplasm**—A new tumor or growth.

**Nerve Block Anesthesia**—Anesthesia produced by injecting a drug close to the nerve so that the nerve impulses are interrupted, thereby producing a loss of sensation.

**Network Model**—An HMO that contracts with several providers in a given local, allowing some overlap of geographic area.

**Neuroma**—A tumor arising from the connective tissue of the nerves.

**Neutroclusion**—Occurs when the upper and lower set of teeth come together normally, but the teeth themselves do not occlude properly.

**Night Care Centers**—Care centers which allow the patient to pursue a normal routine during the day such as working, and be treated at the center and maintained there overnight

**Nonaggregate**—A specified number of individual deductibles must be satisfied before the family limit is met.

**Noncontributory Plan**—Insurance where the employer bears the complete cost of the coverage and the employee does not contribute.

**Nondisability Claims**—Claims for minor injuries that will not require the patient to be kept from his/her job.

**Nondisabling or Per Visit Benefit**—In this type of benefit, there is a waiting period, a daily maximum, and a calendar year maximum. For example, the provision may read, "$10 per day payable after seven days and $200 per calendar year."

**Nonparticipating Physicians**—Physicians who treat Medicare-eligible patients but who decide whether to accept assignment on a case-by-case basis.

**Normal Liability (NL)**—The amount payable under the secondary plan's provisions without regard to any other coverage.

**Nuclear Medicine**—The use of radioactive elements and x-rays to image an organ or body part.

**Nursing Homes**—Specialize in custodial care, that is, care that is primarily for the purpose of meeting the personal needs of the patient and that could be provided by personnel without professional skills or training.

**Occlusal (O)**—The biting surface.

**Occlusal X-rays**—X-rays which show the floor of the mouth and the palate.

**Occlusion**—Closure of the teeth.

**Occupational Illnesses**—Any disorders, illnesses, or conditions which arise at work or from exposure to factors at work.

**Offer**—To propose or undertake, to do or give something in exchange for a return promise from the person to whom the act or gift is being offered.

**Office or Other Outpatient Visit**—Office visits or other encounters between a physician and patient that occur outside a hospital setting.

**Onlay**—A gold alloy casting that lies on the occlusal surface but covers one or more cusps.

**Open Enrollment**—A process that allows late applicants to enroll in a plan without having to complete evidence of insurability.

**Ophthalmology Care**—Eye care provided either by an optometrist or an ophthalmologist (M.D.).

**Oppression**—Putting a person through cruel and unjust hardships with the conscious disregard of rights.

**Optional Modifiers**—Denote special conditions. For additional information consult your CPT®.

**Oral Cavity (Cavum Oris)**—An oval-shaped cavity.

**Oral Surgery**—Treatment of the internal structures of the mouth limited to the dental structures and surrounding tissues.

**Order of Benefit Determination Rules (OBD)**—Fourteen rules determining the order of payment.

**Orthodontics**—Correction or prevention of poor or misaligned teeth.

**Orthoptics**—A retraining of the muscles that control vision.

**Orthosis**—An orthopedic appliance which is as effective as the surgery.

**Orthotic Devices**—Prescribed custom-made arch supports that fit inside most shoes and "bring the floor up to your feet."

**Ostectomy**—The surgical excision of all or part of a bone.

**Osteopathic Treatment**—Involves therapy based on the idea that the body can cure itself if it is in a normal state and provided with the proper environmental conditions.

**Outliers**—DRG cases which are atypically expensive (based on the diagnosis) because of complications or an abnormally long confinement.

**Out-of-Network**—Those providers that have not been approved by the plan.

**Out-of-Pocket**—A member's costs, which include the deductible, cost-sharing arising from the operation of the coinsurance clause, and medical expenditures that are deemed by the plan to be in excess of reasonable and customary charges.

**Out-of-Pocket Expense (OOP)**—Expenses for which the insured is held responsible and must pay "out-of-pocket," such as the deductible and coinsurance.

**Outpatient**—"Come-and-go" or outpatient surgery is when the patient is not admitted to the hospital after surgery because it is not medically necessary. There are no room and board charges.

**Overinsurance**—A situation that occurs when a person is covered under two or more policies and is eligible to collect an accumulation of benefits that actually exceeds the amount charged by the provider.

**Palatal Bar**—The support that runs across the top of the palate (roof of the mouth).

**Palliative Treatment**—An emergency treatment performed to relieve pain or prevent a condition from worsening.

**Panel Tests**—Multiple tests that are combined and run from one specimen.

**Papanicolaou or "Pap Smear"**—A diagnostic laboratory test for detecting the absence or presence of infection, viruses, trauma, or cancer.

**Papillae**—Tiny nipple-like protuberances.

**Paramedics**—Specially trained emergency medical personnel who render emergency treatment at the scene of the injury or illness.

**Part A**—The Medicare basic plan or hospital insurance which covers facility charges for acute inpatient hospital care, skilled nursing, home healthcare, and hospice care.

**Part B**—The Medicare medical insurance which covers doctor's services, outpatient hospital services, home healthcare, outpatient speech and physical therapy, and durable medical equipment.

**Partial Credit Adjustment**—An adjustment that partially reverses a claim payment.

**Participating Physicians**—Providers who have signed an agreement with Medicare to accept the Medicare allowed amount, among other things.

**Patient Claim Form**—A form that contains basically the same information as the ADA Dental Claim Form.

**Pended Claims**—Claims that have not been completely adjudicated or closed.

**Per Period of Disability**—Basic Benefit waiting periods and deductibles; may be based on a per illness basis or a waiting period basis.

**Periodontics**—Treatment of the tissues surrounding and supporting the teeth.

**Periodontitis**—Inflammation of the periodontal tissues. It may be caused by bacteria, calcium deposits, or food particles that collect between the tooth and the gum. If not treated, the infection may spread to the bone, possibly causing loss of teeth. Periodontitis is the primary cause of tooth loss in people over the age of 35 years old.

**Periodontosis**—Any degenerative disease of the periodontal tissue.

**Permanent and Stationary**—A term meaning that nothing more can be done and the patient will have the disability for the rest of his or her life.

**Permanent Disability**—When it is determined that the patient will not be able to return to work.

**Personal Items**—Those items that are primarily for the comfort of the patient and are not medically necessary.

**Physical Medicine**—The manipulation and physical therapy associated with the nonsurgical care and treatment of the patient.

**Physical Status Modifiers**—A modifier that used to indicate various physical conditions and is represented by the initial P, followed by a single digit from one to six.

**Physician Hospital Organization (PHO)**—An organization of physicians and hospitals that bands together for the purpose of obtaining contracts from payer organizations.

**Physician's Final Report**—When the physician notifies the WC carrier that no further treatment is needed (or that no further treatment will significantly alter the patient's condition) and that the patient has been discharged.

**Physicians' Current Procedure Terminology (CPT®)**—A systematic listing for coding the procedures or services performed by a physician.

**Physicians' Desk Reference (PDR)**—A manual that provides information on prescription drugs, including usage, dosage, appearance, prescription status, make-up and other factors.

**Pin Retention**—The insertion of a small, thin needle-like pin into the remaining tooth structure to provide extra support for the restoration.

**Podiatry**—An area of medicine that provides services for the feet.

**Policy**—Same as contract.

**Pontic**—The part of a bridge that is suspended between abutments and replaces a missing tooth.

**Positional Bunion**—A bony growth on the side of the metatarsal bone that enlarges the joint, forcing the joint capsule to stretch over it.

**Power Switch**—Turns the monitor on and off.

**Preadmission Testing (PAT)**—Routine laboratory and x-ray tests performed on an outpatient basis before a scheduled inpatient admission.

**Preauthorization**—A number of insurance carriers will require that certain benefits be preauthorized before the services are received. Preauthorization means to gain approval of the services that are to be performed, as well as to obtain an understanding of whether or not the insurance carrier will provide coverage for these services.

**Precertification**—To get preapproval for admission on elective, nonemergency hospitalization.

**Predetermination**—An estimate of maximum benefits that may be paid under the plan for the services. It is not, however, a guarantee that benefits will be paid.

**Preexisting Condition**—A medical condition that existed before an insurance policy was purchased. Depending on the policy, a preexisting condition may be defined based on when it originated, when symptoms first appeared, or when treatment was first sought.

**Preferred Provider Organization (PPO)**—A group of healthcare providers who agree to provide services to a specific pool of patients for an agreed fee.

**Prefix**—The beginning portion of a term that modifies the meaning of the root word.

**Premiums**—Fees collected by insurance companies from individuals or companies on a regular basis.

**Premolars (Bicuspids)**—Are located behind the cuspids and have two (bi-) cusps or grinding protrusions.

**Preventive Coverage**—Items such as an annual physical, cancer screening (pap smears, mammograms, etc.), flu shots, immunizations, and well-baby care.

**Preventive Services**—Routine services designed to prevent decay, gum disease, etc., through the care of the dental structures before disease has occurred.

**Primary Care Provider (PCP)**—The provider a member has chosen who is responsible for all their healthcare needs.

**Primary Plan**—The benefit plan that determines and pays its benefits first without regard to the existence of any other coverage.

**Procedure Code**—A five-digit numerical code used to designate medical services according to standardized, industry-accepted methods; usually reflected in a CPT® manual.

**Products**—Items or services offered for sale by a company. In the case of insurance carriers, the products are the various policies they offer.

**Professional Component**—The reading or interpreting of lab results or x-rays.

**Professional Services**—Services performed by a licensed individual such as a medical doctor, physician's assistant, nurse, or chiropractor.

**Prophylaxis**—The removal of bacterioplaque, calculus, stains, and other potentially harmful materials from the teeth by superficial scaling and polishing.

**Prosthetic Devices**—Devices designed to replace a missing body part or to restore some function to a paralyzed body part.

**Prosthodontics, Permanent**—Replacement of the natural teeth through the use of a permanent appliance.

**Prosthodontics, Removable**—Replacement of the natural teeth through the use of a removable appliance.

**Provider of Service (often just Provider)**—The physician, chiropractor, dentist or other healthcare professional or establishment (hospital, nursing home, etc.) that provides healthcare services.

**Pulp**—Made up of connective tissue that contains a network of capillaries.

**Pulp Capping**—The placing of a covering over an exposed tooth pulp.

**Pulp Cavity**—The extreme center of the tooth.

**Pulpectomy**—The complete or partial removal of the pulp.

**Pulpotomy**—See Pulpectomy.

**Punitive Damages**—Damages which are intended primarily to punish a wrongdoing defendant and set him up as an example to help deter such actions in the future.

**Qualified Beneficiary**—Anyone who, on the day before the Qualifying Event, is covered under the health coverage plan as an employee, a dependent spouse, or a dependent child.

**Qualifying Event**—Refers to an event which results in the loss of eligibility under the employer sponsored health plan.

**Radiation Oncology**—The use of radiation to treat a condition.

**Radiographs**—X-rays of the mouth and teeth.

**Reasonable Charges**—The amounts approved by the Medicare carrier based on what is considered reasonable for the geographic area in which the doctor practices.

**Reasonableness**—This evaluates the soundness and practicality of the DME approach.

**Rebase**—see **Jump**.

**Rebundling**—The process in which component parts of the procedure are to be denied as already included within the allowable charge for the single procedure.

**Reconstruction**—Procedures performed to aesthetically rebuild or restore a part of the body that was damaged or became defective as a result of an illness or injury.

**Red Book and Blue Book**—Are manuals which list drug product information, along with prevailing wholesale prices.

**Referral**—To send a claim to be reviewed by a technical claims person.

**Region**—The geographic region of the country that is assigned a specific conversion factor. More expensive cost-of-living areas are assigned higher conversion factors than less expensive cost-of-living areas. Some states or cities are divided into multiple or different regions, whereas other states or cities may have only one area or may even be combined with other states or cities.

**Regional Anesthesia**—Anesthesia that produces the loss of sensation of a part of the body due to the interruption of nerve conduction.

**Rehabilitation Benefit**—A benefit that provides for retraining of the employee in a physical ability which will help him or her to seek future employment (i.e., proper use of a wheelchair, use of the left hand when a person loses their right hand).

**Rehabilitation Facilities**—Specialize in long-term, postsickness, or postinjury care.

**Reinsurance**—An insurance that covers expenses when the benefit payments on a self-funded plan exceed a certain amount.

**Relative Value Study (RVS)**—Another reference book used for coding physician services, using the studies that assign unit values to a particular procedure.

**Relative Value Units (RVU's)**—Represent the total RVS for components of the schedule.

**Removal of Exostosis**—The removal of a bony growth that arises from either the maxilla or mandible.

**Renewal**—Paying a premium in order to continue coverage after the initial policy period has expired.

**Request for Additional Information Form**—A form used when more information is needed from the provider of services or the patient regarding the services that were performed or the necessity for those services.

**Reservation of Rights**—Allows the payer to assert a general denial, but to also retain the authority to suspend or pend the claim if so warranted.

**Restoration**—Procedures used to restore a natural tooth.

**Restorative**—Treatment involving the use of fillings or crowns to save or restore dental structures.

**Résumé**—A summary of employment experience and qualifications.

**Retainer**—A device used for maintaining the teeth and jaws in an appropriate position.

**Retrospective Review**—Used to determine after discharge whether the hospitalization and treatment were medically necessary and covered by the terms of the benefit program. This type of review may be used as a substitute for admission and concurrent reviews when the failure to notify the UR program of an admission prevents the regular review procedures.

**Return Receipt Requested**—Upon delivery, a receipt is issued and mailed back to the sender of the package. This allows the sender to have proof of the delivery and the name of the person who signed for it.

**Root**—The portion that is embedded in the bone.

**Root Canal**—The portion of the pulp chamber that carries the blood vessels from the tooth socket to the tooth itself.

**Root Canal**—The removal of the entire root pulp, sterilizing of the chamber, and filling of the chamber with sealing material.

**Root Word**—Usually found in the center of a term and identifies the organ or body part involved.

**Saddle Block**—Another type of spinal anesthetic in which the injection produces a loss of feeling in the region of the body that corresponds to the area that makes contact with a riding saddle (buttocks, perineum, and thighs).

**Saliva**—Consists of salivary amylase and mucus.

**Salivary Amylase**—An enzyme that helps to break down food molecules.

**Salutation**—A form of greeting the letter recipient.

**Scheduled Dental Plan**—Usually no conversion factors are involved. Instead, each ADA code has a specified dollar amount assigned to it.

**Sealants**—A plastic-like coating placed on a healthy tooth to prevent decay.

**Seating**—Placement of the finished crown.

**Second Opinion** or **Confirmatory Consultation**—Designed as a benefit to the patient by confirming the need for surgeries that have a reputation for being done needlessly.

**Second Surgical Opinion (SSO)**—A review of a proposed surgery by a second physician/surgeon to determine the necessity of the planned services.

**Secondary Plan**—The plan that pays after the primary plan has paid its benefits.

**Self-funded Plan**—When the total and ultimate responsibility for providing all plan benefit payments rests solely with the employer, group, or association.

**Sequestrectomy for Osteomyelitis**—The isolation of a portion of bone due to inflammation.

**Serial Surgery**—A surgery on several individual toes or joints with one surgical procedure being performed in a single operative visit.

**Sialodentitis**—Inflammation of a salivary gland.

**Signature**—The name of the person writing the letter or for whom the letter has been written.

**Simple Cavities**—Involve only one surface of a tooth.

**Soft Palate**—Along with the hard palate forms the roof of the mouth. It is located in the rear portion of the mouth and is composed mostly of muscle.

**Space Maintenance**—The placement of wires or a retainer in the mouth to prevent the wrongful movement of teeth into a space where a tooth has been lost.

**Speech Therapy**—Therapy to correct speech impairments.

**Spinal Anesthesia**—A specialized type of nerve block where the spinal nerves are blocked in either the subarachnoid or the epidural space.

**Staff Model**—An HMO that hires physicians or providers to work at the HMO's own facility.

**Stat Fees**—A charge for DXL services performed on an expedited priority basis.

**Statistical Adjustment**—An adjustment that changes the claim data but does not increase or decrease the original claim payment.

**Stomatitis**—Inflammation of the mouth. This can include cold sores, fever blisters, or canker sores.

**Stomatoplasty**—Plastic surgery or repair of the mouth.

**Stoploss**—An attempt to limit payments by an insured person or a Group/IPA in the case of a catastrophic illness or injury to a member.

**Stoploss Insurance**—Insurance that covers plans when their benefit payments exceed a certain amount.

**Structural Bunion**—A condition that occurs when the angle between the first and second metatarsal bones increases to a point at which it is greater than normal.

**Subjective Findings**—Findings that cannot be discerned by anyone other than the patient (i.e., pain, discomfort).

**Subpoena**—A written legal order directing a person or document to appear in court to testify.

**Subrogation**—The right for a portion of the recovery that the claimant may obtain from a third party.

**Suffix**—The ending portion of a term. Suffixes also alter the root word, usually by indicating a state of being.

**Summary Plan Description**—Same as contract.

**Supplemental Adjustment**—An adjustment that increases the original claim payment.

**Surgery**—The branch of medicine that treats diseases, injuries, and deformities by operative or invasive methods.

**Surgical Excision**—Includes excision of reactive inflammatory lesions, scar tissue, or localized congenital lesions.

**Take-Home Prescriptions**—Medications to be taken after the patient is released from the hospital.

**Taste Buds**—Sensory end organs that help carry the sensation of taste to the brain.

**Tax Equity and Fiscal Responsibility Act of 1982 (TEFRA)**—A Federal Act that redirected the financial responsibility for medical coverage of active employees age 65 years and older and their spouses aged 65 years and older to Medicare.

**Technical Component**—Collection of a specimen or taking of an x-ray.

**Telemetry Charges**—Charges for the use of a specialized observation equipment. May be billed separately from the base room and board amount.

**Temporary Dentures**—Sometimes used until the permanent dentures have been constructed.

**Temporary Disability**—Claims for when the patient is not able to perform his or her job requirements until he or she recovers from the injury involved.

**Temporomandibular Joint**—A sliding joint that hinges the lower and upper jaw together.

**Temporomandibular Joint (TMJ) Dysfunction**—A manifestation of an abnormality of the joint where the lower jaw hinges to the upper jaw.

**Tenotomy**—Same as capsulotomy.

**Termination of Coverage**—Cessation of eligibility for benefits under the plan.

**Therapeutic Procedures**—Procedures performed to remove or correct the functioning of a body part that is diseased or injured.

**Third Party Liability (TPL)**—See Acts of Third Parties.

**Third-Party Administrator (TPA)**—A plan administration firm that deals solely with administering the eligibility and claim payment services (along with various other administrative services) for self-funded plans.

**Three-Month Carryover Provision (C/O)**—Eligible charges incurred in the last quarter of the calendar year and applied toward the member's deductible will also count toward the following year's deductible.

**Tickler Files**—Expanding file folders that help you remember items that need to occur on a specific date. Basically a tickler file helps tickle your memory.

**Tissue Conditioning**—A method of correcting tissue irritation resulting from the wearing of dentures.

**Tongue**—A muscular organ that lies on the floor of the mouth and continues partway into the pharynx.

**Topical Anesthesia**—An anesthetic that is applied directly to the surface of the area to be anesthetized.

**Treatment Authorization Request (TAR)**—A form used to request authorization for services which are the financial responsibility of the HMO.

**Treatment-Free Period**—With this provision, if the patient can go without treatment for a specified period of time (often 90 days), then the insurance carrier will no longer consider the condition to be preexisting and will cover the illness or condition under the normal terms of the contract.

**TRICARE (formerly CHAMPUS)**—Provides a comprehensive program of healthcare benefits for active duty and retired services personnel, their dependents, and the dependents of deceased military personnel.

**Tumors**—Abnormal (possibly cancerous) growths in the body.

**Type of Treatment**—The type of service performed, which is usually classified by the following categories: surgery, medical, x-ray, laboratory, and anesthesia.

**UB-92**—The claim form most commonly used to bill for hospital services.

**UCR Calculation**—The process of determining the fee usually charged by similar providers for the same procedure in the same geographic area during a specified period of time.

**Ultrasonography**—A diagnostic imaging technique that uses sound waves to create images of internal organs.

**Unbundling**—When a provider bills separately for each test performed even though all the tests came from the same specimen and were done simultaneously.

**Unit Value**—A numerical value assigned by a relative value study to a procedure code. The unit value is multiplied by the conversion factor to determine the UCR allowance or a basic allowance.

**Unnecessary Surgery**—Surgery recommended as an elective procedure when an alternative method of treatment may be preferable for a number of reasons.

**Unusual Services**—Services that are rarely provided, unusual, or variable and may warrant an additional anesthesia fee.

**Urgent Care Centers**—A facility that provides urgent or emergency treatment.

**Usual, Customary, and Reasonable (UCR)**—An amount usually charged by most providers within a geographic region for a specified service.

**Utilization Review (UR)**—A process whereby insurance carriers review the treatment of a patient and determine whether or not the costs will be covered.

**Van Transportation Units**—Vehicles specially equipped to handle wheelchairs and patients who are unable to get in and out of a regular vehicle.

**Vestibule**—The outer, smaller portion surrounded by the lips, cheeks, gums, and teeth.

**Vestibuloplasty**—Surgery involving the vestibule of the mouth.

**Vocational Rehabilitation**—Retraining in a different job field when the employee is unable to return to their former position.

**Voluntary Program**—Encourages participants to have an SSO, but there is no automatic reduction of benefits if the patient does not comply.

**Wart**—A growth caused by a virus.

**Withhold**—The MCP may retain a portion of the monthly capitation amount to protect the HMO from inadequate patient care or financial management by the PCP.

**Work Hardening**—A program wherein an employee is assigned therapy similar to their work in an attempt to strengthen them and build up their endurance toward a full day's work.

**Workers' Compensation (WC)**—A separate medical and disability reimbursement program which provides 100% coverage for job related injuries, illnesses, and/or conditions arising out of and in the course of employment.

**X-Rays**—Flat or two-dimensional images of a particular body part or organ.

# Credits

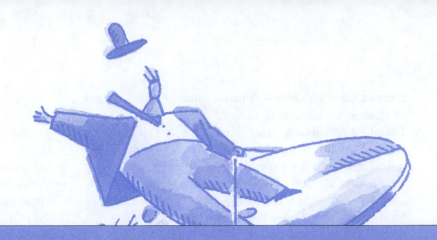

# Index

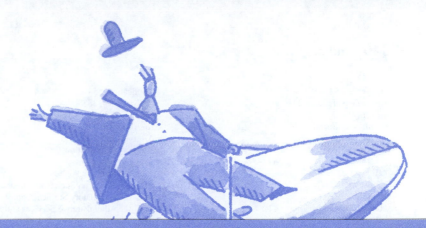